The Patella

Giles R. Scuderi
Editor

The Patella

With a Foreword by John N. Insall

Illustrations by Lydia V. Kibiuk

With 265 Figures

Springer-Verlag
New York Berlin Heidelberg London Paris
Tokyo Hong Kong Barcelona Budapest

Giles R. Scuderi, M.D.
The Insall Scott Kelly Institute for Orthopaedics and Sports Medicine
Beth Israel Medical Center-North Division
New York, NY 10128 USA

Cover illustration: The sulcus and view of the distal end of the femur of a left knee. This illustration appears on p. 15 of the text.

Library of Congress Cataloging-in-Publication Data
The patella / [edited by] Giles R. Scuderi.
p. cm.
Includes bibliographical references and index.
ISBN 0-387-94371-4. — ISBN 3-540-94371-4
1. Patellofemoral joint—Wounds and injuries. 2. Patellofemoral joint—Diseases. 3. Patellofemoral joint—Surgery. 4. Patella—Wounds and injuries. 5. Patella—Diseases. 6. Patella—Surgery.
[DNLM: 1. Patella—physiopathology. 2. Patella—surgery. 3. Knee Joint—physiopathology. WE 870 P2945 1995]
RD661.P37 1995
617.5′82—dc20
DNLM/DLC
for Library of Congress 94-29936

Printed on acid-free paper.

Production coordinated by Impressions, Inc., and managed by Terry Kornak; manufacturing supervised by Rhea Talbert.
Typeset by Impressions Inc., Madison, WI.
Printed and bound by Maple-Vail, York, PA.
Printed in the United States of America.

9 8 7 6 5 4 3 2 1

ISBN 0-387-94371-4 Springer-Verlag New York Berlin Heidelberg
ISBN 3-540-94371-4 Springer-Verlag Berlin Heidelberg New York

Foreword

The problems of the patellofemoral joint remain a challenge to the orthopaedic surgeon. In spite of many articles in scientific journals, an outstanding monograph, and several excellent textbook chapters, the patella is still an enigma in many respects. The etiology of patellar pain is controversial, and there is no completely satisfying explanation for its cause or its relationship to chondromalacia. Curiously, neither the widespread use of arthroscopy nor the advent of newer diagnostic tests such as CT scanning and magnetic resonance imaging have cast much light.

Without a better understanding of why patellar disorders occur it is not surprising that there is no consensus on how to fix them. Arthroscopy has contributed little except to the patient's psyche. The currently most popular surgical treatment for recurrent dislocation of the patella was first described 50 years ago. One concrete advance, albeit a small one, is a better understanding of the role of anatomical abnormalities and patellofemoral dysplasia in patellar instabilities.

It gives me great pleasure that many of the contributors are, like Dr. Scuderi himself, members of the "Insall Club," an organization of my former residents and fellows of which I am inordinately proud. It is truly appropriate that the subject of this volume is the patellofemoral joint because at one time in my career I too struggled to unravel its puzzles. I did not have much success in the end, and perhaps there are no answers to be had. What we have here in this book is a clearly written, accurate, and up to date review of the current state of knowledge without which no orthopaedic surgeon can diagnose or treat patellar disorders.

John N. Insall, M.D.

Preface

The patella has always been an intriguing structure. Located in the front of the knee, it serves several functions. Yet, as the largest sesamoid bone in the body, this structure, along with the supporting extensor mechanism, has been the source of disability and pain in many patients and has puzzled many treating physicians. Together with my esteemed colleagues, we have attempted to establish a comprehensive and practical approach to the management of disorders of the patella and the extensor mechanism of the knee. Hopefully, this book will provide an updated source of reference for orthopaedic surgeons and residents in training who have special interests in disorders of the knee.

At this time, I would also like to acknowledge the tutelage and guidance of my mentors, John N. Insall and W. Norman Scott, who have enlightened me in the practice of knee surgery. Many of my ideas and principles, which are put forth within this text, have been formulated through their instruction.

Finally, this book is dedicated to my wife, Gerrie, and my children, Sean, Ali, and Scott, whose love and support have always been unyielding.

Giles R. Scuderi, M.D.

Contents

Contributors

William S. Adsit, M.D. Department of Orthopaedic Surgery, Naval Hospital Camp Pendleton, Camp Pendleton, CA 92055, USA

Paolo Aglietti, M.D. Department of Orthopaedic Surgery, Florence University, Florence 50139, Italy

Jose A. Alicea, M.D. Insall Scott Kelly Institute for Orthopaedics and Sports Medicine, Beth Israel Medical Center-North Division, New York, NY 10128, USA

James V. Bono, M.D. Department of Orthopaedic Surgery, New England Baptist Hospital, Boston, MA 02120, USA

David D. Bullek, M.D. Private Practice, Westfield, NJ 07090, USA and Insall Scott Kelly Institute for Orthopaedics and Sports Medicine, Beth Israel Medical Center-North Division, New York, NY 10128, USA

Robert Butters, M.S., A.T.C. Garden City Physical Therapy Associates, Garden City, NY 11530, USA

Glen Carlin, B.S. Garden City Physical Therapy Associates, Garden City, NY 11530, USA

Fred D. Cushner, M.D. Insall Scott Kelly Institute for Orthopaedics and Sports Medicine, Beth Israel Medical Center-North Division, New York, NY 10128, USA

Freddie Fu, M.D. Department of Orthopaedic Surgery, University of Pittsburgh School of Medicine, Center for Sports Medicine, Pittsburgh, PA 15213, USA

Bernard Ghelman, M.D. Department of Radiology and Nuclear Medicine, The Hospital for Special Surgery, New York, NY 10021, USA

Steven B. Haas, M.D., M.P.H. The Knee Service, Department of Orthopaedic Surgery, The Hospital for Special Surgery, New York, NY 10021, USA

David C. Hillsgrove, M.D. The Orthopaedic Specialty Hospital, Salt Lake City, UT 84107, USA

John N. Insall, M.D. Insall Scott Kelly Institute for Orthopaedics and Sports Medicine, Beth Israel Medical Center-North Division, New York, NY 10128, USA

Michael A. Kelly, M.D. Insall Scott Kelly Institute for Orthopaedics and Sports Medicine, Beth Israel Medical Center-North Division, New York, NY 10128, USA

James M. Kipnis, M.D. The Orthopaedic and Sports Medicine Institute of Long Island, Rockville Centre, NY 11570, USA

Kevin R. Math, M.D. Department of Radiology and Nuclear Medicine, The Hospital for Special Surgery, New York, NY 10021, USA

Suanne S. Maurer, M.S., A.T.C. Department of Health, Physical Education and Recreation, Hofstra University, 230 Hofstra University, Hempstead, NY 11550, USA

Pier Paolo M. Menchetti, M.D. Department of Orthopaedic Surgery, Florence University, Florence 50139, Italy

Daniel Morgan, M.D., Department of Orthopaedic Surgery, Kingsbrook Jewish Medical Center, Brooklyn, NY 11203, USA

Alan Nagel, M.D. Insall Scott Kelly Institute for Orthopaedics and Sports Medicine, Beth Israel Medical Center-North Division, New York, NY 10128, USA

Jeffrey Y. Ngeow, M.D. The Hospital for Special Surgery, New York, NY 10021, USA

Lonnie E. Paulos, M.D. The Orthopaedic Specialty Hospital, Salt Lake City, UT 84107, USA

Hollis G. Potter, M.D. Department of Radiology and Nuclear Medicine, The Hospital for Special Surgery, New York, NY 10021, USA

W. Norman Scott, M.D. Insall Scott Kelly Institute for Orthopaedics and Sports Medicine, Beth Israel Medical Center-North Division, New York, NY 10128, USA

Giles R. Scuderi, M.D. Insall Scott Kelly Institute for Orthopaedics and Sports Medicine, Beth Israel Medical Center-North Division, New York, NY 10128, USA

K. Donald Shelbourne, M.D. Methodist Sports Medicine Center, Indiana University School of Medicine, Department of Orthopaedic Surgery, Indianapolis, IN 46202, USA

Andrew I. Spitzer, M.D. Kerlan-Jobe Orthopaedic Clinic, Inglewood, CA 90301, USA

Joseph M. Stefko, M.D. Department of Orthopaedics, University of Pittsburgh School of Medicine, Pittsburgh, PA 15213, USA

Alfred J. Tria, Jr., M.D. Department of Orthopaedic Surgery, Robert Wood Johnson Medical School, University of Medicine and Dentistry of New Jersey, New Brunswick, NJ 08854–5635, USA

Vincent J. Vigorita, M.D. Department of Pathology, Lutheran Medical Center, Brooklyn, NY 11220, USA

Kelly G. Vince, M.D., F.R.C.S.(C) University of California–Irvine, Department of Orthopaedic Surgery, and Kerlan-Jobe Orthopaedic Clinic, Inglewood, CA 90301, USA

Jeffrey H. Yormak, M.D. Insall Scott Kelly Institute for Orthopaedics and Sports Medicine, Beth Israel Medical Center-North Division, New York, NY 10128, USA

1

A Historic Review of Patellar Pain

James M. Kipnis and Giles R. Scuderi

Afflictions of the patella have received a great deal of attention over the years. As early as 1906, in the German literature, Budinger described traumatic fissuring of patellar articular cartilage as a source of anterior knee pain.[1] Ludloff[2] and Axhausen[3] reported similar changes on the patellar articular surface, and in an attempt to treat this lesion, in 1910, Ludloff described scraping the articular cartilage. In 1917, Aleman introduced the term *chondromalacia of the patella,* when he observed degeneration of the patellar articular cartilage at the time of arthrotomy.[4,5] By 1924 this term was accepted and popularized in the literature by Koenig.[6] In 1933, Kulowski[7] reported the first U.S. case of chondromalacia patellae in a 21-year-old woman in whom Kulowski observed excessive lateral patellar mobility.

In 1936, Owre[6] detailed the incidence and anatomic location of changes in the patellar articular surface in 125 cadaveric patellae. Commonly, edema and fissuring of the articular cartilage were noted straddling the patellar crest. These changes appeared to be age related, with a higher incidence in specimens that originated from patients older than 60. Using the term *chondromalacia patellae,* Owre proposed that anterior knee pain was caused by degenerative changes in the articular cartilage. Similarly, Heine[8] also found an 88% incidence of chondromalacia patellae in older patients. It had become a general belief that chondromalacia was the precursor to degenerative arthritis of the patella. Later, cadaveric studies by Bennett (1942),[9] Emery (1973),[10] and Casscells (1978)[11] supported these early studies and reported that fibrillation of the patellar articular surface in most middle-aged patients progressed to fasciculation and erosive changes with age. In 1976, Goodfellow[12] further gave credence to this observation by claiming in his classic article that "chondromalacia almost becomes the rule in old age."

Realizing that chondromalacia patellae was not an uncommon finding at arthrotomy, investigators began studying the natural history of this pathologic entity. In 1939, Karlson[5] was the first to report on the natural history of chondromalacia. Observing 67 men with a clinical diagnosis of chondromalacia for as long as 21 years, Karlson found that 10 knees were symptom free, 41 had mild symptoms, and 16 were worse. Since only 23% of patients with proven chondromalacia had progression of symptoms with age, this challenged the theory that symptoms worsen as one ages. Wiles et al.[13] also cast doubt on the issue of symptoms and aging. Although they did describe chondromalacia patellae as the precursor to osteoarthritis, Wiles et al. did find it difficult to estimate how often chondromalacia gave rise to symptoms. More recently, Kelly and Insall[14] reported that the natural history of this condition remains unclear and that the degree of chondromalacia does not always correlate with symptoms.

In 1961, Outerbridge[15,16] reported his observations on the condition of the patellar articular surface in 196 patients undergoing open meniscectomy. He found that the number of patellae showing healthy articular cartilage was approximately equal to the number showing pathologic changes, a much lower incidence than Wiles et al.[13] or Owre[6] reported. In many individuals these pathologic changes were only an incidental finding without a clear correlation to pain. Based on these observations, Outerbridge concluded that chondromalacia was far more common than was generally believed, and when present, usually was asymptomatic. He also observed that the chondromalacic changes were most frequently present on the medial facet of the patella and not along the central ridge, as Owre reported. Other investigators also confirmed Outerbridge's observations of the early changes on the medial articular facet of the patella.[10,17,18] Because these changes on the patella articular surface were not uniform, Outerbridge established a classification system (Table 1.1). Grade I is described as softening and swelling with an intact articular cartilage. Grade II is fragmentation and fissuring of the articular surface within the softened area, while grade III is described as fibrillation or breakdown of the articular surface with a "crab meat" appearance. Grade IV is erosive changes with exposure of the subchondral bone.

Although investigators began noting these various pathologic changes on the articular surface, the exact cause was elusive. Early theories regarding the etiology of chondromalacia fell into three main groups.[15] The first and most popular theory was trauma, either direct or indirect.[4,6,19,20] It was speculated that a direct blow to the patella would impact the articular surface against the femur, causing cracks or fissures, which would progress to further articular damage. A second theory postulated that a metabolic or endocrine condition alone,[21] or in combination with an injury,[2,7] predisposed the articular cartilage to degeneration. Wiberg proposed a third theory for the etiology of chondromalacia[22] and theorized that increased patellofemoral contact forces lead[5] to articular degeneration. In an extensive study of the patellofemoral joint, Wiberg classified variations in the patellar shape. He suggested that the convex shape of the medial facet subjects its articular cartilage to greater localized stresses, especially with flexion beyond 90°. With repetitive injury, this could subsequently lead to painful symptoms. This theory of abnormal patellar contact stress leading to articular lesions was supported in part by the work of Baumgartl (1944),[23] who noted a correlation between patellar type and pathologic changes, including osteochondritis dissecans.

TABLE 1.1. Outerbridge's grading of chondromalacia patellae.

Grade	Description
I	Softening and swelling
II	Fissuring
III	Fibrillation ("crab meat" appearance)
IV	Erosive changes and exposure of the subchondral bone

Although Wiberg's concept of abnormal pressure or friction in extreme flexion was appealing and seemed to come the closest to explaining the etiology of chondromalacia patellae, Outerbridge[15] took some exception to it. The reason for this skepticism was that chondromalacia was not common in Oriental people, who, because of cultural requirements, spend a great deal of time kneeling and squatting. This skepticism was further supported in a later study by Marrar and Pillay,[24] who reported chondromalacia patellae to be an infrequent finding among the Chinese people. Doubt was therefore cast on Wiberg's theory.

Further explanation as to the etiology of chondromalacia patellae suggested that the nutritional supply to the patellar articular cartilage was in someway compromised. However, Outerbridge suggested that if this situation actually existed, then the degenerative changes should begin in the central ridge, where the articular cartilage is thickest and would be most susceptible to alterations in nutritional supply.[15] He did propose that an abnormal ridge on the medial femoral condyle—"Outerbridge ridge"—caused repeated injury to the medial patellar facet, leading to the breakdown of the articular cartilage. Outerbridge suggested resecting this ridge when present in order to prevent further destruction. This theory of the abnormal femoral ridge causing chondromalacia patellae was not universally accepted. Abernethy et al.,[25] and Meachim and Emery[17] did note the ridge but found it did not correlate with the presence of chondromalacia patellae.

The morphology of the patellofemoral joint has also been implicated in disorders of the patella. In an effort to better understand the intimate relationship of the patella with the femoral sulcus, investigators began to look more closely at the bony and cartilaginous configuration. In 1964, Brattstrom[26] studied the shape of the femoral intercondylar sulcus and defined the sulcus angle. His work pioneered a better understanding of the relation of the patellar articulation within the femoral sulcus, and as noted by Merchant,[27] these concepts are still valid today.

In 1968, Hughston published an article on subluxation of the patella,[28] which represented a major turning point in the recognition and treatment of patellofemoral disorders. Discussing the association between anterior knee pain and patellar malalignment, Hughston proposed that chondromalacia of the medial facet was due to impingement of the medial facet against the lateral femoral trochlea during relocation of a subluxating patella. Based on this finding, he recommended a combined proximal and distal realignment of the extensor mechanism as treatment of patellar malalignment.

Ficat[29,30,31] further developed the concept of abnormal patella alignment and coined the term "lateral compartment hyperpressure syndrome." Larson[32] also supported this concept of an excessively tight lateral retinaculum contributing to increased patellar compressive forces with knee flexion. In 1977, Ficat and Hungerford[33] wrote the first and classic text devoted solely to the subject of patellofemoral disorders. In this text, they theorized that an excessively tight lateral retinaculum tilts the patella, producing excessive pressure on the lateral facet, leading to chondromalacia and late osteoarthrosis. Several investigations have also observed that lesions of the lateral facet tend to be progressive and are related to later arthrosis.[17,18,34] Abernethy et al.[25] and Stougard[35] noted bony changes associated with chondromalacia, including increased stiffness of the bone beneath the more involved lateral facet.

In 1974, Merchant et al. introduced the 45° tangential radiograph in an effort to better understand patellofemoral mechanics.[36] Based on this radiograph, the observer would be able to define the femoral sulcus angle as well as the congruence angle. Since the congruence angle was an attempt at evaluating patellar subluxation, the observer would be able to separate those patients with patellofemoral pain into two types: (1) those with normal alignment and (2) those with abnormal alignment and lateral subluxation. Also at this time, Merchant and Mercer suggested a lateral retinacular release for recurrent patellar subluxation.[37]

In contrast to excessive lateral patellofemoral pressure as the sole cause of chondromalacia patellae, Ficat et al.[31] theorized that the pathogenesis of chondromalacia patellae and patellofemoral osteoarthritis may be due to medial patellofemoral hypopressure. Laurin et al.[38] have attempted to substantiate this radiographically with an axial view of the patella at 20° of flexion. This view permits the observer to measure the lateral patellofemoral angle and calculate the patellofemoral index. Conceptually, when there is excessive lateral tilt, the patellofemoral angle will open medially. This medial opening denotes hypopressure of the medial facet while the lateral facet would be experiencing increased pressure.

This concept of medial patellar hypopressure was well described by Goodfellow et al. in 1976,[39] when they noted that the most frequent site for articular cartilage fibrillation was the odd facet, at the extreme medial border of the patella. This odd facet came into contact with the femur only in extreme flexion and thus was an area of habitual disuse. Citing work done with Bullough[40] in 1967, Goodfellow described the tendency for cartilage that is habitually out of contact with other articular cartilage to undergo surface fibrillation. Goodfellow further observed that medial lesions were age related, involving the superficial layer of the articular cartilage, and he believed that these changes were not progressive. In the

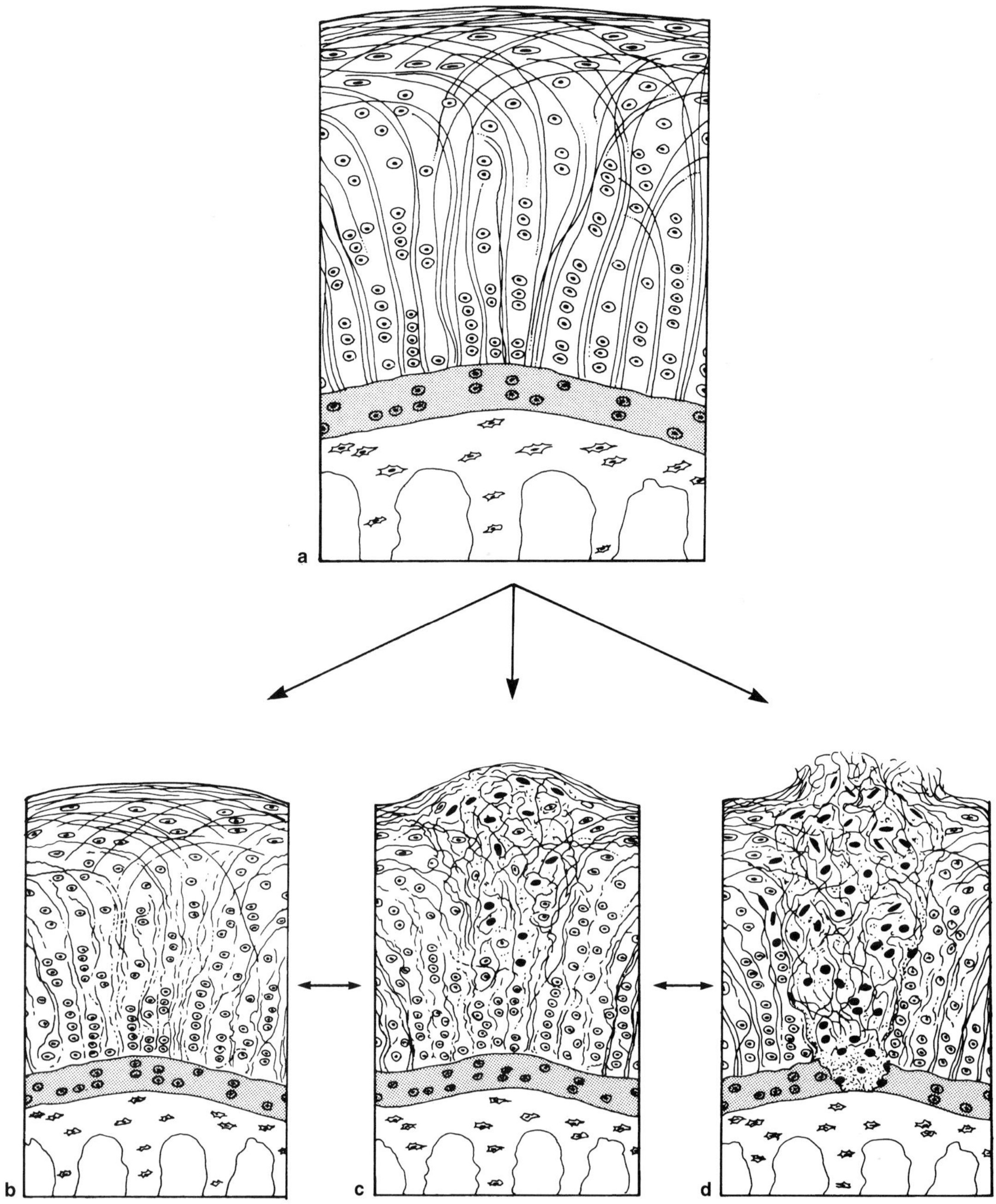

FIGURE 1.1. Stages of basal degeneration. (Adapted from Goodfellow. JBJS 58B:291, 1976 with permission)

younger population, these lesions of the patellar articular surface probably did not cause pain. The previously cited cultural differences reported by Marrar and Pillay[24] supported Goodfellow's observations on the incidence and location of patellar lesions.

Goodfellow et al.[39] also described a second lesion of the articular cartilage, which he termed "basal degeneration." This lesion consisted of fasciculations of collagen in the middle and deep zones of cartilage before affecting the surface layer (Figure 1.1). It was found astride the ridge separating the medial from the odd facet in 23 adolescents complaining of patellofemoral pain. Goodfellow treated this lesion by excision of a disk of cartilage and hypothesized that the pathogenesis was related to the functional anatomy of the patella. Since the basal layer is the origin of chondromalacia, Goodfellow recommended that the entire area of abnormal cartilage be resected to subchondral bone.

Goodfellow et al.,[39] as did others,[25,41,42] rejected the use of the term *chondromalacia patellae* to convey the idea of "pain behind the kneecap," and described the clinical symptoms as *patellofemoral pain.* The term *chondromalacia patellae* should be reserved for the pathologic process in the articular cartilage, which may or may not cause the patellofemoral pain syndrome.

In the 1970s, Insall was instrumental in classifying disorders of the patella according to the condition of the articular cartilage (Table 1.2).[42,43] He also detailed the characteristic findings on physical examination and coined the term "movie sign" to describe the diffuse ache on the anteromedial aspect of the knee when the knee is flexed for a prolonged period of time. The association between the anterior knee pain with patella alta[44,45] and an abnormal Q angle[43,44] was also reported. Similar to Goodfellow et al.,[39] Insall found that chondromalacia frequently involved the midpoint of the patellar crest with equal extension both medially and laterally. It was not unusual to find the upper and lower thirds of the patella spared (Figure 1.2). Because tracking problems and patellar malalignment were implicated in causing patellar pain while incidentally contributing to chondromalacia, Insall recommended and described his technique for proximal patellar realignment. Although the technique has undergone change from its original description as a "tube" realignment,[46] the results continue to be successful.

TABLE 1.2. Insall's classification of patellar disorders.

Condition	Classification
Presence of cartilage damage	Chondromalacia Osteoarthritis Direct trauma and osteochondral fractures Osteochondritis
Variable cartilage damage	Malalignment syndromes Synovial plicae
Usually normal cartilage	Peripatellar causes: bursitis and tendinitis Overuse syndromes Reflex sympathetic dystrophy Patellar anomalies

Numerous techniques have been described for distal realignment of the patella since Hauser's early description.[47] Hauser's method became unpopular because of reports of late osteoarthritis[48] caused by excessive distal or medial transfer of the patellar tendon. Distal realignment procedures, as described by Hughston and Walsh,[49] as well as Elmslie, have accomplished medialization of the tibial tubercle without posterior displacement. Modifications of the distal realignment have also been described by Trillat et al.,[50] Cox,[51] and Brown et al.[52]

Because chronic patellar malalignment has been implicated in the destruction of articular cartilage and the development of osteoarthrosis,[53] several procedures have been recommended to relieve patellofemoral contact stress. In 1976, Maquet,[54] described the biomechanics of the excessive lateral pressure syndrome that appears to cause subsequent arthrosis. He described his technique of elevating or anteriorizing the tibial tubercle in order to decrease the patellofemoral contact pressure and relieve symptoms.[54–56] Prior to this, patellectomy[57] was often the only alter-

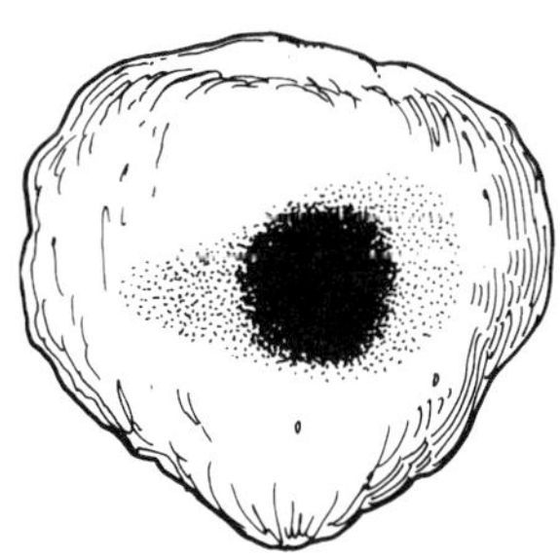

FIGURE 1.2. Patellar map of chondromalacia. (Adapted from Insall. JBJS 58A:1, 1976 with permission)

native for severe patella arthrosis. Also, patellectomy was not without complication as Kelly and Insall[58] have well outlined.

Similar to Maquet,[54] Fulkerson[59] emphasized the importance of relieving patellofemoral joint pressure by anteromedial tibial tubercle transfer. Fulkerson modified the Elmslie–Trillat procedure with a steep oblique osteotomy of the tibial tubercle, allowing 1.0 to 1.5 cm of anterior displacement of the tibial tubercle without supplemental bone graft. The advantage of anteromedialization of the tibial tubercle is that the effects are similar to those of a Maquet osteotomy without the complications of nonunion and skin slough.

Fulkerson and Shea[60] emphasized the importance of patellar malalignment and abnormal stresses of the supporting patellar soft tissues. Fulkerson et al. observed neuromatous degeneration[61] of small nerves in the excessively tight lateral retinaculum and suggested the lateral retinaculum itself as a source of pain in this syndrome. Larson et al.[62] recommended lateral retinacular lengthening as a method to theoretically lessen the compressive forces on the articular surfaces. Lateral releases in combination with various methods of realignment of the patella have been reported as early as 1888 by Roux,[63] 1891 by Pollard,[64] and 1895 by Goldthwait.[65]

Further investigation of the patella has evolved over the years as technology has improved. Schutzer et al.[66] have used computed tomography (CT) images to examine the patellofemoral joint. This technique permitted more precise measurements and established normal criteria for patellar alignment. This information was incorporated into Fulkerson and Hungerford's classification of patellofemoral pain[67] (Table 1.3). In a similar fashion, Shellock et al.[68] used kinematic magnetic resonance imaging (MRI) to assess patellar tracking abnormalities.

Arthroscopy has further enhanced the study of patellofemoral lesions and malalignment. Direct arthroscopic visualization of the patella as it tracks within the femoral sulcus as well as the integrity of the articular surface has proven valuable in the decision-making process.[69] Fulkerson and Shea[53] have reiterated, however, that the arthroscopic examination is not necessary to make the diagnosis of patellar tilt or subluxation because these conditions can be determined by radiographic or CT studies. However, the arthroscopic examination is extremely useful in assessing the extent of damage to the articular cartilage. Realizing that arthroscopic visualization of patellofemoral tracking may provide a direct means of assessing malalignment, Casscells[70] began to report his findings. He noted that when viewed arthroscopically, both the medial and lateral facets normally engage the corresponding surfaces of the femur between 30° and 60° of flexion. In extension, only the lateral patellar facet is in contact with the femur.

Work by Kelly and Mow,[71] as well as by Ateshian et al.[72] using stereophotogrammetry, has quantitated the topography of the patellofemoral articular surface and cartilage thickness (Figures 1.3 and 1.4). This technology also identified material property differences between patellar and femoral articular cartilage. These investigations demonstrated a relative mismatch, with the femoral articular cartilage being stiffer than the patellar articular cartilage. The results suggested that the patella may be more vulnerable than the femoral sulcus to the development of articular cartilage lesions.[14]

Our current understanding of patellofemoral pain has evolved over the 20th century. Whereas up until the late 1960s pain in the anterior aspect of the knee was attributed to

TABLE 1.3. Fulkerson's classification of patellofemoral malalignment.

Type	Description
I	Includes subluxation with no articular lesions
	Subluxation with minimal chondromalacia
	Subluxation with osteoarthritis
II	Subluxation with tilt and no articular changes
	Subluxation with tilt and minimal chondromalacia
	Subluxation with tilt and osteoarthritis
III	Patellar tilt with no articular lesion
	Tilt with chondromalacia
	Tilt with osteoarthritis
IV	No malalignment, no chondromalacia
	No malalignment, chondromalacia is evident
	No malalignment, osteoarthritis is present

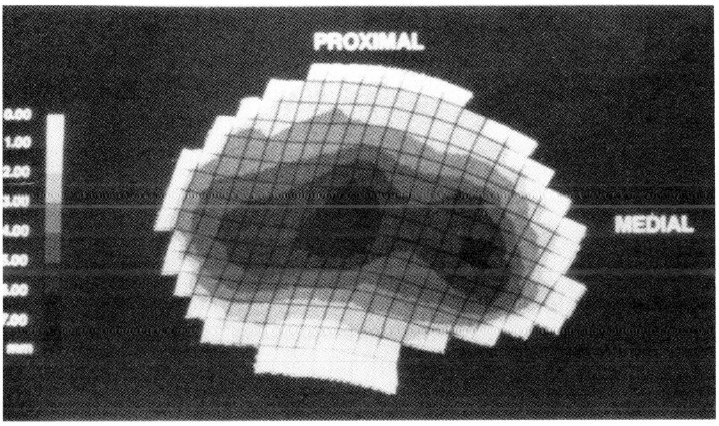

FIGURE 1.3. Stereophotogrammetric mapping of the patellar articular cartilage thickness. (Reprinted from Kelly, M. and Insall, J.: Historical Perspectives of Chondromalacia Patellae. Ortho Clin NA 23(4):517–521, 1992, with permission)

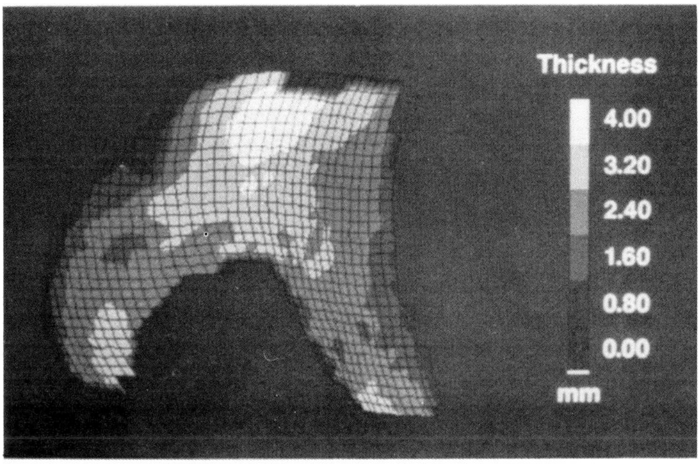

FIGURE 1.4. Stereophotogrammetric mapping of the femoral articular cartilage thickness. (Reprinted from Kelly, M. and Insall, J.: Historical Perspectives of Chondromalacia Patellae. Ortho Clin NA 23(4):517–521, 1992, with permission)

chondromalacia patellae, we now know that such pain frequently is caused by damage to the articular cartilage of the patella and strain on the peripatellar retinaculum brought about by abnormal patella alignment.[47] As new investigative techniques are developed, our understanding of the patellofemoral joint will continue to improve, as will our approach in treating specific maladies of the patellofemoral joint.

References

1. Budinger K: Uber Ablosung von Gelenktulen und Verwandte Prozesse. *Dtsch Z Chir* 1906; 84:311–365.
2. Ludloff: Zur Patholgie der Kniegelenks. *Verh Dtsch Ges Chir* 1910;223.
3. Axhausen G: Umschriebenen Knorpel-knocherlasionen des Kniegelenks. *Berl Klin Wochenschr* 1919;56:265.
4. Aleman O: Chondromalacia post-traumatica patellae. *Acta Chir Scand* 1928;63:149.
5. Karlson S: Chondromalacia patellae. *Acta Chir Scand* 1939;83:347.
6. Owre A: Chondromalacia patellae. *Acta Chir Scand* 1936;77(suppl. 41).
7. Kulowski J: Chondromalacia of the patella: Fissural cartilage degeneration;traumatic chondroplasty; Report of three cases. *JAMA* 1933; 100:1847.
8. Heine J: Arthritis deformans. *Arch Pathol Anat* 1926;260:521.
9. Bennett GA, Waine H, Bauer W: Changes in the knee joint at various ages with particular reference to the nature and development of degenerative joint diseases. New York, The Commonwealth Fund, 1942.
10. Emery IH, Meachin G: Surface morphology

and topography of patello-femoral cartilage fibrillation in Liverpool necropsies. *J Anat* 1973; 116:103.

11. Casscells SW: Gross pathological changes in the knee joint of the aged individual. *Clin Orthop* 1978;132:225.
12. Goodfellow J, Hungerford DS, Zindel M: Patello-femoral joint mechanics and pathology. 1. Functional anatomy of the patello-femoral joint. *J Bone Joint Surg Br* 1976;58B:287–290.
13. Wiles P, Andrews PS, Devas MB: Chondromalacia of the patella. *J Bone Joint Surg Br* 1956;38B:95–113.
14. Kelly MA, Insall JN: Historical perspective of chondromalacia patella. *Orthop Clin North Am* 1992;23(4):517–521.
15. Outerbridge RE: The etiology of chondromalacia patellae. *J Bone Joint Surg Br* 1961; 43B:752–757.
16. Outerbridge RE: Further studies on the etiology of chondromalacia patellae. *J Bone Joint Surg Br* 1964;46B:179.
17. Meachim G, Emery IH: Quantitative aspects of patello-femoral cartilage fibrillation in Liverpool necropsies. *Ann Rheum Dis* 1974;33:39–47.
18. Morscher E: Osteotomy of the patella in chondromalacia. *Arch Orthop Trauma Surg* 1978; 92:139.
19. Chaklin VD: Injuries to the cartilages of the patella and the femoral condyle. *J Bone Joint Surg* 1939;21:133.
20. Cave EF, Rowe CR, Yee LB: Chondromalacia of the patella. *Surg Gynecol Obstet* 1945; 84:446.
21. Hinricsson H: Studies of patellar chondromalacia. An attempt to elucidate its etiology. *Acta Orthop Scand* 1939;10:312–322.
22. Wiberg G: Roentgenographic and anatomic studies of the patello-femoral joint. *Acta Orthop Scand* 1941;12:319.
23. Baumgartl F: Das Knegelenk. Berlin, Springer-Verlag, 1944.
24. Marrar BD, Pillay VK: Chondromalacia of the patella in the Chinese—A post-mortem study. *J Bone Joint Surg Am* 1975;57A:342.
25. Abernethy PJ, Townsend PR, Rose RM, et al.: Is chondromalacia patellae a separate clinical entity? *J Bone Joint Surg Br* 1978;60B:205.
26. Brattstrom H: Shape of the intercondylar groove normally and in recurrent dislocation of the patella. A clinical and x-ray anatomical investigation. *Acta Orthop Scand* 1964; 68(suppl):5–148.
27. Merchant AC: Patellofemoral disorders, in Chapman M (ed): *Operative Orthopaedics.* Philadelphia, JB Lippincott Co., 1988, pp. 1699–1709.
28. Hughston, JC: Subluxation of the patella. *J Bone Joint Surg Am* 1968;50A:1003–1026.
29. Ficat P: Pathologie femoro-patellaire. Paris, Masson et cie, 1970, p. 148.
30. Ficat P, Philipe J, Bizou H: Le defile femoropatellaire. *Rev Med Toulouse* 1970;6:241.
31. Ficat P, Ficat C, Bailleux A: Syndrome d'hyperpression externe de la rotue (S.H.P.E.). *Rev Chir Orthop* 1975;61:39.
32. Larson RL: The patella of the female athlete-subluxation, chondromalacia and patellar compression syndrome. Med Aspect Sport A.M.A. 1974;16:12.
33. Ficat P, Hungerford DS: *Disorders of the Patellofemoral Joint.* Baltimore, Williams & Wilkins Co., 1977.
34. Seeholm BB, Takeda T, Tsubuku M, et al.: Mechanical factors and patellofemoral osteoarthrosis. *Ann Rheum Dis* 1979;38:307.
35. Stougard J: Chondromalacia of the patella-incidence, macroscopical and radiological findings at autopsy. *Acta Orthop Scand* 1975; 46:809–822.
36. Merchant AC, Mercer RL, Jacobsen RH, et al.: Roentgenographic analysis of patellofemoral congruence. *J Bone Joint Surg Am* 1974; 56A:1391.
37. Merchant AC, Mercer RL: Lateral release of the patella: A preliminary report. *Clin Orthop* 1974;103:40.
38. Laurin CA, Dussault R, Levesque HP: The tangential x-ray investigation of the patellofemoral joint; x-ray technique, diagnostic criteria and their interpretation. *Clin Orthop* 1979;144:16–26.
39. Goodfellow J, Hungerford DS, Woods C: Patellofemoral joint mechanics and pathology. 2. Chondromalacia patellae. *J Bone Joint Surg Br* 1976;58B:291–299.
40. Goodfellow JW, Bullough PG: The pattern of aging of the articular cartilage of the elbow joint. *J Bone Joint Surg Br* 1967;49B:175.
41. Radin EL: A rational approach to the treatment of patellofemoral pain. *Clin Orthop* 1979; 144:107.
42. Insall J: Patella pain syndromes and chondromalacia patellae. *Instr Course Lect* 1981; 30:342.
43. Insall J, Falvo KA, Wise DW: Chondromalacia patellae: A prospective study. *J Bone Joint Surg Am* 1976;58A:1.
44. Insall J: "Chondromalacia patellae", patellar

malalignment syndrome. *Orthop Clin North Am* 1979;10:117–127.
45. Insall J, Salvati E: Patella position in the normal knee joint. *Radiology* 1971;101:101.
46. Insall J, Bullough PG, Burstein AH: Proximal "tube" realignment of the patella for chondromalacia patellae. *Clin Orthop* 1979;144:63–69.
47. Hauser EDW: Total tendon transplant for slipping patella. *Surg Gynecol Obstet* 1938;66:199.
48. Chrisman OD, Snook GA, Wilson TC: A long-term prospective study of the Hauser and Roux-Goldthwait procedures for recurrent patella dislocation. *Clin Orthop* 1979;144:27.
49. Hughston JC, Walsh WM: Proximal and distal reconstruction of the extensor mechanism for patella subluxation. *Clin Orthop* 1979;144:36.
50. Trillat A, Dejour H, Covette A: Diagnostic et traitement des subluxations recidivantes de la rotule. *Rev Chir Orthop* 1964;50:813.
51. Cox JS: Evaluation of the Roux-Elmslie-Trillat procedure for knee extensor realignment. *Am J Sports Med* 1982;10:303–310.
52. Brown DE, Alexander AH, Licheman DM: The Elmslie-Trillate procedure: Evaluation in patellar dislocation and subluxation. *Am J Sports Med* 1984;12:104.
53. Fulkerson JP, Shea KP: Current concepts review, disorders of patellofemoral alignments. *J Bone Joint Surg Am* 1990;72A:1424–1429.
54. Maquet P: Advancement of the tibial tuberosity. *Clin Orthop* 1976;115:225–230.
55. Bandi VW: Zur operativen therapie der chondromalacia patellae. *Zentralbl Chir* 1977; 102:1297–1301.
56. Radin EL: Anterior tibial tubercle elevation in the young adult. *Orthop Clin North Am* 1986; 17:297–302.
57. Jones JB, Francis KC, Mahoney JR: Recurrent dislocating patella, a long term follow up study. *Clin Orthop* 1961;20:230.
58. Kelly MA, Insall JN: Patellectomy. *Orthop Clin North Am* 1986;17:289–295.
59. Fulkerson JP: Anteromedialization of the tibial tuberosity for patellofemoral malalignment. *Clin Orthop* 1983;177:176–181.
60. Fulkerson JP, Shea KP: Mechanical basis for patellofemoral pain and cartilage breakdown, in Ewing JW (ed.) *Articular Cartilage and Knee Joint Function: Basic Science and Arthroscopy.* New York, Raven Press, 1990.
61. Fulkerson JP, Tenant R, Jaivin JS, et al.: Histologic evidence of nerve injury associated with patellofemoral malalignment. *Clin Orthop* 1985;197:196.
62. Larson RL, Cabaud HE, Slocum DB, et al.: The patellar compression syndrome. Surgical treatment by lateral retinacular release. *Clin Orthop* 1978;134:158–167.
63. Roux C: Recurrent dislocation of the patella: Operative treatment. *Rev Chir* 1888.
64. Pollard B: Old-standing (congenital) dislocation of patella;reduction of patella after dividing the vastus externus and chiseling a new trochlear surface on the femur; restoration of function of the limb. Lancet May 1891;1203.
65. Goldthwait JE: Dislocation of the patella. *Trans Am Orthop Assoc* 1895;8:237.
66. Schutzer SF, Ramsby GR, Fulkerson JP: Computed tomographic classification of patellofemoral pain patients. *Orthop Clin North Am* 1986; 17:235–248.
67. Fulkerson J, Hungerford D: Disorders of the patellofemoral joint. Baltimore, Williams & Wilkins Co., 1990.
68. Shellock FG, Mink SH, Fix JM: Patellofemoral joint: Kinematic MR imaging to assess tracking abnormalities. *Radiology* 1988;168:551–553.
69. Lindberg U, Hamberg P, Lysholm J, et al.: Arthroscopic examination of the patellofemoral joint using a central one-portal technique. *Orthop Clin North Am* 1986;17:263–268.
70. Casscells SW: The arthroscope in the diagnosis of disorders of the patellofemoral joint. *Clin Orthop* 1979;144:45–50.
71. Kelly MA, Mow VC: Stereophotogrammetry and the patellofemoral joint. Presented at the combined Japanese American Sports Medicine Association meeting, Kawai, HI, January 1991.
72. Ateshian GA, Soslowsky LJ, Mow VC: Quantitation of articular surface topography and cartilage thickness in knee joints using stereophotogrammetry. *J Biomech* 1991;24:761.

2

Embryology and Anatomy of the Patella

Alfred J. Tria, Jr. and Jose A. Alicea

Embryology

The human knee dates back 320 million years in the evolutionary scale to Eryops, the common ancestor of reptiles, birds, and mammals (Figure 2.1). The Eryops knee was bicondylar, with a femorofibular articulation, cruciate ligaments, and asymmetric collateral ligaments. The patella was not yet present. As evolution continued, the fibula migrated distally, away from the joint line; and the bicondylar femur rotated internally and developed a medial offset, bringing the joint progression closer to the midline. The osseous patella developed separately in birds, some reptiles, and in mammals about 70 million years ago. This was a late development compared with the cruciates or the condylar surfaces. The anterior femoral articular surface extended proximally beneath the patella to form the sulcus and completed the development of the patellofemoral joint (Figure 2.2).[1,2]

Streeter outlined a staging system for embryologic development that depended upon the external appearance of the embryo and not upon the length or the age of the embryo.[3] He proposed 23 stages or horizons from the single cell through the end of the embryonic period, when the nutrient vessel enters the humerus. The leg bud appears during horizon 13 (28 days). In horizon 18 (37 days), the chondrification of the femur, tibia, and fibula begins, along with early differentiation of the patella and the patellar ligament. At horizon 22 (45 days), chondrification of the patella begins along with the differentiation of the cruciate ligaments and the menisci. Thus, at the end of the embryonic period, the knee resembles the adult structure (Table 2.1).[4]

There are three primary synovial plicae of the knee: (1) the suprapatellar, (2) the medial, and (3) the infrapatellar (Figure 2.3). The knee joint at 12 weeks of gestation is a single syovial cavity. Between 11 and 20 weeks of gestation a suprapatellar plica forms in approximately one third of the fetuses and goes on to separate the suprapatellar pouch from the primary knee joint by the fourth month of gestation. This plica then develops into four variants in the adult knee: (1) a full septum, (2) a fenestrated septum, (3) a medial shelf, or (4) a fully involuted structure.[5] The medial synovial plica develops during the same gestational period in approximately one third of the fetuses, and the infrapatellar plica develops in 50% of the fetuses.[6] The pathologic conditions of the plicae of the knee can mimic many of the symptoms related to the patellofemoral articulation and should be included in any thorough differential diagnosis. The epiphyses of the distal femur and the proximal tibia are both present at birth. The proximal fibular epiphysis and the patellar ossification center are not present until age 3 years for the female and age 4 or 5 years for the male (Table 2.2).[7]

Patellar Dysplasias

There are several types of patellar dysplasias, including aplasia, hypoplasia, partial hypopla-

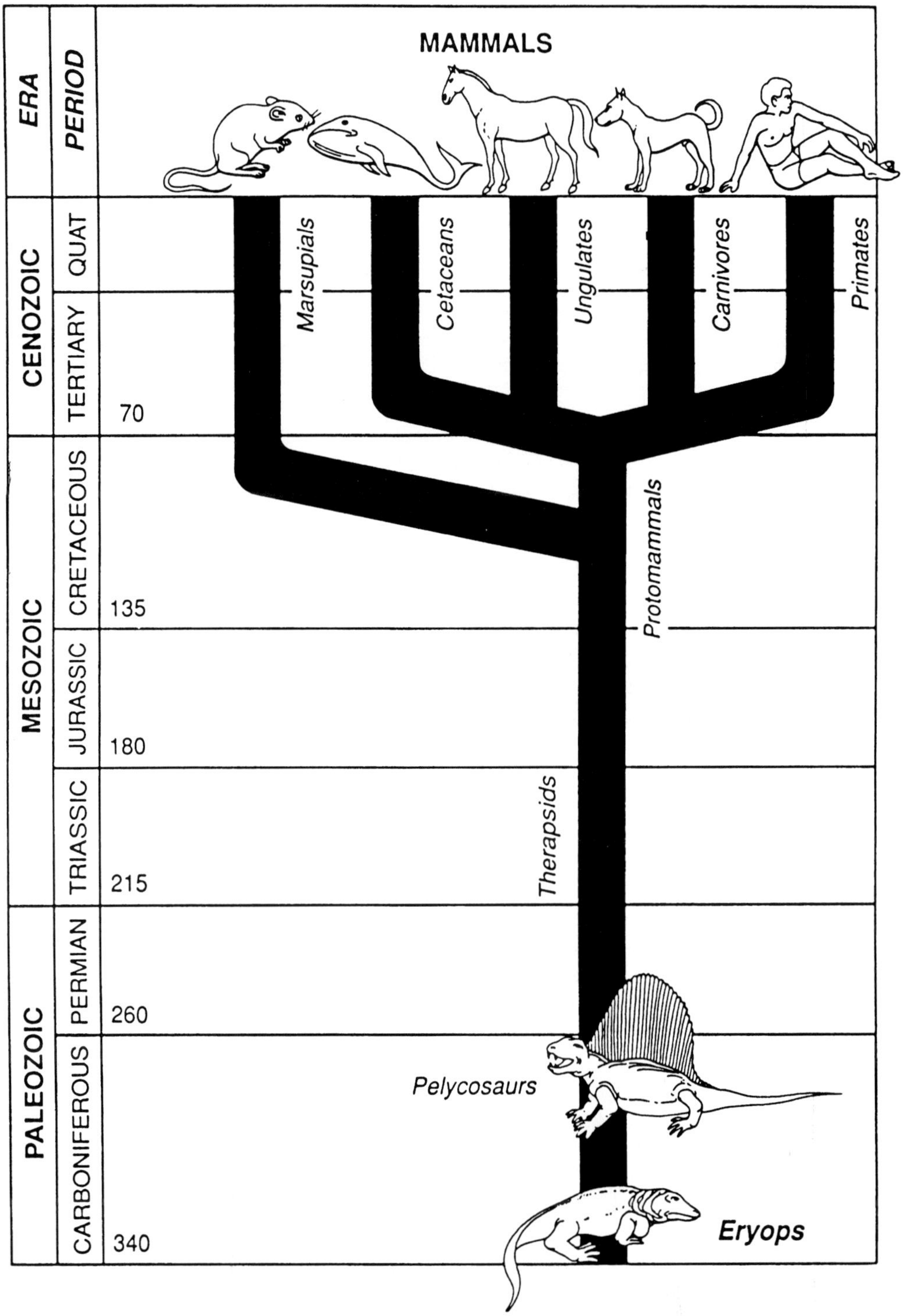

FIGURE 2.1. The relationship of Eryops to mammals as depicted by Mossman and Sarjeant (Adapted from the footprints of extinct animals, Mossman DJ, and Sarjeant WAS. *Sci Am* 250:78–79, 1983 with permission. Copyright © 1983 by Scientific American, Inc. All rights reserved.)

TABLE 2.1. The chronology of limb development in the human embryo.

Horizon	Age* (days)	Crown-rump (mm)	Morphologic event
I			One-cell egg
II			Segmenting egg
III			Free blastocyst
IV	6		Implanting ovum
V	9–10		Ovum implanted but avillous
VI	11–15		Primitive villi, distinct yolk sac
VII	16–20		Branching villi, axis of germinal disk defined
VIII	20–21		Hensen's node, primitive groove evident
IX	21–22		Neural folds, elongated notochord
X	23		Early somite stage
XI	24		13–20 somites
XII	26	3–4	21–29 somites, arm bud appears
XIII	28	4–5	Leg bud appears
XIV	29	6–7	Leg bud finlike
XV	31	7–8	Early mesenchymal skeleton formation
XVI	33	9–10	Foot plate appears, mesenchymal skeleton complete
XVII	35	11–13	Rotation of leg bud in counterclockwise direction
XVIII	37	14–16	Early chondrification of femur, tibia, and fibula; early differentiation of patella
XIX	39	17–20	Formation of femoral condyles
XX	41	21–23	Knee joint interzone formation
XXI	43	22–24	Joint capsule formation complete
XXII	45	25–27	Condrification of patella, appearance of cruciate ligaments and menisci
XXIII	47	28–30	Knee clearly resembles that of adult End of embryonic period

*Age approximate, based on menstrual age.
Adapted from Sledge CB: Some morphologic and experimental aspects of limb development. *Clin Orthop* 1966; 44:241.

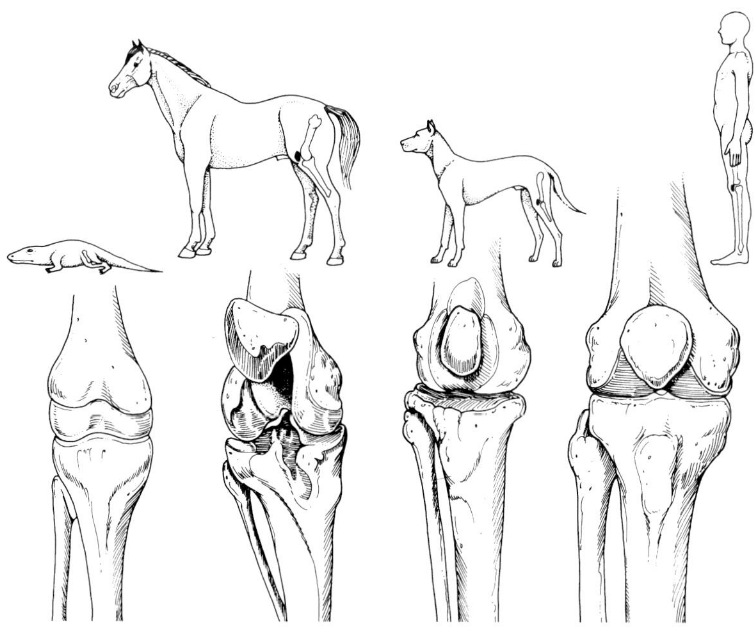

FIGURE 2.2. The development of the knee from Eryops to humans.

TABLE 2.2. The appearance and the closure of the epiphyses of the knee.

	Appearance (years)		Closure (years)	
Epiphysis	Male	Female	Male	Female
Distal femur	(36th fetal week)		18/19	17
Proximal tibia	(40th fetal week)		18/19	16/17
Tibial tuberosity	7–15		19	
Proximal fibula	4	3	18/20	16/18
Patella	4/5	3		

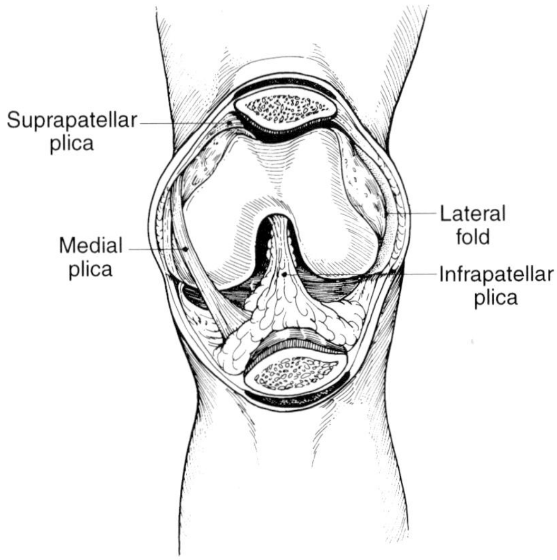

FIGURE 2.3. The synovial plicae of the knee.

sia, bipartite patella, patellar fragmentation, patellar duplication, and patella magna.

In 1897, Little and Mayer independently reported on congenital absence and delayed development of the patella.[8,9] Since then, multiple reports of this condition have appeared in the literature.[10–12] Patellar aplasia, in association with ungual dysplasia and iliac horns, is termed *nail–patella* syndrome.[13]

The patellar ossification center is usually a single entity; however, a secondary center may form simultaneously, leading to a fragmented or fractured appearance. Saupe classified bipartite patellae according to the location of the secondary ossification. Seventy-five percent of

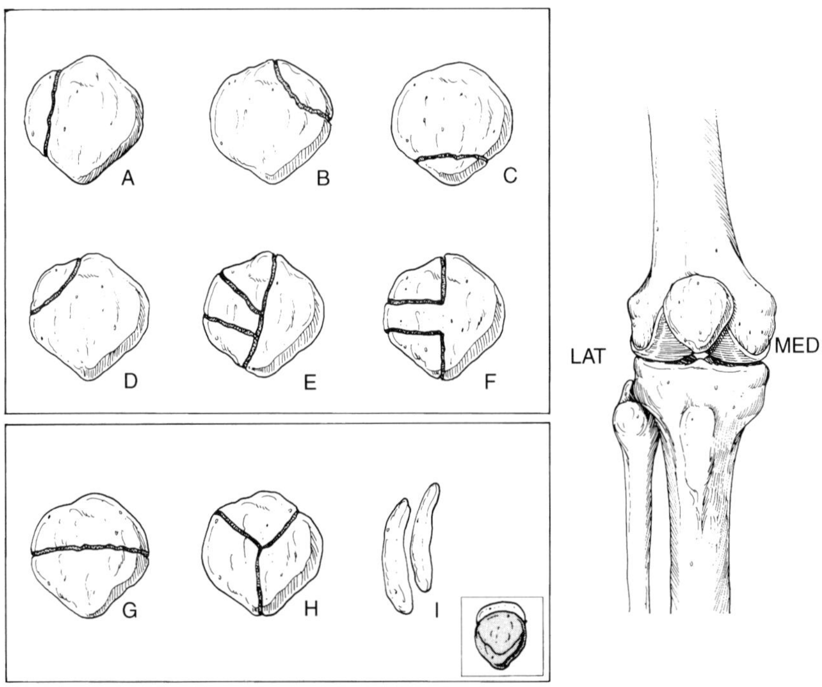

FIGURE 2.4. Patellar dysplasias.

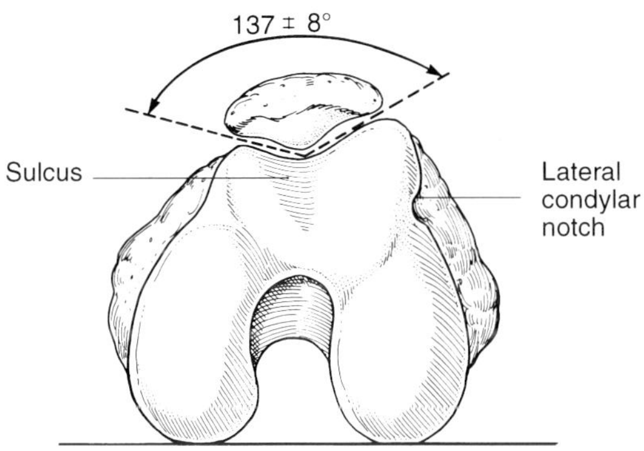

FIGURE 2.5. The sulcus and view of the distal end of the femur of a left knee.

the accessory centers occurred at the superolateral pole (type III), 20% occurred at the lateral margin (type II), and 5% were located at the inferior pole (type I). There is speculation that type I is really asymptomatic Sinding–Larsen–Johansson disease.[14] The incidence of bipartite patella is approximately 1.9%, with a 53% incidence of bilaterality.[15]

There are multiple patellar fragmentations, including tripartite and the extremely unusual patellar duplication (Figure 2.4). The fragmentations represent portions of the original single ossific nucleus that have broken free from the primary patellar bed. Schaer's explanation of a multicentric ossific nucleus would explain the variations in a simpler fashion but the developmental studies do not substantiate this theory.[16]

The patellar fragmentations should not be confused with fractures and can be differentiated from a fracture by the irregularity of the separation space between the main body and the fragments. A vertical fragmentation of the lateral facet has also been reported, and it is commonly interpreted as a fracture because of its linear appearance and rarity of occurrence versus the superolateral secondary ossification center.

A typical fracture line will be clearly visible and distinctly sharp. The fragments of the dysplastic patella are usually larger than the donor beds of the main body. If the fragments are visually approximated to the main bed, the "reconstructed" patella will be larger than the normal patella on the opposite side, whereas separate parts of a fracture will appear to be the same size as the opposite patella when visually joined together.

Another form of fragmentation occurs at the distal pole of the patella. A small calcification may be seen, which sometimes develops into a cup-type shape. Sinding–Larsen–Johansson described this anomaly, which once again should not be confused with a fracture.[17] It is typically seen in the age group from 10 through 15 years, is most commonly bilateral, and fuses to the main body of the patella at maturity.

A fragment of bone across the proximal patella in the adult knee is most commonly seen after a traumatic episode, and represents a disruption of the extensor mechanism and not a patellar dysplasia. Patella magna represents an enlarged patella that is increased in all of its dimensions. The patella is too large for its associated femoral sulcus. This discrepancy is

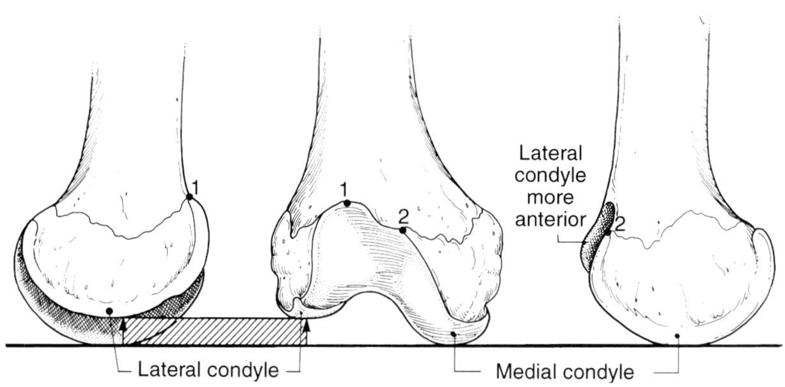

FIGURE 2.6. The anatomic relationship of the medial and lateral femoral condyles. 1, High point of the lateral femoral sulcus; 2, high point of the medial femoral sulcus.

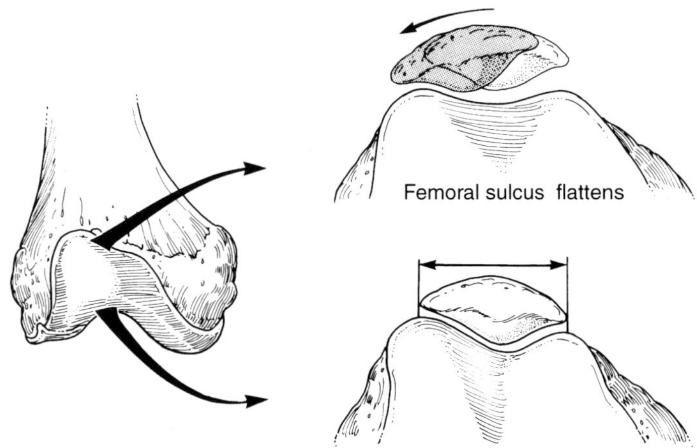

FIGURE 2.7. The femoral sulcus deepens with flexion helping to stabilize the patella.

not commonly associated with clinical symptoms.

Bone Structure

The patellofemoral joint consists of the sulcus of the femur and the patellar articular surface. The normal angle of the femoral sulcus is 137°, with a variation of 8° (Figure 2.5).[18] The lateral condyle of the femur is higher than the medial and helps in preventing lateral subluxation of the patella. The notch on the lateral femoral condyle separates the patellofemoral area from the tibiofemoral contact area. The medial femoral condyle does not have such a distinct dividing mark (Figure 2.6). The sulcus of the femur is flatter at the proximal portion than more distally. Thus, there is a greater possibility for the patella to sublux laterally near full extension of the knee than in flexion because the sulcus deepens distally and provides greater conformity for the patella (Figure 2.7).

The articular surface of the patella is situated on the proximal two thirds of the underlying bone; thus, the extraarticular distal pole attaches to the patellar tendon. There are seven patellar facets: three medial; three lateral; and one extra, nonarticulating facet on the medial side (the odd facet). The medial facets are slightly smaller in overall size than the lateral facets. The medial facet surfaces are also more convex in shape. The odd facet is a nonarticulating facet, except in deep flexion (Figure 2.8).

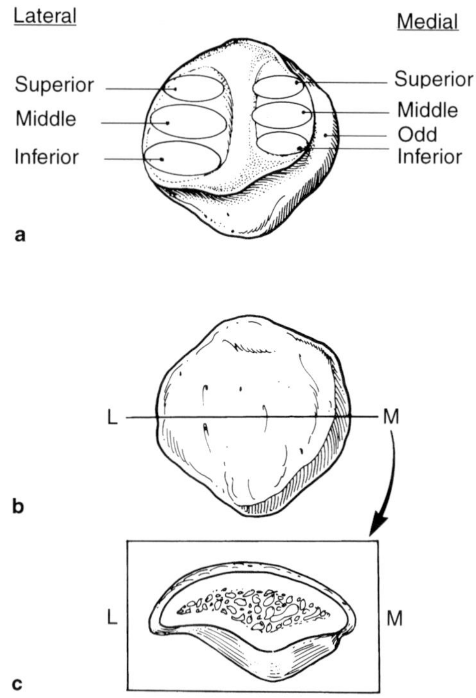

FIGURE 2.8. The seven facets of the patella (a), with an anterior surface view (b), and a cross section showing a typical Wiberg type II patella (c).

Wiberg described three configurations of the patellar facet sizes and felt that the shapes would correlate with patellar pain.[19] The Wib-

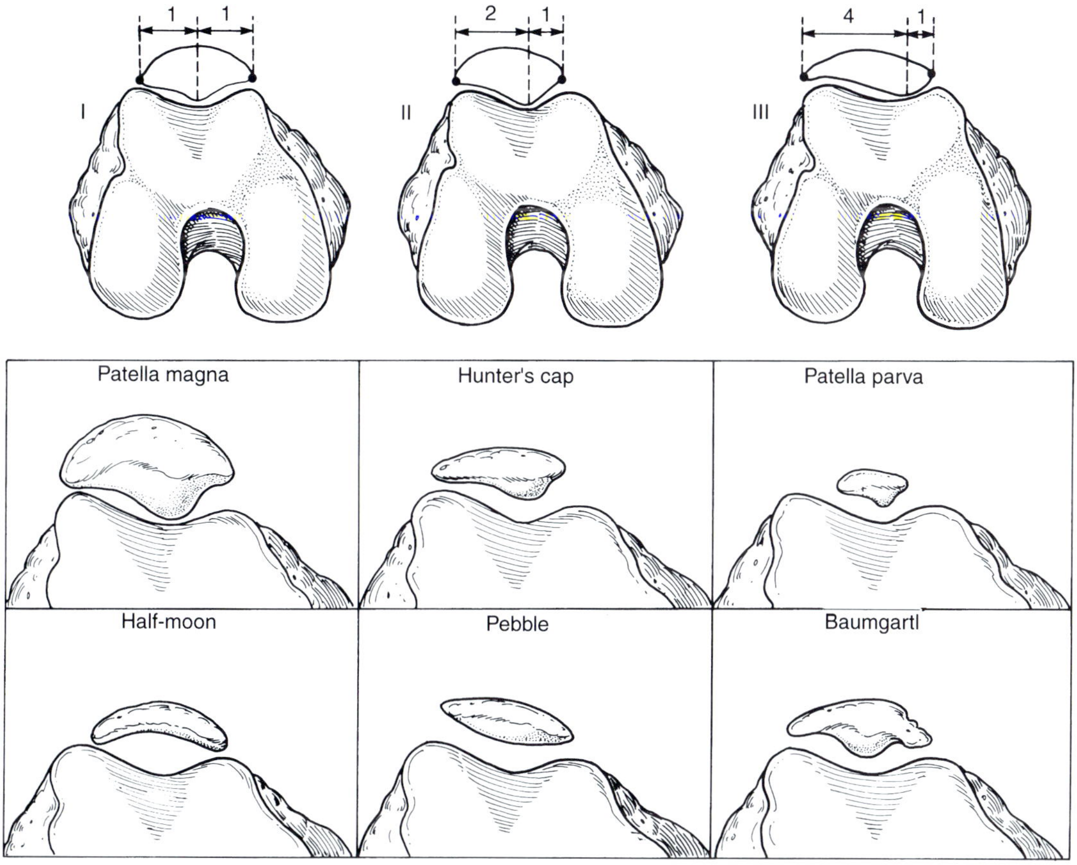

FIGURE 2.9. The Wiberg classification and some typical anatomic variations of the patella.

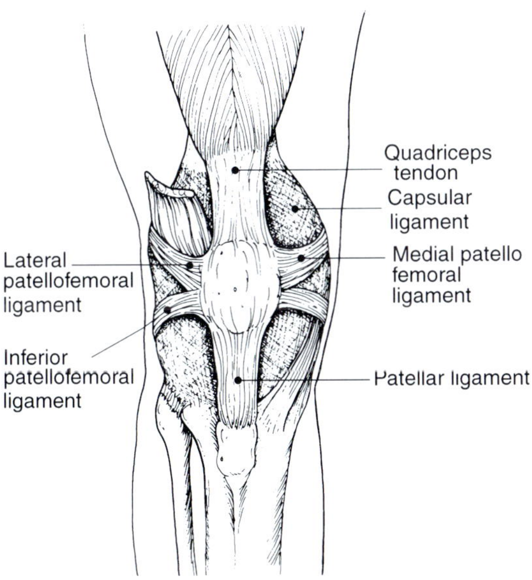

FIGURE 2.10. The patellofemoral ligaments.

erg type I patella has equal medial and lateral facets that are concave. The Wiberg type II patella has a smaller medial facet that is either flat or slightly convex and represents the most common patellar anatomy. The Wiberg type III has a considerably smaller medial facet that is convex. Baumgartl described a protuberant medial facet as a variant on the type III.[20] Wiberg felt that the type III configuration led to chondromalacia and that the type I shape was the ideal. This theory did not become well accepted because the clinical presentations of chondromalacia did not correlate with these anatomic parameters; however, the variations are still of anatomic importance and historic significance. Figure 2.9 includes many of the common variations of patellar anatomy.

FIGURE 2.11. The Q angle of the knee increases with increasing femoral neck anteversion and with increasing external tibial torsion.

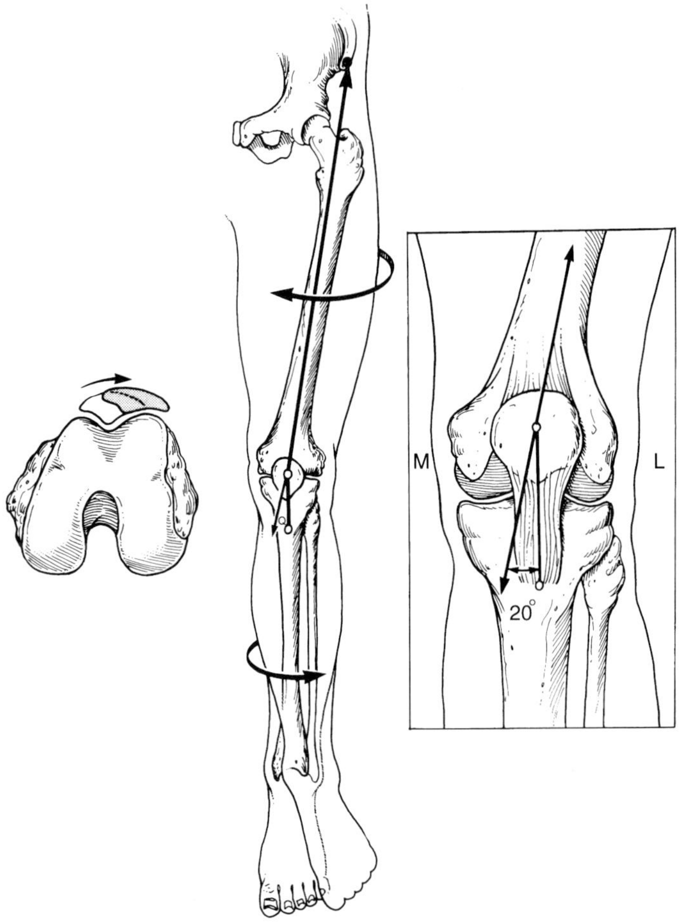

Ligaments and the Extensor Mechanism

The extensor mechanism of the knee consists of the quadriceps muscle group, the patella, the patellar ligament, and the tibial tubercle. The mechanism is responsible for the extension of the knee and relies upon the patella as a fulcrum for a mechanical advantage. The patellofemoral articulation centralizes the entire mechanism on the anterior surface of the femur.

The quadriceps muscle group is composed of four muscles: (1) the rectus femoris, (2) the vastus lateralis, (3) the vastus medialis, and (4) the vastus intermedius. These muscles join in a trilaminar fashion to form the quadriceps tendon. The rectus femoris originates from two attachments on the ileum, it courses in the anterior thigh just deep to the sartorius and it joins the quadriceps tendon 3 to 5 cm above the patella. The vastus lateralis originates from the lateral aspect of the femur and coalesces into the quadriceps tendon through the lateral retinaculum 3 cm from the superolateral aspect of the patella. The vastus medialis arises from the superomedial aspect of the femur and includes two groups of fibers: (1) the medialis obliquus and (2) the medialis longus. The fibers become tendinous a few millimeters prior to inserting into the superomedial aspect of the patella and some extend distally to blend into the medial retinaculum. The vastus intermedius lies deep to all three muscles. Its tendinous fibers blend medially and laterally with the medialis and lateralis, and insert distally into the superior border of

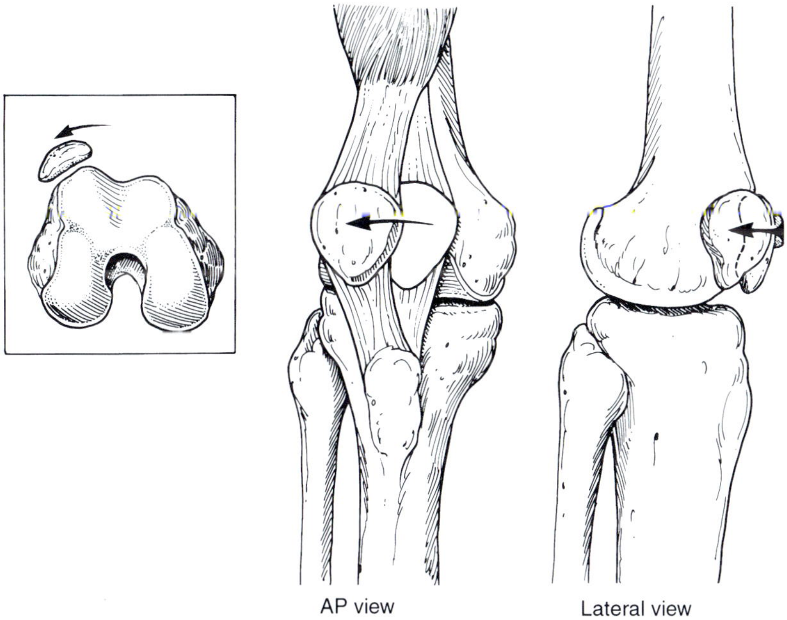

FIGURE 2.12. Congenital subluxation of the patella with a secondary articulating facet on the lateral aspect of the femur.

the patella. The fibers of the quadriceps tendon extend across the anterior surface of the patella and blend distally with the patellar tendon.

The patella is held centrally by the conformity of the facets with the sulcus of the femur and by the patellofemoral ligaments. These ligaments represent a conformation of the capsule into thickened structures on the medial and lateral side of the patella. They are located superiorly and inferiorly on either side, and extend from the anterior surface of the patella posteriorly to the side of each femoral condyle (Figure 2.10).

The patellar ligament extends from the inferior pole of the patella to the tibial tubercle. The ligament is 25 to 40 mm wide and 4 to 6 cm long in the adult. The quadriceps tendon inserts into the proximal pole of the patella and directs the pull of the vastus medialis, the vastus lateralis, the vastus intermedius, and the rectus femoris. The *Q angle* is the angle formed by a line drawn from the anterior superior iliac spine of the pelvis to the center of the patella and from the center of the patella to the center of the tibial tubercle. This angle is influenced by the femoral neck anteversion, the patellar position in the femoral sulcus, and the tibial tubercle position as affected by the lower-extremity tibial torsion.

Patellar tracking is affected by the rotational relationships of the tibia and the femur, the conformation of the patellofemoral articulation, and the directional pull of the quadriceps mechanism. As the femoral neck anteversion and the external tibial torsion increase, the Q angle increases and there is a greater possibility of lateral patellar subluxation (Figure 2.11). The quadriceps mechanism is imbalanced, with the rectus femoris, the vastus lateralis, and the vastus intermedius muscles having a mechanical advantage over the smaller medialis muscle that also has an oblique insertional pull. The quadriceps line of pull is in line with the femoral shaft and is not in line with the anatomic axis of the leg, which lies medial to the axis of the femur. This also leads to an overall lateral force away from the midline. Patellar tracking can also be affected by trochlear dysplasias. Hypoplasias and aplasias of both the medial and the lateral aspects of the trochlea have been described.[21–23]

These changes lead to a flattening of the normal sulcus angle of the femur and a loss of the patellofemoral bone congruity. Without this congruity, stability of the patella becomes dependent on the soft-tissue restraints that anatomically favor lateral subluxation.

Congenital dysplasia of the entire extensor mechanism of the knee causes the patella to articulate with the lateral aspect of the lateral femoral condyle. An articulating facet is formed along the outer aspect of the lateral femoral condyle and the patella loses its right of domain on the anterior aspect of the knee (Figure 2.12).

The contact surfaces between the patellaand the femoral sulcus change continually throughout the range of motion. In full extension, the distal pole of the patella contacts the proximal femoral sulcus in the midline. As flexion begins, the contact areas shift to the medial and the lateral sides, and progress proximally on the patella and distally on the femur (Figure 2.13). Lateral subluxation or dislocation commonly occurs during the initial 30° of flexion, when the patella can be shifted laterally in the sulcus and the contact surface can be shifted in the same direction. As flexion continues, the conformity between the patella and the femur increases, and lateral dislocation becomes almost impossible. The stability in flexion can be contributed both to the contact surfaces and to the deepening of the femoral sulcus (discussed previously).

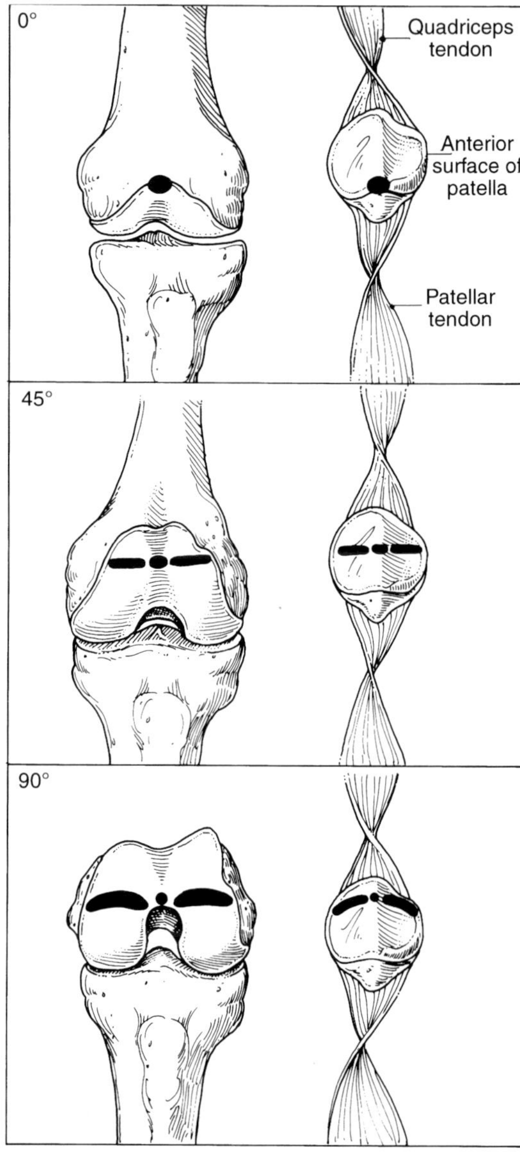

FIGURE 2.13. The patellofemoral contact surfaces showing the progression with flexion of the knee. On the patellar side, the surface contact moves from distal to proximal. On the femoral side, the surface contact moves from proximal to distal. With flexion, the contact spreads from the central area to the medial and the lateral sides.

Vascular Supply

The patella is surrounded by a plexus of blood vessels that is fed by six major arteries. The supreme geniculate is a branch from the superficial femoral artery. The vessel originates at the level of the adductor canal and proceeds distally and laterally to join the circle about the patella. There are four geniculates from the popliteal artery. The superolateral geniculate is the most superior of the four. It divides from the popliteal artery just above the tibial joint line, and proceeds laterally and anteriorly to join the patellar circle at the most superior point on the lateral side. The superomedial geniculate also originates from the popliteal artery just above the tibial joint line, and then proceeds medially and anteriorly to join the patellar circle at the midpoint of the patella on the medial side. The inferolateral genicu-

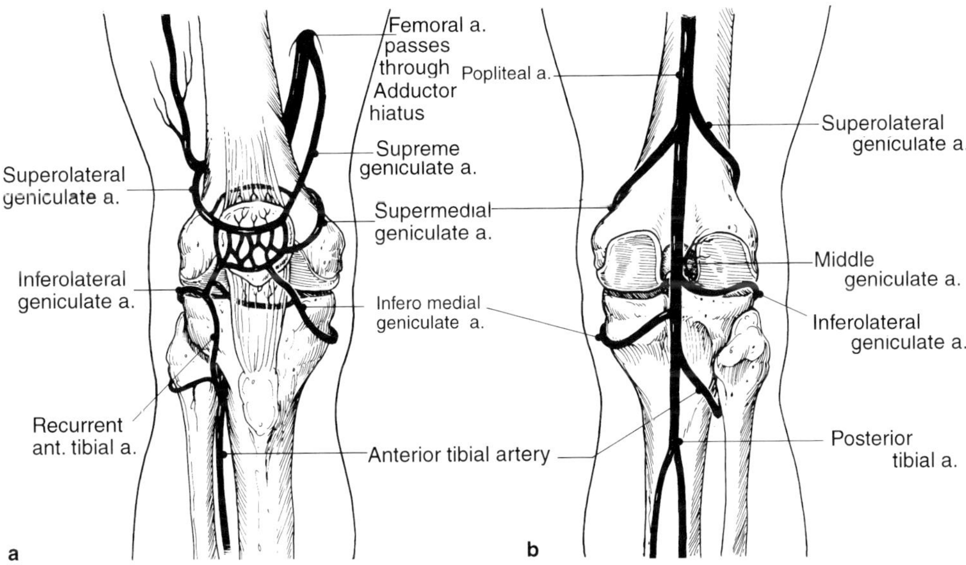

FIGURE 2.14. The vascular supply of the patella shown from the anterior aspect (a) with the insert depicting the posterior view (b) with the origin of the vessels.

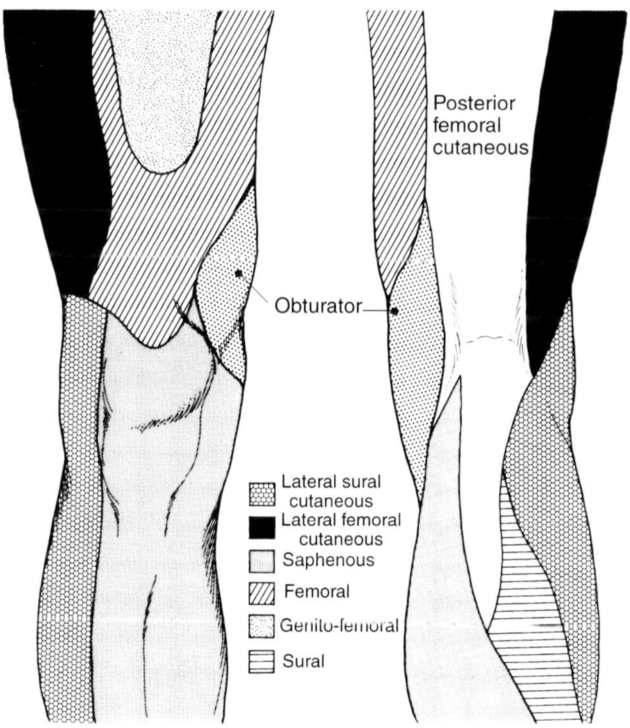

FIGURE 2.15. The cutaneous innervation of the knee from the anterior and the posterior aspects.

late divides from the popliteal artery just below the tibial joint line and proceeds anteriorly along the lateral joint line adjacent to the lateral meniscus. The vessel then turns superiorly to join the patellar circle. The inferomedial geniculate is the most inferior of the four main vessels. It also arises from the popliteal artery just below the tibial joint line and proceeds anteromedially along the side of the tibial metaphysis about 2 cm distal to the joint line. As it proceeds further anteriorly, the vessel turns superiorly and joins the patellar circle. The final vessel is the recurrent anterior tibial artery. This vessel arises from the anterior tibial artery as it penetrates the intraosseous membrane between the proximal tibia and fibula 1 cm below the proximal tibiofibular joint. It then proceeds superiorly to join the patellar circle (Figure 2.14). Scapinelli showed that the blood supply to the patella is predominantly from the distal to the proximal aspect.[24,25] Although the circular ring of vessels about the patella may appear to be symmetrically arranged, the functional blood supply is derived from the inferior aspect of the patellar circular plexus.

Innervation

The anterior cutaneous innervation of the knee includes the nerve roots from L2 through L5. The genitofemoral, femoral, obturator, and saphenous nerves account for the anteromedial innervation of the knee. The lateral femoral and the lateral sural cutaneous nerves innervate the anterolateral aspect (Figure 2.15). No nerve root endings have been identified within the knee joint itself and especially within the body of the patella or the sulcus of the femur. The explanation for patellofemoral pain remains unclear. One can establish anatomic aberrations that correlate with the symptoms of pain; however, the anatomic explanation for the pain remains uncertain.

References

1. Dye SF: An evolutionary perspective of the knee. *J Bone Joint Surg Am* 1987;69A:976–983.
2. Gardner E, O'Rahlilly R: The early development of the knee joint in staged human embryos. *J Anat* 1968;102:289.
3. Streeter GL: Developmental horizons in human embryos (fourth issue): A review of the histogenesis of cartilage and bone. Contrib Embryol No. 220, 1949;33:151.
4. Sledge, CB: Some morphologic and experimental aspects of limb development. *Clin Orthop* 1966;241:44.
5. Zidorn, T: Classification of the suprapatellar septum considering ontogenetic development. *J Arthroscopic Rel Surg* 1992;8(4):459–464.
6. Ogata S., Uhthoff HK: The development of synovial plicae in human knee joints: An embryologic study. *J Arthroscopic Rel Surg* 1990; 6(4):315–321.
7. Tria AJ Jr., Klein KS: An illustrated guide to the knee, in *Anatomy,* New York, Churchill Livingstone, 1992, p. 4.
8. Little EM: Congenital absence or delayed development of the patella. Lancet 1897;2:781–784.
9. Mayer HN: Congenital absence or delayed development of the patella. Lancet 1897;2:1384–1385.
10. Jones B: Congenital absence of both patellae. *J Bone Joint Surg Br* 1955;37B:352.
11. Bernhang AM, Levine SA: Familial absence of the patella. *J Bone Joint Surg Am* 1973;55A; 1088–1090.
12. Rubin G: Congenital absence of patellae and other patellar anomalies in three members of the same family. *JAMA* 1915;64:2062.
13. Drut RM, Chandra S, Latorraca R, et al.: Nail-patella syndrome in a spontaneously aborted 18-week fetus: Ultrastructural and immunofluorescent study of the kidneys. *Am J Med Genet* 1992;43:693–696.
14. Saupe H: Primare Knowchmark Seilerung der Kneiescheibe. *Dtsch Z Chir* 1943;258:386.
15. Scuderi GR, Scuderi DM: Patellar fragmentation. Presented at the AAOS, New Orleans, 1994.
16. Schaer MF: Die Patella Bipartita. *Ergeb Chir Orthop* 1934;27:1.
17. Sinding- Larsen MF: A hitherto unknown affection of the patella in children. *Acta Radiol* 1921;171–173.
18. Aglietti P, Insall JN, Cerulli, G: Patellar pain and incongruence. I. Measurements of incongruence. *CORR* 1983;176:217–224.
19. Wiberg G: Roentgenographic and anatomic studies on the femoro-patellar joint. *Acta Orthop Scand* 1941;12:319–410.
20. Baumgartl F: Das Kniegelenk. Berlin, Springer-Verlag, 1964.
21. Maldague B, Malghem J: Apport du cliche de profil du genou dans le depistage des instabi-

lites rotuliennes: Rapport preliminaire. *Rev Chir Orthop* 1985;71(suppl. II):5.
22. Malghem J, Maldague B: Patellofemoral joint: 30 degree axial radiograph with lateral rotation of thc lcg. *Radiology* 1989;170:566.
23. Dejour J, Walch G. Neyret P, Adeleine P: La dysplasie de la trochlee femorale. *Rev Chir Orthop* 1990;76:45.
24. Scapinelli, R: Blood supply of the human patella. Its relation to ischemic necrosis after fracture. *J Bone Joint Surg Br* 1967;49B:563–570.
25. Shim S, and Leung G: Blood supply of the knee joint. A microangiographic study in children and adults. *Clin Orthop* 1986;208:119–125.

3

Biomechanics of the Patellofemoral Joint

Paolo Aglietti and Pier Paolo M. Menchetti

Functions of the Patella

The main biomechanical function of the patella is to improve the quadriceps efficiency by increasing the lever arm of the extensor mechanism. The patella displaces the patellar tendon away from the femorotibial contact point throughout range of motion, therefore increasing the patellar tendon moment arm.[1-3] There are other important functions. The patella is necessary to centralize the divergent forces coming from the four heads of the quadriceps, and to transmit tension around the femur, in a frictionless way, to the patellar tendon and tibial tuberosity. The hyaline articular cartilage provides an insensitive (aneural), thick, avascular tissue that is specifically adapted to bearing high compressive loads.[2,3]

The patella also functions as a bony shield, not only for the trochlea, but also for the distal femoral condyles with the knee in flexion. Finally, the patella plays an important role in the cosmetics of the knee. This can be readily appreciated by observing the squared appearance of the flexed knee in patellectomized patients.

Knee Extension

The patella is an important contributor to knee extension power. An important mechanical study designed to define and quantitate the extensor function of the patella and the effects of its removal was performed on cadaver limbs by Kaufer (1971–1979).[4,5] The extension moment arm was determined at 120°, 90°, 60°, 30°, and 0° of flexion before patellectomy; after patellectomy, performed through a longitudinal tendon-splitting incision, and before tendon repair; after patellectomy and longitudinal repair, and after patellectomy and transverse repair of the quadriceps tendon to the patellar ligament. The force required for full extension of the knee was applied with a rope sutured to the quadriceps tendon. The rope was passed over a pulley positioned to simulate the direction of the quadriceps pull and traction weights were added until full extension was reached.

The intact knee had a longer quadriceps moment arm than the patellectomized knee (Table 3.1). In the intact knee, the quadriceps moment arm and the contribution of the patella increased almost linearly with knee extension. At 120°, the patella accounted for 0.4 cm (approximately 10%) of the quadriceps moment arm. At full extension, the patella's contribution increased to 1.8 cm (approximately 30%) of the quadriceps moment arm. The longitudinal repair after patellectomy had no effect on the quadriceps moment arm. The transverse repair slightly increased the quadriceps moment arm.

The force necessary for full extension of the intact knee, an average of 21 kg, was termed the 100% force. After patellectomy and longitudinal closure, this same force failed to produce full extension by almost 30°; full extension required an average force of 28.5 kg

TABLE 3.1. Knee extension moment arm.*

Knee Flexion Angle (degrees)	Intact Knee	Postpatellectomy: No Repair	Patellar Effect	Postpatellectomy: Longitudinal Repair	Postpatellectomy: Transverse Repair
120	3.9	3.5	0.4	3.5	3.7
90	4.1	3.6	0.5	3.7	3.9
60	4.5	3.9	0.6	3.9	4.2
30	5.0	3.9	1.1	4.0	4.3
0	5.8	4.0	1.8	4.1	4.4

*Calculated average knee extension moment arm expressed in centimeters.
Source: From Kaufer, *J. Bone Joint Surg. Am.* 1971, 53A(8), 1551–1560. Reproduced with permission.

(130%). After patellectomy and transverse repair, the 100% force failed to produce full extension by almost 20°; full extension required an average force of 25.9 kg (115%). Therefore, full extension after patellectomy required between 15% and 30% increase in quadriceps pull, depending on the type of repair.

Results from this experimental study indicate that the patella provides a mechanical advantage to the extension moment arm by two separate mechanisms. The patella functions as a linkage, providing continuity between the quadriceps tendon and the patellar ligament. After patellectomy and longitudinal repair, the pull on the patellar ligament by the quadriceps is diverted from the central portion of the extensor mechanism into the medial and lateral patellar retinacula. Pull upon retinacula produces less extension torque because the retinacula have a shorter moment arm than the patellar ligament. Transverse repair after patellectomy restores tension to the patellar ligament, which is further from the knee flexion axis and therefore increases the extension moment arm observed with longitudinal repair. Moreover, a transverse repair will slightly lengthen the quadriceps muscle fibers, thus increasing the quadriceps force according to the length–tension relationship.

The patella provides a mechanical advantage beyond mere linkage. Its action is analogous to a pulley that displaces the quadriceps anteriorly, thus increasing its moment arm. In flexion, the patella sinks into the intercondylar notch and produces little anterior displacement of the quadriceps tendon. Therefore, in flexion, the patella has little effect on the extensor moment arm beyond its linking effect. Towards full extension, the patella rises out of the intercondylar groove and produces significant anterior displacement of the quadriceps tendon, accounting for the rapidly increasing length of the quadriceps moment arm.

Patellofemoral Joint Reaction Force

In understanding the biomechanics of the patellofemoral joint and its clinical relevance, it is important to calculate the compressive forces that the patella experiences.

In a study based on vectorial calculations, Hehne[6] demonstrated that the forces acting on the quadriceps tendon and patellar tendon are not the same as often assumed. It is perhaps biomechanically significant that the quadriceps tendon and the patellar tendon are fixed to the patella at different levels. The quadriceps tendon is inserted in the bone in a broader form and closer to the joint surface than the patellar tendon. Therefore, not only does the direction of the force change, as in a simple pulley model, but different forces on the patellar and the quadriceps tendons are also required to maintain the torque equilibrium. Torque equilibrium, considering a rigid body that moves in a roller, requires $F1 \times a1$ to be equal to $F2 \times (a1 + b)$, where $F1$ = quadriceps force; $F2$ = patellar tendon force, $a1$ = lever arm of $F1$, and $a1 + b$ = lever arm of $F2$ (Figure 3.1). This implies that $F2$ acting on the patellar tendon is smaller than $F1$ acting on the quadriceps tendon. The lever arm of $F2$ is longer than the lever arm of $F1$.

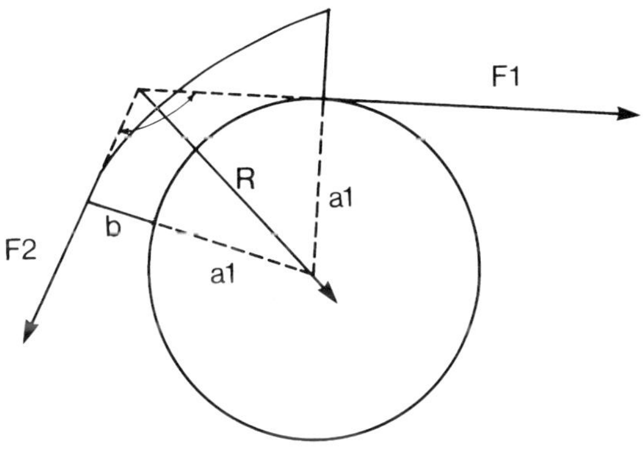

FIGURE 3.1. The force transmitted by a rigid body with different lever arms. *F1* is the quadriceps force; *F2* is the patellar tendon force; *R* is the resulting pressing force of *F1* and *F2*; *a1* is the lever arm of *F1*; and *a1* + *b* is the lever arm of *F2*. (Adapted from Hehne, Clin. Orthop. 1990; 258:75, with permission of JB Lippincott Co.).

In an experimental study on cadaver knees, Buff et al.[7] found that the ratio between the tensions in the quadriceps tendon and the patellar tendon (*Fq*/*Fp*) is different from 1 through the entire range of motion, and that this ratio increases with flexion of the knee. Tensions in the quadriceps tendon and the patellar tendon were measured as a function of flexion angle of the knee (from full extension to 90°) in eight fresh cadaver knees. The femur and the tibia were sectioned 17 cm from the joint space; a femoral intramedullary rod was used to fix the knee to a rigid table. A clamp attached to the sectioned quadriceps tendon was connected by a cable through an adjustable pulley to the load cell of a material tester. The knee was extended by the upward motion of the crosshead of the material tester and the quadriceps force was measured by the load cell. A bone block with the attached patellar tendon was removed from the tibia and then reattached in its original position with two Kirschner wires (K-wires). A spring balance through a hole drilled in the block was attached to measure the patellar tendon force. The quadriceps force and the patellar tendon force increased with decreasing angle of flexion between 90° and 0°, but were not identical for each angle of flexion. The ratio *Fq*/*Fp* ranged from 1.56 at 70° of flexion to 0.86 at 10° of flexion (Figure 3.2).

These direct measurements of the differences between the quadriceps force and the patellar tendon force for most angles of flexion, confirm the mathematical analysis of Maquet[8] of the forces transmitted to the patella. Maquet makes the assumption that the patellofemoral joint reaction (PFJR) force is always perpendicular to the point of contact. If this assumption is correct, the PFJR force does not bisect the angle between the quadriceps force and the patellar tendon force, and *Fq* and *Fp* are not equal. Using the law of cosines, the PFJR force could then be calculated through the construction of the parallelogram of forces, with the following equation:

$$\text{PFJR force} = \sqrt{Fq^2 + Fp^2 + 2\ FqFp \cos \gamma}$$

where Fq = quadriceps force, Fp = patellar tendon force, γ = angle between the quadriceps and patellar tendon force. From the experimental data mentioned previously, it appears that Maquet's mathematical calculation reflects what is actually occurring in the joint. Therefore, the patellofemoral joint seems to act more like a lever than a frictionless pulley. The patella is unconstrained in the sagittal plane and it is free to rock onto a more proximal or distal contact area, changing the ratio *Fq*/*Fp* through the range of motion.

The experimental data that Buff et al.[7] found also confirm the findings that Van Eijden et al.[9] obtained using a mathematical model. Van Eijden's group also studied the ratio between the PFJR force and the quadriceps force (*Fq*) in a range of motion from 0° to 120° of flexion (Figure 3.3). It found that the PFJR force is approximately 50% of the quadriceps force at full extension, and increases to 100% of the quadriceps force at flexion angles between 70° and 120°. This study has important implications in the rehabilitation of patellofemoral pain syndromes. Rehabilitation programs designed to minimize the PFJR force should avoid a range of motion between 70° and 120°, where the PFJR force is 100% of the quadriceps force. In order to minimize the PFJR force, it may be advisable to restrict knee rehabilitation in a range of motion be-

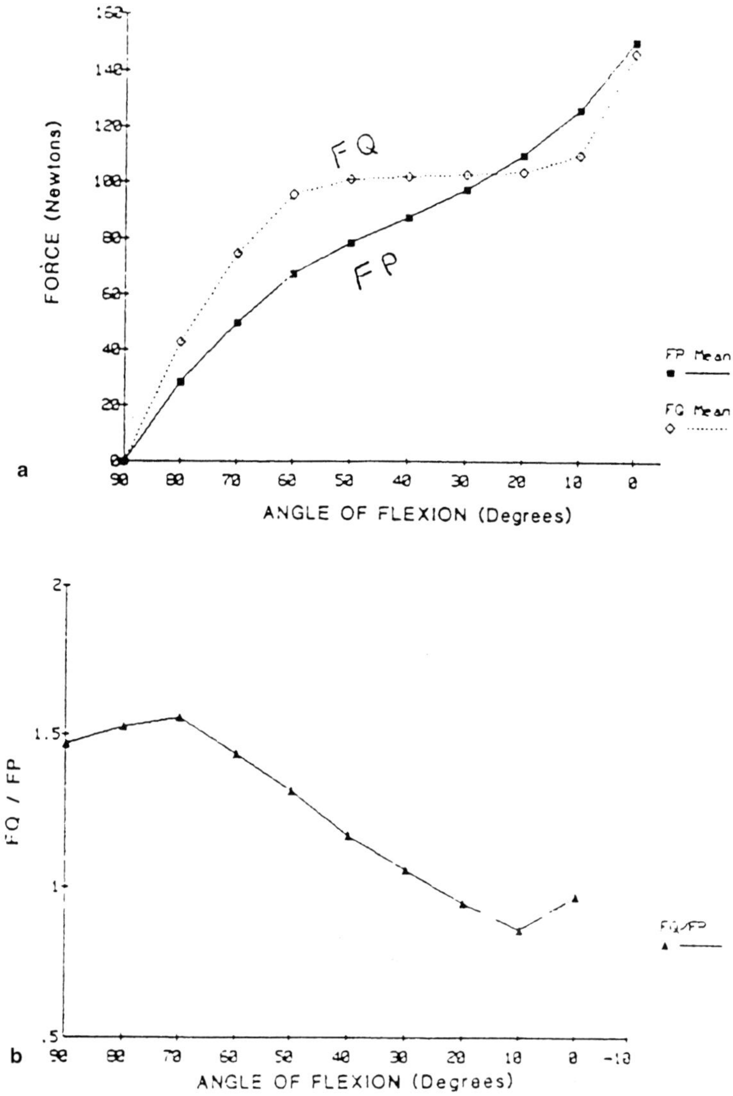

FIGURE 3.2. (a) The curves generated by plotting quadriceps force (*Fq*) and patellar tendon force (*Fp*) for each angle of flexion were not identical. (b) The ratio between the quadriceps force (*Fq*) and the patellar tendon force (*Fp*) in a range of motion between 90° and 0° of flexion. Reprinted from *J Biomech 21*. Buff et. al., Experimental determination of forces transmitted through the patellofemoral joint, p. 17–23, Copyright 1988, with kind permission of Elsevier Science Ltd, The Boulevard, Langford Lane, Kidlington 0X5 1GB, UK.

tween 0° (where the PFJR force is 50% of *Fq*) and 40° (where the PFJR force is 90% of *Fq*).

The PFJR force is the result of the tension in the quadriceps tendon and the patellar tendon due to contraction of the quadriceps. It is the resultant vector of the quadriceps tendon force (M_1) and the patellar tendon force (M_2). These forces can be studied on the sagittal plane. Since the patella is assumed to act as a frictionless pulley, the forces M_1 and M_2 have been supposed in the past to be equal, even if in their recent studies Hehne,[6] Buff et al.,[7] and Van Eijden et al.[9] demonstrated that the patellar tendon force and the quadriceps force are not really equal.

The knowledge of the quadriceps force (*Fq*), and of the angle between the quadriceps force and the patellar tendon force (γ) permits calculating (Figure 3.4) the PFJR force with the following equation:[3]

$$\text{PFJR force} = 2\, Fq \cos(\gamma/2)$$

where γ is the angle between the quadriceps tendon and the patellar tendon.

The quadriceps force *Fq* has also been calculated according to static principles.[10] Since any flexion moment is balanced by a corresponding extension moment to reach an equilibrium, a free body diagram can be constructed to balance flexion and extension

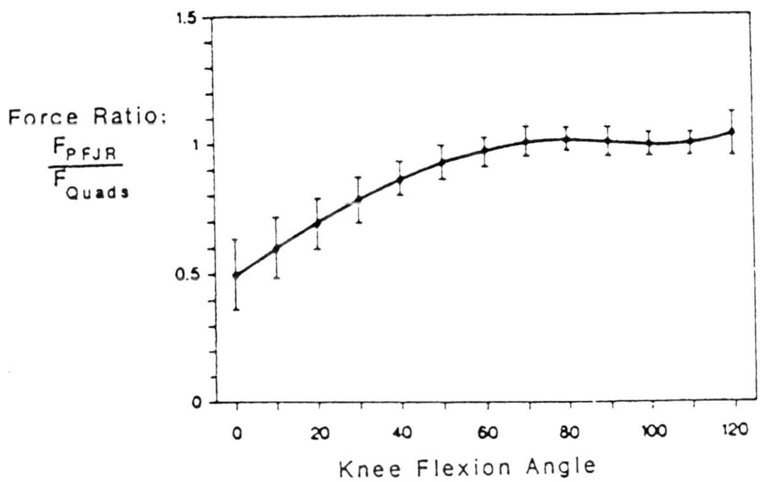

FIGURE 3.3. The ratio between the F_{PFJR} (patellofemoral joint reaction force) and the Fq (quadriceps force) from 0° to 120° of flexion. Between 0° and 70° the F_{PFJR} is less than the force developed by quadriceps contraction. Reprinted from *J Biomech 19.* Van Eijden et al., A mathematical model of the patellofemoral joint, p. 219–228, Copyright 1986, with kind permission from Elsevier Science Ltd, The Boulevard, Langford Lane, Kidlington 0X5 1GB, UK.

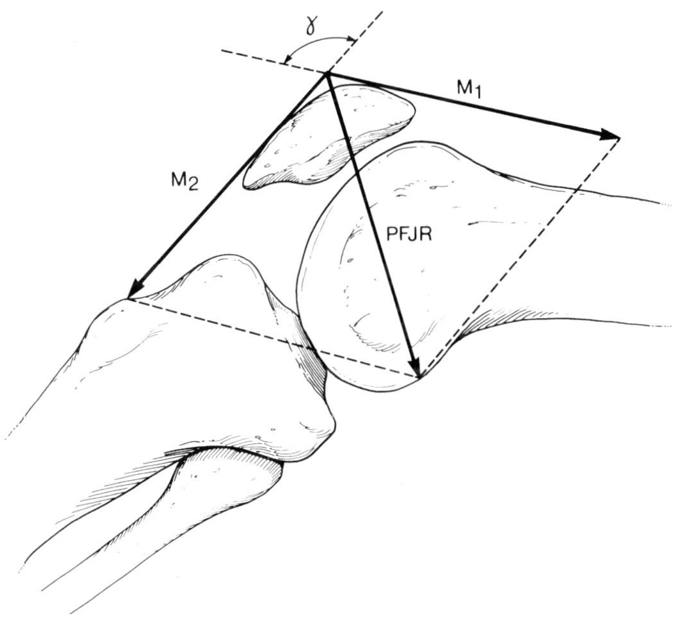

FIGURE 3.4. The patellofemoral joint reaction force is the resultant vector of the quadriceps tendon force (M_1) and the patellar tendon force (M_2). (From Aglietti, Buzzi, Insall in "Surgery of the knee," Churchill Livingstone, New York, © 1993, with permission).

moments (Figure 3.5). This reflects the forces encountered in the static position, the inertial forces of the dynamic situation are ignored. Therefore Fq can be expressed by the following equation:

$$Fq = Fwt\,(f \sin \alpha + t \sin \beta)\,1/r$$

where Fwt is the body weight, r is the extension moment arm from the center of rotation to the patellar tendon, f is the effective length of the femur (from the knee to the vertical line passing through the body's center of gravity), t is the distance from the knee to foot contact with the floor, α is the femoral angle with the vertical, and β is the tibial angle with the vertical.

According to the two equations, it appears that during the act of squatting (as in Figure 3.5), the PFJR force increases with flexion of the knee. Two factors determine the increase of the PFJR force with increasing flexion of the knee. First, $f \sin \alpha$, the flexor moment arm increases with increasing flexion of the knee. This requires an increased Fq (quadriceps

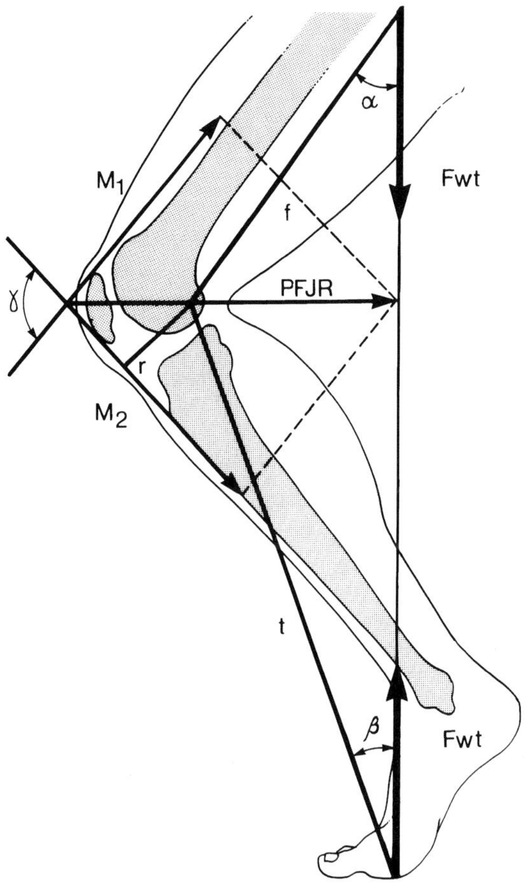

FIGURE 3.5. Standing free body diagram: *Fwt* is the body weight; *r* is the extension moment arm from the center of rotation to the patellar tendon; *f* is the effective length of the femur from the knee to the vertical line passing through the body's center of gravity; *t* is the distance from the knee to the foot contact with the floor; α is the femoral angle with the vertical; and β is the tibial angle with the vertical. In the standing position the main flexing force is the body weight and the PFJR force increases with increasing the knee flexion (see text). (From Aglietti, Buzzi, Insall in "Surgery of the knee," Churchill Livingstone, New York, © 1993, with permission).

force) to maintain an equilibrium. Second, as the angle between the quadriceps force and the patellar tendon force (γ) decreases with increasing flexion, the resultant vector of the PFJR force becomes greater.

Other factors beyond the knee flexion angle may influence the magnitude of the PFJR force and must be taken into account in daily living activities: the inertia of dynamic accelerations and decelerations; the center of gravity of the body that can be displaced forward or backward, respectively decreasing or increasing the flexion moment of the body weight and therefore the PFJR force.[1]

Several authors have investigated the PFJR force during various activities (Table 3.2).

Reilly and Martens[11] studied the PFJR force in level walking, stair climbing, straight leg raising exercises, and deep knee bends. The calculation for the leg raising exercise was a purely mathematical formulation, while the other situations were a combination of a mathematical formulation with experimentally determined parameters. A free body diagram was constructed for the mathematical determination of the patellar tendon force. Only the following forces were considered in the analysis: the tibiofemoral joint reaction force, the weight of the limb, and the weight of the exercise boot. For stair climbing and deep knee bends, the patellar tendon force was determined with a strain gauge instrumented force plate, which produced values for the components of the floor reaction force as the activity was performed. This information was recorded continuously and synchronized with stroboscopic photographs of the subject, and was correlated to various positions of flexion during the activity. During level walking, the angles of flexion are kept low, and a PFJR force of 0.5 times body weight (BW) (at 9° of flexion) was calculated. A PFJR force of 7.6 times BW during deep knee bends (at 120° of flexion) was calculated. During stair climbing or descending, the PFJR force reached a level of 3.3 times BW at 60° of flexion. This value was almost seven times the PFJR force obtained during level walking. A peak PFJR force of 1.4 times BW at 36° of flexion was also determined during the knee extension exercise from 90° of flexion with a 9-kg boot. The straight leg raising exercise against the same resistance resulted in a PFJR force of only 0.5 times BW.

Using an analytic biomechanical model, Kaufman et al.[17] analyzed the PFJR force in five normal subjects during isokinetic exer-

TABLE 3.2. Patellofemoral joint force during various activities.

Authors	Activity	Degrees of Flexion	Force* (× BW)
Reilly and Martens[11]	Walking	9	0.5
	Straight leg raising	0	0.5
	Stairs—up or down	60	3.3
	Squat	120	7.6
Smith[12]	Jumping		20.0
Zernicke et al.[13]	Weight lifting	90	25.0
Ellis et al.[14]	Rising from chair	120	3.1
Dahlkvist et al.[15]	Squat–rise	140	6.0
	Squat–descent	140	7.6
Huberti and Hayes[16]	Isometric extension	90	6.5
Kaufman et al.[17]	Isokinetic exercise	70	5.1

*BW = body weight.
Adapted from Kaufman, Nan, Litchy et al., Dynamic joint forces during knee isokinetic exercise. Am. J. Sports Med. 1991, 19(3), 305–316.

cises. A Cybex-II isokinetic dynamometer was used to provide load at a constant angular velocity with accommodating resistance. Each subject was instructed to exert a maximal voluntary effort during flexion and extension. Two speeds of 60° and 180°/s were used. In order to predict the joint forces, a three-dimensional model of the knee joint was constructed. The inputs to the model were the motion of the lower leg and the forces applied to the shank. The three-dimensional motion of the lower limb was measured with a triaxial electrogoniometer mounted on the subject's knee. The patellofemoral compressive force during isokinetic exercise was low at knee flexion angles of less than 20° and was maximum at 70° of flexion. The peak PFJR force performing isokinetic exercises was 5.1 BW at 60°/s and 70° of flexion, and 4.9 BW at 180°/s and 70° of flexion. This is greater than the force estimated for certain daily activities such as going up or down stairs (3.3 BW at 60° of flexion)[11] or rising from a chair (3.1 BW at 120° of flexion),[14] but less than squatting (7.6 BW at 120° of flexion)[11] or during athletic activities involving jumping (20 BW)[12] (Table 3.2).

Finally, while collecting cinematographic data on weight lifters for the analysis of the knee joint forces and moments of force, Zernicke et al.[13] observed a human patellar-tendon rupture during an actual competition. In this situation, the moment of force at the knee joint reached a maximum of 550 nm at 90° of flexion (Figure 3.6) and a PFJR force of as much as 25 BW at 90° of flexion was estimated.

The biomechanics of the knee extension exercise with the subject being seated has been also investigated. This situation can be illustrated by a free body diagram (Figure 3.7). The flexion moment arm due to gravity now increases, decreasing the angle of knee flexion. This means that the required quadriceps force and the PFJR force must increase with extension, which is the reverse of what happens during squatting.

Patellofemoral Contact Area

Using different techniques, several authors studied the patellofemoral (PF) contact areas[3,18–20] (Table 3.3).

Aglietti et al.[18] used a casting technique with injection of acrylic cement into the knees of cadavers in order to study the normal PF contact areas (Figure 3.8). The normal contact areas were determined using different loads (from 0 to 250 lb [0 to 112.5 kg]) applied to the vastus intermedius and rectus anterior tendons, and at different degrees of flexion (from

FIGURE 3.6. During the weight lifting, the moment of force at the knee joint can reach a maximum of 550 nm at 90° of flexion and cause the patellar tendon to rupture. In this situation, the peak PFJR force is as much as 25 BW (body weight) at 90° of flexion. (From Zernicke, Garhammer, Jobe, J. Bone Joint Surg., 1977; 59A(2): *181*, with permission).

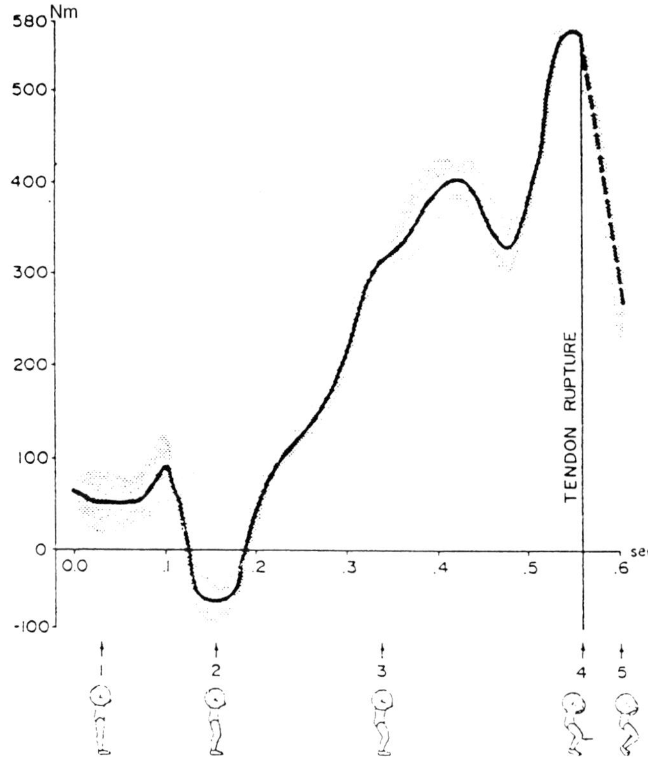

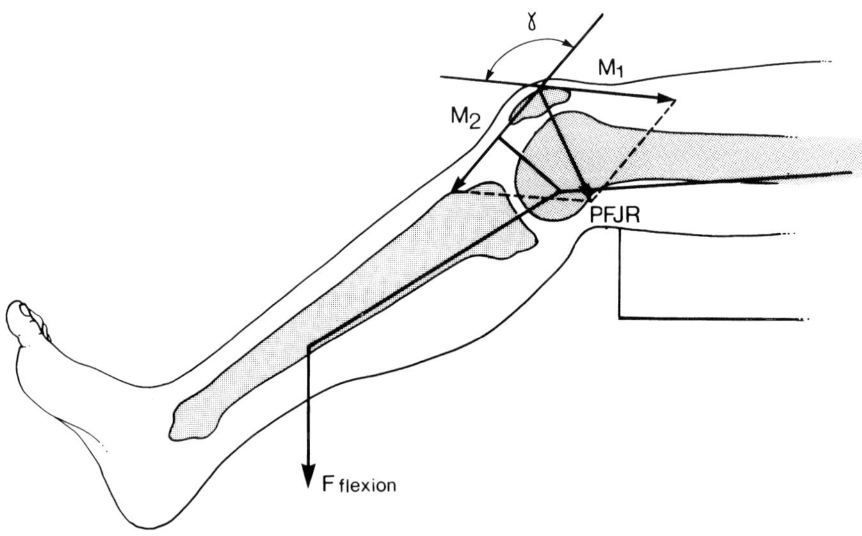

FIGURE 3.7. Free body diagram of the extension exercise. The flexion moment increases towards extension and increasing quadriceps force is required to reach full extension. This is the reverse of flexion under body weight in the standing position, where more quadriceps force is required, increasing flexion. (From Aglietti, Buzzi, Insall in "Surgery of the knee," Churchill Livingstone, New York, © 1993, with permission).

TABLE 3.3. Patellofemoral contact area.

Authors	Degrees of Flexion				
	20	30	60	90	120
Aglietti et al.[18]		2.95 cm²	4.72 cm²	5.0 cm²	
Hungerford and Barry[3]		2.1 cm²	3.2 cm²	3.5 cm²	
Huberti and Hayes,[16] Hayes et al.[20] (normal knees)	2.6 cm²	3.1 cm²	3.9 cm²	4.1 cm²	4.6 cm²
(tendofemoral contact)					3.4 cm²

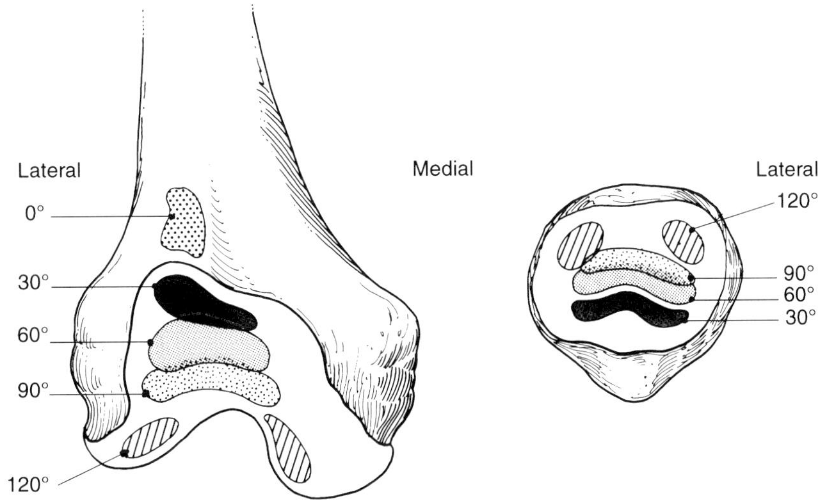

FIGURE 3.8. The patellofemoral contact areas at various knee flexion angles. From Aglietti, Insall, Walker et al. Clin. Orthop. 1975; 107:175 with permission of J.B. Lippincott Co.

0° to 120°). At 0° of flexion, the patella was completely above the femoral articular surface for the full range of loads. At 30° of flexion, the inferior aspect of the patella contacted the uppermost portion of the femoral condyles. Contact began between the lateral femoral condyle and the lateral patellar facet, but by 30° was evenly distributed on both sides. At 60° of flexion, the contact was between the central portion of the patellar surface and the femoral groove, slightly inferior to the contact area at 30°. At 90° of flexion, the contact was between the superior aspect of the patellar articular cartilage and an area of the femoral groove just above the notch. At 120° of flexion, contact was between the superior aspect of the patella and the two areas surrounding the notch on the femur. Using a load of 150 lb (67.5 kg), the contact area at 30°, 60°, and 90° was 2.95, 4.72, and 5.0 cm², respectively. The contact area increased by increasing flexion from 30° to 90°.

In an experimental study on cadaver knees, Goodfellow et al.[19] determined the PF contact areas under load throughout the range of motion by a dye technique, making a sequence of four contact prints at 20°, 45°, 90°, and 135° of flexion. From extension to 90° of flexion, a band of contact sweeps across the patella from the inferior to the superior pole, except the "odd facet" of the patella that makes no contact. From full extension to 90° of flexion, the patella is the only component of the extensor mechanism that makes contact with the articular surface of the femur. In this range of motion the patella holds the quadriceps tendon away from the femur, but beyond 90° of flexion the posterior surface of the quadriceps tendon is brought into contact with the trochlear facets of the femur. Between 90° and 135° of flexion the patella rotates and the odd facet engages the medial femoral condyle.

Hungerford and Barry[3] found in their experimental studies on cadaver knees that the first PF contact is made between 10° and 20° of flexion along the inferior margin of the patella in a continuous band across both medial and lateral facets. As flexion proceeds, the contact area moves proximally on the patella, extending from the ridge separating the medial from the odd facet to the lateral border of the lateral facet. The contact area increases with increasing flexion. From 20° to 90° of flexion, all the zones of the patellar articular cartilage, with the exception of the odd facet, are brought into contact with femoral articular cartilage. After 90° of flexion, the medial facet begins to come into the intercondylar notch, while the odd facet makes contact with the lateral margin of the medial condyle.

Using pressure-sensitive films and a special knee-joint loading fixture, Hayes et al.[20] measured the PF contact area in normal cadaveric knees and in chondromalacic cadaveric patellofemoral joints (Table 3.3). In normal knees the PF contact area changed with the flexion angle and was 2.6 cm^2 at 20°, 3.1 cm^2 at 30°, 3.9 cm^2 at 60°, and 4.1 cm^2 at 90°. Increasing flexion from 20° to 90°, the contact area moved from the distal third of the patellar cartilage to the proximal half. The contact area reached the proximal margin of the cartilage only at 120° of flexion. At 120° of flexion, the PF contact area was 4.6 cm^2. At 120° of flexion, there was also a tendofemoral contact between the posterior surface of the quadriceps tendon and the trochlear facets of the femur. The tendofemoral contact area was 3.4 cm^2 (approximately 75% of the corresponding PF contact area at the same degree of flexion). In the study on chondromalacic patellofemoral joints, the following grading system was used to indicate the severity of the lesions: I = swelling and softening, II = fissures, III = erosions, and IV = erosions with bone exposure. In chondromalacic patellofemoral joints, the PF contact area was 1.69 cm^2 at 20°, 1.81 cm^2 at 30°, 3.12 cm^2 at 60°, and 2.52 cm^2 at 90°. Contact area did not differ significantly between grades I–II and III–IV lesions, but a great reduction, increasing flexion of the knee, in chondromalacic patellofemoral joints compared with normal knees was observed.

Patellofemoral Contact Pressure

In the biomechanics of the patellofemoral joint, more important than the absolute value of the PFJR force is the PF contact pressure. This is the ratio of the PFJR force to the contact area. Throughout the range of motion of the knee both the contact area and the PFJR force vary significantly. The increase of the contact area in flexion compensates for the increasing PFJR force.

Using pressure-sensitive films, Hayes et al.[20] measured the PF contact pressure in normal knees and in chondromalacic cadaveric patellofemoral joints. Knee moments corresponding to one third of the values reported in the literature for maximum isometric voluntary quadriceps contraction were applied at 20°, 30°, 60°, and 90° of flexion: 23.6, 30.7, 47.2, and 35 nm, respectively. At 120° of flexion, two thirds of the reported maximum moments were applied.

In normal knees the pressure distribution was remarkably uniform over the entire contact area (±0.25 MPa). The pressures on both the lateral and the medial facets were approximately the same. The average PF contact pressure ranged from 2.0 MPa at 20° to 4.4 MPa at 90°, showing the steepest increase from 2.4 MPa at 30° to 4.1 MPa at 60°. At 120°, the average PF contact pressure decreased to 3.5 MPa. At 120°, there was a tendofemoral contact proximal to the patella and the average tendofemoral contact pressure was 1.6 MPa (approximately 50% of the PF contact pressure at the same angle of flexion). Thus, tendofemoral contact plays an important role to reduce PF contact pressures.

Contact pressure in chondromalacic patellofemoral joints was measured with a normal capsule, after capsular plication (both medial and lateral), and after capsular release (lateral and bilateral) at 20°, 30°, 60°, and 90° of flexion. In chondromalacic patellofemoral joints with an intact capsule, the contact pressures depended on the extent and degenerative grade of the lesions. Localized lesions of grades I–II (cartilage swelling and fissures) exhibited great reductions in pressure directly over the lesion. Average pressures over the lesions were 1.6 MPa compared with an average of 3.4 MPa on normal regions of the contact area. This represents a 53% reduction in pressure on grades I–II lesions resulting from the decreased cartilage stiffness of these softened areas. Localized lesions of grades III–IV (cartilage erosions) resulted in nearly a total loss of contact pressure over these areas. The capsular plication procedures resulted in pressure increases on the corresponding facet, whereas lateral and bilateral capsular release procedures do not result in consistent pressure reductions.

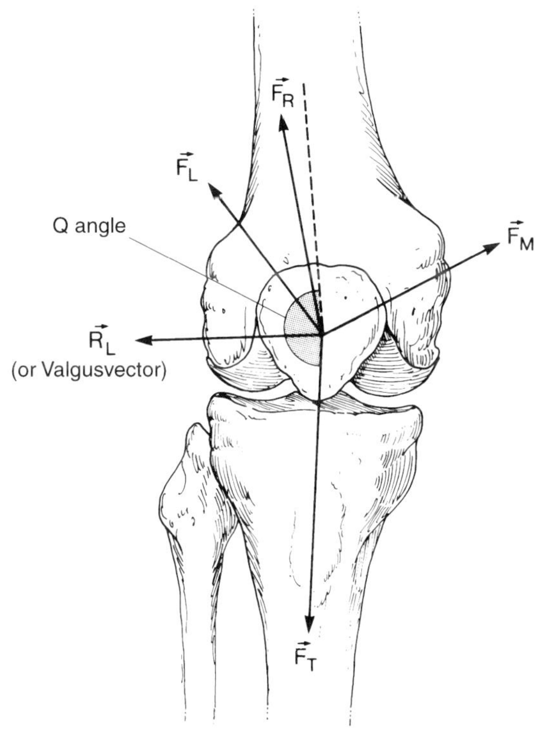

FIGURE 3.9. Orientation of quadriceps force in the coronal plane. F_L is the force exerted by the vastus lateralis muscle; F_R is the force exerted by the rectus femoris muscle; F_T is the patellar tendon force; and R_L is the resulting lateral force given by the Q angle or "valgus vector" as the sum of $F_L + F_R + F_T$. (Adapted from Hehne, Clin. Orthop. 1990; 258:74, with permission of JB Lippincott Co.).

Patellar Tracking

In full extension, the "screw home" mechanism of the tibia, rotating externally in the terminal 30° of extension, displaces the tibial tubercle laterally.[3] This produces the *Q angle*, the angle between the line of application of the quadriceps force and the direction of the patellar tendon (Figure 3.9). Tension on the quadriceps will tend to produce a lateral displacement vector of the patella on the frontal plane. This lateral or "valgus vector" is resisted by the oblique fibers of the vastus medialis obliquus, by the the medial retinacular structures, and by the lateral facet of the trochlea. The vastus medialis obliquus, extending distally and inserting medially in the patella, produces an important medial force. At full extension, the force F_M counteracts the force R_L directed laterally provided by the Q angle (Figure 3.9). In torque equilibrium, the sum of the forces of vastus lateralis and rectus muscles, $F_L + F_R$, is equal to $F_T + R_L$, where F_T is the patellar tendon force and R_L is the resulting lateral force given by the Q angle.[6]

With the knee in full extension and the quadriceps contracted, the patella lies proximal to the trochlea. During the first 20° of flexion, the tibia derotates and this decreases the Q angle, also decreasing the lateral vector. The patella is drawn into the trochlea and the first articular contact is made by 10° knee flexion.[1] Because of the Q angle, the patella enters the trochlea from the lateral side.[3]

Because of the Q angle, the quadriceps force can be divided in the horizontal plane into two components[1] (Figure 3.10). A first component acts on the lateral patellar facet and presses the articular surface against the femoral trochlea. This force can be resolved in two forces: (1) a force normal to the joint surface and (2) a force directed laterally: $F_r = F_n + F_t$. A second component acts medially on the tibial tuberosity and produces an internal tibial rotation.

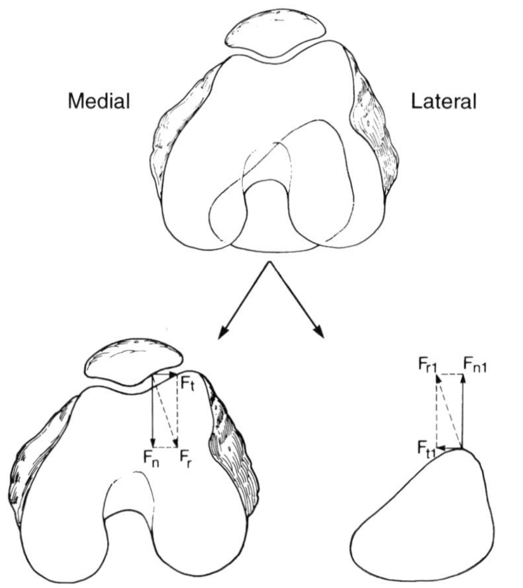

FIGURE 3.10. Vector diagram of forces transmitted in the horizontal plane by the quadriceps muscle on the patella and on the tibial tuberosity. F_r and F_{r1} are the resulting forces of the quadriceps muscle in the horizontal plane (as the sum of $F_t + F_n$, and $F_{t1} + F_{n1}$), acting on the patella and the tibial tuberosity, respectively; F_t is the force directed against the lateral margin of the femoral trochlea; F_{t1} is the tangential force to the tibial tuberosity; F_n is the normal force to the joint surface; F_{n1} is the normal force to the tibial tuberosity.

The articular patellar surface is divided into the medial and the lateral facets by the central ridge. The respective sizes of the medial and the lateral facets are variable. In an extensive radiographic study, Wiberg[21] classified the patellae into three different types, and Baumgartl[22] added a fourth type. Type I has medial and lateral facets of roughly the same size. Type II has a medial facet smaller than the lateral facet. Type III has a greatly reduced medial facet compared with the lateral facet. Type IV was described without the central ridge of the medial facet. According to a recent anatomic study,[23] type II occurs most frequently (57%), followed by type I (24%) and type III (19%).

There is a group of patellofemoral disorders, which can be called patellofemoral malalignment or dysplasia, that include lateral tracking of the patella. It has been disputed which anatomic factor is genetically determined and which is an adaptive change, a product of functional adjustment. From the embryologic point of view, the patella has medial and lateral facets initially equal in size. By the sixth month of gestation the dimensions of the lateral patellar facet exceed those of the medial as it is found in the adult. Therefore, the term *dysplasia* could be put forward to characterize the situation in which the medial facet is smaller or greatly reduced compared with the lateral facet.[6]

A statistical analysis of several measurements of the quadriceps mechanism that Reider[23] obtained in a study on cadaver knees, in an attempt to relate the shape of the patella to the structures and forces acting on it, revealed interesting correlations (Figure 3.11). A correlation was found between Wiberg's classification of the patella and the width of the lateral patellofemoral ligament; the more a patella's profile tended toward Wiberg's type III (where the medial facet is small and convex, while the lateral facet is broad and concave), the broader its lateral patellofemoral ligament tended to be. Other correlation was found between the length of the patellar tendon and the width of the medial patellofemoral ligament. Since a long patellar tendon (patella alta) is associated with lateral deviations of the patella, is not surprising to find that where there are longer tendons there are less robust or absent medial patellofemoral ligaments. Other correlations were found between patellar dimensions (height, width, and thickness) and soft-tissue structures. Patellar height, width, and thickness tended to correlate with the dimensions of the soft-tissue structures and not with each other.

The frontal rotation (the rotatory movement of the patella about the anteroposterior axis) and the tilt of the patella on the coronary plane (rotatory movement of the patella about the superoinferior axis) have been investigated by Fujikawa et al.[24] in an experimental study on eight human cadaveric knee joints. These measurements were performed at 0°, 25°, 45°, 60°, 90°, 115°, and 130° of flexion. A small amount of casting material, silicone rubber, was introduced between the femur and the pa-

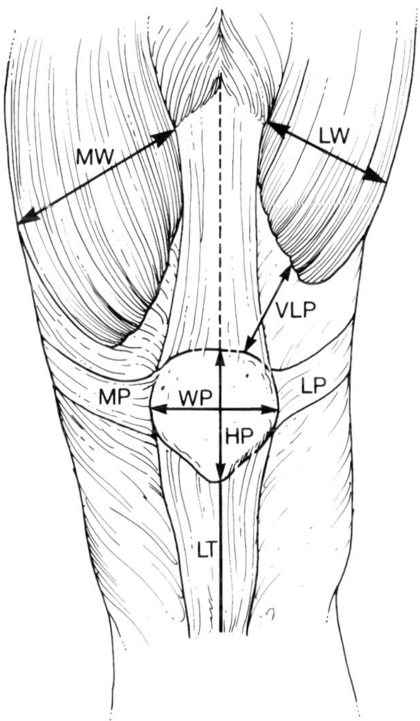

FIGURE 3.11. Parameters evaluated in the statistical analysis of the extensor mechanism in the attempt to relate the shape of the patella to the structures and forces acting on it. MW is the width of the vastus medialis muscle; LW is the width of the vastus lateralis muscle; VLP is the distance between the distalmost muscle fibers of the vastus lateralis and the superolateral angle of the patella; WP is the anterior width of the patella; HP is the anterior height of the patella; LT is the patellar tendon length; MP is the width of the medial patellofemoral ligament; and LP is the width of the lateral patellofemoral ligament. (Adapted from Reider, J. Bone Joint Surg., 1981; 63A(3):352, with permission).

tella to determine the contact area at any angle of flexion. The frontal rotation of the patella was measured by observing the change in the angle made between two K-wires attached to the patella and the femur. The two K-wires were attached such that they made a right angle at 25° of flexion (considered as a reference for the measurements). This procedure was repeated for all the angles of flexion. The patellar tilt was measured using horizontal slices of a patellofemoral contact casting in polymethylmetacrylate, as the change in the *lateral patellofemoral angle* (the angle, measured in an axial view, between a line tangent to the top of the medial and the lateral femoral condyle, and a second line tangent to the lateral patellar facet). This study found that the patella rotates laterally about the anteroposterior axis (the lower pole of the patella turned laterally) by 5.6° to 6.5° as the flexion increases from 25° to 130°. Two thirds of the patellar rotation occurred by 60° of flexion. The lateral patellofemoral angle increased with increasing flexion from 25° (an average of 7°) to 115° (an average of 18°), so that as the knee flexed from 25° to 115°, the patella tilted medially 11°.

Hirokawa[25] calculated the variations of the three-dimensional patellar motions (from full extension to 160° of flexion) with a mathematical model analysis of the patellofemoral joint in normal cadaveric knees. The mathematical description of the shape of the articular surface has been deduced by the application of a computer-aided design theory, and measurements about the positions and areas of attachment of the quadriceps muscle and the patellar ligament were performed on three cadaver knees. The attachment of the quadriceps muscle and the patellar ligament were defined by two points both on the patella and on the tibial tuberosity. A three-dimensional mathematical model was then created, taking into account the geometries of the joint. From the mathematical analysis results that the patella rotates about 70° in the sagittal plane, twists about 15° in the horizontal plane and tilts about 10° in the frontal plane while the knee is flexed from 20° to 160°.

Clinically, patellar tracking is evaluated with the patient seated on the examining table with the knee flexed at 90°. The examiner's hand is placed on the knee so that the medial and the lateral patellar border are palpated with the index and the thumb. The patient is asked to actively extend the knee. Normal patellar tracking is present when the patella glides smoothly into the femoral sulcus, and only a minimal lateral displacement can be appreciated in the final extension when the patella exits the trochlear groove. A more marked lateral displacement is defined as lateralization, while greater degrees of pathologic tracking are defined as subluxation or dislocation. It is also important to evaluate the tilt of the patella. In normal knees the medial border of the patella should be at the same level as the lateral in full extension. The presence of a lateral tilt (lateral patellar border lower than the medial) in extension, which gradually reduces in flexion, is expression of an abnormal patellar tracking. During the physical examination, it is useful to evaluate the various abnormalities of patellar tracking (lateralization, subluxation, and tilt) and to confirm these later with radiographic axial views or computed tomography (CT).

The use of CT imaging has allowed exploration of the patellofemoral relationships in the arc between full extension and 30° flexion. The results confirm that the normal patella is slightly displaced laterally in full extension, but it reduces early in flexion. The patellar tilt, measured as the angle between the lateral patellar facet and the tangent to the posterior condyles, should be open laterally throughout the arc of motion in normal knees. Values less than 8° are thought to be pathologic.[1] In subluxating or dislocating patellae there is an excessive lateral patellar displacement and lateral patellar tilt, which are more evident in extension but tend to reduce in flexion.

An important parameter to evaluate using CT scan is the lateral displacement of the tibial tuberosity in relationship to the deepest point of the trochlear groove. The tibial tuberosity–sulcus femoralis (TT-SF) distance gives a measure of the valgus vector imposed on the extensor mechanism at a given degree of flexion. Since the tibial tuberosity lies laterally to the sulcus femoralis, the greater the TT-SF distance, the higher the valgus vector of the extensor mechanism. The CT scanning permits measuring the TT-SF distance in full extension or in flexion. The tibial cut is made through the tibial tuberosity and at 90° to the tibial axis. The femoral cut is oriented to pass through midpatella, which corresponds to the lower third of the articular surface, and the posterior femoral condyles. By superimposing the femoral and the tibial cut, the TT-SF can be measured (Figure 3.12). The average TT-SF distance of a normal knee in extension is 12.7 mm, while in a knee with patellar instability, the average TT-SF distance is 19.8 mm.[26] Values nearly or greater than 20 mm with the knee in extension are considered pathologic.

The use of imaging techniques has allowed a better understanding of the patellofemoral joint in normal and pathologic knees. The normal patellar motion during the first 30° of flexion was also investigated by magnetic resonance imaging (MRI) in an experimental study performed by Kujala et al.[27] in young patients without knee symptoms (Figure 3.13). Midpatellar sagittal and axial sections were employed with the knee flexed 0°, 10°, 20°, and 30°. The sulcus angle, the lateral patellofemoral angle, the lateral patellar displacement, the lateral patellar tilt, and the congruence angle were measured. The sulcus angle was greater at full extension than at 30° of flexion. The lateral patellofemoral angle increased from 0° to 30° of flexion. The lateral patellar displacement decreased from 0° to 30° of flexion. Lateral patellar tilt decreased during the first 30° of knee flexion. The congruence angle, measured in an axial view, is the angle between the line that bisects the sulcus angle to establish a zero reference line and a line projected from the apex of the sulcus angle to the lowest point on the articular patellar ridge. If the apex of the patellar articular ridge is lateral to the zero line, the congruence angle is positive; if it is medial, the angle is negative. The congruence angle in extension was positive (open laterally) and shifted medially during the first 30° of knee flexion.

These measurements, obtained from normal knees, were compared with knees affected by recurrent patellar dislocations. Knees with recurrent patellar dislocations showed higher values of sulcus angle, lateral patellar displacement, and congruence angle; they showed lower values of the lateral patellofemoral angle, which indicates that dislocating patellae were more lateralized and tilted laterally.

Clinical Relevance

The understanding of the biomechanics of the patellofemoral joint has an important clinical

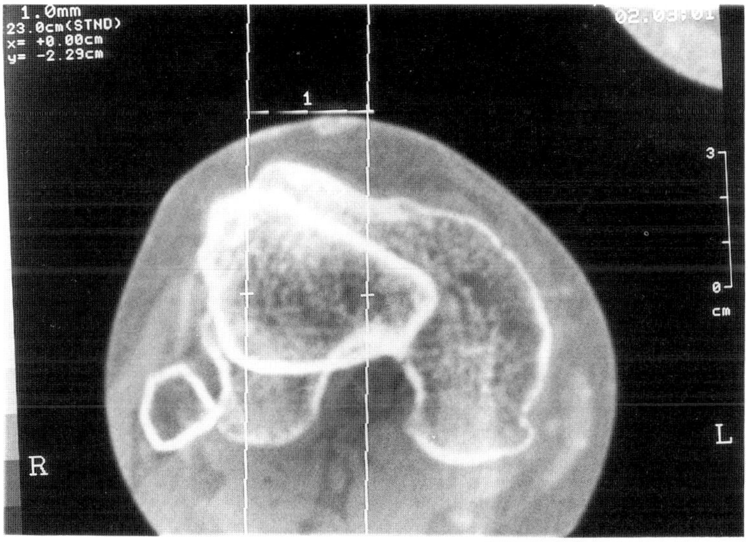

FIGURE 3.12. Measurement of the tibial tuberosity–sulcus femoralis distance (TT–SF distance) in full extension. By superimposing the femoral cut and the tibial cut, the distance between the tibial tuberosity and the deepest point of the sulcus can be measured. Values greater than 20 mm are considered pathologic.

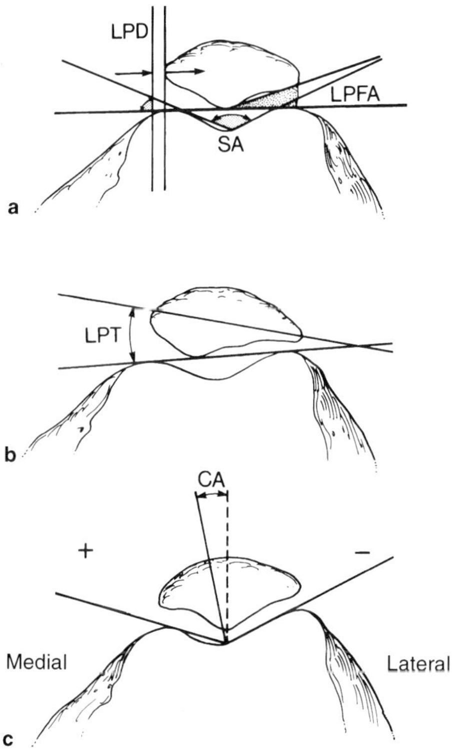

FIGURE 3.13. Patellofemoral joint imaged axially with the knee flexed at 30°. (a) SA is the sulcus angle, LPFA is the lateral patellofemoral angle, LPD is the lateral patellar displacement; (b) LPT is the lateral patellar tilt; and (c) CA is the patellofemoral congruence angle.

relevance on both surgical treatment and rehabilitation.

Surgical Treatment

Surgical treatments commonly used in patellofemoral joint disorders include patellectomy, and tibial tubercle elevation and medial or medial and distal tibial tubercle transposition.

Patellectomy

In the past, patellectomy has been used in the treatment of various patellofemoral disorders. These include patellar fractures, recurrent dislocation–subluxation of the patella, chondromalacia, and patellofemoral arthritis. With the improved patellar realignment procedures, the successful development of total knee replacement and the improved understanding of the patellofemoral biomechanics, the indication for patellectomy has narrowed.[28]

The patella has an important function displacing the patellar tendon away from the center of rotation of the knee and thus lengthening the patellar tendon moment arm. The patella's contribution to the extensor moment arm was demonstrated by Kaufer[4,5] to increase from 14% at 120° of flexion to 31% at full extension.

In his study, Kaufer also demonstrated that a longitudinal repair after patellectomy performed through a longitudinal tendon-splitting incision is less efficient than a transverse repair. The transverse repair restores tension to the patellar ligament and therefore increases the extension moment arm observed with longitudinal repair, where a significant part of the tensile force may be transferred to the tibia through the retinacula, which have shorter moment arms.

In a retrospective study, Stougard[29] examined 72 patients patellectomized for recurrent patellar dislocation, patellar fractures, chondromalacia of the patella, and patellofemoral osteoarthritis. After an average of six-years followup, moderate alleviation of the pain was found, even if patellectomy had caused an insufficiency of the quadriceps muscle and did not appear able to arrest existing tibiofemoral osteoarthritic processes.

Sutton et al.[30] performed an interesting study on the effect of partial and complete patellectomy. Thirty-three patients were examined after patellectomy for patellar fractures, patellofemoral arthritis, or chondromalacia of the patella. After both partial and complete patellectomy, an average loss of 18° of range of motion was found. Complete patellectomy resulted in greater ligament instability, quadriceps atrophy (an average of 2 cm), and loss of quadriceps strength (a 49% reduction in strength of the extensor mechanism) compared with partial patellectomy. Knee motion during walking was evaluated in the knee operated on and in the opposite, normal knee. The excursion did not differ from normal for the group with partial patellectomy. Significant differences in the group with complete patellectomy revealed less stance-phase flexion (average, 7°), less flexion going up stairs (average, 18°), and less flexion going down stairs (average, 16°) were found.

In examining 44 patellectomized patients (50 knees), Steurer et al.[31] noted that patellectomy alters the normal knee joint mechanics. All the patellectomized knees showed radiographic changes. The severity of these changes could be correlated to the biomechanical abnormalities as characterized by a sharp variation in the instant center pathway. The change in the instant center pathway signaled the conversion of sliding forces between the femur and the tibia to plowing forces noted particularly during the last 60° extension. These plowing forces may cause damage to the tibiofemoral articular cartilage, and this well explains the degenerative changes caused by patellectomy and the increase in tibiofemoral arthritis in these patients.

Watkins et al.[32] have clinically confirmed decreased quadriceps strength with Cybex-II isokinetic examination of 12 patellectomized patients. A Cybex-II isokinetic dynamometer, at the speed of 30°/s and 180°/s, has been used to measure quadriceps and hamstrings function (in a range of motion between 90° and 0° of flexion) and the results were compared with the untreated limb. When compared with the untreated side, the peak quadriceps torque of the knee with patellectomy was decreased by an average of 54% at the test speed of 30°/s and by 49% at the speed of 180°/s. Quadriceps torque values were decreased throughout the range of motion, except near full extension. At the test speed of 30°/s, the peak values for the torque of the hamstrings in the patellectomized knees were not significantly different from the untreated side, but were significantly less on the patellectomized side than in the untreated side at the test speed of 180°/s. These data indicate a great deficiency in the quadriceps strength of the patellectomized knee and agree with the clinical findings.

Wendt and Johnson[33] evaluated the relationship between quadriceps excursion and torque in ten cadaver knees. Excursion of the patella and quadriceps, with a constant load on the quadriceps, were measured from 0° to 90° of flexion. Wendt and Johnson found that the mean excursion of the quadriceps was 66.2 ± 5 mm from 0° to 90° of flexion and, with 10° intervals, the maximum excursion of the quadriceps (9.49 mm) occurred between 30° and 40° of flexion, while the minimum excursion (5.40 mm) was found between 80° and 90° of flexion. Patellectomy decreased quadriceps excursion from an average value of 66 mm to 51 mm from 0° to 90° of flexion, and also decreased the maximum excursion of the quadriceps from 9.49 mm between 30° and 40° of flexion to 6.55 mm in the same range of motion. Finally, a correlation was found between the quadriceps torque and the increments of excursion, with the highest torque being at 30° of flexion.

Tibial Tubercle Elevation and Transposition

Several authors recommended the elevation of the tibial tubercle as a method to reduce patellofemoral contact pressures.[8,10,16,20,34–37] Elevation of the tibial tubercle has been considered as an adequate treatment for severe patellofemoral chondromalacia or early osteoarthritis.

An advancement of the tibial tuberosity decreases the patellofemoral contact pressures by:

1. Increasing the lever arm of the patellar tendon, which is the perpendicular distance between the center of rotation of the knee and the tendon
2. Increasing the angle between the quadriceps tendon and the patellar tendon (Figure 3.14)

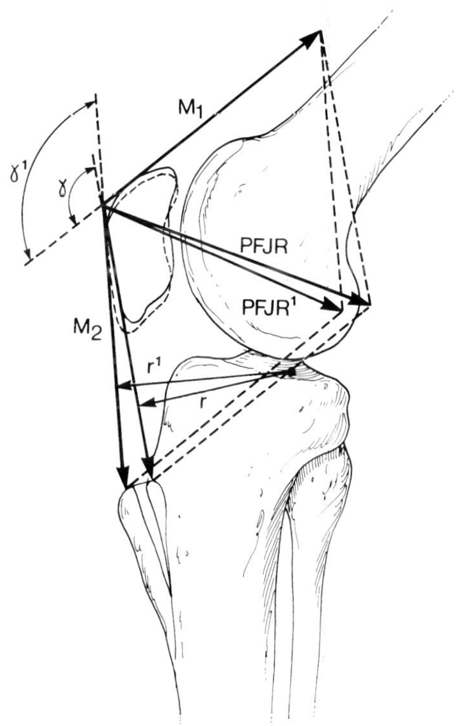

FIGURE 3.14. Biomechanical effects of advancement of the tibial tuberosity. M_1 is the quadriceps tendon force; M_2 is the patellar tendon force; γ is the angle between M_1 and M_2. An advancement of the tibial tuberosity decreases the PFJR force to the value of PFJR^1 by increasing the angle between the quadriceps tendon and the patellar tendon from γ to γ^1 and by increasing the lever arm of the patellar tendon from r to r^1 (so that less force is required in the patellar tendon to produce the same torque). (Adapted from Aglietti, Buzzi, Insall in "Surgery of the knee," Churchill Livingstone, New York, © 1993, with permission).

Maquet[8,34] calculated that a 2-cm elevation of the tibial tubercle yielded up to a 50% reduction in the patellofemoral compressive forces. According to Maquet, a 2- to 2.5-cm advancement was the maximum obtainable without jeopardizing the skin over the tibial tubercle.

Since Maquet's[8] original description, many experimental studies have been performed on the elevation of the tibial tubercle.

Ferguson et al.[35] implanted six miniature contact stress transducers in the retropatellar cartilage of cadaver knees and subjected them to isometric quadriceps contraction. The study demonstrated that elevation of the tibial tubercle relieved the contact stress at 0°, 45°, and 90° of flexion, and the effects were more pronounced at 90°. Most of the relief was achieved with a 0.5-in (1.3 cm) tubercle elevation. A 1- or a 1.5-in (2.5 to 3.8 cm) elevation provides no additional mechanical benefits beyond those available with the 0.5-in (1.3 cm) elevation. In fact, with the anterior displacement of the tibial tubercle there is an anterior rocking of the distal margin of the patella and a shift of the contact area to the superior patellar pole. Since this transfer of stress to the proximal pole occurs increasingly with increasing elevation of the tubercle, it follows that elevation of more than 0.5 in (1.3 cm) should be used cautiously.

Fulkerson[36] has described a technique that allows anteromedialization of the tibial tuberosity without the need of a bone graft.

Through an anterolateral skin incision, a lateral retinacular release is performed, and the patella is everted to perform shaving of loose cartilage flaps or abrasion of areas of exposed subchondral bone. The osteotomy plane is oblique in a posterior and lateral direction. The osteotomy should taper distally, so that a 2- to 3-mm bone pedicle is left 5 to 7 cm distal to the tuberosity. Once the osteotomy is completed, the bone fragment is displaced in an anteromedial direction along the osteotomy plane by rotating around the intact distal pedicle, and is locked in place with cortical screws engaging into the posterior cortex of the tibia.

Fulkerson et al.[37] have evaluated the biomechanical effects of anteromedialization of the tibial tubercle in five cadaver knees, using pressure-sensitive films. Before anteromedialization of the tibial tubercle the loads on the lateral facet exceeded those on the medial facet from 0° up to 60° of flexion. At 0° of flexion the average load on the lateral facet was 3.6 MPa compared with 0.5 MPa on the medial facet, and three of the five knees exhibited no load on the medial facet. At 10° of flexion the patellae remained lateralized, but by 20° of flexion the patellae were engaged in the trochlea with significant loads on the medial facets. Displacement of the tibial tuberosity in an anterior (average, 14.8 mm) and medial (average, 9.2 mm) direction, while causing little difference in the loads of the medial facet, greatly decreased (average, 65%) the loads on the lateral facet between 0° and 30°. Beyond 30° of flexion patellofemoral pressures were not reduced over preoperative values, although they remained balanced between the medial and the lateral facets.

In an experimental study on cadaver knees, Nakamura et al.[38] demonstrated that advancement of the tibial tuberosity influences both the PF contact area and the forces acting on the patellofemoral joint. The contact area was studied with casting techniques. The geometry of the joint was studied with lateral radiographs of the knee in a flexion range from 0° to 110°. Metal wedges of 1, 2, and 3 cm were used to elevate the tuberosity. The length of the split down the anterior crest of the tibia also varied from 5, 10, and 15 cm. A mathematical model was adopted to calculate the forces acting on the patellofemoral joint.

The study by Nakamura et al. indicates that the patellar tendon moment arm was changed by a minor extent by metal wedges of increasing thickness. The decrease of the PFJR force was mainly due to the increase of the angle between the quadriceps tendon and the patellar tendon. The PF contact area decreased progressively with increasing thickness of the wedge and became gradually concentrated on the proximal part of the patellar surface. The forces at the patellofemoral joint decreased with increasing thickness of the wedges at 0°, 30°, and 60° of flexion. At 90° and 110° of flexion the forces decreased with a wedge thickness of 1 cm, but they tended to increase paradoxically with greater thicknesses. In conclusion, to minimize the distal shift of the patella caused by advancement of the tibial tuberosity, Nakamura et al. suggest that the split in the tibia should be at least 10 cm long, because the longer the split, the smaller the downward shift of the patella, and that the elevation should be about 1 cm and no more.

Using pressure-sensitive films, Huberti and Hayes,[16] and Hayes et al.[20] measured the PF contact areas and pressures in chondromalacic cadaveric knees at 30°, 60°, and 90° of flexion, with intact capsule and after a 1.25- and a 2.5-cm elevation of the tibial tubercle. With an intact capsule the PF contact area ranged from 1.8 cm^2 at 30° of flexion to 3.3 cm^2 at 90° of flexion, while the peak PF contact pressure increased from 4.2 MPa at 30° to 8.9 MPa at 90° of flexion. The mean contact area was significantly reduced by a 1.25-cm elevation at 90° of flexion, and by a 2.5-cm elevation at both 60° and 90° of flexion. Mean and peak contact pressures did not show a significant decrease, going from a 1.25- to a 2.5-cm elevation of the tibial tubercle. Huberti and coworkers also measured the effects of Q angle variation on the PF contact pressure patterns in normal cadaveric knees. The Q angle was varied by changing the direction of the quadriceps tendon. A 10° increase in Q angle increased the PF contact pressure of about 45% at 20°; a 10° decrease in Q angle also increased the PF contact pressures of 53% at 20°, 29% at 30°, 41% at 60°, and 23% at 90°. Therefore, operations involving tibial tubercle transposition should be attempted with caution.

Rehabilitation

In order to administer an appropriate rehabilitation program it is important to have a basic understanding of the patellofemoral biomechanics. The influence of PF contact area, PF contact pressures, and pataller tracking should be taken into consideration as a program is selected.

Patellofemoral Pain

In their studies, Reilly and Martens[11] calculated a peak PFJR force of 120 kg (1.4 BW) at 36° of flexion during the knee extension from 90° of flexion with a 9-kg boot. The straight leg raising against the same resistance resulted in a PFJR force of only 0.5 BW. Patients with pain referable to the patellofemoral joint can hardly tolerate the knee extension exercises against resistance: straight leg raising exercises are a more suitable alternative for an appropriate rehabilitation.

Using an analytic biomechanical model, Kaufman et al.[17] measured the PFJR force during isokinetic exercise at 60°/s and 180°/s. The patellofemoral compressive force performing isokinetic exercises was low at knee flexion angles of less than 20° and maximum at 70° of flexion. The peak PFJR force during isokinetic exercise has been calculated to be 5.1 BW with 60°/s at 70° and 4.9 BW with 180°/s at 70° of flexion. From this study, results indicate that at low flexion angles, the PFJR force is low. Therefore, in patients with patellofemoral symptoms, isokinetic exercise should be contraindicated, or if performed, should be limited to those flexion angles and velocities in which the PFJR force is low.

Doucette and Goble[39] have recently investigated the influence of a physical therapy program on pain and patellar tracking clinically and radiologically in 51 knees with lateral patellar compression syndrome. Radiologic parameters were measured with axial views, before and after the treatment, with the congruence angle and the *patellofemoral index* (the ratio between the thickness of the medial patellofemoral interspace and the lateral patellofemoral interspace: in normal knees the medial interspace is equal or slightly wider than the lateral, and the index is 1.6 or less). The patients performed individualized, five-stage physical therapy programs, recording before and after physical therapy the following information: subjective pain, duration of physical therapy, stage of treatment, circumference of the thigh difference, hamstrings and iliotibial band flexibility, Q angle, sulcus angle, congruence angle, and patellofemoral index. In stage 1, ice, electric galvanic stimulation, ultrasound, and anti-inflammatory medication can be used to decrease patellofemoral pain responsible for the reflex inhibition of the vastus medialis obliquus (VMO), and thus preventing the normal exercise performance.

In stage 2, VMO strengthening exercises, stretching the hamstrings, gastrocnemius, hip flexor (improving flexibility to decrease the patellofemoral compression during dynamic activities), and stretching of the iliotibial band (providing a lateral stabilization) were performed. The VMO strengthening was performed with: (1) isometric quadriceps sets at 20° of flexion; (2) leg raises supine with the femur externally rotated, the knee at 20° of flexion, and the opposite knee bent; (3) short arc quadriceps: patient supine, with roll under thigh, the knee flexed at 50°, and the leg externally rotated, extending the knee to 20°. Stretching of the iliotibial band was performed in the Ober's position, standing with the involved leg posterior and across the opposite leg, and leaning toward the opposite leg.

In stage 3, there was an advanced VMO strengthening with open kinetic chain and closed kinetic chain exercises (such as squat, seated leg press, and resistive walking). After these three phases, an isokinetic strength testing was performed during stage 4. Subjects remained at this stage until they were able to test to 85% of the strength in their uninvolved knees. When both legs were involved, subjects were given a final test when they were pain-free. Eighty-four percent of the subjects were pain-free after an average of eight weeks of rehabilitation. After the rehabilitation, a decrease in the congruence angle of the patients (average, 6.6°) was demonstrated, indicating a more medial tilt of the patella. The results of this study indicated that patellar tracking was improved with vastus medialis strengthening, iliotibial band and lateral retinaculum stretching, and joint mobility exercises.

Steinkamp et al.[40] demonstrated that patients with patellofemoral joint arthritis may tolerate rehabilitation with the leg press exercise better than with the leg extension exercise in the functional range of motion because of lower patellofemoral joint stresses. Knee moments, PFJR force, and patellofemoral joint stresses (compressive force per unit of contact area) were calculated in 20 normal subjects at 0°, 30°, 60°, and 90° of flexion during the leg press and the leg extension exercises.

All three parameters (knee moment, patellofemoral joint reaction force, and patellofemoral joint stress) were greater in the leg extension exercise than the leg press exercise at 0° and at 30° of flexion. At 60° and 90° of flexion, they were greater in leg press than leg extension exercises (Figure 3.15). Considering that the functional range of motion for most activities of daily living is in the lower end of knee flexion range, we can see that the leg extension exercise in this range of motion (from 0° to 30°) subjects the patellofemoral joint to a significant amount of stress, more than the leg press.

Werner[41] has performed interesting studies of rehabilitation treatment of patients with patellofemoral symptoms.

In a first study, the effect of patella taping on torque and electromyogram (EMG) activity in concentric and eccentric action of the knee extensor and flexor muscles in 48 patients with patellofemoral pain syndrome was considered. Most of the patients had a normal patellar mobility, but there were also patients with a medial patellar hypermobility, others with lateral patellar hypermobility, and a further group with an increased patellar mobility in both directions. The patients were tested concentrically and eccentrically on a Kin-Com dynamometer with simultaneous EMG recording with the patella untaped, or medially or laterally taped. Patients with medial patellar hypermobility showed a sharp improvement in quadriceps performance when their patellae were taped laterally compared with untaped. The greatest improvement was found during eccentric actions, where both the knee extensor torque and the agonist EMG activity showed a significant increase. A decrease in the hamstring/quadriceps ratio during eccentric action at 180°/s when their patellae were taped laterally, due to increased knee extensor torque, was also found. Patients with lateral patellar hypermobility increased their knee extensor torques and decreased their hamstring/quadriceps ratio during both eccentric and concentric actions at 60°/s when their patellae were taped medially compared with untaped. Patients with normal patellar mobility showed a significant decrease of their knee extensor torques and of the agonist EMG activity during most of the knee extension movements when their patellae were taped either laterally or medially. Werner also found that the patients' hamstring performance did not benefit from patella taping. The knee flexor torque decreased greatly at some of the different measurements when the patella was taped either laterally or medially.

In a second study, 30 patients with unilateral patellofemoral symptoms (pain generally associated with patellofemoral joint loading activities such as running or climbing stairs), a hypotrophic vastus medialis muscle, and tight lateral thigh muscles were treated with transcutaneous electric stimulation of the VMO and stretching of the lateral thigh muscles twice daily for ten weeks. Before and after treatment, the position of the patella at 30° of flexion and the area of the vastus medialis and lateralis muscles were studied by CT. The quadriceps torque was measured before and after treatment with a Cybex-II dynamometer at 60°/s and at 180°/s in a range of motion from 0° to 90° of flexion. An evaluation with a functional knee score was also carried out. The healthy contralateral leg was used in all examinations as a control. Clinically, two

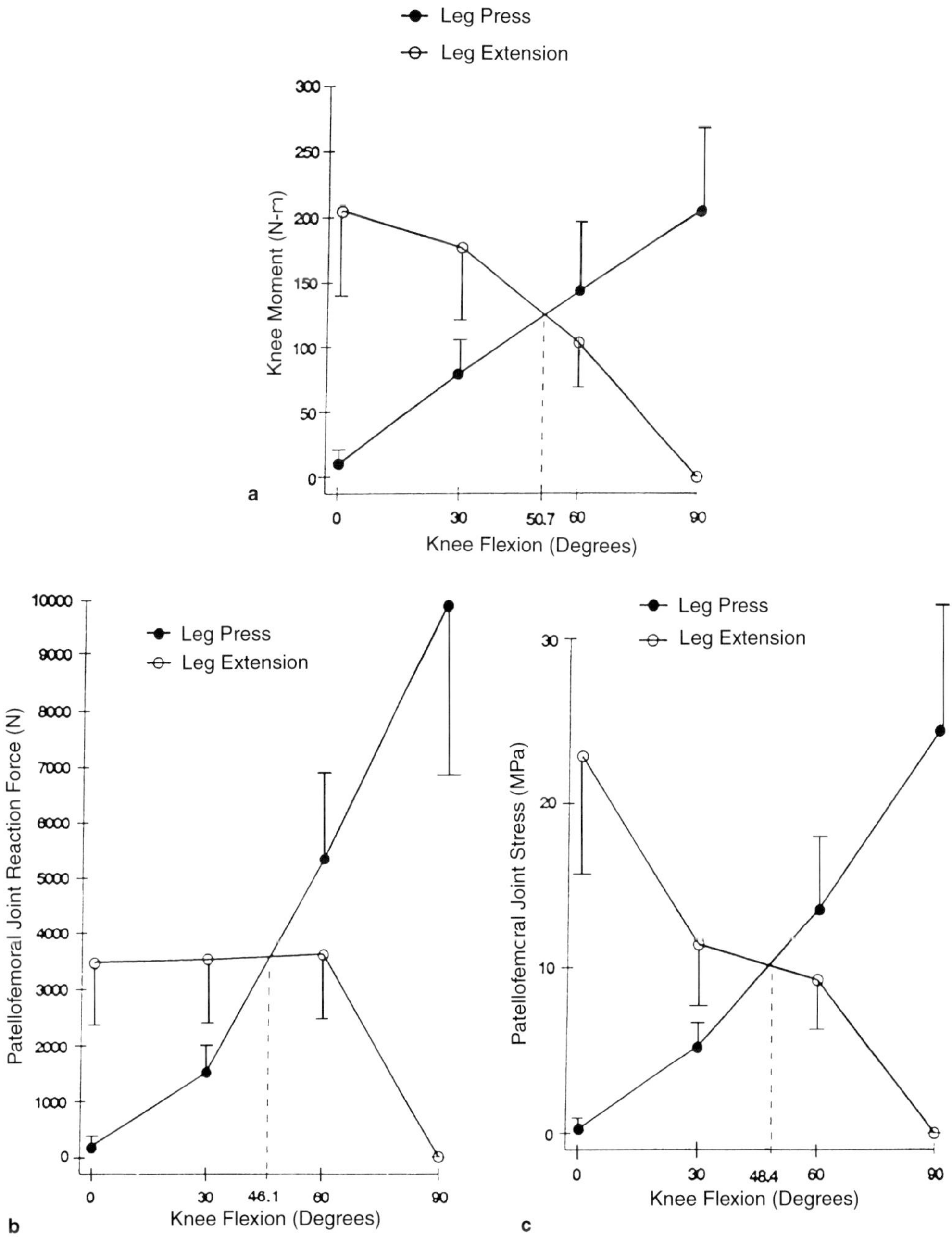

FIGURE 3.15. (a) Knee moment, (b) patellofemoral joint reaction force (PFJR force), and (c) patellofemoral joint stress (compressive force per contact area) evaluated at 0°, 30°, 60°, and 90° of flexion in leg press and in leg extension exercises (see text). (From Steinkamp, Dillingham and Markel, Biomechanical considerations in patellofemoral joint rehabilitation. Am. J. Sports Med., 1993: 21(3):441–442, with permission).

thirds of the patients had improved after ten weeks of treatment and this improvement remained at followup 3.5 years later. Werner attributes this improvement to reduced pain inhibition of voluntary muscle contraction. In addition, the area of the vastus medialis increased significantly (6%) after treatment, while the area of the vastus lateralis and the position of the patella did not change. In the control leg, the areas of both the vastus medialis and the vastus lateralis were unchanged. The quadriceps torque at 180°/s of the electrically stimulated leg improved significantly after treatment (104.7 nm) compared with the value before treatment (98.8 nm).

The Influence of the Posterior Cruciate Ligament

Many authors[42,43,44] recommended nonoperative treatment of a torn posterior cruciate ligament. Although reports of series with relatively short-term followup have indicated good results, recent long-term studies have shown that the function of the knee tends to slowly deteriorate with time.[43] This is probably due to abnormal forces adversely affecting the articular surfaces of all three components of the knee, as a result of increased posterior tibial translation. Tibone et al.[45] observed that, with the posterior cruciate ligament torn, flexion of the knee is increased in the midstance phase of gait. In an in vivo biomechanical study, Castle et al.[46] observed that the rupture of the posterior cruciate ligament results in posterior tibial subluxation during activities of daily living performed with more flexion (such as the ascent and descent of stairs).

Skyhar et al.[47] studied the articular contact pressures in a non-weight-bearing cadaver-knee model before and after sequential sectioning of the posterior cruciate ligament and posterolateral complex. Using pressure-sensitive film, they found a significant increase in the patellofemoral compartment pressures after isolated or combined sectioning of the ligament.

When the posterior cruciate ligament is torn, the patella and the patellar ligament assume a prominent role in the resistance to posterior tibial translation. The abnormal posterior tibial sag produces a shortened moment arm of the quadriceps with a reduced mechanical advantage. Rehabilitation after posterior cruciate ligament lesions should emphasize strengthening of the quadriceps and minimize posterior tibial translation.

Exercise for the quadriceps can be performed in an open kinetic chain, such as the leg extension (in which the foot is mobile and motion at the knee joint occurs independently from the motion of the hip and ankle joints), in a range of motion from 70° to 0° of flexion because in that arc posterior tibial translation is minimized.

This is confirmed in a study that Hirokawa et al.[48] performed on 12 cadaveric knees. In this study, the anterior–posterior displacement and rotation of the tibia elicited by isolated loading (from 0 to 12 kg at 2-kg intervals) of the quadriceps was determined as a function of the flexion angle (from 0° to 120°) and muscle load using a computerized radiographic technique. Quadriceps contraction can result in a significant anterior displacement of the tibia in the range of 0° to 80° of flexion and in a mild posterior displacement in the range of 80° to 120° of flexion. Peak anterior displacements of 6.3 mm resulted at 30° of flexion with a 12-kg load in the quadriceps, while a constant 1.5-mm posterior displacement was observed throughout flexion angles exceeding 80°. Quadriceps loading resulted in internal rotation of the tibia in the range of 0° to 90° of flexion (with a peak value of 7° at 15° of flexion with a 12-kg load) and in external rotation of the tibia in the range of 90° to 120° (with a peak value of 1.28° at 120° of flexion with a 12-kg load in the quadriceps).

For rehabilitation after posterior cruciate ligament lesions, when an isokinetic quadriceps exercise is performed, the resistance pad should be placed at the distal level to minimize articular contact pressure,[46] and to reduce posterior tibial translation.

Lutz et al.[49] analyzed the forces at the tibiofemoral joint during open and closed kinetic chain exercises in five healthy subjects performing maximum isometric contractions at

30°, 60°, and 90° of knee flexion during open kinetic chain extension, open kinetic chain flexion, and closed kinetic chain exercises. Electromyographic activity of the quadriceps and hamstrings was also recorded. A two-dimensional biomechanical model was adopted to calculate the tibiofemoral shear and compression forces. During the open kinetic chain extension exercise, maximum posterior shear forces of 285 N occurred at 30° of flexion and maximum anterior shear forces of 1,780 N occurred at 90° of flexion. The closed kinetic chain exercise produced less posterior shear forces at all angles when compared with the open kinetic chain extension exercise and less anterior shear forces at all angles, except 30°, when compared with the open kinetic chain flexion exercise. In addition, during the closed kinetic chain exercise, the tibiofemoral compression force decreased, increasing flexion of the knee.

References

1. Fulkerson JP, Hungerford DS: Biomechanics of the patellofemoral joint, in *Disorders of the patellofemoral joint*. Baltimore, The Williams & Wilkins Co, 1990, pp 25–41.
2. Aglietti P, Buzzi R, Insall JN: Disorders of the patellofemoral joint, in Insall JN (ed.): *Surgery of the Knee*. Churchill Livingstone, New York, 1993, pp. 246 251.
3. Hungerford DS, Barry N: Biomechanics of the patellofemoral joint. *Clin Orthop* 1979;144:9–15.
4. Kaufer H: Mechanical function of the patella. *J Bone Joint Surg Am* 1971;53A:1551–1560.
5. Kaufer H: Patellar biomechanics. *Clin Orthop* 1979;144:51–54.
6. Hehne HF: Biomechanics of the patellofemoral joint and its clinical relevance. *Clin Orthop* 1990;258:73–85.
7. Buff HU, Jones LC, Hungerford DS: Experimental determination of forces transmitted through the patellofemoral joint. *J Biomech* 1988;21:17–23.
8. Maquet P: Advancement of the tibial tuberosity. *Clin Orthop* 1976;115:225–228.
9. Van Eijden TMGJ, Kouwenhoven E, Verburg J, et al.: A mathematical model of the patellofemoral joint. *J Biomech* 1986;19:219–229.
10. Bandi W: Chondromalacia patellae and femoro-patellare arthrose. *Helv Chir Acta* 1972; 1(suppl.):3–70.
11. Reilly DT, Martens M: Experimental analysis of the quadriceps muscle force and patellofemoral joint reaction force for various activities. *Acta Orthop Scand* 1972;43:126–137.
12. Smith AJ: Estimates of muscle and joint force at the knee and ankle during jumping activities. *J Hum Movement Stud* 1975;1:78–86.
13. Zernicke RF, Garhammer J, Jobe FW, et al.: Human patellar-tendon rupture. *J Bone Joint Surg Am* 1977;59A(2):179–183.
14. Ellis ML, Seedhom BB, Amis AA, et al.: Forces in the knee joint whilst rising from normal and motorized chairs. *Eng Med* 1979;8:33–40.
15. Dahlkvist NY, Mayo P, Seedhom BB: Forces during squatting and rising from a deep squat. *Eng Med* 1982;11:69–76.
16. Huberti HH, Hayes WC: Patello femoral contact pressures. The influence of Q angle and tendofemoral contact. *J Bone Joint Surg Am* 1984;66A:715–724.
17. Kaufman KR, An K, Litchy WJ, et al.: Dynamic joint forces during knee isokinetic exercise. *Am J Sports Med* 1991;19(3):305–316.
18. Aglietti P, Insall JN, Walker PS, et al.: A new patella prosthesis. *Clin Orthop* 1975;107:175–187.
19. Goodfellow J, Hungerford DS, Zindel M: Patellofemoral joint mechanics and pathology. 1. Functional anatomy of the patellofemoral joint. *J Bone Joint Surg Br* 1976;58B:287–291.
20. Hayes WC, Huberti HH, Lewallen DG, et al.: Patellofemoral contact pressure and the effects of surgical reconstructive procedures, in Ewing JW (ed.): *Articular Cartilage and Knee Joint Function. Basic Science and Arthroscopy*. New York, Raven Press, 1990, pp. 57–77.
21. Wiberg G: Roentgenographic and anatomic studies on the patellofemoral joint. *Acta Orthop Scand* 1941;12:319–410.
22. Baumgartl F: *Das Kniegelenk*. Berlin, Springer-Verlag, 1944.
23. Reider B, Marshall JL, Koslin B, et al.: The anterior aspect of the knee joint. *J Bone Joint Surg Am* 1981;63A(3):351–356.
24. Fujikawa K, Seedhom BB, Wright V: Biomechanics of the patellofemoral joint. Part I: A study of the contact and the congruity of the patellofemoral compartment and movement of the patella. *Eng Med* 1983;12:1, 3–11.
25. Hirokawa S: Three-dimensional mathematical model analysis of the patellofemoral joint. *J Biomech* 1991;24:659–669.
26. Dejour H: Factor responsible for patellar in-

stability, in *Fifth European Congress of Knee Surgery and Arthroscopy.* Stockholm, June 1990.
27. Kujala UM, Osterman K, Kormano M, et al.: Patellar motion analyzed by magnetic resonance imaging. *Acta Orthop Scand* 1989;60(1): 13–16.
28. Kelly MA, Brittis DA: Patellectomy. *Orthop Clin North Am* 1992;23(4):657–663.
29. Stougard J: Patellectomy. *Acta Orthop Scand* 1970;41:110–121.
30. Sutton FS, Thompson CH, Lipke J, et al.: The effect of patellectomy on knee function. *J Bone Joint Surg Am* 1976;58A(4):537–540.
31. Steurer PA, Gradisar IA, Hoyt WA, et al.: Patellectomy: A clinical study and biomechanical evaluation. *Clin Orthop* 1979;144:84–90.
32. Watkins MP, Harris BA, Wender S, et al.: Effect of patellectomy on the function of the quadriceps and hamstrings. *J Bone Joint Surg Am* 1983;65A(3):390–395.
33. Wendt PP, Johnson RP: A study of quadriceps excursion, torque, and the effect of patellectomy cadaver knees. *J Bone Joint Surg Am* 1985;67A(5):726–732.
34. Maquet P: Mechanics and osteoarthritis of the patellofemoral joint. *Clin Orthop* 1979;144:70–73.
35. Ferguson AB, Brown TD, Fu FH, et al.: Relief of patellofemoral contact stress by anterior displacement of the tibial tubercle. *J Bone Joint Surg Am* 1979;61A:159–166.
36. Fulkerson JP: Anteromedialization of the tibial tuberosity for patellofemoral malalignment. *Clin Orthop* 1983;177:176–181.
37. Fulkerson JP, Becker GJ, Meaney JA, et al.: Anteromedial tibial tubercle transfer without bone graft. *Am J Sports Med* 1990;18(5):490–497.
38. Nakamura N, Ellis M, Seedhom BB: Advancement of the tibial tuberosity. A biomechanical study. *J Bone Joint Surg Br* 1985;67B:255–260.
39. Doucette SA, Goble EM: The effect of exercise on patellar tracking in lateral patellar compression syndrome. *Am J Sports Med* 1992;20(4): 434–440.
40. Steinkamp LA, Dillingham MF, Markel MD, et al.: Biomechanical considerations in patellofemoral joint rehabilitation. *Am J Sports Med* 1993;21(3):438–444.
41. Werner S: *Patello Femoral Pain Syndrome—An Experimental Clinical Investigation,* thesis. Konel Carolinska Medico Chirurgiska Institutet, Stockholm, 1993.
42. Dandy DJ, Pusey RJ: The long-term results of unrepaired tears of the posterior cruciate ligament. *J Bone Joint Surg Br* 1982;64B:92–94.
43. Dejour H, Walch G, Peyrot J, et al.: Histoire naturelle de la rupture du ligament croisé postérieur. *Rev Chir Orthop Reparatrice Appar Mot* 1988;74:35–43.
44. Keller PM, Shelbourne KD, McCarrol JR, et al.: Nonoperatively treated isolated posterior cruciate ligament injuries. *Am J Sports Med* 1993;21:132–136.
45. Tibone JE, Antich TJ, Perry J, et al.: Functional analysis of untreated and reconstructed posterior cruciate ligament injuries. *Am J Sports Med* 1988;16:217–223.
46. Castle TH, Noyes FR, Grood ES: Posterior tibial subluxation of the posterior cruciate deficient knee. *Clin Orthop* 1992;284:193–202.
47. Skyhar MJ, Warren RF, Ortiz GJ, et al.: The effects of the sectioning of the posterior cruciate ligament and the posterolateral complex on the articular contact pressure within the knee. *J Bone Joint Surg Am* 1993;75A:694–699.
48. Hirokawa S, Solomonow M, Lu Y, et al.: Anterior-posterior and rotational displacement of the tibia elicited by quadriceps contraction. *Am J Sports Med* 1992;20(3):299–306.
49. Lutz GE, Palmitier RA, An KN, et al.: Comparison of tibiofemoral joint forces during open kinetic chain and closed kinetic chain exercises. *J Bone Joint Surg Am* 1993;75A:732–739.

4

Pathology of the Patella

Vincent J. Vigorita and Daniel Morgan

The pathology of the patella is best understood by reviewing the synovium, articular cartilage, and bone, and those disorders predilected to pathologic alterations of these tissues.

The Synovium

The *synovium* consists of a thin intimal layer of synovial cells or synoviocytes, which lies above a richly fibrovascular zone, the subintimal layer, that contains arterioles, fat, and other connective tissue cells such as fibroblasts, histiocytes, and occasionally mast cells[1] (Figure 4.1). This loose connective tissue zone layer becomes gradually more fibrous at capsular insertions. The intimal zone consists of an admixture of cell types, broadly classified as those demonstrating macrophage function (synovial A cells) and those more synthesizing in function (synovial B cells). Ultrastructural studies demonstrate abundant mitochondria, Golgi apparatus, vacuoles, lysosomes, phagosomes, vesicles, and surface undulations are characteristics suited to macrophage activity in type A cells, and rough endoplasmic reticulum, free ribosomes, and smoother profiles are characteristics suited to synthetic activity in type B cells. As might be expected, synoviocytes may be "intermediate" in nature, featuring organelle functions of both type A and type B. Although the synovial cells lack desmosomes or tight junctions, characteristic of epithelial tissue, the complexity of this cell structure is evident in the changes seen in various pathologic states. Hyperplasia (Figure 4.2) may be limited to a mild increase in intimal cell number, or there may be a dramatic change, including large, bizarre cells such as the Grimley–Sokoloff giant cells of rheumatoid arthritis or even striking mucin-producing cells. In this latter condition (mucinous hypertrophy of the synovium), the copious amount of material secreted testifies to the great secretory capacity of this membrane.

Synovial Disorders

Normally, the synovium appears pale pink in color and architecturally covers all surfaces of the joint space, excluding the articular cartilage and fibrocartilage of the meniscus. However, the synovium does cover peripheral aspects of the meniscus, and synovial intima-type cells do coat parts of the cruciate ligamentous insertions. Only in abnormal conditions does the synovium encroach upon the surface of articular cartilage, a change classically seen in the reddish "pannus" or inflammatory synovial invasion of the articular cartilage in rheumatoid arthritis.

The villous appearance of the synovium is not necessarily abnormal, but rather it is nonspecific and may be seen in a broad range of conditions. In general, traumatic synovitis and degenerative joint disease (osteoarthritis) are attended by edematous change and mild villous hypertrophy. Inflammatory arthritis (classically rheumatoid arthritis) shows a dramatically reddish hyperplastic synovium with

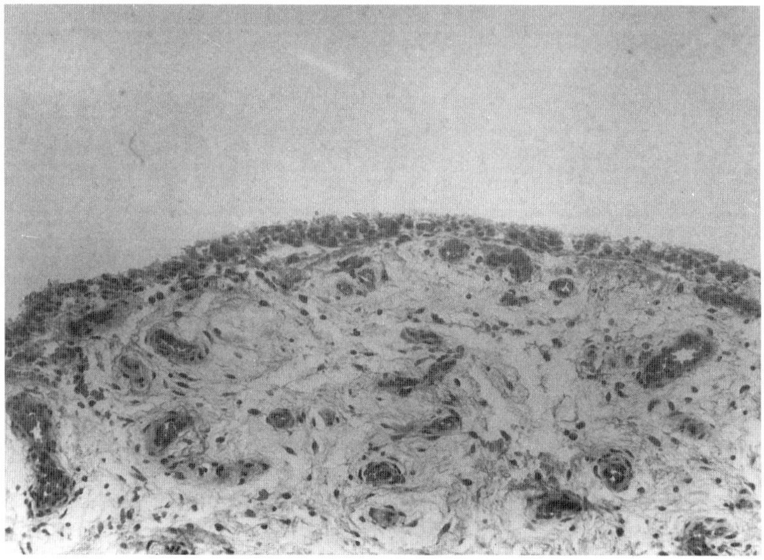

FIGURE 4.1. Normal synovium. The most superficial zone (or intima) consists of a one- to two-cell layer of synoviocytes below which is a fibrovascular zone (subintima) containing fibroblasts, histiocytes, and mast cells.

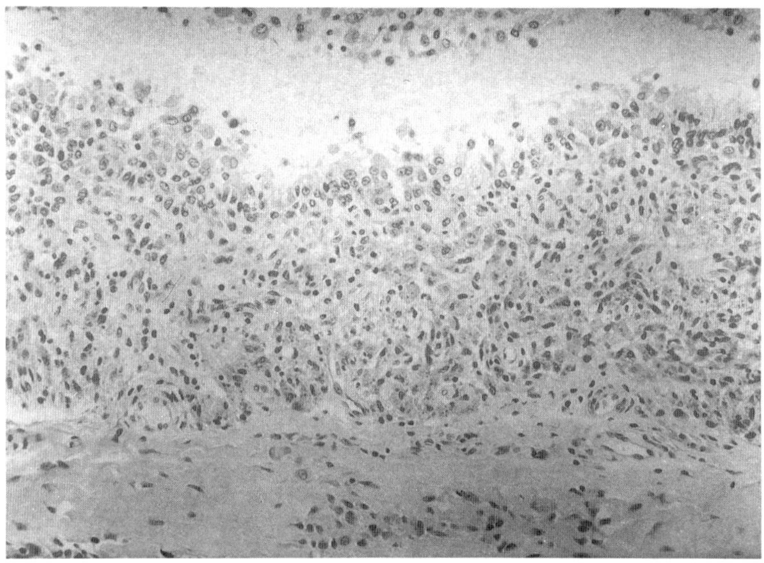

FIGURE 4.2. Hyperplastic synovium. The synovioctye layer (intima) shows increased size and numbers of cells.

fibrinous exudation characterized by abundant tan fibrinous loose bodies called *rice bodies.*

Normally, the intimal superficial cellular layer of the synovium appears smooth and transparent, but it turns thick, dull, and opaque with pathologic change. With hemorrhage, synovium becomes obviously bloody, but in chronic hemarthrosis it turns a rusty reddish brown, owing to hemosiderin deposition and the release of iron from red blood cells. In severe cases, a dark purple may be seen. The appearance of a rusty or reddish purple synovium indicates bleeding and may be seen in trauma, bleeding disorders such as hemophilia, and pigmented villonodular synovitis. Whereas in ochronosis (alkaptonuria) the synovium may appear a dull gray, fibrocartilage and articular cartilage will be discolored black. Darkening or blackening may also be seen when there is extensive release of metallic debris. White foci in the synovium usu-

usually indicate gout (urate deposition), pseudogout (calcium pyrophosphate crystal deposition), or soft-tissue calcifications (deposits due to trauma or calcinosis syndromes). Cement debris may also lead to pallor.

The subintimal fibrovascular layer is the zone containing the ubiquitous fibrohistiocytic cells, and the zone infiltrated by lymphocytes and plasma cells in rheumatoid arthritis. The various components and cells of the synovial subintima explain the source of tumors reported in the knee, such as:

- Hemangiomas (arterioles)
- Hemangiopericytomas (the pericyte of the arteriole)
- Fibromas (fibroblast)
- Leiomyomas (smooth muscle of arteriole wall)
- Lipomas, Hoffa's disease (fat)
- Pigmented villonodular synovitis (fibrohistiocyte)

The etiology of the rare malignant tumors arising near joints, called synovial sarcoma and epithelioid sarcoma, is less well known. These latter tumors are highly malignant and are characterized by aggressive and destructive local growth and metastatic potential.

Functions of the Synovium

The functions of the synovium are best appreciated by understanding the characteristics of its cellular components and microarchitectural structure.[2] For example, the synovial A cells are suited to phagocytic (or macrophage) activity and ingest native or foreign material, such as hemosiderin in chronic bleeding conditions (hemophilia) or iatrogenically introduced substances (gold in the treatment of rheumatoid arthritis). The phagocytic potential of the synovium is probably best illustrated by the great foreign body giant cell and histiocytic reaction in some cases of loosened prostheses, or in the resorption of bone and cartilage debris in rapidly destructive joint disease or neuropathic joints. On the other hand, the synovial B cell is suited to synthetic function and most characteristically secretes the hyaluronate protein of the synovial fluid. However, type A and type B cells both appear to have secretory and phagocytic potential. Other functions in conjunction with the vascular and lymphatic systems of the synovium include the regulation of movement of physiologically important proteins and electrolytes.

Iron Synovitis: Hemarthrosis and Hemophilia

Considering the rich vascularity of the subintimal layer of the synovium, microscopic bleeds from normal daily use of the joint may be expected. In fact, a few red blood cells are considered normal in joint fluid analysis. Trauma to the knee, however, is often accompanied by significant hemarthrosis, an important association since bleeding—or perhaps more specifically the release of iron from ruptured red blood cells—stimulates clinically significant synovial change, that is, a synovitis characterized by pain and swelling.

In chronic hemarthrosis, iron will accumulate in the synovium.[3] Histopathologic localization includes both the synovial intimal cells and histiocytic cells of the subintimal zone. Experimental evidence suggests that iron adversely affects synovial function. Chronic hemarthrosis, for example, actually may increase the synthetic function of the otherwise macrophagic synovial type A cell. Hemophilia represents this situation in a clinical extreme.[4]

Classically, hemophilia A is characterized by inadequacy of factor VIII. It primarily affects males, with substantial intra-articular bleeds into the joints, especially the knees. Grossly, the joint becomes brown. Synovial hyperplasia is significant, iron accumulation in the joint is profound, and secondary destruction of the articular surface and the bone is dramatic. The use of factor VIII concentrates as therapy has slowed considerably the progression of arthropathy but, unfortunately, it has created one of the significant early-risk groups for the acquired immunodeficiency syndrome (AIDS). Genetically engineered factor VIII replacements have been developed but remain prohibitively expensive. Large tumorlike masses of blood coagulum sealed off by fibrous tissue may ensue, termed *pseudotumor of hemophilia,* and should be removed surgically if possible. Although in its clinical extreme hemophilia represents an inexorable vicious cycle, the hemarthrosis associated with trauma is obviously less significant. However, chronic bleeding of whatever etiology will lead to iron-associated synovial change (iron synovitis). At what point this becomes clinically significant is unclear. It is of interest that experimental models of hemarthrosis pathologically mimic hemophilia more than pigmented villonodular synovitis, which is associated with iron secondarily.

Crystal-Induced Synovitis

There are essentially two synoviotropic crystal deposition disorders of the knee: (1) gout and (2) CPDD (calcium pyrophosphate deposition disease, chondrocalcinosis, or pseudogout). Although the two are often considered together, they are distinct etiologically, clinically, and pathologically.

Gout is a severe and painful arthritis of the first metatarsophalangeal joint, but virtually any joint or part of the body may be affected. The patella is an uncommon site.[5] In general, gout should be suspected in painful episodes of arthritis in one or more joints of the lower extremity, with the patient showing significant, if not complete, improvement between episodes. Although the diagnosis should be suspected with elevated serum uric acid (roughly >8.0 mg/dL in men and >6.5 mg/dL in women), normouricemic episodes of gout are well documented.

In gout, attacks of severe pain may last up to several days. The joint may appear erythematous and the patient is ill with chills and fever. Initially, radiographs are unremarkable with only soft tissue swelling. With progressive attacks and more urate crystal deposition, tophi, which are granulomatous aggregates of crystals, accumulate in the joint tissue, causing discrete radiolucent marginal erosions of the articular bone. Despite significant bone destruction, joint preservation may be well maintained until late in the disease.

The intraoperative appearance of gout is dramatic: on cut section, tophi show chalk-white aggregates of a soft texture. Microscopically, the crystal aggregates are surrounded by a great mononuclear and giant cell inflammatory reaction (Figure 4.3). Surgical removal of large tophi may improve joint function. Confirmation requires demonstration of the crystals, which can be done using compensated polarized light microscopy (Figure 4.4). This technique requires a light microscope, polarizing lenses, and a red compensator filter. Fluid aspirated from the joint is submitted to the laboratory in a test tube; the fluid is centrifuged and the sediment is spread onto a glass slide for microscopic examination.

Calcium Pyrophosphate Deposition Disease (CPDD, Chondrocalcinosis, or Pseudogout)*

Calcium pyrophosphate deposition disease (CPDD) is a polyarticular deposition of calcium pyrophosphate crystals in fibrocartilage, articular cartilage, and synovial tissue in the knee, hip, symphysis pubis, wrist, and intervertebral disk.[6] Anatomic studies have demonstrated a predilection for the fibrocartilage of the meniscus and the synovium, and less so for the superficial zones of the articular cartilage. Although CPDD may be seen microscopically in at least 15% of osteoarthritic knees examined at joint replacements, the characteristic white, flecklike deposits observed intraoperatively are seen less frequently (Figure 4.5).

The prevalence of CPDD in degenerative joint disease is consistent with the accumulation of pyrophosphates by release from articular cartilage. Since chondroid metaplasia has been observed with deposits of calcium pyrophosphate, local activation of certain enzymes, such as alkaline phosphatase or inorganic pyrophosphatases, leading to inactivation of cal-

---

*CPDD designates the crystals (calcium pyrophosphate) deposited in this disorder. Pseudogout refers to the occasional painful occurrence of CPDD-induced arthritis, mimicking gout. Chondrocalcinosis refers to the fine linear radiopaque densities seen in the joint spaces of involved cases.

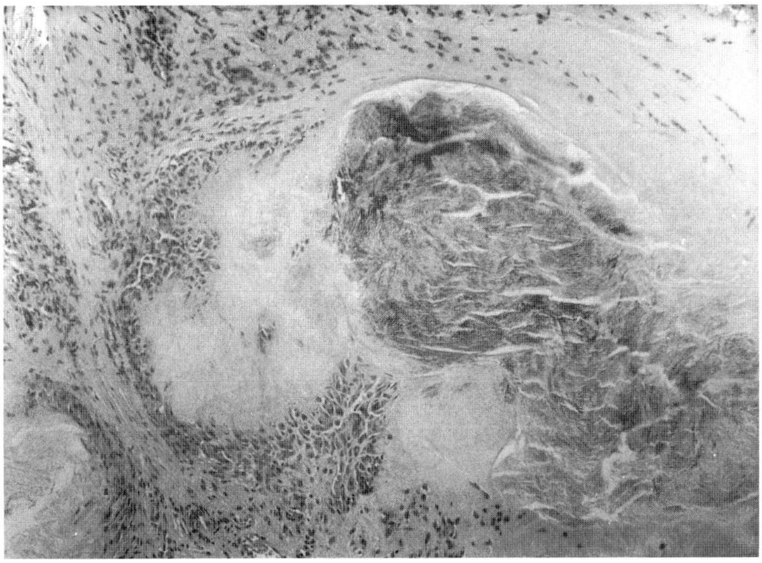

FIGURE 4.3. The mononuclear and giant cell granulomatous reaction to gout crystals. When dissolved, as in routine fixation, crystals appear as amorphous pale zones (left).

cification inhibitors, may be important. It is significant that symptomatic arthritis, due specifically to CPDD, is unusual and much less common than gout. CPDD is usually less painful than gout but shares similarities of exacerbation during surgery and relief between episodes. Joints, especially the knees, are bilaterally and symmetrically involved. Radiographs show fine, radiopaque linear densities appearing along the joint space. The meniscus, articular and synovial tissues, and superficial articular cartilage are all involved. Unlike gout, the clinically apparent disease does not necessarily correlate with the extent of roentgenographically detectable disease. Microscopically, the crystals are rhomboidal, less birefringent, and less inflammatory than in gout (Figure 4.6). Treatment is directed at relief during painful attacks and includes salicylates, indomethacin, and other nonsteroidal anti-inflammatory agents.

Prosthesis Pathology

Debris generated by total knee replacement arthroplasty can lead to a significant inflammatory reaction and extensive osteolysis. The inflammatory reaction often consists of multinucleated giants cells or histiocytes engulfing particulate matter—histiocytes being bone marrow monocyte-derived macrophages or phagocytes. Wear debris with significant associated foreign body-type inflammation is well described with metallic debris, polyethylene, and methyl methacrylate cement. Although metal and polyethylene do not dissolve during tissue processing, cement may. Nontheless, arthroplasty wear debris is usually diagnosed grossly as discoloration of the synovium. With metal debris, tissue becomes dusky gray or black, and with polyethylene and cement, tissue becomes pale tan or whitish. Microscopically, under polarized light, metal and polyethylene particles are refractile, that is, they give off light. Evidence of dissolved cement is usually noted as intracellular cytoplasmic residual irregularly shaped vacuoles. Tissue damage and osteolysis is believed to be due to local tissue cytokines such such as interleukin-1, prostaglandic PGE_2, and neutral proteinases produced by activated synovial cells and macrophages. Similar mechanisms are thought to explain adverse tissue reactions with artificial ligament materials. In ligament replacements, material, dose, and probably size are also factors in eliciting an adverse tissue response.[7]

Synovial Plicae

Synovial plicae are a common incidental finding at autopsy (20% to 50%) and have been

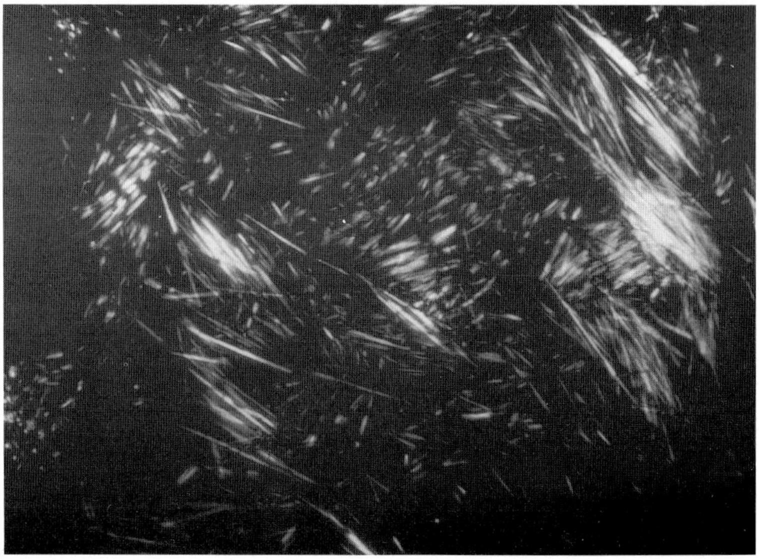

FIGURE 4.4. With polarized light, gout crystals are seen to be fine, slender, needlelike, and brilliantly refractile.

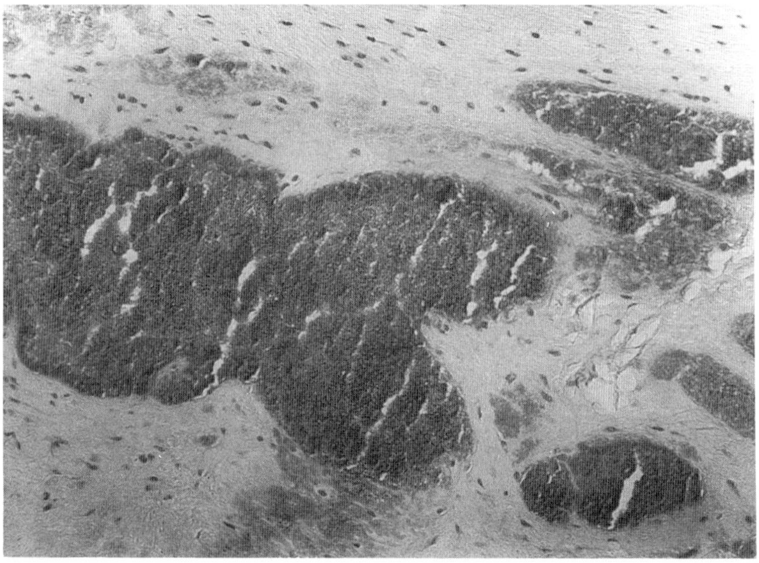

FIGURE 4.5. Unlike sodium urate crystals, calcium pyrophosphate crystals appear as purple depositions on routine tissue processing. The lack of an inflammatory response is in contrast to that of gout.

reported in as high as 80% of knees coming to arthroscopic surgery.[8] First described in 1916 by Fullerton, synovial plicae are thought to represent incomplete remnants of the normally cavity-forming synovial mesenchyme. Many types of plicae have been reported, reflecting various reabsorption defects. Histologically, resected plicae are relatively nondescript, consisting of a connective tissue band covered with a thin layer of synovial-like cells. In plicae removed during arthroscopy for knee pain, the tissue may show some inflammation or fibrosis.

Hoffa's Disease

Since 1906, when Hoffa called attention to excess fatty tissue in the knee, hypertrophy of the synovium and fat in the infrapatellar fat pad have been appreciated as a pathologic entity. The fat pad normally fills the intracapsular extrasynovial pyramidal space between

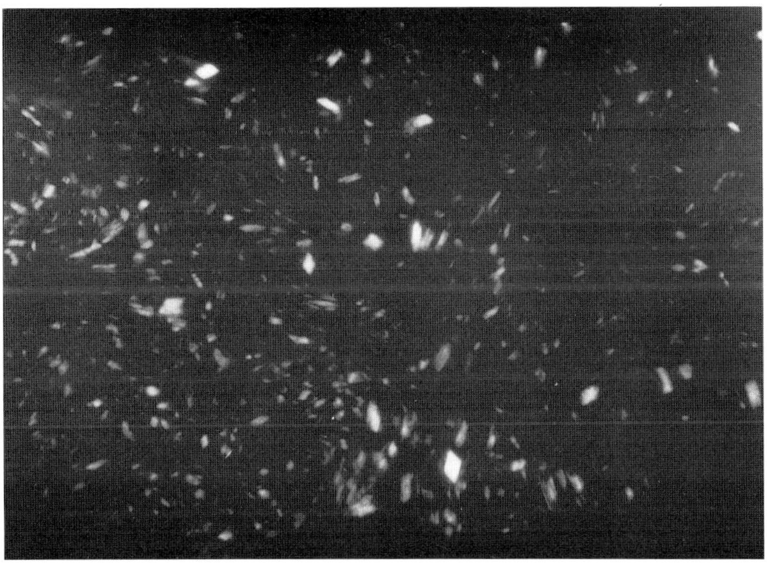

FIGURE 4.6. Calcium pyrophosphate crystals are less refractile on polarized light and have a rectangular or rhomboid shape.

the patella tendon, and the femoral and the tibial condyles. It is known to be rich in pain-sensitive neurovascular tissue and therefore is potentially a cause of symptomatic knee pain. Hoffa's disease may be due to trauma, edema, or other space-occupying lesions that lead to exacerbation of the normal projection of the fat pad into the joint cavity, particularly an extension of the knee. The histopathology is usually a combination of (excess) fat tissue, often morphologically normal, lined by synovium of varying degrees of hyperplasia and mild chronic inflammation. *Lipoma arborescens* is a term preferred by some and is similar pathologically.[9] Here, villous fatty synovial tissue projects into the joint. It is associated with degenerative joint disease, rheumatoid arthritis, or diabetes.

Synovial Chondromatosis (Synovial Osteochondromatosis)

The synovium, capable of undergoing metaplasia to cartilage in a broad range of conditions including trauma and degenerative joint disease, may produce multiple cartilaginous and chondro-osseous loose bodies throughout the joint[10] (Figure 4.7). The latter condition, synovial chondromatosis (synovial osteochondromatosis), is best characterized as a benign tumorous proliferation. Initially embedded in the synovium, the nodules may dislodge from the synovium and become free loose bodies ranging in number from a few to hundreds.

Synovial chondromatosis is a monoarticular condition of the third, fourth, and fifth decades of life with predilection for the knee. It is usually associated with swelling and may be associated with pain, limitation of motion, and occasionally clicking or locking. Radiographically, the condition is easily recognized if the cartilaginous bodies have undergone calcification or ossification, which they often do. The numerous radiopaque densities range in size from a millimeter to centimeters, varying considerably in the extent of calcification. Arthrography is useful in diagnosing the noncalcified bodies. Grossly, the synovium shows flakelike bodies, or it may possess an irregular nodular contour. Whitish or translucent bluish-gray nodules, ranging greatly in size and shape, may be more obviously attached on the membrane or floating in the joint space.

Histopathologic differences of these bodies have supported a distinction between a secondary synovial chondromatosis associated with degenerative joint disease and a primary synovial chondromatosis not associated with any underlying disorder. The loose bodies in the secondary condition classically may show more organized cellular growth such as layers

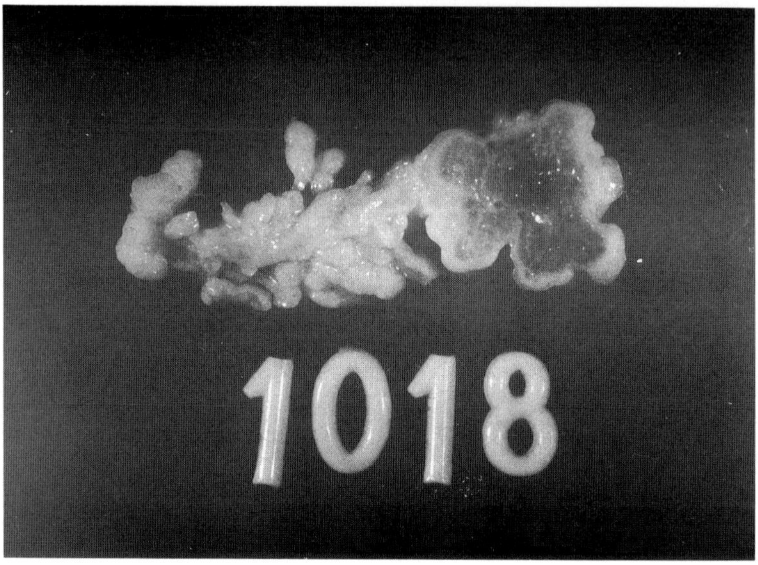

FIGURE 4.7. In traumatic knees or degenerative joint disease, the synovium may undergo chondroid or chondro-osseous metaplasia, as seen in this synovium that has undergone the formation of a centrally ossified cartilaginous nodule.

of calcification (Figure 4.8). However, in primary synovial chondromatosis, a more disorganized growth of cartilage cells is often apparent (Figure 4.9).

Surgical removal of all the nodules is important in preventing recurrence. If the chondro-osseous bodies are entirely free loose bodies within the joint, a thorough cleaning of the joint may suffice. However, the disorder may involve chondro-osseous change within the synovial subintimal connective tissue, a fact that may require synovectomy to prevent recurrence. In rare instances, chondrosarcomas may arise in the setting of synovial chondromatosis. They are characterized by extracapsular involvement and should be distinguished from a de novo primary synovial chondrosarcoma of the joint.

Pigmented Villonodular Synovitis

Although sometimes considered an inflammatory reaction, pigmented villonodular synovitis (PVNS) is a tumorous proliferation of stromal mononuclear and multinucleated giant cells of fibrohistiocytic origin[11] (Figure 4.10). The nodular growth pattern, the occasionally observed mitotic activity of the stroma, the relative lack of inflammatory cells, and the ability to erode local tissue support the classification of PVNS as a tumor. The name is fitting for only some of the lesions. PVNS may show little pigmentation; is often a solitary nodular growth with little villous hyperplasia; and, as mentioned, shows little inflammatory activity (Figure 4.11).

The joint fluid color is variable, ranging from normal to brownish-red. The synovium may appear diffusely pigmented or, more commonly, focally so. The pigment is due to both hemosiderin accumulation from microscopic synovial hemorrhage (brown) and aggregations of lipid-laden macrophages (yellow) in the periphery of expanding nodules. Hyperplastic and pigmented changes mimicking those of chronic hemarthrosis in the adjacent synovium are secondary in nature and do not represent the lesion proper.

At least five clinical types of PVNS are identified in the knee:

1. Loose body
2. A localized nodule (pedunculated or embedded in the synovium)
3. Aggregates of nodules confined to one compartment
4. A truly diffuse involvement of the synovium
5. Synovial PVNS extending into the bursa

Localized nodular and nodular aggregate types are the most common types of PVNS.

Typically, PVNS is a monoarticular arthri-

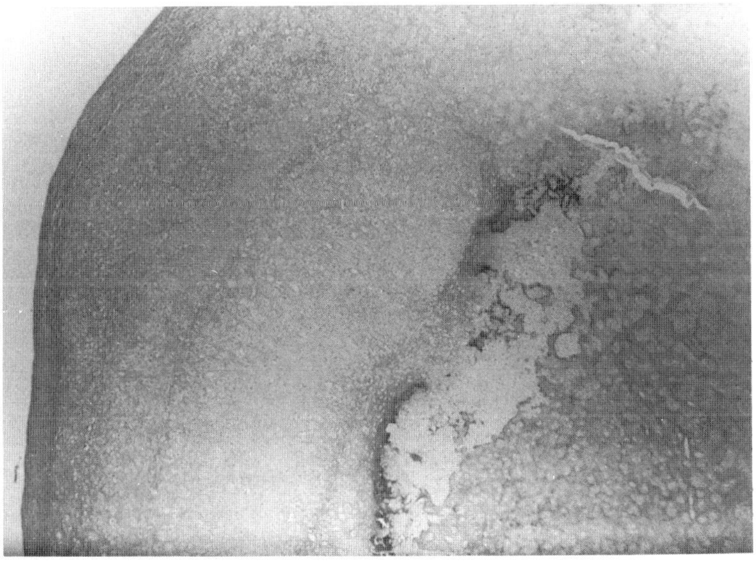

FIGURE 4.8. In chondromatosis associated secondarily with joint disease, the layers of calcification may appear distinct, as seen in this microscopic transection of a radiopaque loose body.

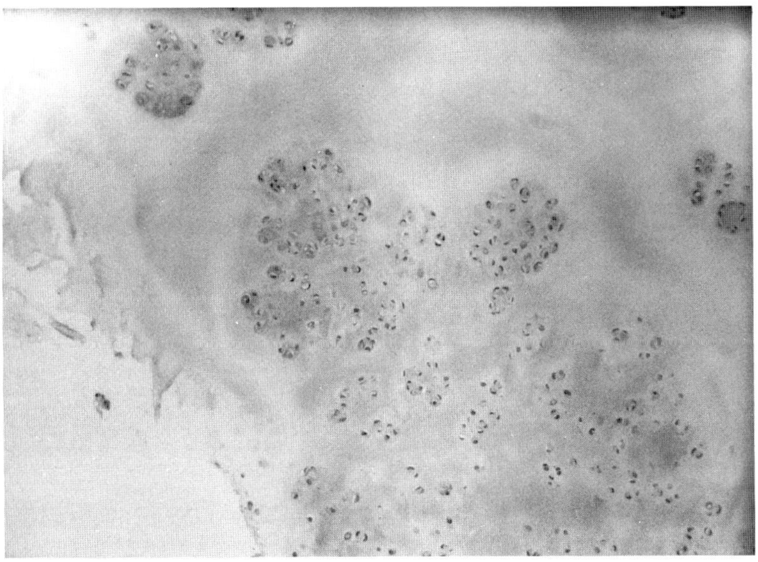

FIGURE 4.9. The classic microscopic appearance in primary synovial chondromatosis is that of a lobular proliferation of chondrocytes: the microscopic chondrocytic aggregation.

tis usually observed in the early and middle adult period, rarely at the extreme ends of life. Symptoms may be gradual in onset. Clinically, patients may present with discomfort or pain. Swelling, stiffness, locking, or even instability of the knee may occur. Torsion of a pedunculated nodular form of PVNS has been associated with the unusual clinical presentation of acute pain.

The most common x-ray findings in the knee are soft tissue swelling. Arthrograms may best demonstrate the nodules as discrete pitting defects. Bone changes are less frequent, but they may include erosions and degenerative changes.

The treatment of PVNS is surgical. If an isolated loose body or nodule is confirmed, arthroscopic surgical excision may be attempted. However, the propensity of the lesions to recur (in up to one third of cases) requires careful examination of the remainder of the joint to exclude multiple foci. Smaller

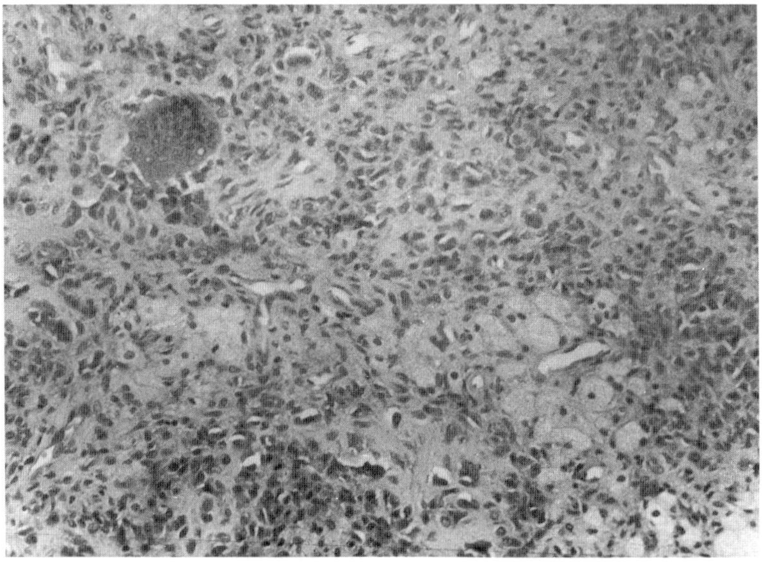

FIGURE 4.10. Microscopically, the collagenous stroma is awash in mesenchymal mononuclear and giant cells. Inflammation is sparse. Xanthomatous cells are usually focal in distribution.

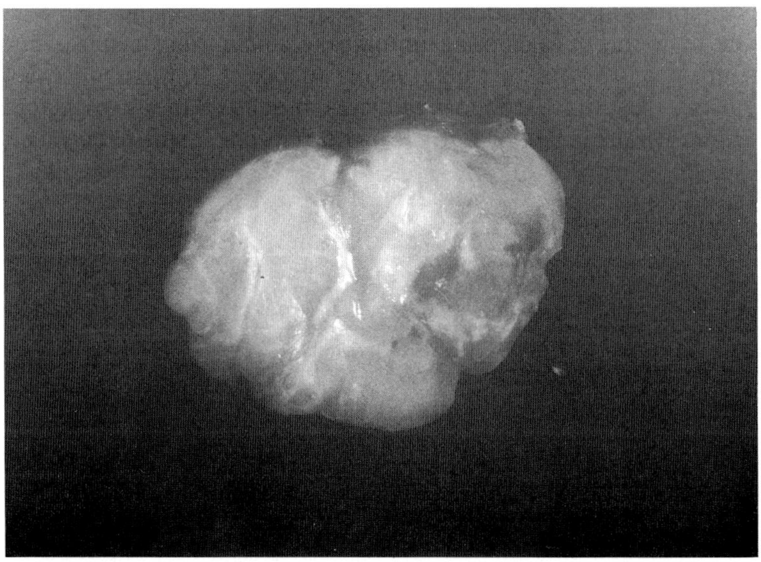

FIGURE 4.11. On cross section, the nodules of pigmented villonodular synovitis (PVNS) usually show the pigment of the peripheral. Here the central silk-colored region of collagenous stroma is surrounded by a rim of pigment (lipid-laden macrophages, or xanthoma cells and hemosiderin).

nodules may be missed, embedded as they are in the subintimal synovial layers. The diffuse form of PVNS is more problematic and requires total synovectomy. If not removed, PVNS will continue to grow and erode into the articular bone. Bursal PVNS also requires adequate surgical excision and may extend deeply into surrounding soft tissue.

Malignant Tumors

Malignant tumors of the synovium are extremely rare. Synovial sarcoma, despite its name, does not arise within the joint, although it has been described in the bursa. It is a malignant mesenchymal tumor that usually arises in structures adjacent to the joint, most often in tenosynovial lining anatomic structures.[12] It derives its name from its microscopic appearance, which mimics the histologic appearance of the embryonic synovium. Synovial sarcoma occurs in close association with tendon sheaths, bursae, and joint capsules, and has a propensity to differentiate toward a spindle cell, or fibroblastlike mesodermal cell population, as well as an epithelial population, giving it, in its classic presentation, a biphasic microscopic appearance. Approximately 70% of the tumors occur in the lower extremity, and 15% occur above the knee. It is the fourth most common soft-tissue sarcoma, accounting for approximately 10% of all malignant mesenchymal neoplasms. It is most prevalent between the ages of 15 and 35 years, and the characteristic presentation is that of a painful, palpable soft-tissue mass. Roentgenographically, the synovial sarcoma presents as a soft-tissue mass, with about half the cases demonstrating calcification. There may be local bone changes secondary to a mass effect of an adjacent growing lesion. These malignant lesions recur locally, and spread by both regional lymph node and pulmonary metastic routes. Histologically, the tumor is diagnosed by the identification of a biphasic cell population (Figure 4.12).

Immunocytochemical and immunohistologic staining have demonstrated a mesenchymal tissue in one component and epithelial differentiation in the other. Descriptions in the literature of monophasic variants of synovial sarcoma, with a predominance of one of these two cell types, have raised questions about classification. Prognosis may be related to gross anatomic and histologic findings, with a better prognosis in younger patients with tumors less than 5 cm, tumors located in the lower extremity with an epithelial gland cellularity greater than 50%, and a mitotic activity of less than 15 mitoses/10 high-power field (HPF).[13] A recent multimodality approach involving surgery, radiotherapy, and combined chemotherapy may improve survival in this highly malignant tumor.

Articular Cartilage

Chondromalacia Patella

Chondromalacia patella, although frequently used interchangeably with "anterior knee pain," is a controversial entity from the pathologist's perspective. Autopsy studies have shown chondromalacia to be a common incidental finding occurring in more than 50% of the population at age 30 and almost 100% by age 60.[14]

The gross appearance of chondromalacia and its location have been extensively studied and reported in the literature. Outerbridge felt chondromalacia most frequently started on the medial facet of the patella.[15] His staging system for the gross appearance of chondromalacia at arthrotomy remains useful in the arthroscopic description. Insall et al. mapped the location of chondromalacia in young adults and found the lesions centered primar-

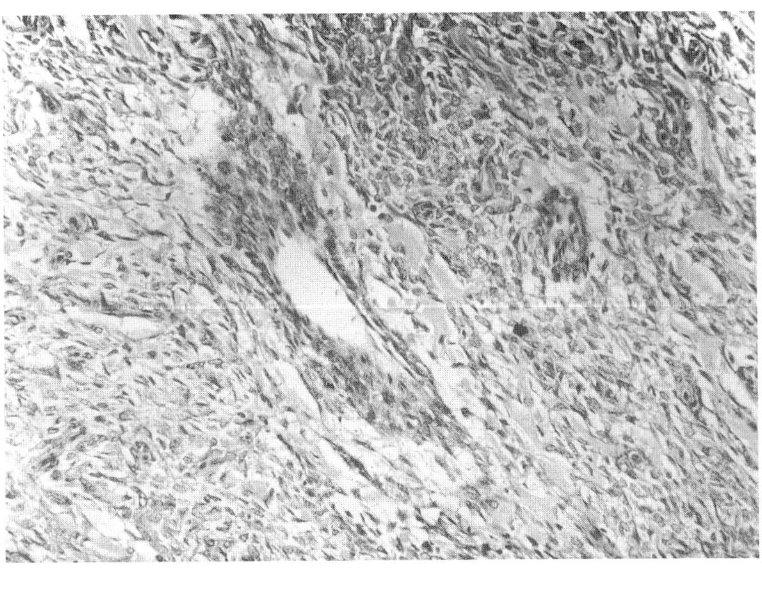

FIGURE 4.12. Synovial sarcoma demonstrating a biphasic pattern: glandular arranged epithelial cells (center) with spindle cell stromal background.

ily around the medial raphe and on the lateral facet.[16] In older patients with osteoarthritis, the lateral facet is almost universally affected.

In a cross-sectional autopsy study, Emery and Meachim reviewed the age distribution and progression of chondromalacia.[17] They felt chondromalacia starts in the periphery of the patella, next affects the medial facet, spreads to the lateral facet, and the lateral facet cartilage erodes to the bone. Eburnation of the lateral facet was common, but rarely was the medial facet eburnated, even in severe cases.

The gross appearance of grade I (closed) chondromalacia ranges from minimal, detectable only by probing, to a "blistered" appearance. The underlying lesion is edema of the cartilage, explaining the "softness" often associated with the lesion. This edematous cartilage is fragile and prone to further damage. Microscopically small fissures extend to the cartilage surface. Edema is apparent and the chondrocytes appear normal. Ultrastructural studies have shown disorganization and later rupture of the collagen network. Biochemically, the edematous cartilage has an increased water content and a decrease in sulfated mucopolysaccharides. Grades II and III chondromalacia show progressive changes, with more and deeper fissures extending to the subchondral bone. The cartilage matrix becomes fragmented. The chondrocytes are affected—becoming both hyperactive and degenerative. Some chondrocytes undergo fibrous differentiation. These changes represent degeneration and necrosis of the cartilage. Grade IV chondromalacia involves extensive cartilage loss and the bony changes of osteoarthritis–subchondral sclerosis and osteophyte formation.

Arthritis: Degenerative Joint Disease versus Rheumatoid Arthritis

Although a broad range of disorders may give rise to arthritis, de novo arthritis may be readily classified into two groups: (1) degenerative joint disease (DJD) (osteoarthritis) and (2) rheumatoid arthritis. They are distinct etiologically, clinically, roentgenographically, and pathologically (macroscopically and microscopically).

Whereas both DJD (osteoarthritis) and rheumatoid arthritis commonly involve the knee, there are significant differences in the primary component of the joint involved. Notwithstanding recent experimental interest in synovial tissue modulation of cartilage destruction by substances such as catabolin (interleukin-1), the synovium in DJD appears to be an innocent bystander, at least initially. The brunt of damage first involves the articular cartilage (fibrillation and eventual denudement) (Figure 4.13) and second involves the bone (subchondral cyst formation and sclerosis with marginal new bone formation or osteophytosis). Although the synovium may show hyperplasia, this is usually minimal and nonspecific. Rarely does inflammation reach the extent seen in rheumatoid arthritis. In acute rheumatoid arthritis the synovium shows the most significant pathology. Infiltrated by lymphocytes and plasma cells, the synoviocytes become hyperplastic and the surface exudes a fibrinous exudate. Changes in the articular cartilage are truly secondary as the pannus, or inflammatory synovium, invades the surface of the joint, causing chondrolysis; eventual cartilage denudement; and, in chronic cases, the appearance of a secondary degenerative phenomenon. However, both chondrolysis and osteoporosis characterize rheumatoid arthritis, thus distinguishing it clearly from degenerative joint disease.

This distinction is evident in laboratory diagnosis and monitoring. The inflammatory changes in rheumatoid arthritis are discernible in elevated sedimentation rates and positive rheumatoid factors (an elevated immunoglobulin protein, usually IgM, circulating in the serum). There is no equivalent useful laboratory monitor for DJD.

Degenerative Joint Disease (Osteoarthritis, DJD)

DJD is classically a painful joint condition initially associated with relief at joint rest and later with pain throughout activity, usually increasing with age and commonly involving the knees, especially in obese persons or those with significant previous traumatic damage.

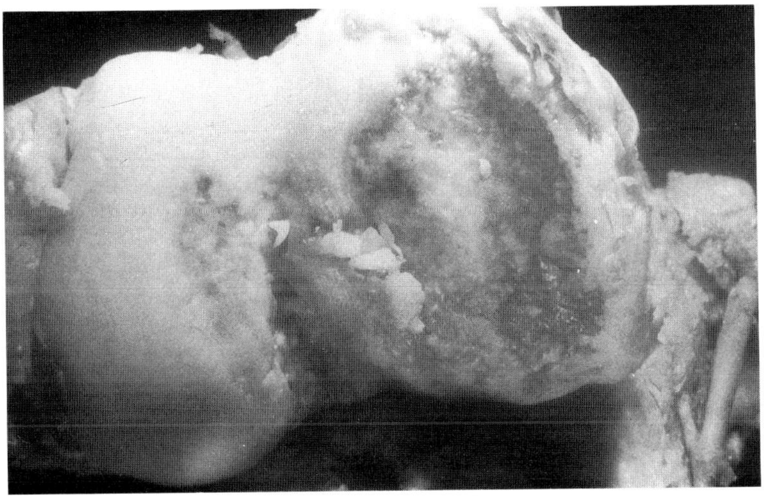

FIGURE 4.13. Fibillated and denuded articular cartilage on a femoral condyle revealing the eburnated hyperemic exposed subchondral bone.

There is no specific laboratory abnormality in DJD. Radiographic changes in the knees initially show joint space narrowing and subchondral sclerosis. Eventually, new bone forms at the margins of articular cartilage (osteophytosis), which may give rise to villous synovial hypertrophy and metaplasia leading to chondro-osseous loose bodies. Loose bodies may arise from either dislodged fragments of cartilage, bone or synovium, or metaplasia of the synovium to cartilage and, often, bone by endochondral ossification. Loose bodies vary considerably in size and shape, and obviously in radiodensity, depending on the degree of calcification and ossification. Variants of DJD include an inflammatory type, characterized by more lymphocytic infiltration and hyperplasia of the synovium, and a rapidly destructive joint process that shows accelerated clinical and roentgenographic joint damage correlated pathologically by extensive cartilage and bone debris throughout the joint.

Rheumatoid Arthritis

Rheumatoid arthritis is classically a chronic, symmetric, persistent arthritis that often affects the knees, and may be associated with systemic symptoms and rheumatoid nodules (classically subcutaneous). Its etiology remains obscure, but laboratory studies and familial history suggest both immunologic and genetic factors in its expression. Most patients with rheumatoid arthritis have a circulating protein in their blood, usually IgM, which is the basis for the *rheumatoid factor test,* a nonspecific but often useful serologic test in corroborating the clinicopathologic diagnosis. Atypical infections may trigger an as yet undetermined genetic predisposition. The presence of rheumatoid factor and elevated sedimentation rates correlate well with the characteristic synovial changes of a hyperemic synovial tissue infiltrated by a pronounced lymphocyte and plasma cell infiltration, often producing a fibrinous exudate (Figure 4.14). The latter proteinaceous exudation may override the articular bone surfaces of the joint, often creating tan friable bodies (rice bodies).

Other disorders have been associated with rheumatoidlike inflammatory joint disease, but these "rheumatoid variants," such as psoriatic arthritis, Reiter's syndrome, and the arthritides associated with colitis, show less inflammatory synovial changes, vary in clinical progression of disease, and usually are not associated with a positive rheumatoid factor.

Bone

Bone tumors are rare, and the patella is an uncommon site for them. Less than 1% of primary bone tumors arise in the patella.[18] Even less common are metastatic tumors of the patella, with only a handful being reported in the

FIGURE 4.14. Rheumatoid synovium becomes hyperplastic and swollen by a lymphocyte and plasma cell infiltration.

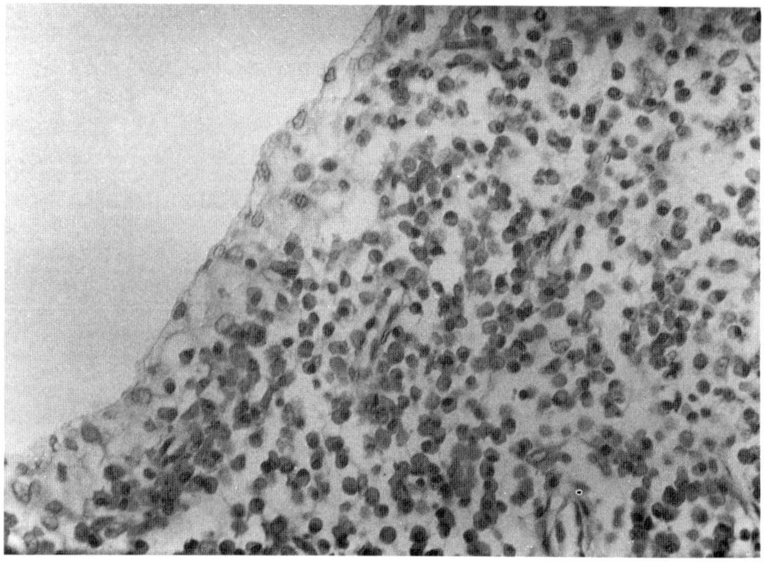

literature.[19] Of the tumors that do arise in the patella, the large majority (90%) are benign. The most common tumors of the patella are chondroblastoma[20] and giant cell tumor.[21] Simple bone cysts are occasionally seen.[22] Other diagnoses are rare. Hemangioma,[23] enchondroma,[24] osteochondroma, intraosseous lipoma, osteoblastoma,[25] aneurysmal bone cyst,[26] and intraosseous ganglia[27] are benign.

Developmental, Hamartomatous, and Tumorlike Lesions

Cystic Lesions of the Knee

The most common cystic-type replacement of bone tissue is that which ensues following the remodeling of bone pursuant to degenerative joint disease or trauma. However, there are two well-defined primary cystic lesions of the skeleton that may involve the patella.

Unicameral Bone Cyst

Unicameral or simple bone cyst is a benign replacement of cancellous bone by a serous fluid, the etiology of which is unknown (Figure 4.15). The lesion occurs most frequently in the proximal femur and the proximal humerus. It has been rarely reported in the patella. More than 80% of unicameral bone cysts present between 5 and 20 years of age, with the male-to-female ratio being about 2.5:1. Simple bone cyst may cause an expansion of the cortex on the roentgenogram because of the remodeling effect of the cortical bone. This may result in fractures, and thus pain, which is not an uncommon presentation of these lesions.

Aneurysmal Bone Cyst

The aneurysmal bone cyst (ABC) is a distinct, benign, pseudotumorous lesion of the bone that is usually differentiated from the simple bone cyst by both its roentgenographic and histopathologic appearances. Its exact cause is not known, but it may be the result of the secondary effects of bone remodeling pursuant to areas of intraosseous vascular disturbances. Twenty-four percent of all ABCs occur at the knee, of which 1% occur in the patella. Classically, the ABC was described as an eccentric, trabeculated lesion in the skeleton, and it may occur at any osseous site. Recent studies have shown that numerous bone lesions may be partly complicated by features of an ABC, and therefore the pathologic diagnosis must be carefully correlated with the roentgenographic

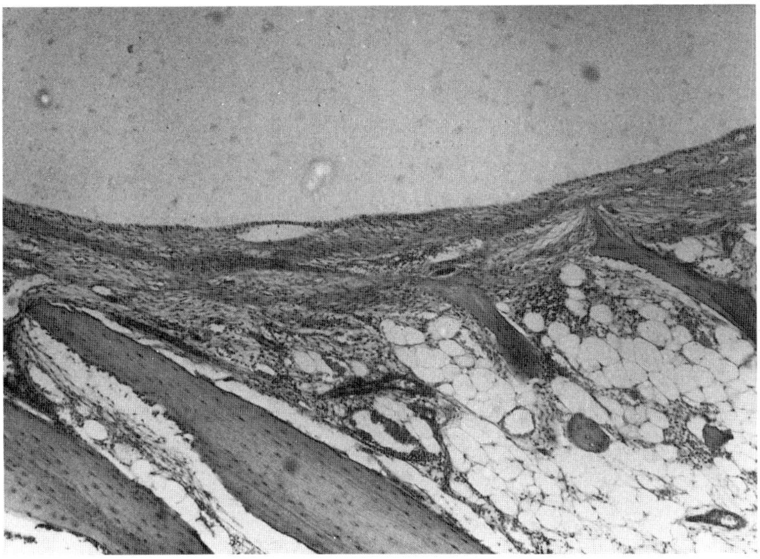

FIGURE 4.15. A fluid-filled cavity lined by a bland fibrous membrane is characteristic of a unicameral bone cyst.

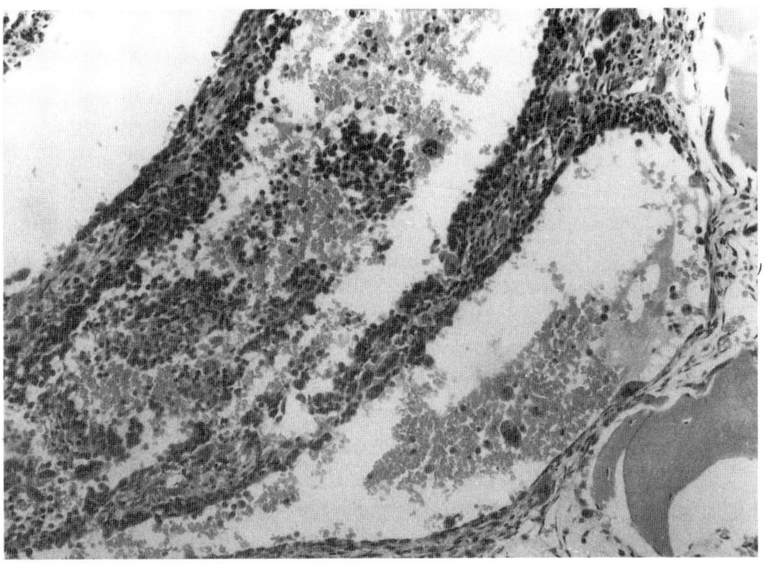

FIGURE 4.16. Sinewy cellular membranes lined by mononuclear cells and giant cells with abundant hemorrhage characterizes the aneurysmal bone cyst (ABC).

appearance to ensure adequate diagnostic accuracy. The peak age of the ABC is between 10 and 20 years, with 75% of cases occurring under 20 years of age. There is a more equal sex distribution to this lesion than that of the simple bone cyst.

Clinically, the most common finding is swelling at the lesion, which may or may not be painful. In a third of the cases, the onset of symptoms may be related to trauma where pathologic fracture may occur. Computed tomography (CT) scanning or magnetic resonance imaging (MRI) may be useful to evaluate the lesions and show mostly a fluid appearance of its contents. Grossly, the periosteum is usually elevated and intact, enveloping a thin rim of reactive bone. The lesion proper may appear bluish because of acute and chronic bleeding, the cavity itself showing hemorrhagic-appearing spongelike cavities filled with blood and other fluid. Although not pulsatile, it is a vascular lesion. Bone tissue

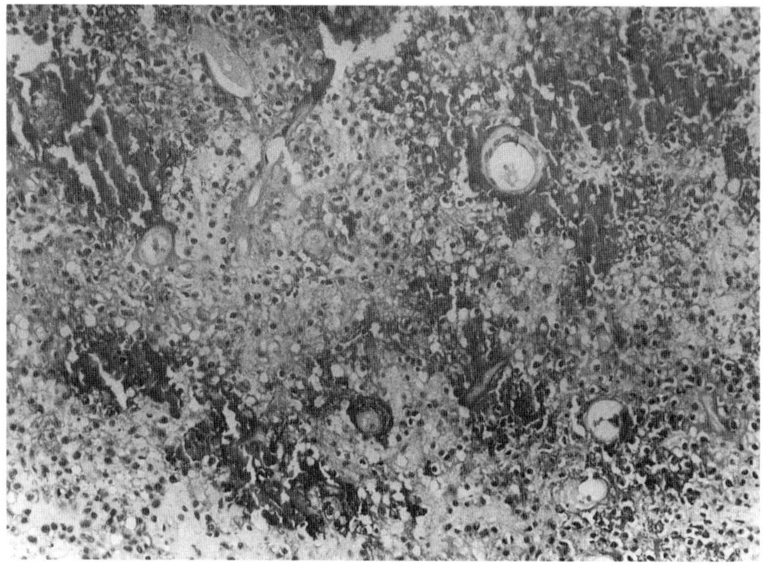

FIGURE 4.17. Cellular chondroblasts merge with zones of calcification, which are often linear and punctate, enveloping individual cells in a chicken-wire pattern.

walls are thin, often with fibrous septa. The tissue itself is histologically different from that of a simple bone cyst, which has a bland membrane as its salient microscopic feature. In an ABC, there is a cellular cavity, often with the membranes filled with giant cells (Figure 4.16). The clinical course is variable but may show progression. Others may spontaneously cease and may slowly ossify, repairing themselves, as is the case with simple bone cysts. The ABCs may recur and, as mentioned, may be a complicating feature to several other neoplasms such as giant cell tumor, chondroblastoma, chondromyxoid fibroma, and other lesions.

Osteochondroma (Exostosis)

Osteochondroma is a benign developmental tumorlike condition that represents an eccentric mass growing away from the joint space, most likely representing the independent growth of the skeleton. These eccentric lesions may be sessile or pedunculated, and usually present as a mass. They may or may not be symptomatic, depending on the pressure effects on the nerves or fracture of the stalk. It is the second most common tumor or tumorlike lesion of the knee, making up approximately 19% of all reported cases, but less than 1% occur in the patella. Osteochondromas peak in the 10- to 18-year-old age range, with growth being greatest during puberty. Osteochondromas usually cease growth after skeletal maturation. Any solitary osteochondroma that continues to grow after skeletal maturation, as well as those changing in size in multiple hereditary exostosis (MHE), should be considered carefully for the diagnosis of chondrosarcomatous transformation. There is a slight male predominance for osteochondroma. The gross pathologic appearance is that of a mature piece of bone capped by a thin cartilaginous cap. Histologically, an examiner sees a band of periosteum covering a proliferating zone of organized columns of chondrocytes that are undergoing endochondral ossification. The cap may be variable in thickness and fragments of the cap may fall off after trauma, developing separate growths similar to osseocartilaginous loose bodies seen in synovial loose bodies.

Benign Tumors

Chondroblastoma

Chondroblastoma characteristically occurs as a slowly growing benign lytic lesion over the epiphysis in a skeletally immature person. Thirty-six percent of all chondroblastomas occur in the knee. It is the 12th most commonly reported primary osseous tumor of the knee, and occurs with almost equal distribution in the proximal tibia (48%) and the distal femur (45%). Five percent of knee chondroblastomas occur in the patella, with the fibula being the least common site (2%). The peak age of occurrence is between 10 and 20 years (85%) with a 1.8:1 male-to-female ratio. The lesion usually presents with pain and may rarely involve the articular cartilage, causing symptoms primarily associated with the joint. A fracture into the chondroblastoma may lead to loose bodies, and may even mimic osteochondritis dissecans roentgenographically and clinically. The origins of chondroblastoma are not known, but ultrastructural studies have suggested that the major cell in this tumor has some similarities to a primitive cartilaginous cell. Histologically, chondroblastoma is characterized by a polygonal cell population with focal areas of calcification noted in approximately 50% of cases, the calcification often appearing in a linear fashion enveloping individual cells (Figure 4.17). The lesion may be cellular and may be confused microscopically with a malignant tumor.

Osteoblastoma

Osteoblastoma is a benign tumor that is characterized histologically by its similarity to osteoid osteoma in which there is abundant osteoblast cellularity with production of osteoid and bone in an irregular organization. Only 10% of reported osteoblastomas occur in the knee, constituting less than 1% of primary bone tumors of the knee (proximal tibia, 64%; distal femur, 22%). The patella accounts for a surprisingly high percentage of knee cases (14%). Approximately 90% of these tumors occur between ages 5 and 30 years, with a 3:1 male predominance. These lesions are usually larger than 2 cm and have a roentgenographic appearance, which may vary from one of pure lysis to one in which there is detectable bone formation.

Giant Cell Tumor

Giant cell tumor, or osteoclastoma, occurs at the end of the bones as a well-circumscribed lytic lesion, usually abutting the articular cartilage. It derives its name from the microscopic appearance in which there is a sea of multinucleated giant cells enmeshed in a noninflammatory mesodermal mononuclear cell matrix of uncertain histogenesis. Although most giant cell tumors are benign, the lesion may metastasize. Giant cell tumors that are fully malignant from the start and act in a sarcomatous fashion are also well documented in the literature. The peak occurrence for giant

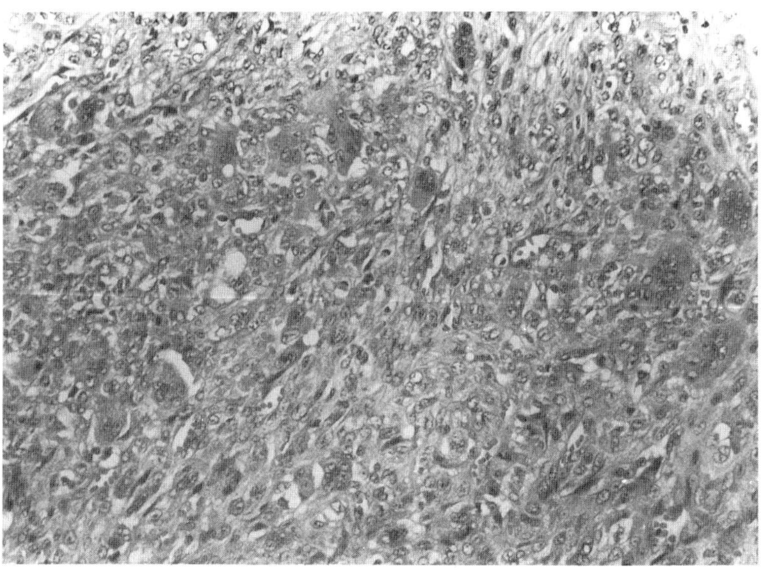

FIGURE 4.18. Giant cell tumor. A sea of mononuclear cells with multinucleated giant cells in a typical admixture.

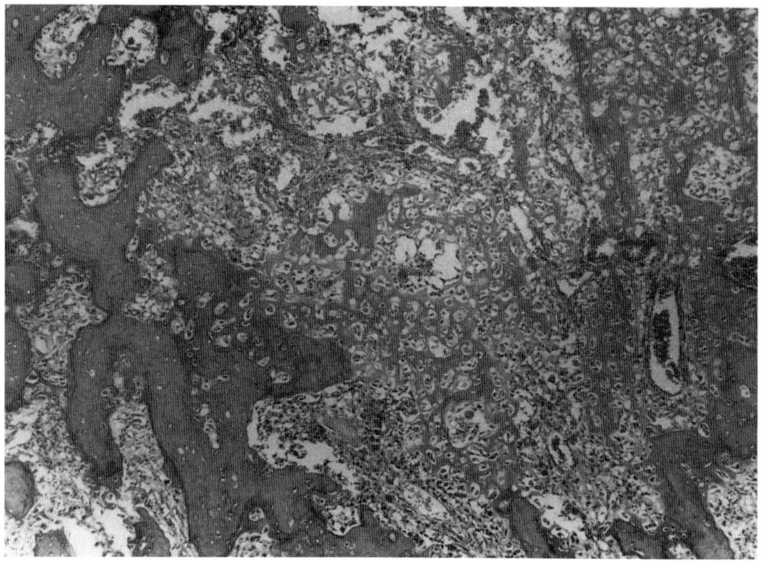

FIGURE 4.19. Osteosarcoma showing malignant cells producing abundant disorganized osteoid and mineralized matrix.

TABLE 4.1. Patella tumors.

Tumor type	No.	Age	Male: female
Benign			
Chondroblastoma	16	23*	13:3
Giant cell	8	26	6:2
Simple bone cyst	6	25	5:1
Hemangioma	3	15	2:1
Osteochondroma	2	46	2:0
Lipoma	2	16*	1:1
Osteoblastoma	1	25	0:1
Malignant			
Lymphoma	3	49*	1:1*
Hemangioendothelioma	1	20	1:0

*Unknown in one patient.
From Kransdorf et al.[18]

cell tumor is in the young adult, with 80% of cases occurring between 20 and 40 years of age. Giant cell tumor is rare prior to puberty. Thus, lytic lesions at the end of the bone prior to skeletal maturation favor the diagnosis of chondroblastoma, and after skeletal maturation, giant cell tumor. There is a slight female predilection in reported cases.

Clinically, the major symptom is pain, usually in the joint, with decreased range of motion often because of effusion or expansion of the bone. Although the tumor abuts the articular cartilage, it rarely extends into the joint space. There may be swelling, and pathologic fracture is not uncommon. Characteristically, there is a well-defined radiolucent mass on the roentgenogram, with well-defined borders. It is usually situated eccentrically at the metaphyseal–epiphyseal areas. Classification of giant cell tumors roentgenographically has been proposed and is reputed to be of prognostic value. In the Enneking staging system, stage I "quiescent" lesions appear small and slowly expand with an intact cortex and well-defined borders. Active lesions (stage II) usually show a thinned or missing cortex, but have an intact periosteum. Borders are less clear. This is the most common form encountered. In stage III, or the aggressive giant cell tumor, the cortex is destroyed. The tumor is not confined by the periosteum. Here a large expansive lesion, possibly extending to the articular cartilage, suggests rapid growth.

Grossly, giant cell tumors appear usually as solid lesions with a light brown to red color, uniform, without bone or calcification. There may be associated hyperemia and significant bleeding at incision. Histologically, the characteristic uniform and even distribution of giant cells is diagnostic (Figure 4.18). Histologic study alone and even flow cytometry studies of the DNA content of the nuclei of cells from giant cell tumors are unable to predict which of these lesions metastasize.

The clinical course of giant cell tumors is highly variable, ranging from local growth over years, to more rapid invasion in brief periods of time. Although malignant transformation has been reputed in 5% of cases, one cannot exclude that these malignant giant cell tumors are not sarcomas from the beginning. Malignant giant cell tumors may have fibrosarcomatous, malignant fibrous histiocytomatous, or osteosarcomatous areas, raising the possibility of initial diagnostic accuracy. Radiation treatment is contraindicated because of the potential for sarcomatous stimulation. Local recurrence has been reported in less than 10% with appropriate surgical treatment, and usually occurs within three years of surgery. Patients with pulmonary metastases may survive with the appropriate treatment.

Malignant tumors of the patella are extremely rare. Osteosarcoma[28] (Figure 4.19), lymphomas, hemangioendothelioma, and malignant fibrous histiocytoma have all been reported. Metastases are also extremely uncommon in the patella, even in disseminated metastatic disease[19,29] (Table 4.1).

Acknowledgements The authors wish to acknowledge the assistance of Rose Bracero in preparing the manuscript.

References

1. Hasselbacher P: Structure of the synovial membrane. *Clin Rheumatol Dis* 1981;7(1):57–69.
2. Vernon-Roberts B: Structure and function of joints, in Currey HLF (ed.): *Mason and Currey's Clinical Rheumatology*. ed. 4. Edinburgh, Churchill Livingstone, 1986, pp. 1–15.
3. France MP, Gupta SK: Nonhemophilic hemosiderotic synovitis of the shoulder. A case report. *Clin Orthop* 1991;262:132–136.
4. Arnold WD, Hilgartner MW: Hemophilic arthropathy: Current concepts of pathogenesis and management. *J Bone Joint Surg Am* 1977;59A: 287–305.
5. Walot I, Staple T: Case report 539. *Skeletal Radiol* 1989;18:233–236.
6. Markel SF, Hart WR: Arthropathy in calcium pyrophosphate dihydrate crystal deposition disease. *Arch Pathol Lab Med* 1982;106:529–533.
7. Olson EJ, Kang JD, Fu FH, et al.: The biochemical and histological effects of artificial ligament wear particles: In vitro and in vivo studies. *Am J Sports Med* 1988;16(6):558–569.
8. Johnson DP, Eastwood DM, Witherow PJ: Symptomatic synovial plicae of the knee. *J Bone Joint Surg Am* 1993;75A(10):1485–1496.
9. Martinez D, Millner PA, Coral A, et al.: Case report 745. *Skeletal Radiol* 1992;21:393–395.
10. Milgram JW. Synovial osteochondromatosis: A histopathologic study of 30 cases. *J Bone Joint Surg Am* 1977;59A:792–801.
11. Rao AS, Vigorita VJ: Pigmented villonodular synovitis (giant cell tumor of the tendon sheath and synovial membrane). *J Bone Joint Surg Am* 1984;66A:76–94.
12. Wright PH, Sim FH, Soulc EH, ct al.: Synovial sarcoma. *J Bone Joint Surg Am* 1982;64A:112–122.
13. Rooser B, Willen H, Hugoson A, et al.: Prognostic factors in synovial sarcoma. *Cancer* 1989;63:2182–2185.
14. Owre A. Chondromalacia patellae. *Acta Chir Scand* 1936;77(suppl. 41):1–156.
15. Outerbridge RE. Further studies on the etiology of chondromalacia patellae. *J Bone Joint Surg Br* 1964;46B:179–190.
16. Insall J, Falvo KA, Wise DW: Chondromalacia patellae: A prospective study. *J Bone Joint Surg Am* 1976;58A:1–8.
17. Emery IH, Meachim G: Surface morphology and topography of patellofemoral cartilage fibrillation in Liverpool necropsies. *J Anat* 1973; 116(1):103–120.
18. Kransdorf MJ, Moser RP, Vinh, TN, et al.: Primary tumors of the patella. A review of 42 cases. *Skeletal Radiol* 1989;18:365–371.
19. Stoler B, Staple TW: Metastases to the patella. *Radiology* 1969;93:853–856.
20. Bloem JL, Mulder JD: Chondroblastoma: A clinical and radiological study of 104 cases. *Skeletal Radiol* 1985;14:1–9.
21. Kelikian H, Clayton I. Giant cell tumor of the patella. *J Bone Joint Surg Am* 1957;39A:414–420.
22. Schultz E, Greenspan A: Case report 378. *Skeletal Radiol* 1986;15:405–407.
23. Bansal VP, Singh R, Grewal DS, et al.: Haemangioma of the patella: A report of two cases. *J Bone Joint Surg Br* 1974;56B:139–141.
24. Lammot TR. Enchondroma of the patella. *J Bone Joint Surg Am* 1968;50A:1230–1232.
25. De Coster E, Van Tiggelen R, Shahabpour M, et al.: Osteoblastoma of the patella. Case report and review of the literature. *Clin Orthop* 1989; 243:216–219.
26. Faris WF, Rubin BD, Fielding JW. Aneurys-

mal bone cyst of the patella: A case report. *J Bone Joint Surg Am* 1978;60A:711.
27. Carter TE, Detenbect LC. Intraosseous ganglion cyst of the patella: Report of a case. *Tex Med* 1974;70(4):95–96.
28. Goodwin MA. Primary osteosarcoma of the patella. *J Bone Joint Surg Br* 1961;43B:338–341.
29. Ashby MR, Dappen N. Esophageal carcinoma metastatic to the patella: A case report. *JAMA* 1976;235:2519–2520.

5

Physical Examination of the Patellofemoral Joint

Jeffrey H. Yormak and Giles R. Scuderi

Disorders of the patellofemoral joint have often posed a diagnostic dilemma for the treating physician. Typically, patients with patellofemoral disorders present with anterior knee pain, but these patients also often complain of aching pain medially as well as posteriorly. The pain can be aggravated by prolonged sitting with the knee in a flexed position (*movie sign*), stair climbing, or a sudden change in activity level. The nature of these symptoms as well as others such as catching, locking, or giving way are nonspecific and often lead to difficulty differentiating patellofemoral disorders from other internal derangements of the knee. Careful attention to detail during the history and physical examination will normally allow the examiner to isolate the patellofemoral joint as the source of the problem. It is important to also recognize that the patellofemoral joint can be affected by local as well as remote conditions.[1] Common local conditions about the knee include such entities as bursitis, tendonitis, torn menisci, ligamentous instability, or degenerative joint disease. Remote conditions such as femoral anteversion and body habitus can alter the biomechanics of the patellofemoral joint as well and present as anterior knee pain (Table 5.1).

TABLE 5.1. Causes of patellofemoral pain.

Local	Acute trauma
	Repetitive trauma/overuse syndrome
	Posttraumatic sequelae
	Patellofemoral dysplasia
	Osteochondritis dissecans
	Synovial plica
Distant	Increased Q angle
	Gynecoid pelvis
	Femoral anteversion
	Genu valgum
	Genu varum
	Genu recurvatum
	Tibia vara
	External tibial torsion
	Pronated forefoot
Systemic	Congenital hyperlaxity
	Obesity

Although careful examination of the lower extremity, including limb alignment, patellofemoral soft-tissue support, and patellofemoral morphology, enables the examining physician to identify the etiology of the patellofemoral disorder, a comprehensive evaluation system relating diagnosis and treatment has not yet been developed. To date, the Merchant classification system is the most comprehensive.[2] This system defines the etiology and pathomechanics of patellofemoral disorders, and categorizes the diagnoses such that treatment plans may be initiated (Table 5.2). Section I of this classification categorizes traumatic conditions and the late effects of trauma on the otherwise normal knee. Section II classifies patellar instability, while section III includes chondromalacia patella for which no underlying etiology has been defined. Sections IV and V include osteochondritis dissecans and synovial plicae, respectively. The most recent classification includes a new section—iatrogenic disorders. A pitfall of the

Merchant classification is that it inadequately represents conditions affecting the pediatric knee, especially congenital disorders.

Although a comprehensive classification system does not yet exist, the concept of relating specific physical findings to diagnosis and treatment is vital. The purpose of this chapter is to describe the details of performing an examination of the patellofemoral joint. The physical examination provides the groundwork from which the diagnosis is made and treatment is initiated.

Standing Examination

For the physical examination to be properly performed, the patient should be wearing shorts throughout the examination so that both the involved and contralateral limb can be fully inspected. Examination takes place in the standing, sitting, supine, and prone positions, and begins with observation of the standing patient. Substantial information can be gained from this portion of the examination and should be performed carefully. During

TABLE 5.2. The Merchant classification system of patellofemoral disorders.*

I. Trauma (conditions caused by trauma in the otherwise normal knee)
   A. Acute trauma
      1. Contusion (924.11)
      2. Fracture
         a. Patella (822)
         b. Femoral trochlea (821.2)
         c. Proximal tibial epiphysis (tubercle) (823.0)
      3. Dislocation (rare in the normal knee) (836.3)
      4. Rupture
         a. Quadriceps tendon (843.8)
         b. Patellar tendon (844.8)
   B. Repetitive trauma (overuse syndromes)
      1. Patellar tendinitis ("jumper's knee") (726.64)
      2. Quadriceps tendinitis (726.69)
      3. Peripatellar tendinitis (e.g., anterior knee pain of the adolescent caused by hamstring contracture) (726.699)
      4. Prepatellar bursitis ("housemaid's knee") (726.65)
      5. Apophysitis
         a. Osgood–Schlatter disease (732.43)
         b. Sinding–Larsen–Johansson disease (732.422)
   C. Late effects of trauma (905)
      1. Posttraumatic chondromalacia patellae
      2. Posttraumatic patellofemoral arthritis
      3. Anterior fat pad syndrome (posttraumatic fibrosis)
      4. Reflex sympathetic dystrophy of the patella
      5. Patellar osseous dystrophy
      6. Acquired patella infera (718.366)
      7. Acquired quadriceps fibrosis

II. Patellofemoral dysplasia
   A. Lateral patellar compression syndrome (LPCS) (718.365)
      1. Secondary chondromalacia patellae (717.7)
      2. Secondary patellofemoral arthritis (715.289)
   B. Chronic subluxation of the patella (CSP) (718.364)
      1. Secondary chondromalacia patellae (717.7)
      2. Secondary patellofemoral arthritis (715.289)
   C. Recurrent dislocation of the patella (RDP) (718.361)
      1. Associated fractures (822)
         a. Osteochondral (intra-articular)
         b. Avulsion (extra-articular)
      2. Secondary chondromalacia patellae (717.7)
      3. Secondary patellofemoral arthritis (715.289)
   D. Chronic dislocation of the patella (718.362)
      1. Developmental
      2. Acquired

III. Idiopathic chondromalacia patellae (717.7)

IV. Osteochondritis dissecans
   A. Patella (732.704)
   B. Femoral trochlea (732.703)

V. Synovial plicae (727.8916) (anatomic variants made symptomatic by acute or repetitive trauma)
   A. Pathologic medial patellar plica ("shelf") (727.89161)
   B. Pathologic suprapatellar plica (727.89163)
   C. Pathologic lateral patellar plica (727.89165)

VI. Iatrogenic disorders
   A. Iatrogenic medial patellar compression syndrome
   B. Iatrogenic chronic medial subluxation of the patella
   C. Iatrogenic patella infera (718.366)

*Orthopaedic ICD-9-CM Expanded Diagnostic Codes in parentheses.
From: Merchant AC. Clinical classification of patellofemoral disorders. Sports Med and Arthroscopy Rev (Raven Press). Vol. 2, No. 3, Aug 1994. Reprinted with permission.

this portion of the examination the standing axial alignment should be noted since any bony anomalies of the pelvis, femora, tibia, or feet can alter the biomechanics of the knee with resultant patellofemoral pain. With the patient standing, evaluate the pelvic geometry. Women tend to have a broad based or *gynecoid pelvis* that exaggerates the *quadriceps (Q) angle,* resulting in a valgus force on the patella. This type of pelvis is frequently found in patients with symptoms related to maltracking. A flexed pelvis can also be observed and may be the result of a structural anomaly or the result of a tight quadriceps musculature with an associated hip flexion contracture.

Moving distally, the next area of interest is the proximal femur. Variation in this area cannot be directly appreciated but can be inferred from the position of the patellae. Usually, with the feet in a neutral position, the patellae point straight ahead. *Femoral anteversion* or internal rotation contractures of the hip will lead to increased internal rotation of the femur. This, in turn, can result in an inward pointing of the patellae described as the "*squinting patellae*"[3] (Figure 5.1). The accuracy of this finding is predicated on the feet pointing straight ahead and no rotational malalignment of the lower leg existing. Femoral anteversion can also be reconfirmed when the hip range of motion is assessed during the prone examination.

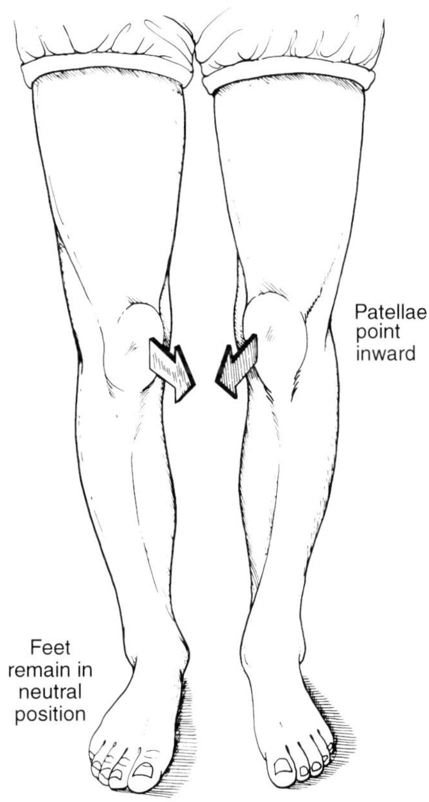

FIGURE 5.1. Squinting patellae. Rotational malalignment of the limb leads to an increased Q angle.

Continuing distally, the alignment of the knee is observed and any abnormalities such as *genu varum* or *genu valgum* are recorded. Both genu varum and genu valgum alter the alignment of the patellofemoral joint. More often, patients with genu valgum have patellofemoral symptoms than those with genu varum. In the genu valgum population, both subluxation and the lateral patella compression syndrome are common. *Genu recurvatum* may be found as well and may be unilateral or bilateral. Therefore, it is important to compare the involved knee with the contralateral limb. Genu recurvatum may be secondary to generalized ligamentous laxity, or possibly to an anterior cruciate or a posterior cruciate ligament injury. With ligamentous laxity, both knees hyperextend equally, whereas in a cruciate injury, side-to-side differences may be observed. Another observation is a *flexion contracture,* which is often missed or forgotten in the evaluation of patellofemoral pain but can be significant. A flexion contracture may result from an untreated, displaced bucket-handle meniscal tear, a contusion, or simply hamstring tightness.

The next area of interest is tibial rotation, which can be evaluated by noting the rotation of the foot as compared with the patella. If the foot is excessively externally rotated, *external tibial torsion* may be present. Diagnosing external tibial torsion raises the possibility of an increased quadriceps angle and an increased lateral displacement vector on the patella. Both subluxation and the lateral patella compression syndrome are diagnoses to consider in this scenario. Internal tibial torsion can also be seen but is not generally associated with patellofemoral disorders.

Finally, look at the patient's feet and ankles. There are two findings here that can be of significance. The first is *hindfoot valgus* with or without pes planus. This may be secondary to malunion of a calcaneus fracture, a ruptured tibialis posterior tendon, ligamentous laxity, or many other conditions. The important point in this scenario is that hindfoot valgus places a valgus force on the knee with gradual elongation of the medial collateral ligament and subsequent valgus position of the knee in stance. This situation is associated with an increased Q angle and may therefore contribute to patellofemoral complaints. The second finding to look for is an *equinous deformity* or tight heel cord, because a small equinous deformity can cause anterior knee pain. The reason for this is that during stance the foot is unable to dorsiflex normally and the knee subsequently compensates by hyperextending.

Following the previously mentioned observations, the patient is asked to perform a half-squat and hold the position for several seconds, or for as long as possible. This test is nonspecific in nature but will re-create anterior knee symptoms in patients suffering from patellofemoral disorders. The *half-squat test* thus simply serves to confirm that the patient is indeed complaining of patellofemoral pain. It does not in any way define the etiology of the pain.

Evaluation of gait is also important. The patient walks up and down the hallway and any abnormalities are noted. Alterations in gait can cause abnormal forces about the knee and can contribute to anterior knee pain. Leg length inequalities can also be observed at this time.

Seated Examination

With the patient seated, both limbs should dangle loosely over the edge of the examination table. The outline of the individual quadriceps and adductor muscle groups can be easily distinguished. Thigh muscle girth should be measured and evaluated for symmetry. This measurement is made at a consistent reference point above the patella for later comparison. Normally, the vastus medialis inserts on the superomedial one third to one half of the patella, where a slight bulge of the muscle can be observed (Figure 5.2). Quadriceps musculature is more prominent on isometric contraction and normally the vastus medialis extends further distally than the vastus lateralis.[3] Atrophy of the vastus medialis, as evidenced by flattening of the muscle in this region, will contribute in a significant way to patellofemoral symptoms. Also, an abnormally high insertion of the vastus muscle into the top one fourth to one third of the patella is indicative of abnormal muscular development and a possible malalignment related disorder.

While in the seated position, normal patellae will point straight out at the examiner. In *patella alta,* the patellae will actually point upward toward the ceiling (Figure 5.3). The

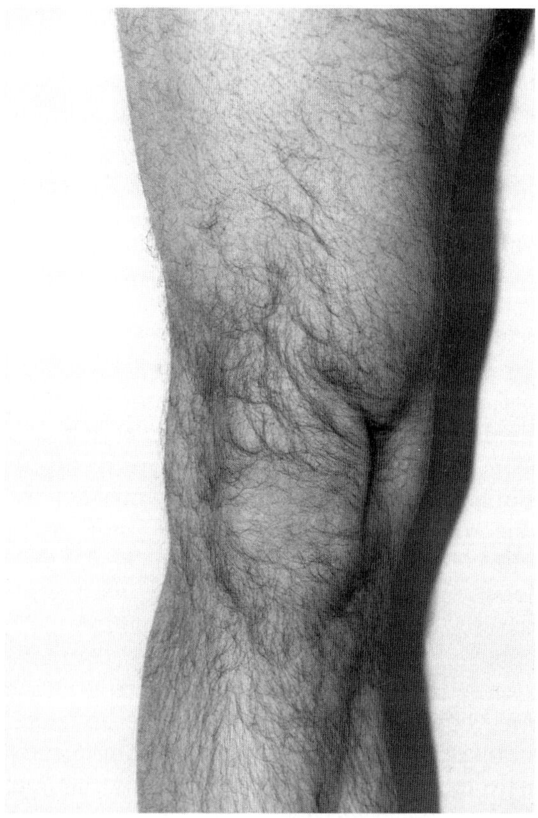

FIGURE 5.2. Quadricep anatomy. Vastus medialis inserts on top one-third to one-half of the patella. The vastus lateralis inserts distal to the vastus medialis.

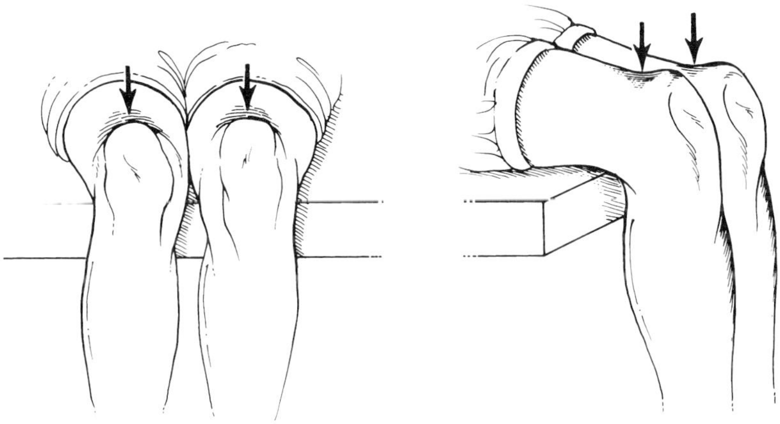

FIGURE 5.3. Patella alta. Patellofemoral instability is often associated with patella alta.

"*camel back*"[4] sign is a prominence of the infrapatellar fat pad also seen with patella alta (Figure 5.4). Several studies have shown a significant relationship between patella alta and patellofemoral symptoms, in particular, instability.[2] One might also note "*grasshopper eyes,*"[4] a situation in which the patellae are both proximally displaced as well as externally (laterally) rotated (Figure 5.5). Grasshopper eyes are consistent with patella alta and lateral patella tilt. The remainder of the examination will serve to confirm these findings and correlate them with the patient's historic complaints.

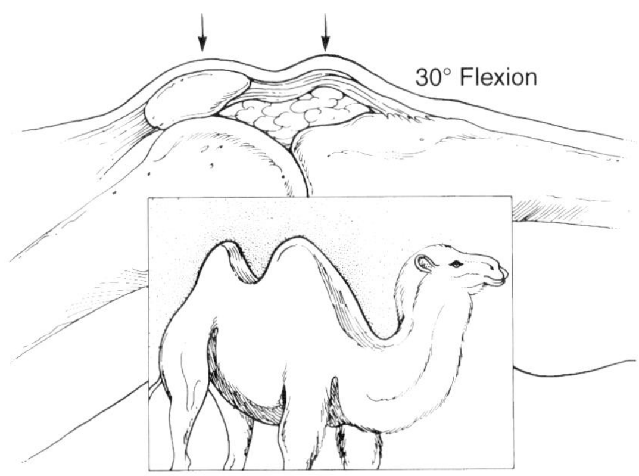

FIGURE 5.4. Camelback sign. Prominence of the infrapatellar fat pad is often associated with patella alta.

While viewing the patella, notice the skin depressions both medial and lateral to the inferior pole of the patella (Figure 5.6). When an effusion is present, these depressions are not visible. This finding is helpful in distinguishing intra-articular disorders, such as a tear of the anterior cruciate ligament, from patellar instability, where more commonly, retinacular soft-tissue swelling is present. Also, while at this level, the examiner may notice a lesion at the joint line such as a meniscal cyst, again indicative of intra-articular pathology. Finally, the examiner may notice swelling directly over the patellar tendon itself, consistent with patella tendinitis or prepatella bursitis.

In the region of the tibial tubercle, an abnormally large prominence may be observed, which is usually indicative of *Osgood–Schlatter disease* (Figure 5.7). This finding can more easily be seen from the side and, as always, comparison with the opposite side is vital. A second area to notice is just medial to the tibial tubercle in the region of the pes anserinus insertion. Swelling, usually subtle in nature, can be seen here and is consistent with *pes anserinus bursitis.* These observations, along with others mentioned previously, define specific pathologic entities that have a known cause, predictable course of development, and known treatment regimen.

Supine Examination

Many of the observations from the standing and seated portion of the examination are

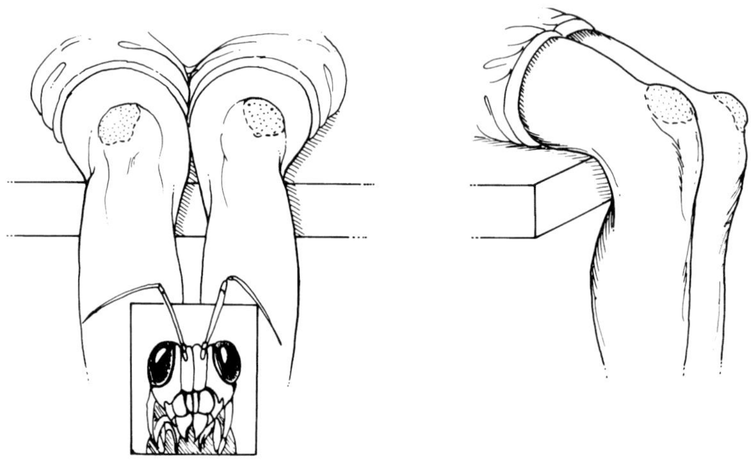

FIGURE 5.5. Grasshopper eyes. Proximal and lateral facing position of the patella associated with patella alta and lateral tilt.

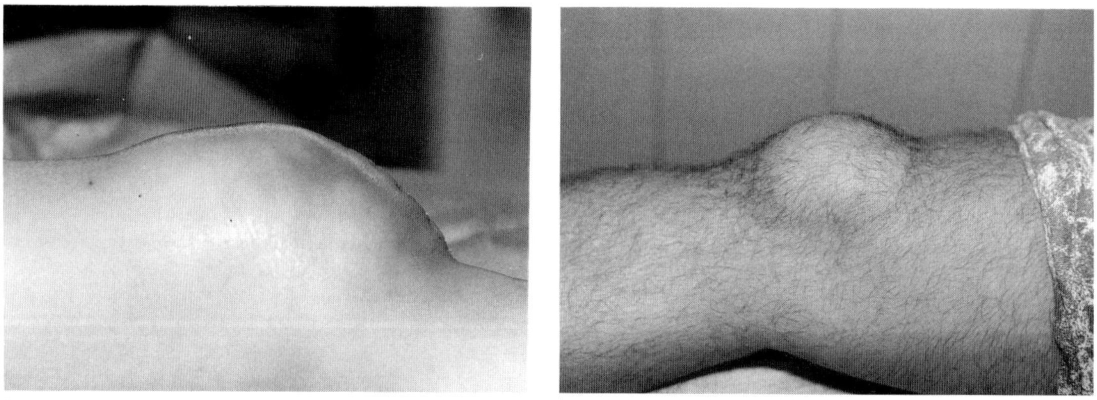

a b

FIGURE 5.6. (a) Diffuse swelling consistent with an intra-articular effusion. (b) Localized swelling with a prepatellar bursitis.

quickly reassessed with the patient supine on the examination table. The *Q angle,* as described by Brattstrom,[5] indicating the relative medial or lateral insertion of the quadriceps mechanism is then measured. This is accomplished by drawing an imaginary line connecting the center of the patella and the anterior–superior iliac spine, marking the line of pull of the quadriceps tendon. A second line is drawn from the center of the patella to the center of the tibial tubercle, marking the line of pull of the patellar tendon. The intersection of these two imaginary lines forms the Q angle (Figure 5.8). In females, the normal Q angle is from 10° to 20°; while in males, the Q angle should normally be from 8° to 10°.[6] Aglietti et al. reported a Q angle of 17° in females and 14° in males, with both sexes having an SD of 3°.[7] Insall considers 14° as normal and above 20° as abnormal.[7] Hughston believes that a Q angle greater than 10° is abnormal and should be corrected.[4] An increased Q angle is not a reliable indicator of patellar malalignment, but it can be found in patients with femoral anteversion, external tibial torsion, and genu valgum.

The Q angle is a reflection of the valgus vector acting on the patella by contraction of the quadriceps. The Q angle is greatest at full extension because of the "screw home" mechanism. This mechanism is characterized by the tibial tubercle moving laterally with ex-

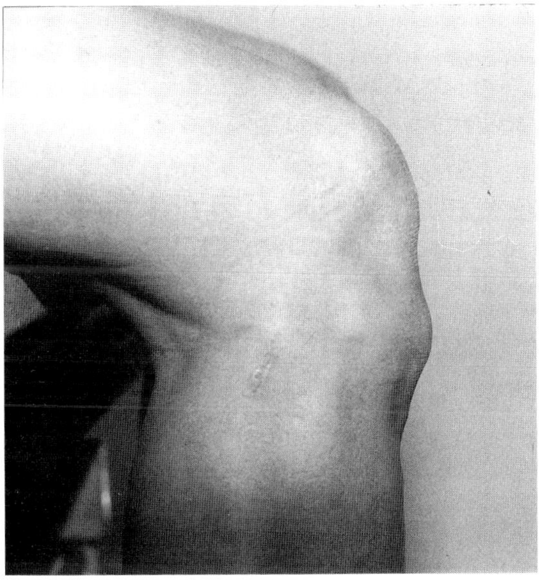

FIGURE 5.7. Osgood–Schlatter disease. A local cause of anterior knee pain.

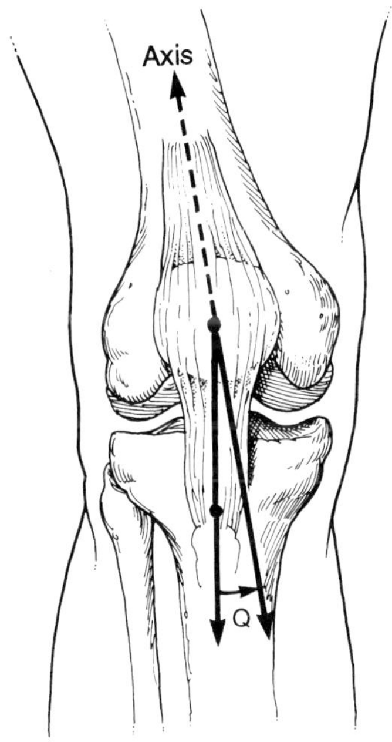

FIGURE 5.8. The Q angle. An assessment of the line of pull of the quadriceps mechanism.

ternal tibial rotation during terminal knee extension. Therefore, as the knee flexes, the Q angle should decrease. At 90° of flexion, the tibial tubercle is directly inferior to the distal pole of the patella. Failure of the tuberosity to rotate directly inferior to the patella suggests lateral placement of the tibial tuberosity.

The Q angle can also be measured with the knee flexed 90°, which Kolowich et al. describes as the *tubercle–sulcus angle (TSA)*. This measurement is defined by a line from the center of the patella to the tibial tubercle and the angle formed with a line perpendicular to the transepicondylar axis passing through the center of the patella (Figure 5.9). A normal TSA is 0°, whereas greater than 10° is considered abnormal.[8] The benefit of this measurement is that the patella is engaged in the sulcus and any rotational anomalies can be observed.

Careful palpation of the peripatellar soft tissue helps delineate areas of tenderness, thickening, or defects. This should include all structures about the knee. Commonly, the patellar tendon or quadriceps tendon may be painful and inflamed. Thickening consistent with an old partially healed quadriceps tendon rupture presenting with extensor lag and patellofem-

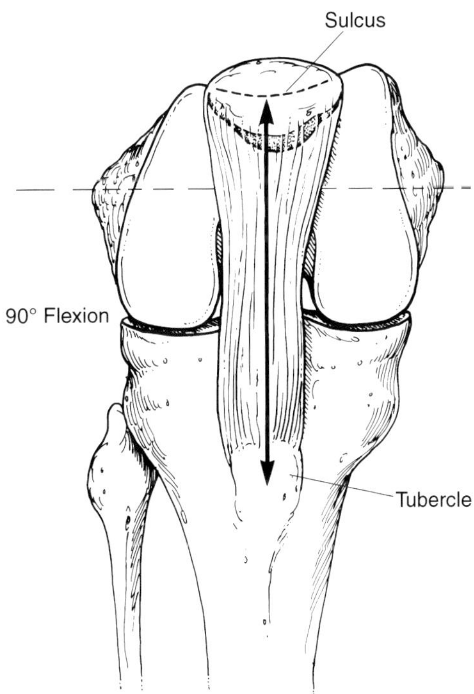

FIGURE 5.9. Tubercle–sulcus angle. An assessment of the line of pull of the quadriceps mechanism with the patella located in the femoral sulcus at 90°.

oral symptoms, or even patellar tenderness from an occult fracture may be differentiated. Palpation continues distally to the tibial tubercle for evidence of tenderness and prominence consistent with Osgood–Schlatter disease, and then medially seeking evidence of pes anserinus bursitis. Of course, these diagnoses normally occur in different age populations, but it is important to be specific when examining a patient so that the exact symptomatic site is noted. Palpate the lateral retinaculum for tenderness, defects, or thickening. Slowly move around posteriorly, palpating the lateral femoral epicondyle, lateral joint line, lateral collateral ligament, and fibular head. Tenderness or change of contour in any of these areas will require further investigation. Possible findings in this portion of the examination include plica, retinacular defect, lateral meniscal tear, or lateral collateral ligament tear. Continuing posteriorly, the popliteal fossa is palpated for hamstring tightness, evidence of Baker's cyst or other mass, and for the presence and quality of a popliteal pulse. Further definition of any posterior abnormalities can be accomplished during the prone portion of the examination. Palpation on the medial aspect of the knee continues in a like fashion and, as with the lateral side, it is important to distinguish distinct areas of tenderness such as retinacular tenderness from joint line tenderness. Defects in the medial retinaculum may also be palpated, especially following acute dislocations (Figure 5.10). These distinctions are sometimes difficult and cannot always be made; however, with time and practice, clinical specificity can improve significantly.

Several tests can be performed to evaluate the static and dynamic forces acting on the patella. First, dynamic evaluation of the patellofemoral joint can be accomplished by assessing active flexion and extension of the knee. Normally, the patella engages the femoral sulcus at 30° to 40° of flexion.[3] At terminal extension, the patella may be observed to sublux laterally out of the femoral sulcus. As the knee resumes flexion, the patella may be noted to jump back into place, indicating a laterally tracking patella. Lateral deviation of the patella in terminal extension has been characterized as the "*J sign*" (Figure 5.11).

The *active quadriceps pull test,*[8] a dynamic evaluation, has been described to actively assess quadriceps activity as well (Figure 5.12). With the knee extended, the quadriceps is contracted and the patella movement is observed. Normally, the patella should be pulled superiorly in a straight line. When the pull is excessive in a lateral direction, the test is considered to be abnormal with an overpull of the vastus lateralis.

The *patellofemoral grind test,*[3] a static examination, is performed next. With the patient supine and the examiner gently compressing the patella in the femoral sulcus, the patient is instructed to contract the quadriceps. The test is positive if the patient complains of pain or discomfort. Pain on compression of the patellofemoral joint is indicative of articular injury and when coupled with crepitus and recurrent effusion, is suggestive of degenerative changes. It is important to differentiate the pain of degenerative changes from that of other sources. At this point, with the patient still supine and the knee extended, palpation of the medial and the lateral facets of the patella can determine specific areas of tenderness. At the same time, the examiner can palpate the femoral condyles for tenderness or osteochondral defects. Care should be taken to differentiate patellofemoral pain from that of impinging synovium or painful retinaculum. Tenderness in the lateral retinaculum may be the result of recurrent stretching or retinacular nerve injury.

The patella *apprehension test* of Fairbanks,[9] indicative of instability, is next performed while the relaxed patient lays supine with the knee flexed to 20° (Figure 5.13). This can easily be done by having the patient cross the affected leg over the contralateral limb. A laterally directed force is applied to the medial border of the patella. As the patella moves laterally, the patient fears a dislocation and resists further displacement by contraction of the quadriceps and extension of the knee. This test is often considered pathognomonic for patella instability.

The *Sage sign,*[10] another static test of pa-

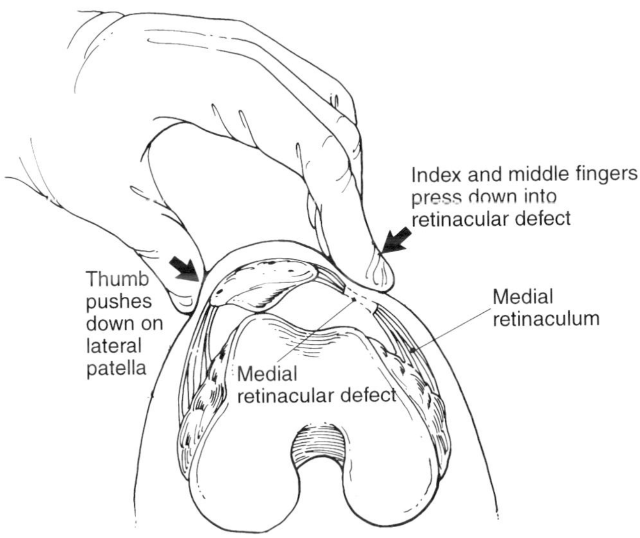

FIGURE 5.10. Palpation of the medial retinacular defect.

tellofemoral disorders, is indicative of a tight lateral retinaculum. This test is done with the patient in the supine position and the relaxed knee flexed to 20°. The examiner attempts to displace the patella medially; medial patella excursion of less than one quarter of the greatest patella width is considered a positive Sage sign. Quantitatively, 10 mm of medial displacement is considered normal, whereas 5 mm or less is considered abnormal and consistent with a tight lateral retinaculum.

Kolowich et al. have described the *passive patella glide test,*[8] a further extension of the Sage sign, which is indicative of the tension of both the medial and lateral retinacular structures. With the quadriceps relaxed, the patella is displaced medially or laterally while the knee is supported in 20° to 30° of flexion (Figure 5.14). Considering the patella as four longitudinal quadrants, a lateral glide of three or more quadrants is indicative of an incompetent medial retinaculum. A medial glide of one quadrant or less is consistent with a tight lateral retinaculum, similar to a positive Sage sign. When the patella displaces medially three or more quadrants, a hypermobile patella is diagnosed.

The *passive patella tilt test*[8] is another test that evaluates the tightness of the lateral retinaculum (Figure 5.15). With the patient supine, the knee fully extended, and the quadriceps fully relaxed, the examiner gently lifts the lateral edge of the patella away from the lateral femoral condyle. A neutral tilt angle is one in which the axis is parallel to the floor. A negative tilt is when the lateral edge of the patella is below the horizontal. A neutral or negative tilt angle is consistent with an excessively tight lateral retinaculum. The degree of passive patella tilt should always be compared with the asymptomatic side.

In addition to glide and tilt, a *rotational malalignment* of the patella may also exist. This is determined by assessing the position of the inferior pole of the patella in relationship to the superior pole. The most common finding is external rotation of the patella, which is seen when the inferior pole is lateral to the superior pole. Patellar displacement may also have an *anteroposterior* component. If the inferior pole is posterior to the superior pole, an inferior tilt is present. The opposite relationship, a superior tilt, is rarely found.

Patellofemoral mechanics can also be altered by a tight iliotibial band (ITB). Normally, the ITB is drawn posteriorly with flexion. An abnormally tight retinaculum between the patella and the ITB will draw the patella into a laterally tilted position, and will compress the lateral facet. The *Ober's test*[11] is used to evaluate contracture of the ITB. To perform Ober's test, the patient is turned onto the side with the affected limb uppermost. With the hip in neutral flexion/extension, the limb is

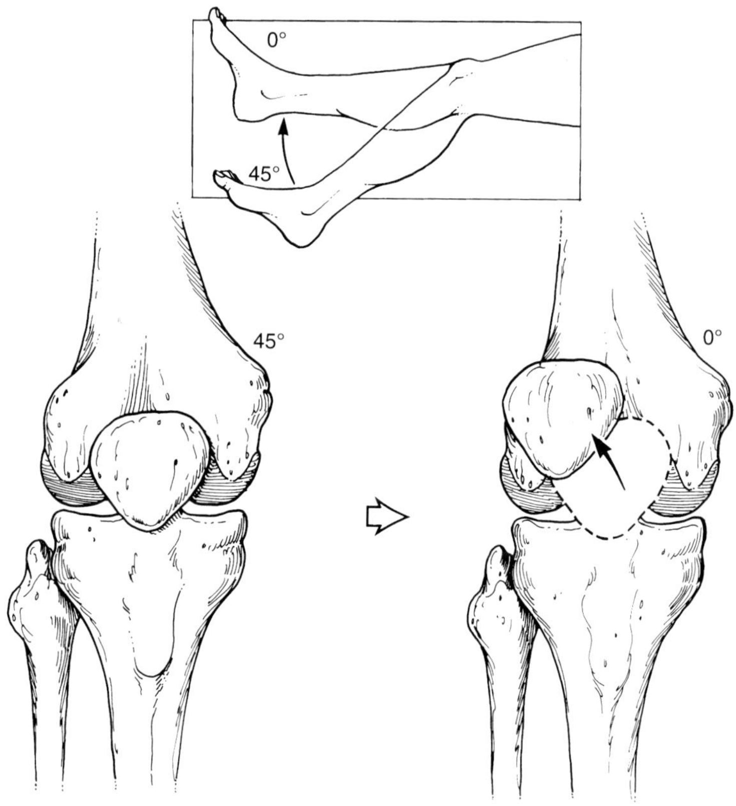

FIGURE 5.11. The J sign. Lateral deviation of the patella with terminal extension rather than the normal straight proximal line of pull.

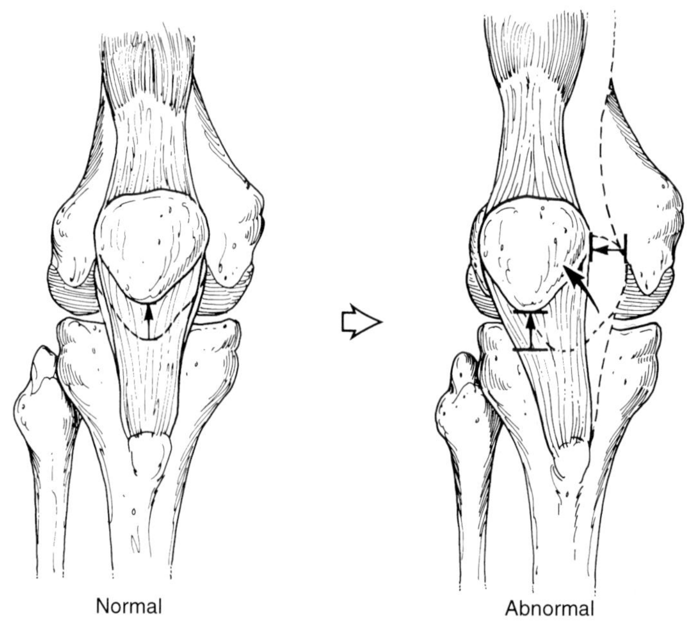

FIGURE 5.12. The active quadriceps pull test. With the knee extended, active contraction of the quadriceps causes the patella to shift laterally rather than proximally toward the anterior–superior iliac spine. (A, lateral pull; B, proximal pull).

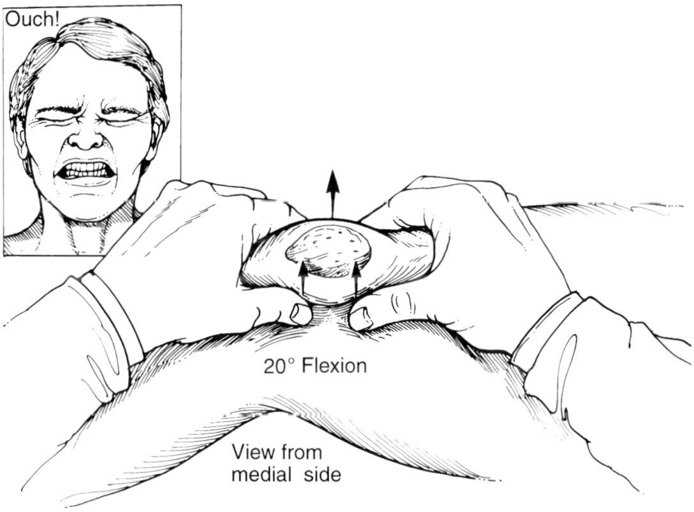

FIGURE 5.13. The apprehension test. Fear of patella subluxation/dislocation or quadricep contraction with lateral deviation of the patella characterizes this sign.

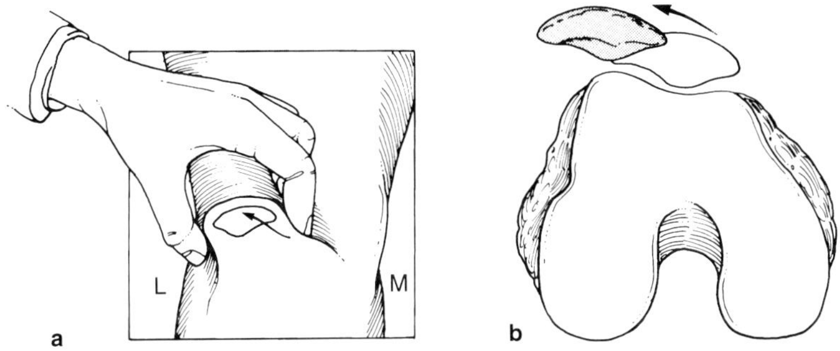

FIGURE 5.14. The passive patella glide test. With the knee flexed to 30° and the quadricep relaxed, the patella is pushed medially (a) and then laterally (b). Medial deviation of one quadrant or less is consistent with a contracted lateral retinaculum. Lateral deviation of greater than two quadrants is consistent with a lax or ruptured medial retinaculum.

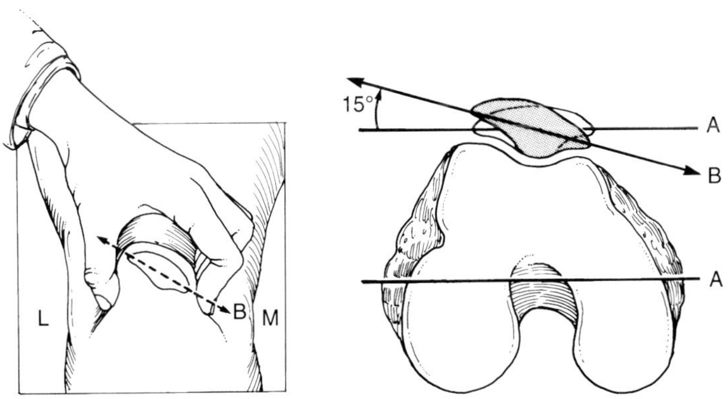

FIGURE 5.15. The passive patella tilt test. The inability to tilt the patella beyond a line parallel to the transepicondylar axis is consistent with a contracted lateral retinaculum (A′ transepicondylar axis; A, patella horizontal to transepicondylar axis; B, patella tilted beyond horizontal).

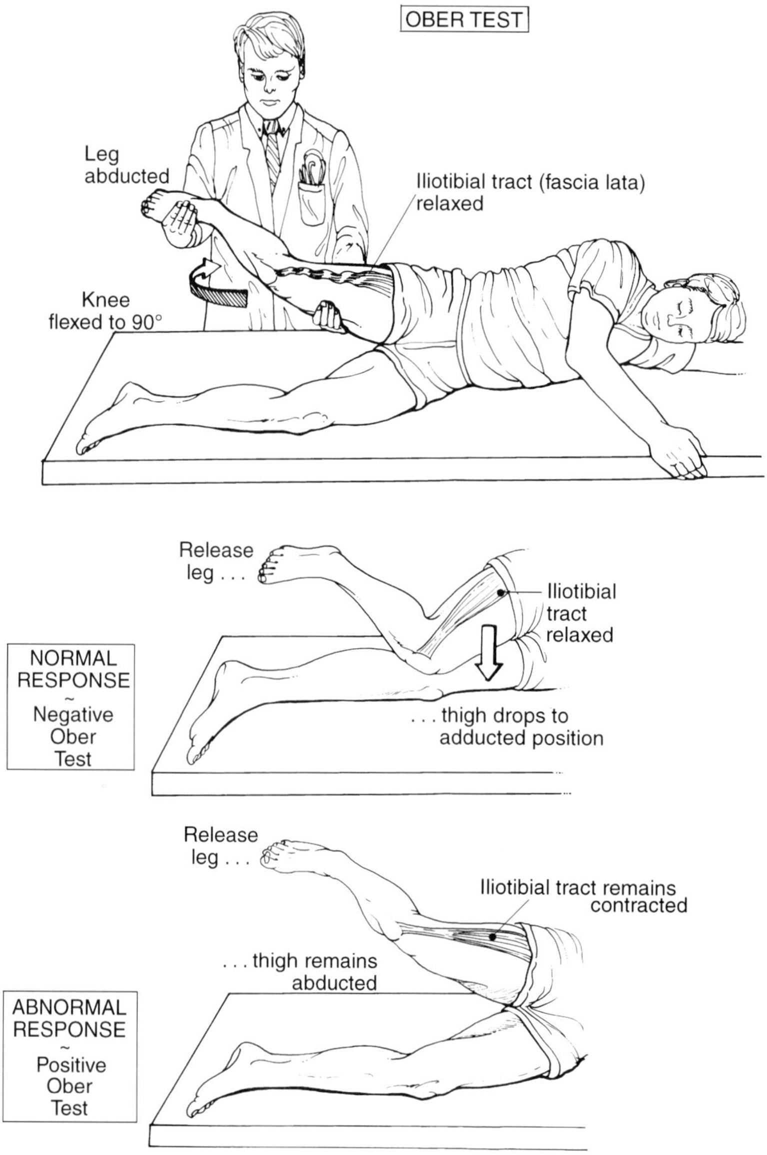

FIGURE 5.16. Ober's test. Tests for contraction of the iliotibial band (ITB).

maximally abducted and the knee flexed to 90°. The abducted limb is then gently released (Figure 5.16). A positive Ober's test is noted when the leg fails to fall to the adducted position and the limb remains suspended in a partially abducted position, indicating a contracted ITB.

Finally, the range of motion of the hip, the knee, and the ankle are tested. Ankle range of motion needs to be tested with the knee in both extension and flexion to evaluate for gastrocnemius tightness. Likewise, knee motion needs to be checked with the hip in extension and 90° of flexion to evaluate for hamstring tightness. *Hamstring tightness* is quantified using the *popliteal angle* (Figure 5.17). Hamstring tightness can increase patellofemoral forces by acting as an antagonist against the quadriceps musculature. For completion of the motion examination, the patient is

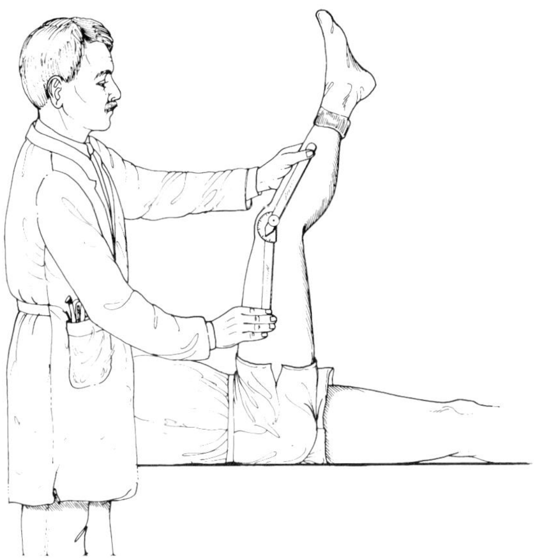

FIGURE 5.17. The popliteal angle. With the hip flexed to 90° to place the hamstrings under tension, the knee is extended and the tibiofemoral angle is measured.

turned prone to evaluate hip internal and external rotation, as well as for further evaluation of tibial rotation. As discussed earlier, limitation of external rotation or abnormal tibial rotation can contribute to maltracking disorders by increasing the functional Q angle. With the patient remaining prone, any final inspection and palpation of the posterior structures can be completed.

Summary

After performance of the previously mentioned maneuvers, the physical examination as well as the patient's history are completed. Hopefully, a diagnosis has been reached. Again, it needs to be stressed that the concept of chondromalacia or anterior knee pain syndrome as a diagnosis should be discarded. When examining the patellofemoral joint, specific diagnoses should be sought, thereby allowing problem-specific treatment. The list in Table 5-1 of possible causes of patellofemoral pain should be carefully reviewed. In most cases, a distinct diagnosis can be defined. A successful result, with a satisfied patient, will come from the correlation of a good history with the performance of a structured and directed physical examination.

References

1. Haas SB, Scuderi GR: Examination and radiographic assessment of the patellofemoral joint. *Semin Orthop* 1990;5(3):108–114.
2. Merchant AC: The classification of patellofemoral disorders. *Arthroscopy* 1988;4:235–240.
3. Scuderi GR: Surgical treatment for patellar instability. *Orthop Clin North Am* 1992;23(4):619–630.
4. Hughston JC: Subluxation of the patella. *J Bone Joint Surg Am* 1968;50:1003–1026.
5. Brattstrom H: Patella alta in non-dislocating knee joints. *Acta Orthop Scand* 1970;41:578.
6. Freeman BL: Recurrent dislocations, in Crenshaw AH (ed): *Campbell's Operative Orthopaedics,* ed 7. St. Louis, CV Mosby Co., 1987, pp. 2173–2218.
7. Aglietti P, Insall JN, Cerulli G: Patellar pain and incongruence. I. Measurements of incongruence. *Clin Orthop* 1983;176:217–224.
8. Kolowich PA, Paulos LE, Rosenberg TD, et al.: Lateral release of the patella: Indications and contraindications. *Am J Sports Med* 1990;18(4):359–365.
9. Fairbank HA: Internal derangement of the knee in children. *Proc R Soc London* 1937;3:11.
10. Fulkerson JP, Shea KP: Disorders of patellofemoral alignment. *J Bone Joint Surg Am* 1990;72A:1424–1429.
11. Ober FR: The role of the iliotibial band and fascia lata as a factor in the causation of low-back disabilities and sciatica. *J Bone Joint Surg Am* 1936;18A:106.

6

Imaging of the Patellofemoral Joint

Kevin R. Math, Bernard Ghelman, and Hollis G. Potter

The rapidly expanding technologic improvements in diagnostic imaging have afforded radiology an increasingly important role in the diagnosis and management of musculoskeletal disorders. For the past two decades, cross-sectional imaging with computed tomography (CT) and magnetic resonance imaging (MRI) have supplemented conventional radiography, arthrography, and the radionuclide bone scan, to provide important information about biomechanic structure and function of the bones and the joints. This chapter will address the utility of the various imaging modalities in the radiologic assessment of the patellofemoral joint.

Conventional Radiography

The routine radiographic examination of the knee at The Hospital for Special Surgery (HSS) includes standing anteroposterior, lateral, and axial (Merchant) views. The examination may be supplemented by the "tunnel" view, which depicts the medial and posterior femoral condyles and intercondylar notch. Normal AP, lateral, and Merchant views are depicted in Figure 6.1.

AP View

The AP view of the knee may be obtained with the patient supine or standing. The latter technique will more accurately reflect femoral tibial alignment and maintenance of the medial and the lateral joint spaces in the normal standing position. Physiologic valgus angulation of approximately 7° exists with the knee fully extended.[1] Joint space narrowing is often secondary to loss of articular cartilage, as occurs in arthritis and chondromalacia. Mild degrees of cartilage loss and interval progression of cartilage loss may not be detected if weight-bearing stress is not applied to the knee.[2]

The AP view provides little information about the patellofemoral joint space and the patella tracking, which is best obtained on tangential views. With the knee extended, there is a physiologic mild degree of lateral displacement of the patella, which should not be misinterpreted as subluxation on the AP view. This view is useful in assessing the morphology of the patella (width and length), anatomic variations (e.g., multipartite patella, dorsal defect of the patella), patella fracture, and size and symmetry of the femoral condyles.[3] Hypoplasia of the lateral femoral condyle may be associated with recurrent lateral patella subluxation.[4]

The vertical position of the patella, though best assessed on the lateral view, may also be subjectively estimated on the AP view. Brattstrom has advocated measuring the distance between the lower pole of the patella and a line drawn across the distal femoral condyles on the AP view, suggesting that patella alta should be suspected if this measurement exceeds 20 mm.[5] However, technical variations such as x-ray beam angle and patient positioning limit the utility of this measurement.

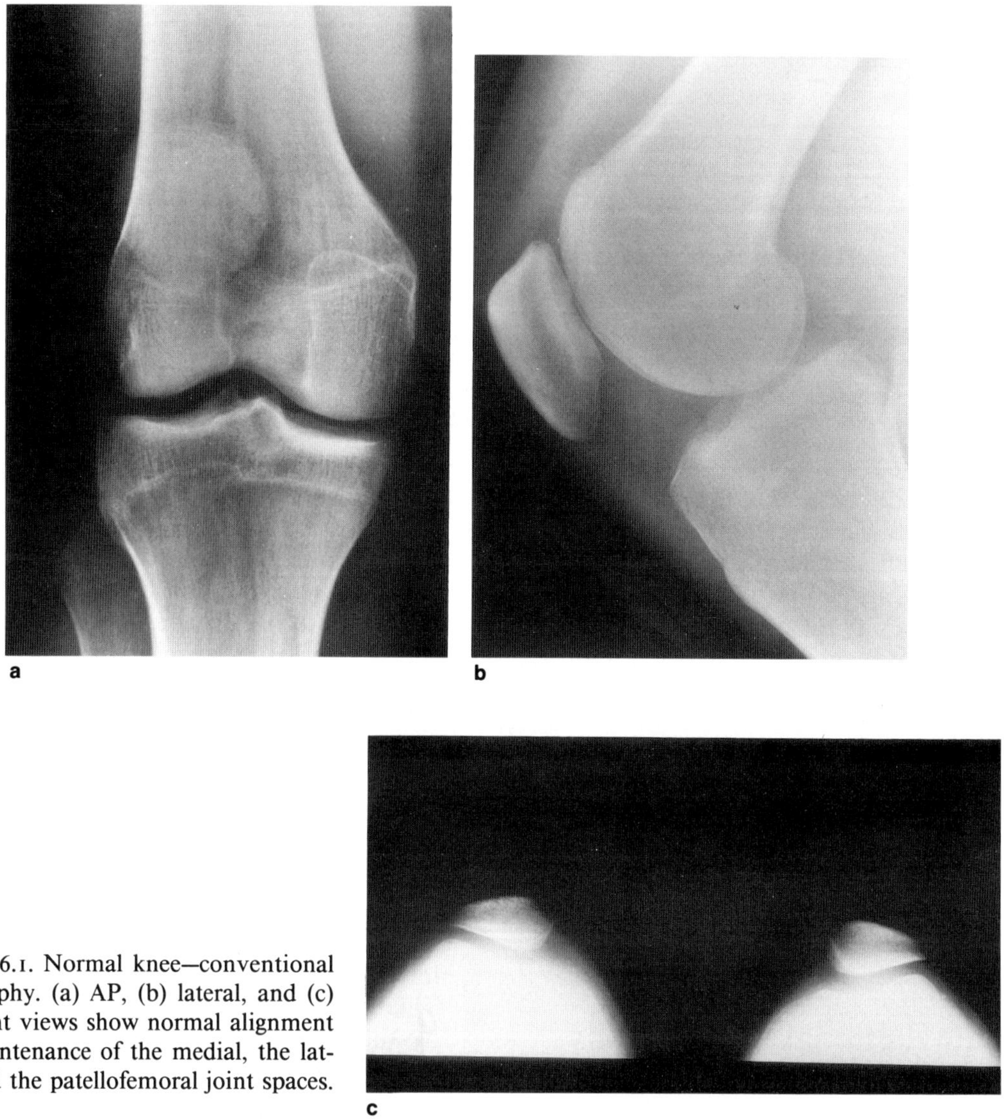

FIGURE 6.1. Normal knee—conventional radiography. (a) AP, (b) lateral, and (c) Merchant views show normal alignment and maintenance of the medial, the lateral, and the patellofemoral joint spaces.

Absolute measurements of patella height on the AP view are unreliable and this parameter is best assessed on the lateral view.[6]

Lastly, inasmuch as the supporting structures of the knee and biomechanic stresses at the knee contribute to chronic patellofemoral disorders, measurement of the valgus angulation at the knee, as ascertained by the quadriceps (Q) angle, give another parameter whereby patella balance may be assessed. This angle, which Brattstrom[5] described, is assessed on physical examination by drawing one line from the anterior superior iliac spine to the center of the patella and a second line from the center of the patella to the center of the tibial tubercle. The angle formed by these lines gives an estimation of the angle of pull between the quadriceps and the patella tendons. The normal Q angle in men is between 8° and 10°; in women the angle is between 10° and 20°. An increased Q angle (greater than 20°) may predispose to patella subluxation.[7]

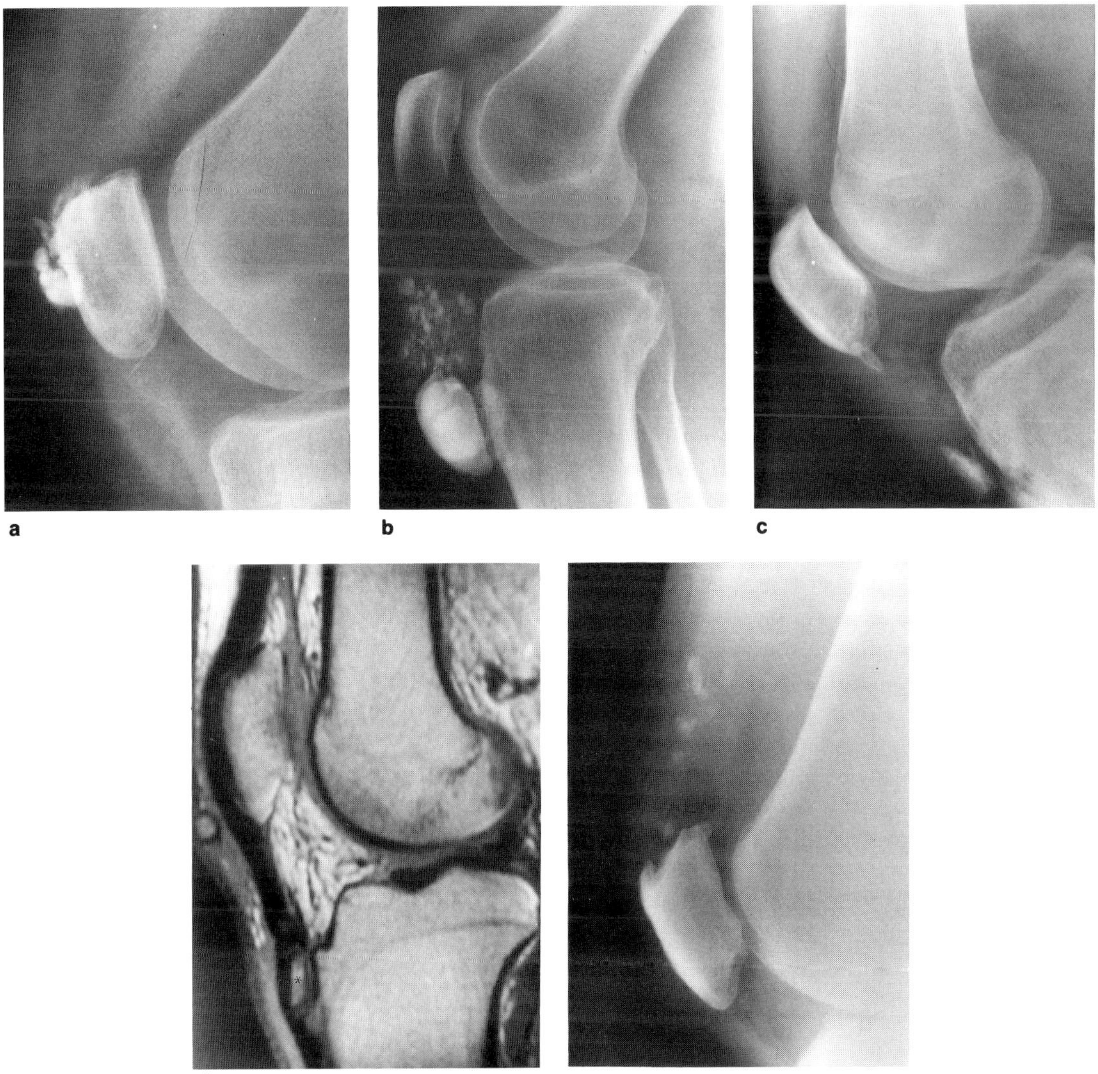

a b c d e

FIGURE 6.2. Abnormal soft-tissue calcification/ossification about the patellofemoral joint. (a) prepatellar bursitis ("housemaid's knee") and (b) pretibial bursitis ("preacher's knee")—coarse bursal calcifications are identified at sites of recurrent pressure injury. (c) Osgood–Schlatter disease (OSD) and Sinding–Larsen–Johansson (SLJ) disease: lateral radiograph shows ossification at the patella and tibial tubercle insertions of the patella tendon, secondary to concomitant SLJ disease and OSD in the same patient. (d) OSD (different patient): sagittal proton density (TR/TE = 2000/16) MRI demonstrates ossification at the tibial patella tendon insertion (asterisk). (e) Chronic quadriceps tendon injury: there are multiple foci of calcification within a thickened, poorly defined quadriceps tendon.

Lateral View

The standard lateral view of the knee is made with the knee in 30° of flexion, the patient supine, and the lateral aspect of the knee against the cassette. The x-ray beam is angled 90° to the table and centered at the knee joint.

The extensor mechanism of the knee is well visualized on the lateral view, and the tendons, the regional bursae, and the fat pads can be inspected for edema, inflammation, and abnormal calcifications. Abnormal soft-tissue calcification or ossification may be seen in the quadriceps and the patella tendons, the regional bursae, the muscles (myositis ossificans), and the infrapatellar fat pad (Hoffa's disease). Medial collateral ligament calcification, as seen in Pelligrini–Stieda disease, is best seen on the AP view. Although these calcifications are usually posttraumatic in etiology, other causes of soft-tissue calcification such as metastatic calcification in patients with renal failure and secondary hyperparathyroidism should be considered (Figure 6.2). Osgood–Schlatter disease[8,9] and Sinding–Larsen–Johansson disease[10,11] are manifested by abnormal calcification and surrounding edema at the patella tendon insertions on the tibial tubercle and the inferior patella, respectively. Bursitis is manifested by soft-tissue swelling and occasional calcification; in the knee, the prepatellar bursa ("housemaid's knee") and the pretibial bursa ("preacher's knee") are commonly involved. The suprapatellar region should be inspected for a joint effusion, manifested as an oval area of soft-tissue density in the suprapatellar bursa, which communicates with the joint (Figure 6.3). This is a nonspecific finding, and may be seen with synovial effusion, hemarthrosis, or infection. In the setting of acute trauma, a cross-table lateral view, obtained with the patient supine and the x-ray beam angled parallel to the table, may demonstrate a fat-fluid level, indicating intra-articular fracture with leakage of marrow fat, (i.e., lipohemarthrosis) (Figure 6.4). This sign is useful in osteoporotic patients in which intra-articular fractures are often occult, prompting further radiologic evaluation, such as additional views or other imaging modalities. The patellofemoral joint space can be examined on the lateral view, although because of the usual triangular configuration of the patella, it is better demonstrated on axial (Merchant) views.

The condylopatellar femoral sulcus, located at the articular surface of the lateral femoral condyle, can be visualized on the lateral view. Cobby et al.,[12] using the method of Warren,[13] measured the depth of the condylopatellar sulcus of the lateral femoral condyle, correlating it with MRI and arthroscopic findings. They suggest that a correlation between anterior cruciate ligament (ACL) injury and a deep sulcus, concluding a depth of greater than 1.5 mm (3 SD above the mean), is a reliable indirect conventional radiographic sign of a torn ACL.[12]

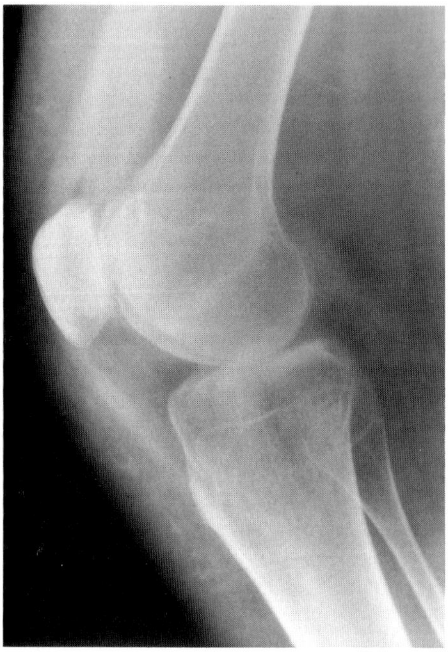

FIGURE 6.3. Joint effusion. There is an oval soft-tissue density in the suprapatellar pouch, corresponding to the infected joint fluid in this patient with recurrent septic arthritis. (Compare with normal suprapatellar region in Figure 6.1.)

Assessment of vertical patella position or patella height can readily be made on the lateral view, and several methods of measurement have been advanced to discern cephalad or caudal displacement of the patella (patella alta and patella baja, respectively) (Figures 6.5 and 6.6). Patella alta is commonly associated with patellofemoral pain and instability. Causes include spastic neuromuscular diseases such as cerebral palsy, in addition to prior Osgood–Schlatter[14] or Sinding–Larsen–Johansson disease and patella tendon rupture. Patella baja is often seen in achondroplastic dwarfs[15] in whom it is usually asymptomatic. Other more common causes include posttraumatic quadriceps rupture[16,17] and the postoperative patella (following tibial tubercle trans-

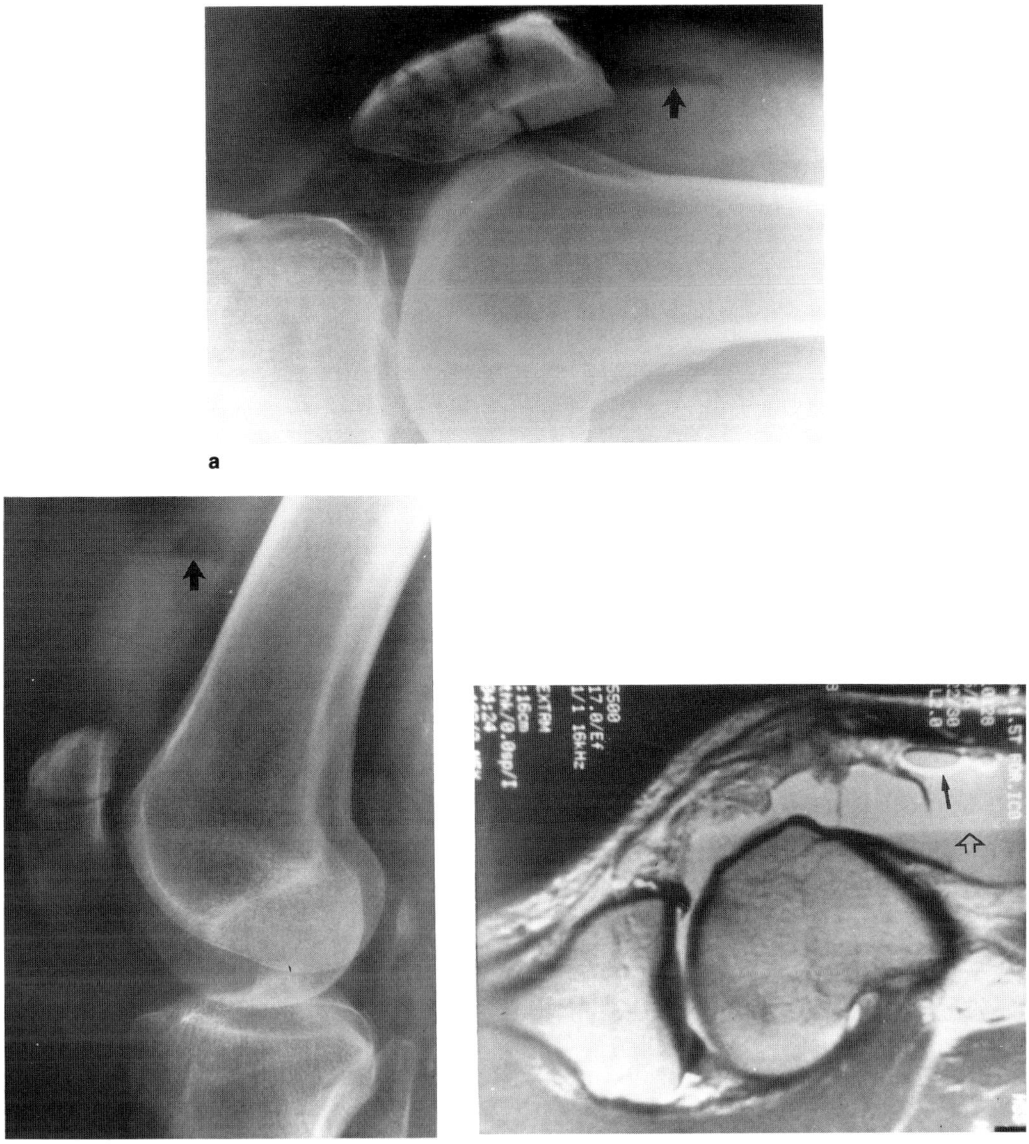

FIGURE 6.4. Fat-fluid level (lipohemarthrosis). (a) Cross-table lateral radiograph with horizontal x-ray beam and patient supine shows a comminuted patella fracture. The fat is seen anteriorly in the nondependent portion of the suprapatella pouch (arrow). (b) Lateral radiograph (different patient) obtained with patient standing—fat is seen in nondependent superior portion of suprapatellar pouch (arrow). (c) Sagittal proton density (TR/TE 5500/17) MRI: Patient sustained a patellar fracture from traumatic patellar dislocation. Fat globules are seen "floating" anteriorly (black arrow). A band of bright or dark signal can be seen on either side of the fat-fluid interface secondary to chemical-shift artifact. The fluid-fluid level interface (open arrow) is due to hemarthrosis with blood degradation products settling dependently.

fer or ACL reconstruction), as well as flaccid neuromuscular diseases such as polio.

Vertical patella height is important in the overall biomechanics and stability of the extensor mechanism and patellofemoral joint. The commonly used methods of assessment of patella height will be described.

1. *Blumensaat's Technique* (Figure 6.7).[18]

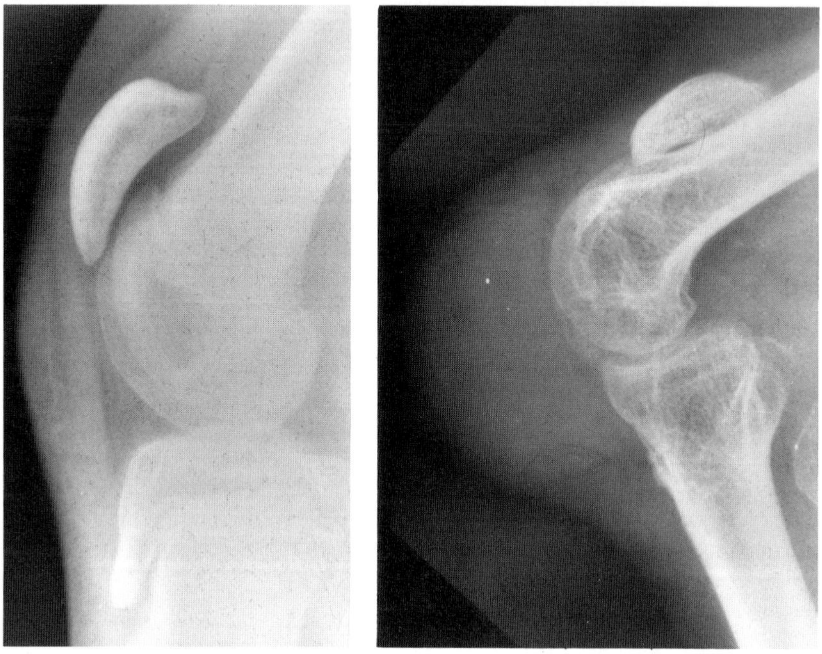

a b

FIGURE 6.5. Patella alta—secondary to cerebral palsy. (a) The patella is elongated and high-riding secondary to chronic spastic disease. (b) Different patient—marked patella alta with massive soft-tissue swelling in the region of the anatomic prepatellar bursa. Pronounced prepatellar bursitis in this spastic quadriplegic was due to crawling.

On a standard lateral view of the knee with the knee flexed 30°, a line is projected anteriorly from the dome of the intercondylar notch. According to Blumensaat, the inferior pole of the patella should be approximately at this level (Blumensaat's line). On the lateral view, the patella usually lies between Blumensaat's line and a line projected anteriorly from the distal femur growth-plate scar (see Figure 6.3). This technique has proved to be unreliable, owing to technical inconsistencies in obtaining the lateral view as well as anatomic variations in the angle of Blumensaat's line with respect to the long axis of the femur.[3,5] Insall and Salvati have shown this line to be an inaccurate assessment of patella position, with all normal patellae in their series positioned above this line.[19]

2. *Insall–Salvati* (Figure 6.8).[19] Insall and Salvati have described the most widely employed method for assessing patella height based on the length of the patella tendon (LT) divided by the greatest diagonal length of the patella (LP). LT is measured from the tendon origin at the inferior patella to its insertion at the tibial tubercle. The length of the patella tendon should be roughly equal to the length of the patella; the normal LT/LP ratio was calculated to be 1.02, with an SD of 0.13. An LT/LP ratio of less than 0.80 or greater than 1.20 is considered indicative of patella infera or patella alta, respectively. Of note, this technique remains accurate in virtually all degrees of flexion and extension of the knee; the Insall–Salvati index obtained with the knee maximally extended is nearly identical to that calculated in 30° of flexion.[20]

3. *Blackburne–Peel* (Figure 6.9).[21] Similar to the previously described method, a ratio of LT to LP is constructed. By this method, the perpendicular distance from the lower margin of the articular surface of the patella to the level of the anterior tibial plateau is measured (A) and divided by the length of the articular surface of the patella (B). Blackburne and Peel suggested this ratio would be a more accurate

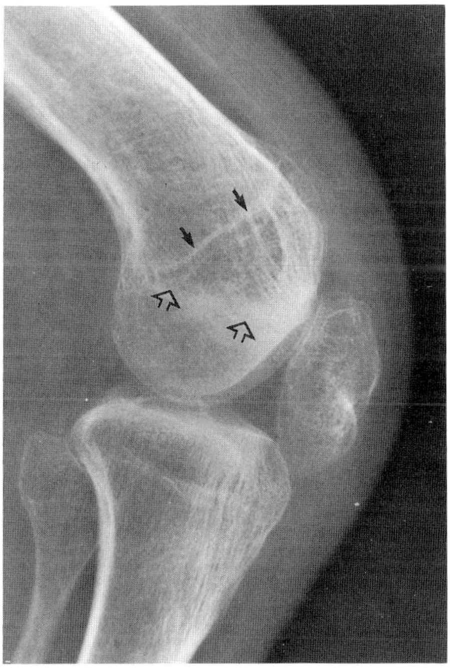

FIGURE 6.6. Patella baja—polio. Low-lying patella owing to flaccid neuromuscular disease. Blumensaat's line (open arrows) and the growth-plate scar (arrows) are demonstrated.

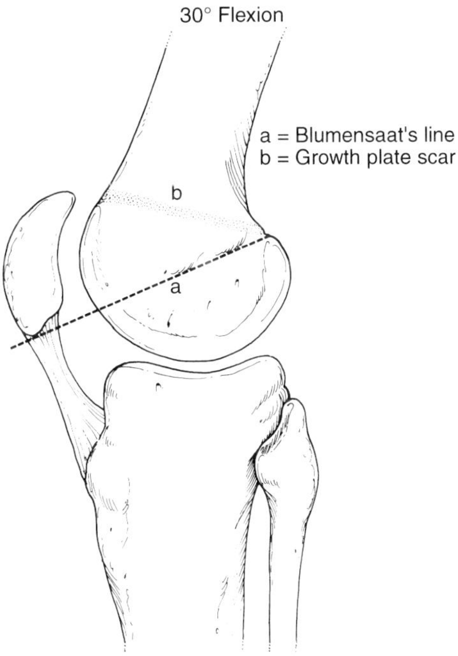

FIGURE 6.7. Blumensaat's technique. The lower pole of the patella lies at the level of Blumensaat's line, with the patella located between this line and a line projected from the growth-plate scar. This is a rough estimate of patella height; anatomic variations and technical inconsistencies limit the utility of this technique.

assessment of patella height, avoiding confounding variables such as anatomic variation in the size of the inferior pole of the patella (nonarticular surface) and difficulty in assessing the location of the tibial tubercle in patients with prior Osgood–Schlatter disease. The normal A/B ratio in their series was 0.80, with an SD of 0.14.

4. *Norman, Egund, and Ekelund* (Figure 6.10).[20] This method assesses the vertical position of the patella on a cross-table lateral view, with the knee maximally extended and the quadriceps muscle contracted prior to exposing the film. The foot is externally rotated by approximately 10° to 15° in order to superimpose the femoral condyles. The vertical position of the patella is assessed relative to a line drawn through the distal femoral condyles rather than relative to the proximal tibia, thereby avoiding the potential confounding variable of individual anatomic variations in the inclination of the tibial plateau. The measured parameters, including vertical position of the patella, length of the patella, and length of the patella tendon are expressed relative to body height in centimeters to calculate a relative height and length of the patella. The vertical position of the patella in relation to body height (vertical index) was found to be identical in males and females (0.21, SD = 0.02). Assessment of patella height by this method provides yet further information on patellofemoral biomechanic relationships.

5. *Caton–Linclau* (Figure 6.11).[22,23] Vertical patella height is assessed by dividing the distance between the anterosuperior rim of the tibia and the lowermost end of the patella articular surface by the total length of the patella articular surface. This method is similar to that of Blackburne–Peel in that it relies on easily identifiable and reproducible landmarks, and both express the ratio relative to the length of the patella articular surface,

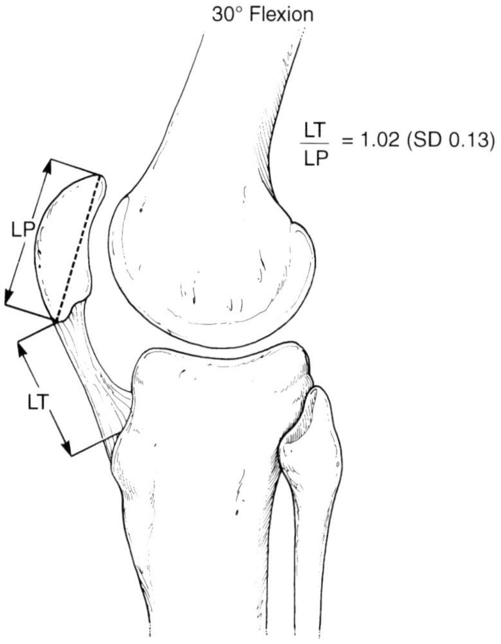

FIGURE 6.8. Insall–Salvati. Patella height is expressed as a ratio of patella tendon length (LT) to the greatest diagonal length of the patella (LP). This method is the most widely used and is useful for assessing patella height in virtually all degrees of flexion.

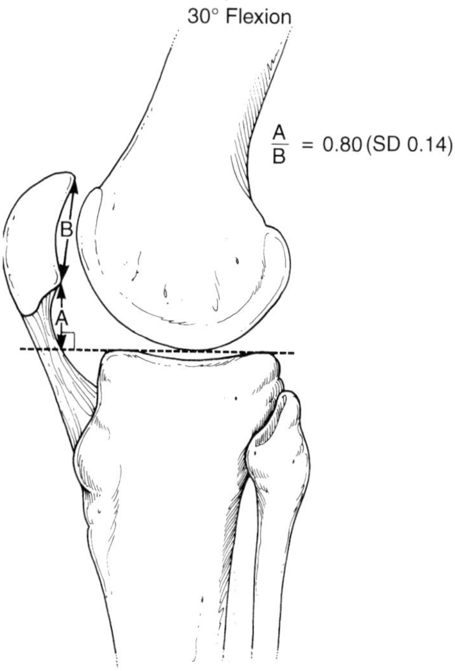

FIGURE 6.9. Blackburne–Peel. Patella height is expressed as a ratio of the perpendicular distance from the lower articular surface of the patella to the level of the tibial plateau (A) to the length of the articular surface of the patella (B).

which is less variable than the greatest patella length, as used in the Insall–Salvati method. Scuderi[24] demonstrated the vertical patella height by this method to be 0.97 in males and 0.96 in females, with an SD of 0.14.

Axial Tangential View

The axial tangential view is ideal for assessing the position and the orientation of the patella in the axial plane. Specifically, the view is ideal for evaluating the contour of the patella facets and gives important clinical information regarding the location of the patella with respect to the femoral trochlear sulcus. The subchondral bone of the patella articular surfaces is well demonstrated; however, the apex of the patella on this view does not necessarily correlate with the apex of the patella articular cartilage, as seen on CT arthrography or MRI.

Although several techniques have been described for obtaining tangential or "skyline" views, the Merchant[25] view and the Laurin[26] technique are the most widely used axial views in assessment of patella subluxation and/or tilt. The Merchant view is the most easily reproducible and is the axial view of choice at HSS.

1. *Merchant View* (Figure 6.12). The Merchant view is obtained with the patient in the supine position and the knees flexed 45°, the lower legs resting on an angled platform. The x-ray beam is angled toward the feet, 30° from the horizontal and the film cassette set is positioned 30 cm below the knees, resting on the shins. The x-ray beam strikes the cassette at a 90° angle, imaging both knees simultaneously.

Two angles are measured on this view: (1) the sulcus angle (measuring femoral trochlear depth) and (2) the congruence angle (measuring patellofemoral relationship). Brattstrom[27] defined the *sulcus angle* as the angle formed

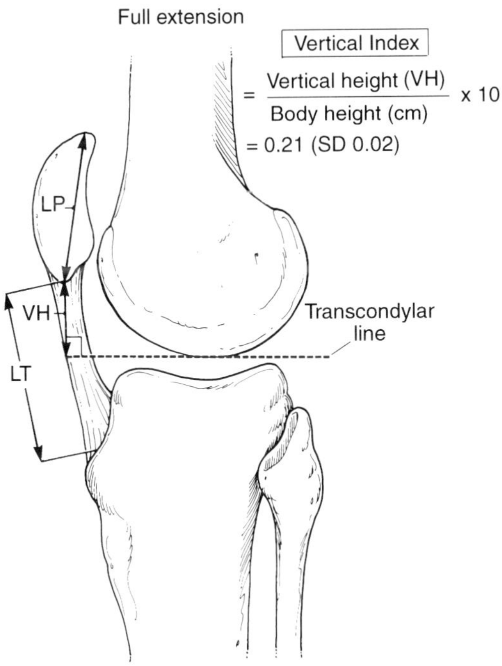

FIGURE 6.10. Norman, Egund, and Ekelund. Patella height is assessed on a cross-table lateral view with the knee fully extended. The parameters are expressed relative to body height. LT, patella tendon length; LP, greatest diagonal length of the patella.

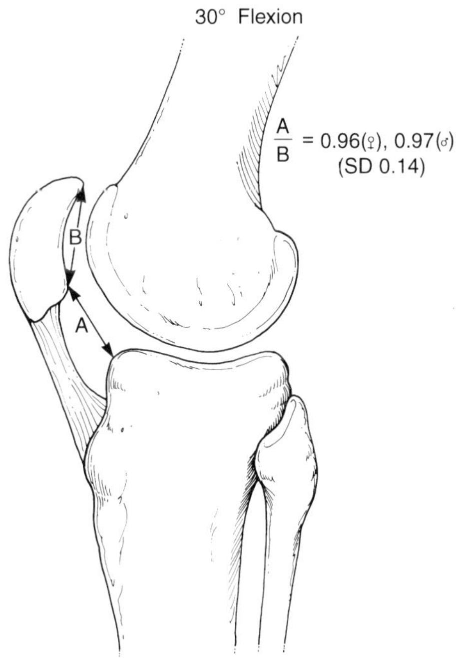

FIGURE 6.11. Caton–Linclau. Patella height is expressed as the ratio of distance between the lower articular surface of the patella and the anterosuperior tibial plateau (A) to the length of the patella articular surface (B).

by lines drawn from the deepest point of the intercondylar groove to the highest point on the medial and the lateral femoral condyles. This measurement reflects relative depth of the intercondylar sulcus; the greater the sulcus angle, the less lateral buttressing the lateral condyle imparts, and the greater the tendency toward lateral patellar tilt and subluxation.[3] The average sulcus angle on the Merchant view is 138° (SD 6°) and is equal in males and females.[25] The congruence angle is measured by bisecting the sulcus angle to construct a reference line, and projecting a second line from the apex of the sulcus angle to the lowermost point of the subchondral articular surface of the patella (apex). If the line drawn through the patella apex is lateral to the reference line, the angle is assigned a positive value; if it is medial to this line, a negative value is assigned. The normal congruence angle averages −6°, with an SD of 11°. According to Merchant, a congruence angle of greater than +16° is considered abnormal, indicating lateral patella subluxation. In fact, Merchant measured the average congruence angle of patients with recurrent lateral patella dislocation to be increased at +23°. Aglietti et al.[28] confirmed these measurements, calculating average congruence angles for normal persons and those with recurrent lateral subluxation of −8° (SD 6°) and +16°, respectively. The average sulcus angle in their study was also greater in subluxing patellae (147° versus 137° for normals). In addition, Aglietti et al. consider the upper limit of normal for the congruence angle to be a more conservative +4°, different from that described by Merchant (+16°).[28]

2. *Laurin Technique* (Figure 6.13).[26] Laurin and others studied the orientation of the patella on an axial image obtained with the knee in 20° of flexion rather than the 45° of flexion on the Merchant view. The rationale for viewing the patella in mild flexion is based on the

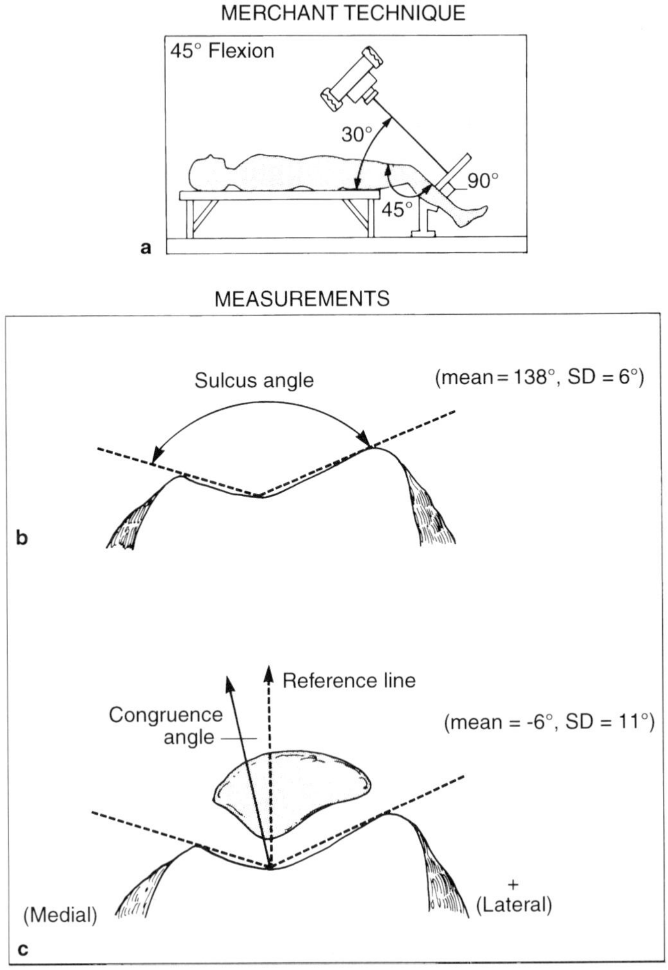

FIGURE 6.12. (a) Merchant view in which the knee is flexed 45° and the x-ray beam is angled toward the feet. (b) Sulcus angle–assesses the relative depth of the sulcus. The angle between lines drawn from the deepest point of the sulcus to the anterior aspects of the medial and the lateral femoral condyles. (c) Congruence angle–angle between reference line (bisecting sulcus angle) and line drawn from sulcus to patella apex.

fact that most patella subluxation and dislocations occur within the first 20° to 30° of flexion.[29,30] With flexion greater than 30°, the patellar is drawn caudally into the intercondylar groove, tending to center directly over the groove.[31] Tension of the flexor mechanism of the knee in 45° of flexion on the Merchant view can provide stability for the patella, which can conceivably lead to misinterpretation of subluxable patellae as being in the normal position (i.e., false-negative). Measurements obtained on the Laurin view also assess patella "tilt" in addition to subluxation.

The image is obtained with the patient sitting and the knee flexed 20°. The film cassette is held approximately 12 cm proximal to the patella and pushed against the anterior thighs. The x-ray beam is directed cephalad and superior, 20° from the horizontal. Two measurements are made on this view: (1) the lateral patellofemoral angle and (2) the patellofemoral index. The lateral patellofemoral angle is formed by the intersection of one line drawn across the anterior femoral condyles and a second line drawn tangent to the lateral facet of the patella. This angle should be open laterally. If the lines are parallel or diverge medially, there is thought to be a tendency towards subluxation or dislocation. Laurin et al. reported 97% of normal controls to have an angle open laterally and in 3%, the lateral facet is parallel to the anterior femoral condylar line. In contrast, in patients with patella subluxation, 60% of the lines were parallel and 40% had angles that were divergent medially. No case of patella subluxation in

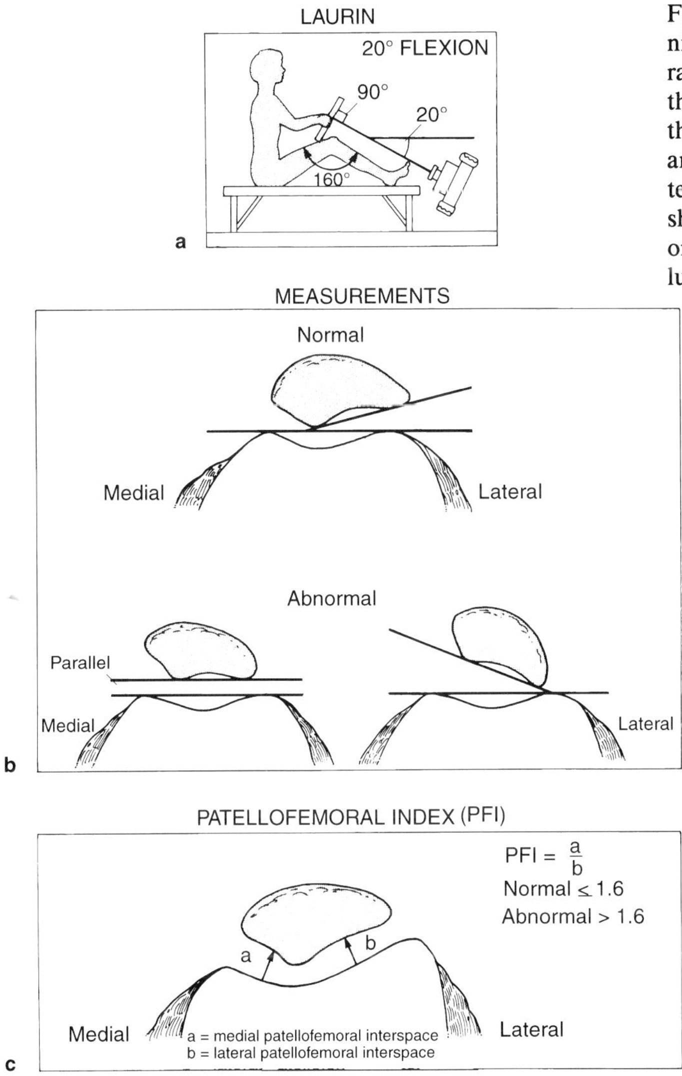

FIGURE 6.13. Laurin technique. (a) Technique—the knee is flexed 20° and the x-ray beam is directed cephalad, exposing the film held by the patient against the thighs. (b) Lateral patellofemoral angle—angle between lines drawn tangent to anterior condyles and lateral patella facet should diverge laterally. (c) Patellofemoral index—assesses for patella tilt/subluxation by the lateral interspace.

this series had an angle that diverged laterally, making this sign fairly reliable.

The patellofemoral index (PFI) is the ratio of the thickness of the medial patellofemoral interspace (*a*) and the shortest thickness of the lateral patellofemoral interspace (*b*). All normal patients in the study had a patellofemoral interspace (*a/b*) of less than or equal to 1.6, while all subluxable patellae had an index of greater than 1.6. Therefore, patients with an abnormal patellofemoral articulation, either owing to chondromalacia or predisposition to patella subluxation, may exhibit an increased PFI, despite preservation of the lateral patellofemoral angle. This so-called "minitilt" of the patella can be clinically significant in patellofemoral pain and is only evident on assessment of the PFI.

Anatomic Variations

Normal Patella Development

Ossification of the patella begins in the third year of life and is usually multicentric.[15] Irregular ossification of the patella is commonly seen in young children, resulting in a frag-

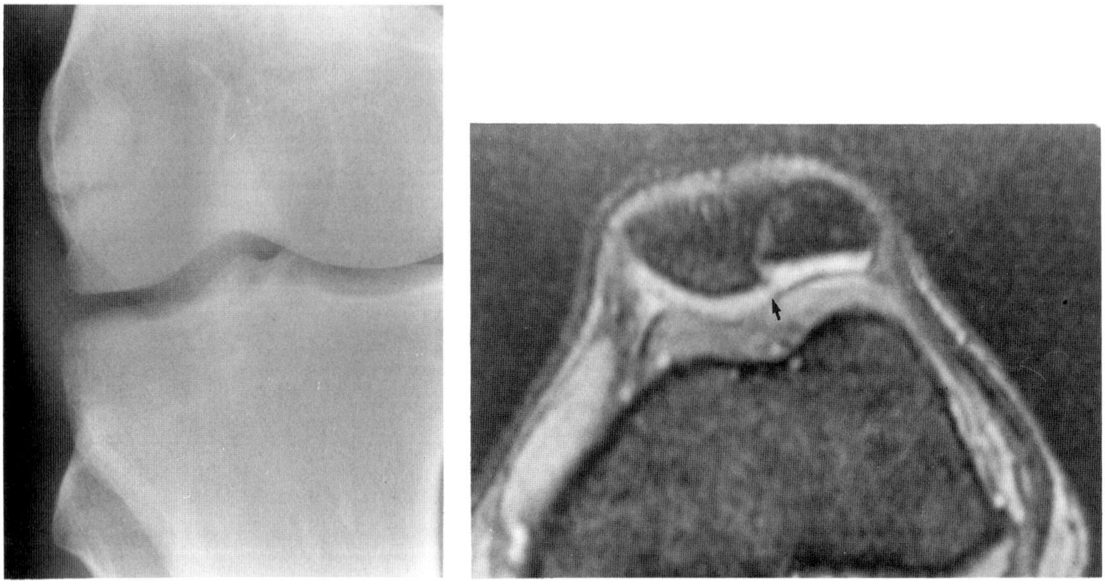

a b

FIGURE 6.14. Bipartite patella. (a) There is a crescentic lucency traversing the superolateral aspect of the patella. The edges do not appear to fit evenly together, as they would in a patella fracture (b) axial gradient echo (TR/TE = 350/18) MRI. There is an irregular area of increased signal intensity (equivalent to articular cartilage) through the lateral patella with maintenance of continuity of the overlying articular cartilage (arrow).

mented appearance that should not be mistaken for osseous injury. Great variability in size and configuration of the patella exists among normal children and adults. Stippled calcification of the patella, the vertebrae, and the triradiate cartilage is seen in infants with Zellweger (cerebrohepatorenal) syndrome, a rare autosomal recessive disorder, also marked by ocular, hepatic, and neurologic abnormalities.[32,33]

Types of Patellae

Three facets are identified on an axial view of the patella: (1) the lateral facet, (2) the medial facet, and (3) the odd facet. The lateral and the medial facets are separated by a median ridge that extends longitudinally along the posterior patella. The odd facet is located most medially and is smaller than the adjacent medial facet. The medial facet is usually shorter and variable in size and configuration than the lateral facet. The lateral facet is longer and usually less steeply angled than the medial facet. Its surface is usually concave, while the surface of the medial facet can be flat or convex.

There is great variability in the configuration of the patella on the axial tangential view in terms of symmetry and size of the facets. These configurations were originally classified by Wiberg[34] and were later modified by others. Although Wiberg's classification is commonly referred to, different patellar configurations may be thought of as a spectrum of normal variants, as there is no definite correlation with the evidence of patellofemoral degenerative disease or chondromalacia.[15]

Wiberg described the following three configurations of the patella,[34] which can be readily assessed on the axial tangential radiographs:

- *Type I.* The medial and lateral facets are

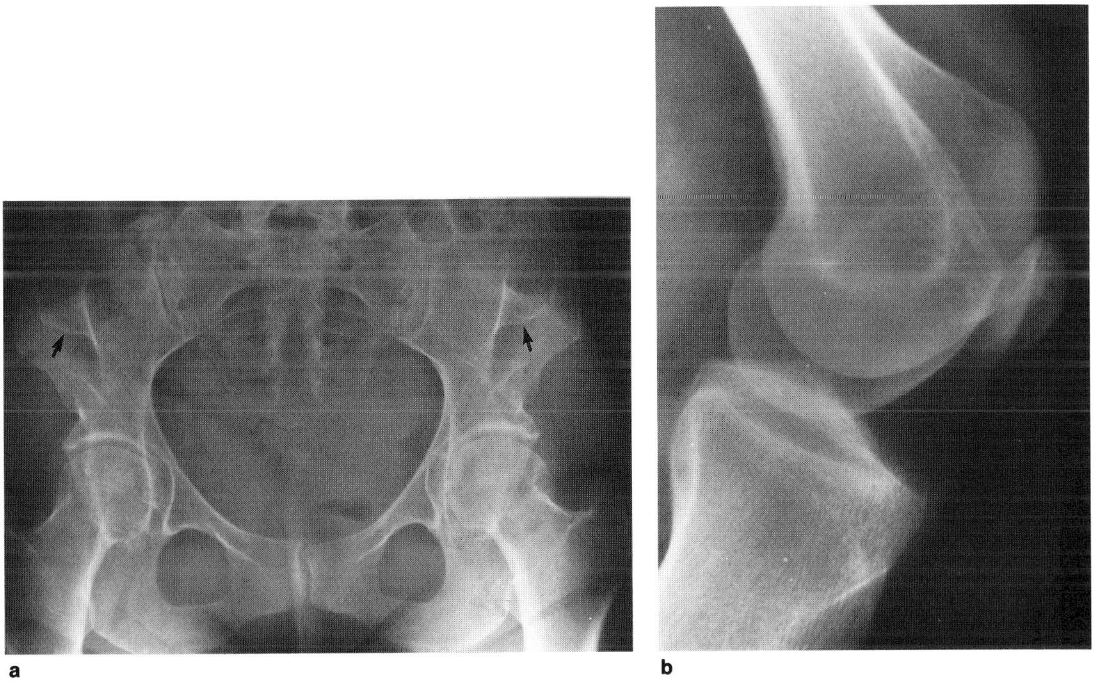

FIGURE 6.15. Fong's disease. (a) AP view of the pelvis demonstrates the bilateral posterior iliac horns (arrows) that are characteristic of the disease. (b) Different patient—the patella is hypoplastic.

both slightly concave and are roughly equivalent in size. This configuration is thought to promote the greatest stability.

- *Type II.* The medial facet is smaller than the lateral facet, and has a flat or concave surface. The lateral facet maintains a concave contour.
- *Type III.* The medial facet is much smaller than the lateral facet and has a convex surface that is nearly at a right angle to the lateral facet.

The incidence of Wiberg's type I, II, and III patellae are approximately 10%, 65%, and 25%, respectively.[35]

Bipartite/Multipartite Patella

Incomplete fusion of patella ossification centers can result in a bipartite or a multipartite patella (Figure 6.14). This variation, occurring in 0.05% to 1.66% of knees,[36,37] typically involves the superolateral patella and is often bilateral. If the incomplete ossification is oriented longitudinally, in the coronal plane, anterior and posterior fragments result (patella duplication)[15]; this appearance would be unusual in fracture. The characteristic appearance, the location, and the common bilaterality of bipartite patella help to distinguish it from patella fracture. Another helpful finding is the slight incongruence of fragments in bipartite patella, while fracture fragment edges typically fit evenly together. In equivocal cases, CT and MRI can be helpful in differentiating this normal variant from traumatic injury. Radionuclide bone scan may also be helpful, demonstrating greatly increased activity in fracture and normal symmetric activity in bipartite patellae.

Dorsal Defect of the Patella

Dorsal defect of the patella (DDP) is usually detected incidentally in a patient with knee pain. The lesion is lucent, well defined, and rounded, and is seen at the superolateral border of the patella.[38] This location is identical to that of a bipartite patella, suggesting that it

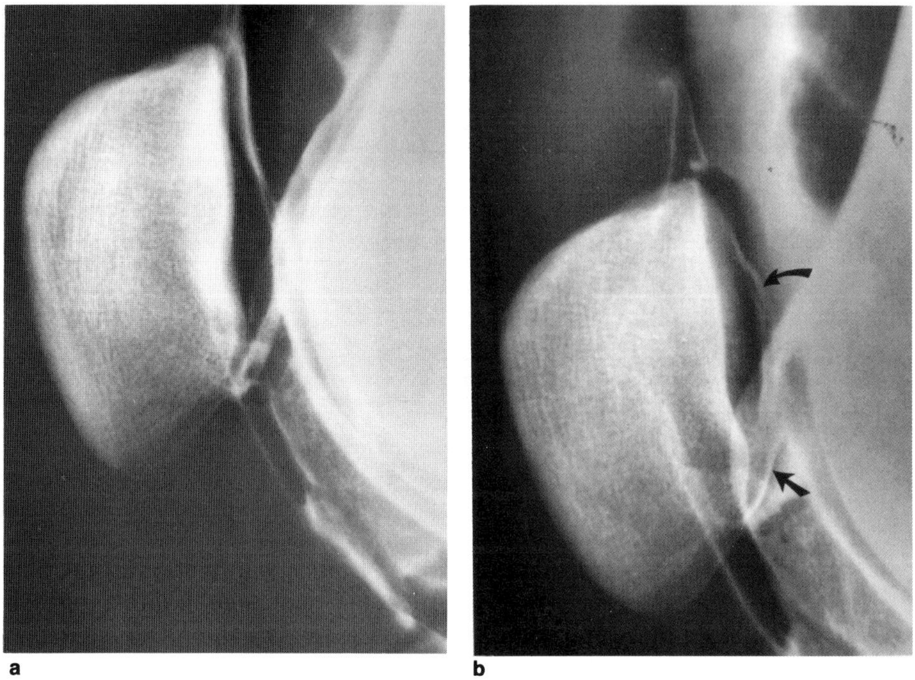

FIGURE 6.16. Normal double-contrast arthrogram. (a) Lateral view of the extended knee demonstrates normal contour and thickness of the articular cartilage of the patella. There is considerable overlap of the medial and the lateral facets. (b) Internal rotation of the knee brings the medial facet into profile (arrows).

is an anomaly of ossification. This lesion is not rare, reportedly occurring in approximately 0.3% to 1.0% of the population.[39,40] Bilaterality exists in 25% to 33%.[39,41] Pathologically, the lesion is composed of nonspecific fibrous tissue and spicules of bone.[38] The cartilage overlying the lesion is usually intact. The lucent appearance of the lesion in a patient with knee pain often incites a lengthy differential diagnosis, including chondroblastoma, osteochondritis dissecans, osteomyelitis, and metastases. However, its distinctive radiographic appearance and location are virtually diagnostic. DDP frequently heals spontaneously by sclerosis.[42]

Fong's Disease (Nail–Patella Syndrome)

This disorder has autosomal dominant inheritance and is characterized by dysplastic fingernails, hypoplastic or absent patellae, characteristic bilateral posterior iliac horns, and additional skeletal and soft-tissue abnormalities (Figure 6.15).[43] In the knee, in addition to hypoplasia of the patella, there is commonly hypoplasia of the lateral femoral condyle, which results in the common clinical presentation of recurrent patellar dislocation.[44] A sloping tibial plateau and prominence of the tibial tubercle have also been described in this syndrome. Incidentally, familial bilateral absence of the patellae is an extremely rare condition, described in two families, which is presumably a separate entity from Fong's disease.[45,46]

Arthrography

Arthrography provides visualization of the intra-articular structures of the knee, including menisci, articular cartilage, ligaments, and synovium through the intra-articular injection of opaque contrast medium and air. Double-contrast arthrography is performed by injecting approximately 4 mL of positive contrast

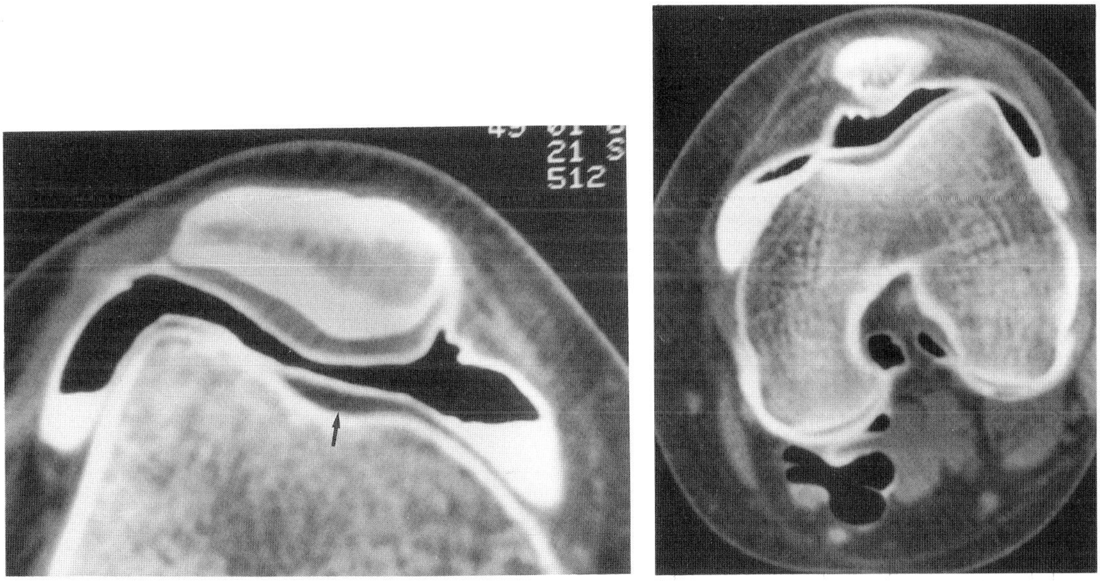

b

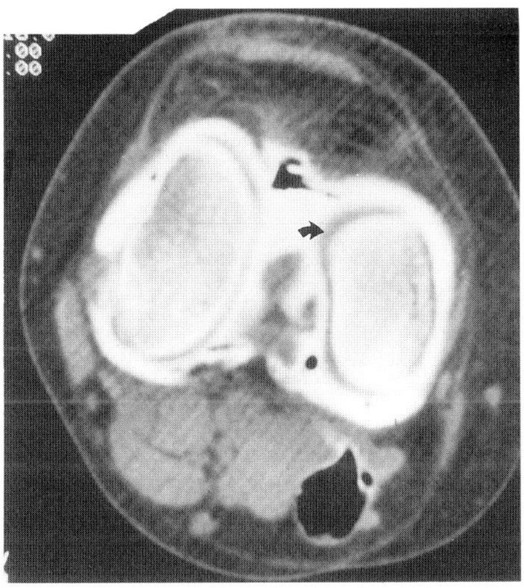

c

FIGURE 6.17. Normal CT arthrogram. (a) Uniform thickness of articular cartilage is seen over the lateral facet, the apex, and the medial facet, with normal relative thinning over the odd facet. Note that the fat anterior to the distal femur (arrow) is lower in density than articular cartilage. (b) Articular cartilage of the femoral trochlea. (c) Articular cartilage of the medial (arrow) and the lateral femoral condyles. An air-filled popliteal cyst is incidentally seen. Soft-tissue density in the intercondylar notch represents the cruciate ligaments.

and 40 mL of room air; the knee is then exercised and multiple radiographs are obtained.[47] Double-contrast arthrography depicts thc hyalinc articular cartilagc of thc patella and femoral condyles; this cartilage is normally lucent and is not visualized on conventional radiographs. Intra-articular pathology, including meniscal tears, loose bodies, synovial disease, plicae, synovial cysts, and articular cartilage abnormalities, are readily demonstrated by this technique. The patellofemoral joint is assessed on the lateral and the Merchant views. On the lateral view, the articular cartilage of the lateral and the medial facets are best visualized on external and internal rotation of the patella, respectively (Figure 6.16). This serves to make the cartilage of these facets tangential to the x-ray beam, demonstrating cartilaginous abnormalities to best advantage.

Double-contrast knee arthrography is seldom performed without subsequent CT scan. CT scan, following arthrography, provides more detailed information of the patella and

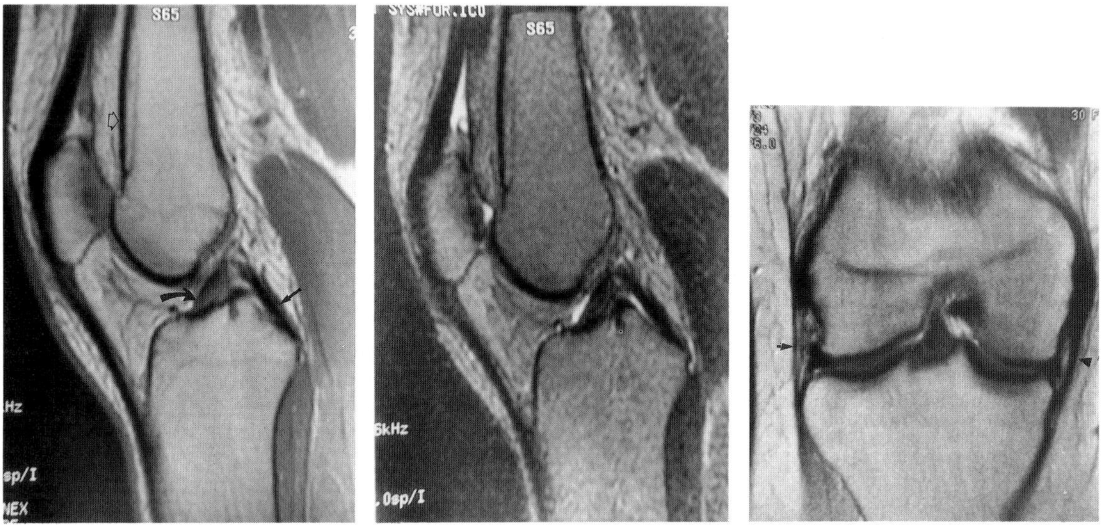

a b c

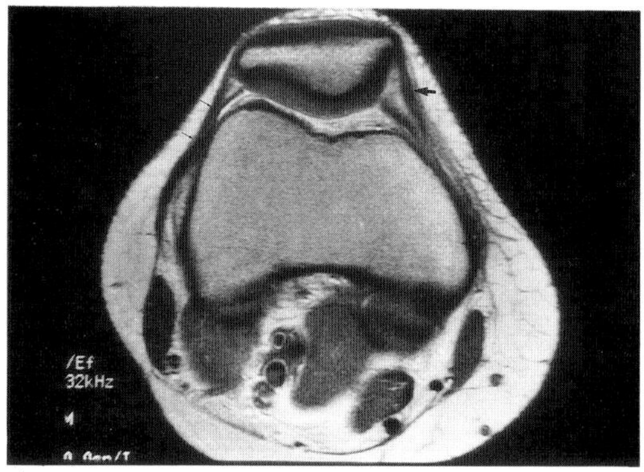

d

FIGURE 6.18. Normal knee—MRI. Sagittal spin echo (a) proton density (TR/TE 2000/16) and (b) T_2-weighted (TR/TE 2000/80) images show the normal low signal intensity quadriceps and patella tendons in addition to the anterior (curved arrow) and posterior (straight arrow) cruciate ligaments. Cortical bone (open arrow) always has low signal intensity. Note the physiologic amount of fluid that has high signal intensity on the T_2-weighted image. (c) Coronal proton density image. The low signal intensity medial collateral ligament (arrowhead) and iliotibial band (arrow) are shown. The cruciate ligaments are visualized in the intercondylar notch. (d) Axial proton density image. Note the normal low signal intensity medial (arrow) and lateral (small arrows) retinacula. The patella cartilage is normal with underlying low signal intensity subchondral bone.

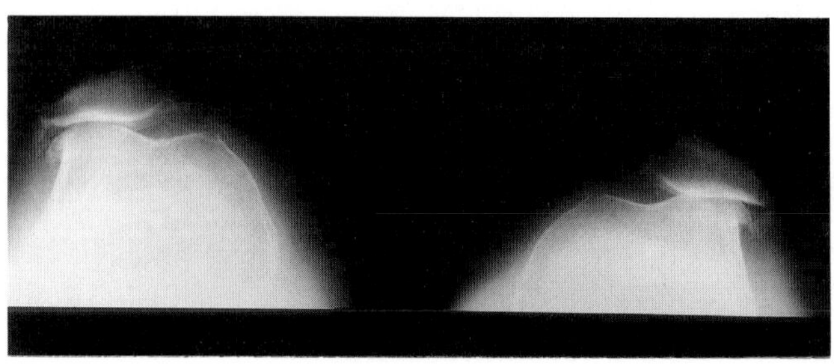

FIGURE 6.19. Bilateral lateral patellar subluxation. Merchant view of both knees demonstrates severe lateral narrowing of both patellofemoral joints. The patellae are subluxed laterally and there are bony proliferative changes in this patient with advanced osteoarthritis.

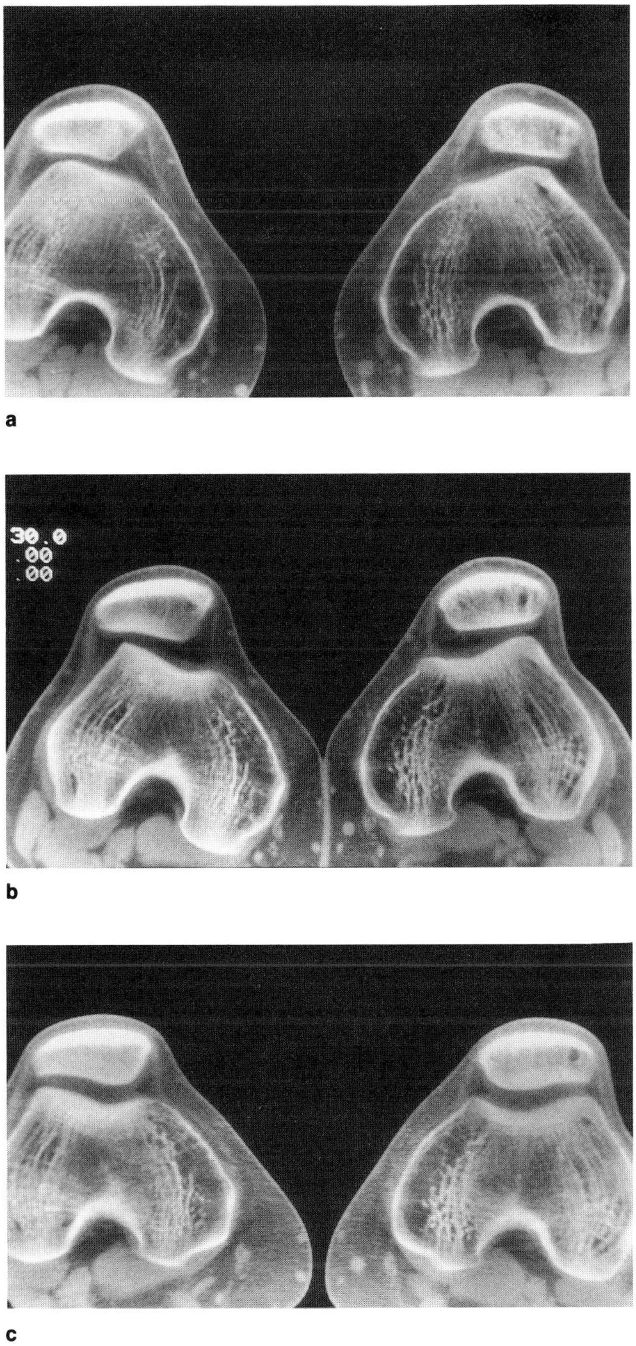

FIGURE 6.20. Transient bilateral lateral patella subluxation. Unenhanced CT through the patellofemoral joints, obtained in (a) full extension, (b) 15° flexion, and (c) 30° flexion. The left patella is subluxed laterally in extension and in 15° flexion; the right patella is subluxed laterally in 15° flexion. Patellofemoral alignment is normal at 30° flexion.

surrounding structures in the axial plane with a high degree of spatial resolution. A small amount of epinephrine is injected intra-articularly during arthrography if CT scan will be subsequently performed, in order to delay resorption of contrast from the joint. Although

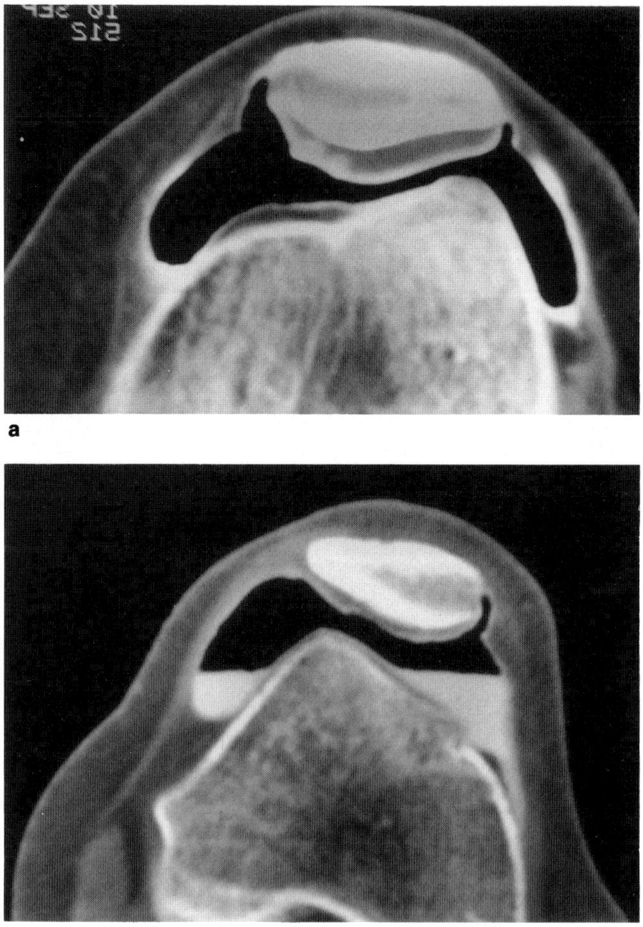

a

b

FIGURE 6.21. Chondromalacia patellae—CT arthrography. (a) There is contrast imbibition and ulceration involving the articular cartilage of the medial facet. (b) Different patient—there is generalized thinning of articular cartilage involving the medial facet of the patella and a large portion of the lateral facet.

MRI has virtually replaced arthrography for examination of the cruciate ligaments and menisci, CT arthrography continues to play an important role in patellofemoral imaging. Its greatest utility lies in imaging patients with suspected plica syndrome, loose bodies, and chondromalacia patella.

CT

CT is used in several ways for assessing the patellofemoral joint. Following double-contrast arthrography, the integrity of the articular cartilage of the patella and the anterior femoral condyles, as well as other structures such as synovial plicae and synovial cysts are well demonstrated on CT (Figure 6.17). For an optimal study, no more than 3 to 5 mL of contrast and no less than 35 to 40 mL of air should be injected intra-articularly.

CT is useful in evaluating intra- or extra-articular calcifications, which can be easily overlooked in MRI, where they appear as foci of diminished signal. Calcified intra-articular loose bodies should be imaged by air arthrogram with CT, without positive contrast material, as the opaque contrast may obscure their visualization. CT is also helpful in assessing patellofemoral tracking, as will be discussed in the section titled Patellofemoral Tracking.

Bone Scan

Radionuclide bone scanning is a nuclear imaging technique whereby a labeled radiophar-

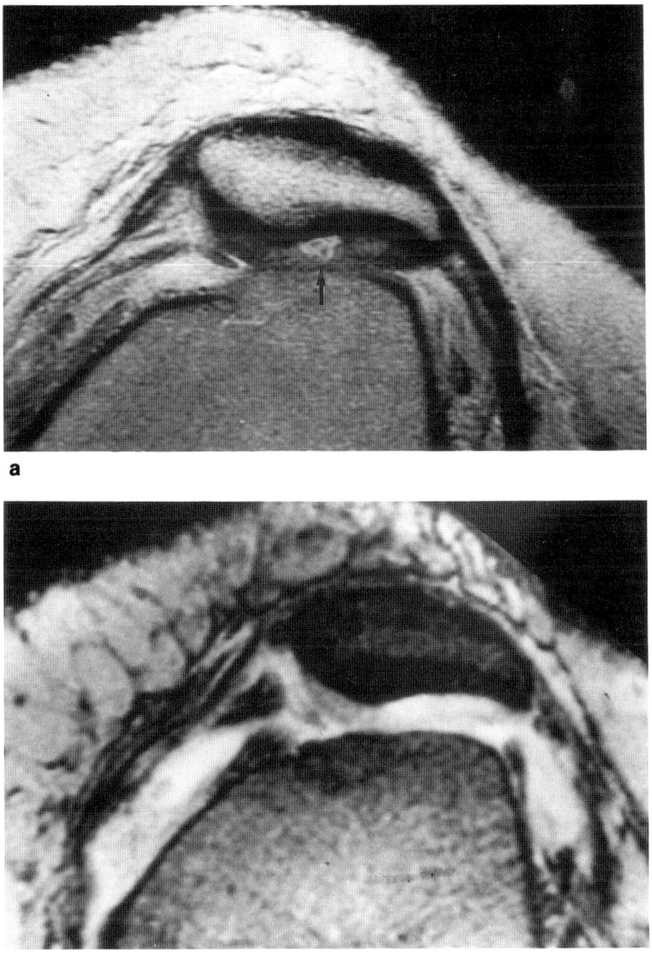

a

b

FIGURE 6.22. Chondromalacia patellae—MRI. Effect of different pulse sequences: (a) axial fast spin echo proton density (TR/TE 5000/19) image and (b) axial gradient echo (TR/TE 500/16) image. There is a large focus of increased signal intensity in the articular cartilage of the lateral facet, extending down to the subchondral bone. The abnormality is more clearly visualized on the fast spin echo image. Lack of intra-articular joint fluid limits evaluation of the chondral surface contour.

TABLE 6.1. The Shahriaree arthroscopic grading system for chondromalacia patellae and the corresponding theoretical MRI findings.

Shahriaree arthroscopic stage	Theoretical MRI findings
I. Softening and "swelling" of articular cartilage	Focal signal intensity changes without contour deformity
II. Blistering of cartilage with intact surface	Focal signal intensity change and contour bulge
III. Surface irregularity/ulceration/fibrillation (not extending down to the bone)	Focal signal intensity change, contour irregularities, cartilage thinning, and fluid extension into cartilage
IV. Similar to stage III but the ulceration extends to the subchondral bone (± subchondral bony changes)	Similar to stage III with defects extending to the cortical bone (± subchondral bony changes)

Adapted from Brown and Quinn.[79]

maceutical (most commonly technetium 99m methylene diphosphonate) is injected intravenously and the skeleton is imaged using a gamma camera. Osseous activity is proportional to the rate of bone turnover/remodeling and regional blood flow. Therefore, any conditions that increase either of these parameters, such as trauma, infection, neoplasm, and arthritis, will increase uptake of the agent, causing these areas to appear "hot." Many pa-

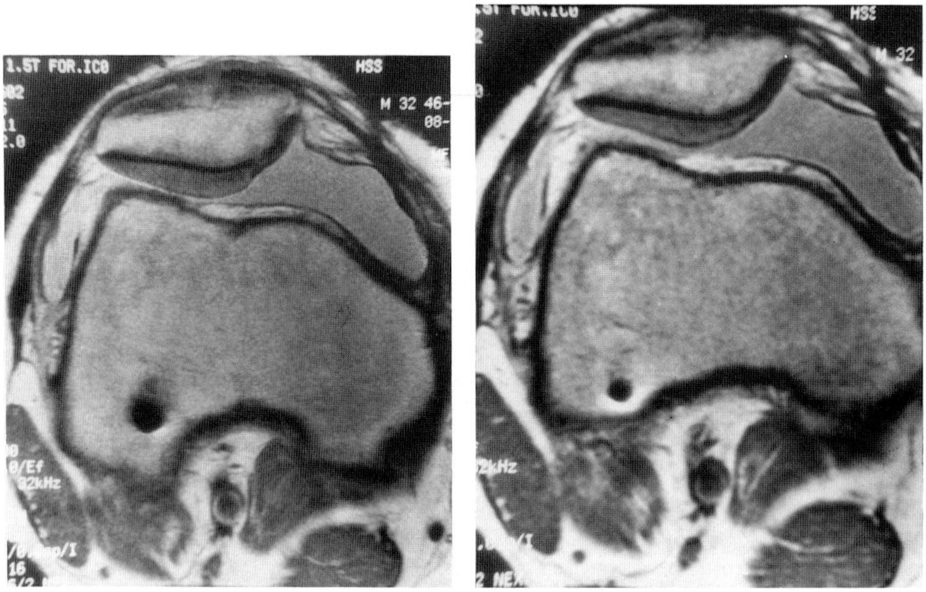

a b

FIGURE 6.23. Chondromalacia patellae—MRI. Effect of different matrix sizes: fast spin echo proton density (TR/TE 4000/19) axial images through the patellofemoral joint (a) matrix size 512 × 256 (2 NEX) and (b) matrix size 256 × 192 (2 NEX). Contour irregularity over the medial facet is better appreciated on the high-resolution image (b). Note that the true apex of the articular cartilage does not correspond to the apex of subchondral bone, which is measured on radiographs.

tients with anterior knee pain will have increased uptake in the knee[48]; however, the exact cause or chronicity of the abnormality cannot be established. Because of the inherent poor specificity of this study and its relatively poor spatial resolution, this technique is of limited use for examining the patellofemoral joint. Although the technique is highly sensitive for subtle osseous pathology (e.g., stress fractures) that may be occult on plain radiographs, other imaging modalities such as CT or MRI are invariably needed for clarification of scintigraphic abnormalities and offer superior anatomic detail.

The primary utility of the bone scan is in its ability to provide physiologic information regarding regional osseous metabolism. Such information can conceivably be used to clarify equivocal abnormalities detected on other imaging modalities; however, in our experience, it is rarely indicated for evaluation of patellofemoral disease. Other nuclear imaging techniques such as Indium-111 labeled leukocyte scans and Gallium-67 citrate scanning are more inflammation-specific and may be useful in cases of suspected infection.

MRI

MRI continues to play an ever increasing crucial role in the evaluation of musculoskeletal disorders. This modality offers the advantages of multiplanar imaging capabilities, noninvasiveness, lack of ionizing radiation, superior soft-tissue contrast, and improved specificity in characterizing pathologic processes based on signal characteristics. In addition, MRI offers superior sensitivity for detection of some pathologic tissue changes that are often occult on other imaging modalities[49]; radiographically occult bone contusion, stress fracture, and early osteonecrosis are often readily detected on MRI.

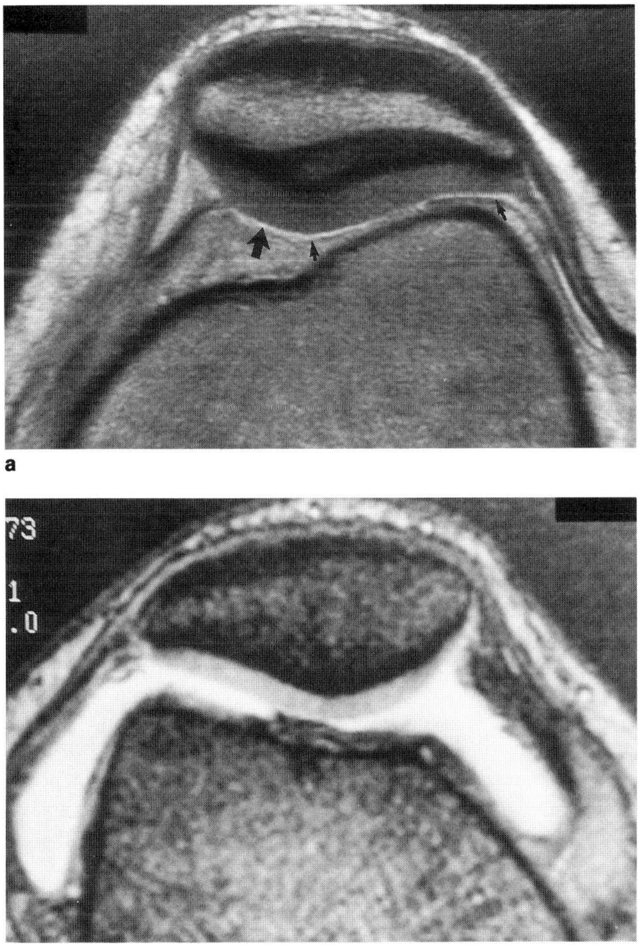

a

b

FIGURE 6.24. Patella articular cartilage—MRI. Evaluation of articular cartilage contour in two different patients is facilitated by (a) a small amount of joint fluid (arrows) and (b) moderate effusion. (Compare with Figure 6.22.)

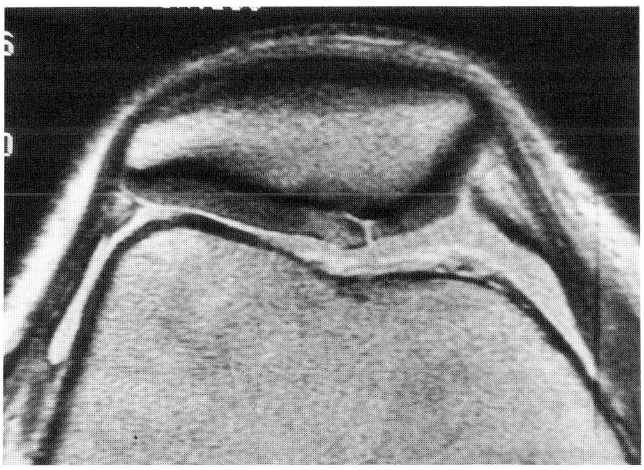

FIGURE 6.25. Advanced chondromalacia patellae—MRI. Axial fast spin echo proton density (TR/TE 5000/19) image through the patella. There is abnormal signal and fissuring involving articular cartilage over the patella apex. There is extension to and early involvement of subchondral bone.

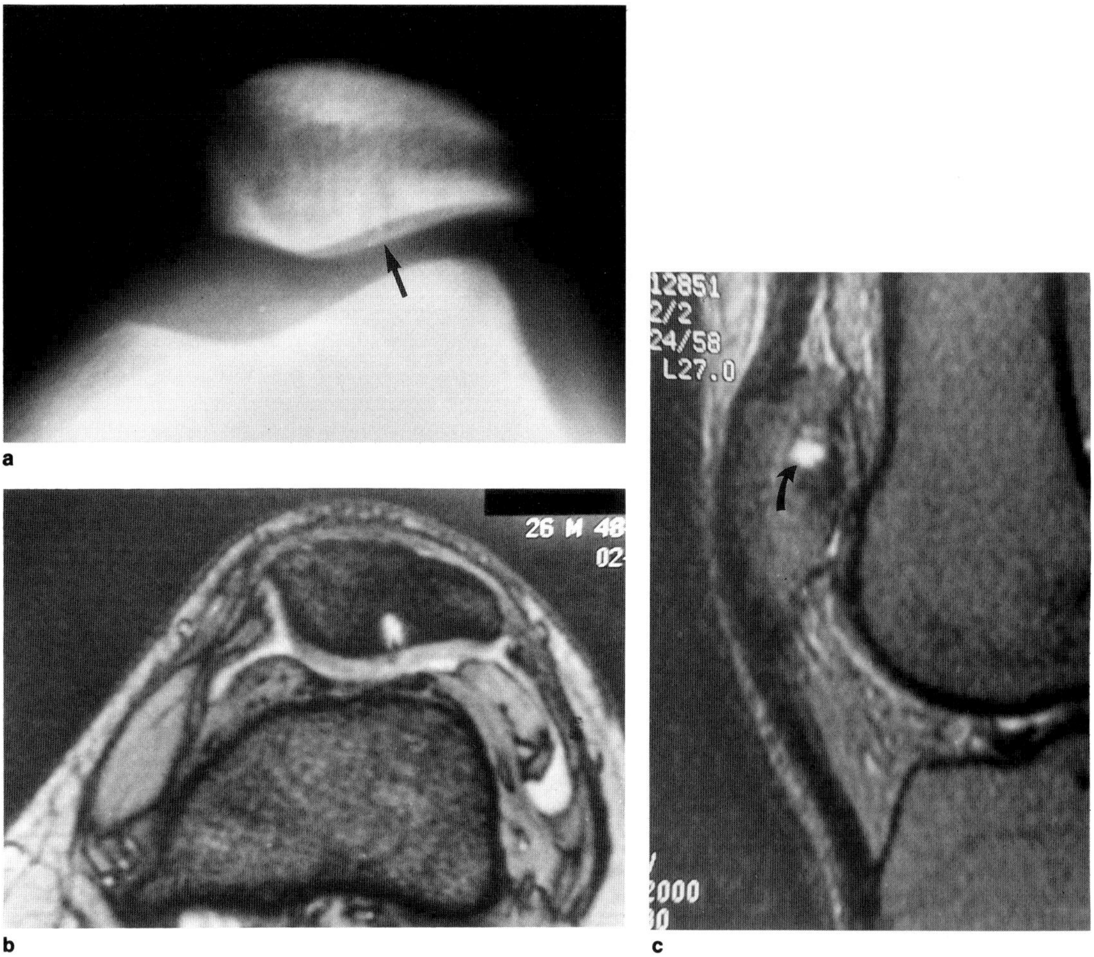

FIGURE 6.26. Advanced chondromalacia patellae. (a) Merchant view shows subtle lucency in the subchondral bone of the lateral facet (arrow), (b) axial, and (c) sagittal T_2-weighted images demonstrate a focal chondral defect and associated subchondral cystic changes in the lateral facet (arrow).

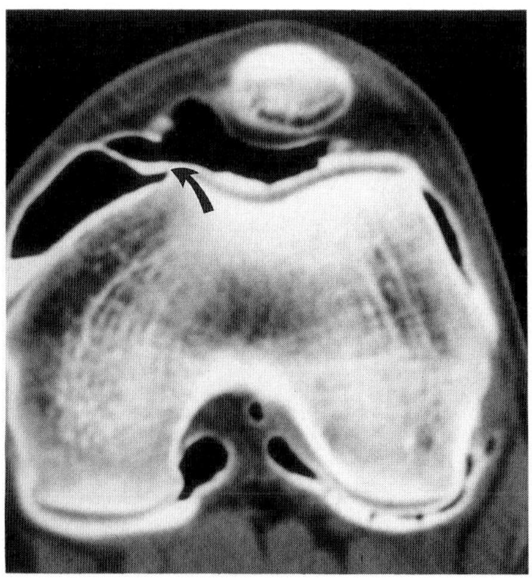

FIGURE 6.27. Synovial plicae. Double-contrast CT arthrogram. There is a normal thin medial plica with contrast pooling near its femoral attachment (arrow).

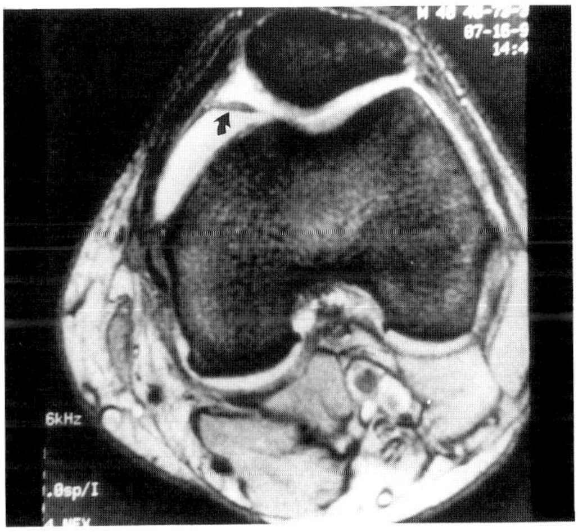

FIGURE 6.28. Plica syndrome. Axial gradient echo (TR/TE 400/16) MRI demonstrates a thickened medial plica (arrow), well delineated against the surrounding synovial fluid. There is concomitant chondromalacia of the medial patella facet.

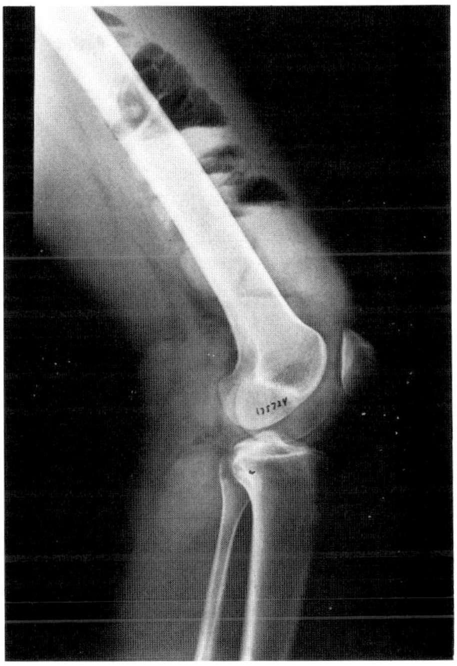

FIGURE 6.29. Pigmented villonodular synovitis. Double-contrast arthrogram demonstrates marked enlargement of the suprapatellar pouch. Joint aspiration yielded a large amount of brown fluid. The numerous septa and corrugated contour was secondary to multiple foci of nodular pathologic synovium.

MRI is particularly useful in the knee for assessment of internal derangement. Conventional spin echo proton density and T_2-weighted images demonstrate the cruciate ligaments, menisci, and collateral ligaments with a high degree of resolution. Fat suppression techniques, whereby the bright signal from marrow fat is suppressed, has facilitated detection of the presence and the extent of abnormal signal from intramedullary processes such as edema, hemorrhage, and infiltrative diseases. Other pulse sequences such as gradient echo imaging are employed for definition of articular cartilage abnormalities such as chondromalacia.

Regarding the patellofemoral joint, MRI offers excellent definition of the extensor mechanism and supporting structures, including the patella, quadriceps, patella tendons, articular cartilage, adjacent bursae, and supporting retinacular structures (Figure 6.18). Contraindications to MRI are few and include cardiac pacemakers, certain types of cardiac prosthetic valves, cochlear implants, and metallic cerebral aneurysm clips. Conventional MRI techniques are limited by metallic orthopedic hardware, including joint prostheses, and metallic plates and screws. However, the advent of fast spin echo imaging permits improved visualization of bone and surrounding soft-tissue structures in such patients, owing to diminished magnetic susceptibility.

Patellofemoral Tracking

As described earlier in this chapter, static assessment of patellofemoral alignment and quantitative measurement of several parameters can be made on conventional tangential radiographs (Figure 6.19).[25,26,50–53] However, the axial views of Merchant and Laurin, on which the measurements are typically made, assess patellofemoral relationships in 45° and 20° of flexion, respectively. Unfortunately, adequate assessment of patellofemoral tracking by these methods is limited by difficulty in consistent positioning on the tangential views and occasional superimposition of important structures such as the patella and the femoral

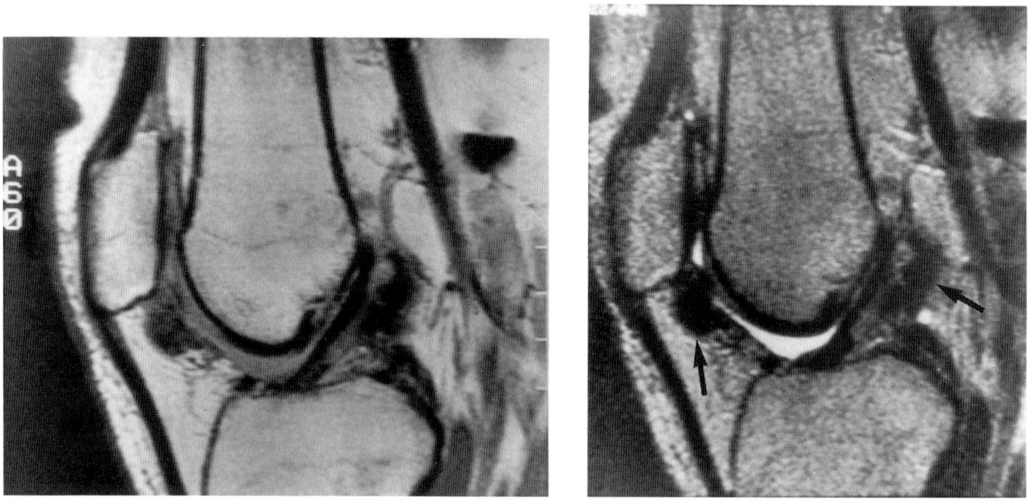

a b

FIGURE 6.30. Pigmented villonodular synovitis. (a) Proton density (TR/TE 2300/20) and (b) T_2-weighted (TR/TE 2300/80) sagittal MRI. There are multiple foci of diminished signal intensity on the proton density images that decrease in intensity with T_2-weighting (arrows). Note the normal increased signal intensity of joint fluid on the T_2-weighted image.

trochlear groove. In addition, and perhaps most importantly, it is imperative to image the patellofemoral joint in the first 30° of flexion,[26,51] where patella malalignment may be maximal. With increasing degrees of flexion, the patella is drawn caudally into the center of the femoral trochlear groove, which may completely or partially reduce a subluxing patella (Figure 6.20). Clearly, assessment of patellofemoral tracking by conventional axial radiographs alone is of limited sensitivity for detection of patella malalignment; imaging by these techniques alone may incorrectly label as "normal" a symptomatic patient with mild patellofemoral malalignment.

Further information regarding patellofemoral tracking may be provided by CT[31,52–54] and MRI.[55–60] These methods have been studied using both static and dynamic imaging. On static imaging, axial sections are obtained through the patellofemoral joint in incremental increased degrees of flexion. With dynamic scanning, axial images are obtained through active or passive flexion and computer software is used to construct a cine loop.

CT and MRI have the distinct advantage of evaluating the patellofemoral joint during the initial degrees of flexion. Incremental or kinematic axial images can demonstrate the degree of flexion where patella malalignment is maximal and assess whether or not it reduces. Static CT images through the patellofemoral joint in varying degrees of flexion (0°, 15° 30°, and 45°) readily demonstrate the degree of patella tilt or subluxation[61,62]; the parameters normally measured on the Merchant view can be similarly assessed. MRI offers the additional advantage of imaging the supporting structures and surrounding soft tissues of the patellofemoral joint such as the retinacula, cartilage, and quadriceps and patella tendons, which are also important in patellofemoral tracking.

Cine video (kinematic) analysis of patellofemoral alignment, obtained through a range of motion (0° to 90° on CT, 0° to 30° on MRI) provides qualitative information on patellofemoral relationships.[54–62] This can be a useful clinical adjunct to the usual quantitative parameters that are obtained. However, special-

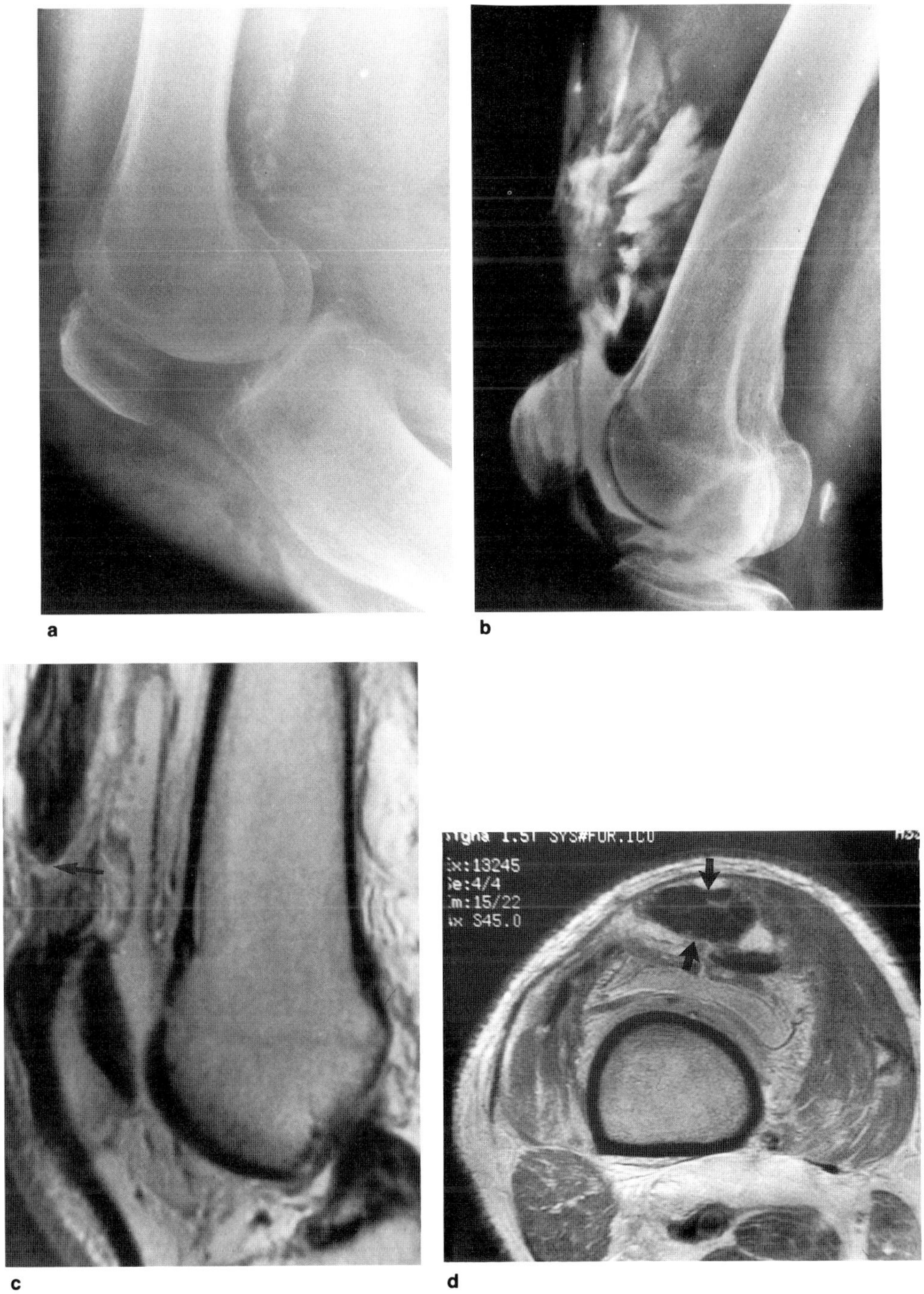

FIGURE 6.31. Quadriceps tendon tear. (a) Lateral plain film shows patella baja and poor definition of the distal quadriceps tendon. There is subcutaneous soft-tissue swelling in the infrapatellar region. (b) Arthrogram (different patient) demonstrates contrast extension through the tear into the regional soft tissues and the quadriceps muscle. (c) Sagittal and (d) axial fast spin echo proton density (TR/TE 2300/20) MRI demonstrates a complete tear. The retracted enlarged free tendon edge is seen superior to the patella (arrows), with surrounding edema and hemorrhage around the tendon and in the quadriceps muscle.

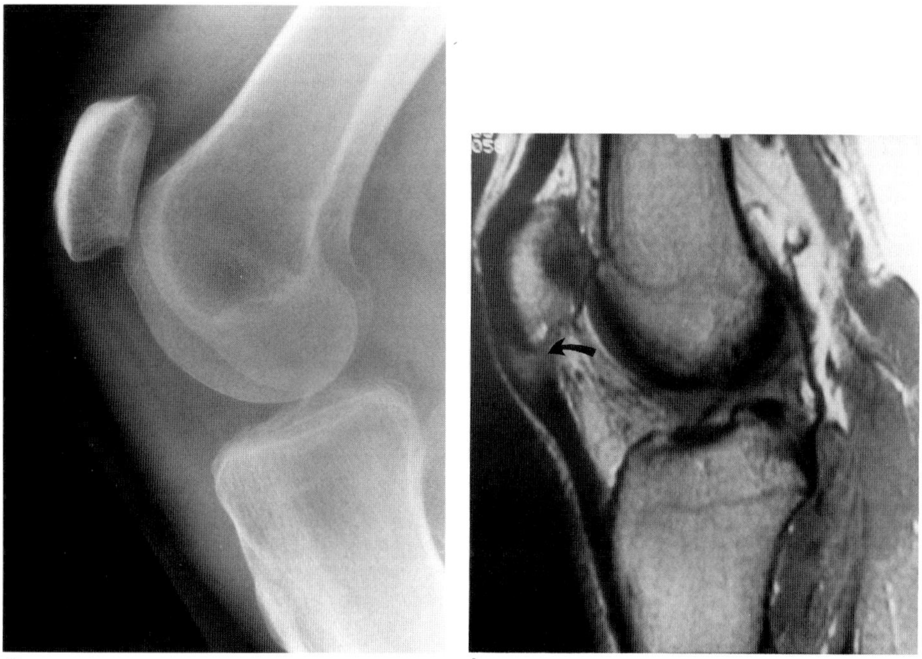

a b

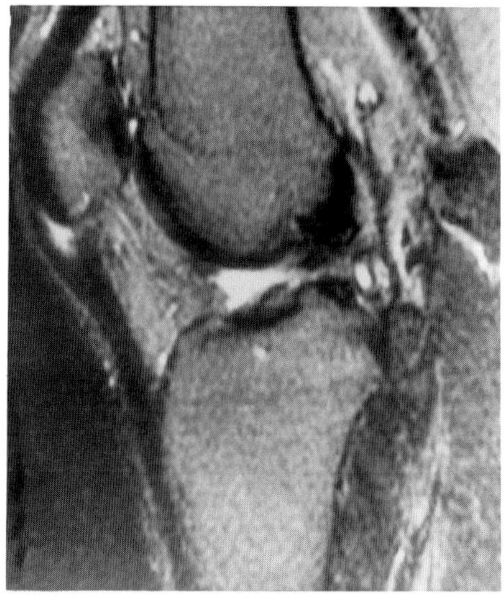

c

FIGURE 6.32. Patella tendon tear. (a) Lateral plain film demonstrates traumatic patella alta in this patient with a complete tear. There is concomitant generalized thickening of the tendon. (b) Sagittal proton density (TR/TE 2000/16) image and (c) T_2-weighted (TR/TE 2000/80) MRI of a different patient demonstrate a focus of abnormal signal in the proximal tendon (arrow), which gets brighter on T_2-weighted images in this patient with traumatic partial patella tendon tear.

ized computer software and positioning devices, as well as increased examination time are necessary for this type of analysis, limiting its availability and feasibility for routine imaging.

Chondromalacia Patellae

The patella articular cartilage is the thickest articular cartilage in the body[63] and it is subject to a variety of degenerative and traumatic disorders. Evaluation of the integrity of this cartilage and that of the femoral trochlear

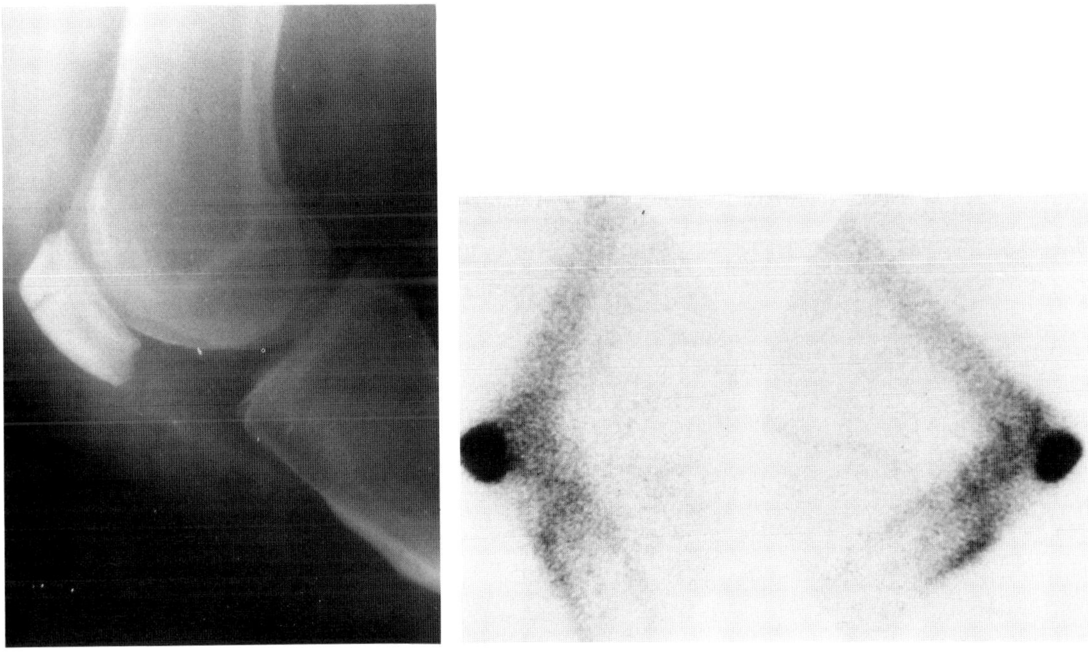

a b

FIGURE 6.33. Bilateral patella stress fractures: young athlete with chronic bilateral anterior knee pain. (a) Lateral view of the right knee shows a fracture of the superior patella. Radiographic examination of the left knee was normal. (b) Bone scan—lateral view of both knees shows bilateral increased activity in the patellae. The patient had bilateral patellar stress fractures, although only one was detected on plain films.

articular surface are important in the evaluation of patellofemoral pain. With the advent of MRI, imaging of articular cartilage has received much attention in the radiology literature.[64–70] Imaging characteristics of chondromalacia patellae (CMP) by the various modalities will be described.

Conventional Radiography

The articular cartilage is indirectly imaged by assessing maintenance of patellofemoral joint space on the lateral and tangential axial views. However, this technique is not specific, as several disorders such as degenerative joint disease and inflammatory arthritis can result in thinning of the articular cartilage. Also, focal cartilage defects or internal cartilage abnormalities with preservation of cartilage thickness and subchondral bone will not be detected, thereby limiting the sensitivity of plain radiography.

CT Arthrography

Findings of CMP on CT arthrography are identical to those of arthrography alone; however, they are seen to much better advantage on cross-sectional techniques. Arthrographic findings reflect the morphologic cartilaginous changes that progress during the natural history of the disease: cartilage edema and swelling progress to ulceration and contour irregularity, which may, in turn, lead to denuded cartilage and exposure of subchondral bone in advanced stages.[71–73] These findings include (in order of increasing severity of disease) articular cartilage contour irregularity ("blistering"), fibrillation ("crab meat" appearance), ulceration and cartilage thinning, and subchondral bony changes.[74,75] These findings may involve the patellar articular cartilage, femoral condylar, or trochlear articular cartilage or both. The important arthrographic sign of CMP for which CT arthrography is highly

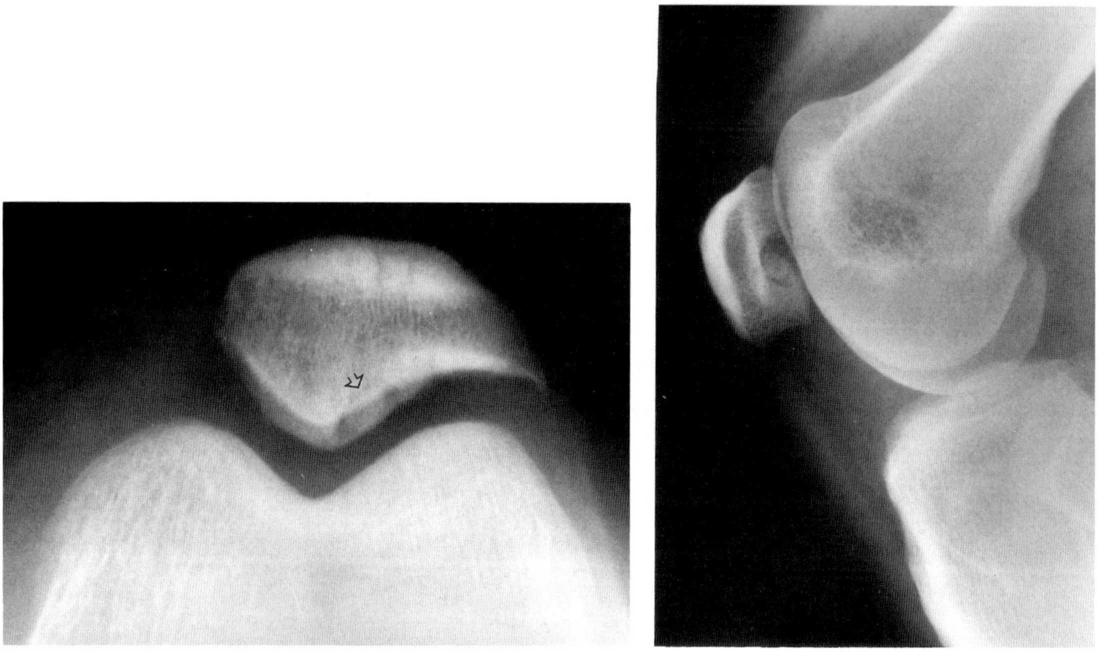

a b

FIGURE 6.34. Osteochondritis dissecans (OCD)—patella. (a) Merchant and (b) lateral views of the patella. There is a focus of OCD involving the lateral facet (arrow). The lesion is adjacent to the convexity of the apex, a common site in the patella.

sensitive is contrast imbibition. This is manifested by extension of contrast into the articular cartilage, which may be focal or diffuse. CT arthrography is definitively more sensitive for cartilage irregularity and imbibition of contrast than arthrography alone (Figure 6.21).[53,76,77] As with MRI, advanced stages of CMP are more reliably detected than early cartilage changes (subtle blistering or surface irregularity). Articular cartilage over the femoral condyles and trochlear surfaces can be visualized on CT arthrography (see Figure 6.17); however, the rounded contour of these surfaces limits optimal evaluation, as all axial sections image obliquely, resulting in volume-averaging artifacts.[64]

MRI

MRI not only depicts the integrity of the articular cartilage by defining its thickness, contour, and presence of focal defects, but MRI can also use internal signal changes within the articular cartilage to theoretically detect earlier stages of CMP. Morphologic cartilage changes are similar to those seen on CT arthrography and include contour irregularity, cartilage swelling or thinning, and subchondral bony abnormality. The Shahriaree arthroscopic grading system for CMP[78] and the corresponding theoretic MRI findings have been summarized by Brown and, Quinn[79] (Table 6.1).

Several authors[64,65,80–82] have studied the sensitivity of several different pulse sequences for detection of early and late stages of CMP. Although several imaging sequences have been investigated, including conventional T_1- and T_2-weighted spin echo techniques, gradient echo imaging, and fat suppression, there is no clear consensus as to which is the most reliable. At HSS, the patellofemoral joint is imaged using axial gradient echo (GRE) and high-resolution fast spin echo axial images (Figure 6.22). These are supplemented by the standard dual echo sagittal images. The goal of whichever pulse sequence is chosen is to distinguish subchondral bone from articular cartilage and to demonstrate the smoothness

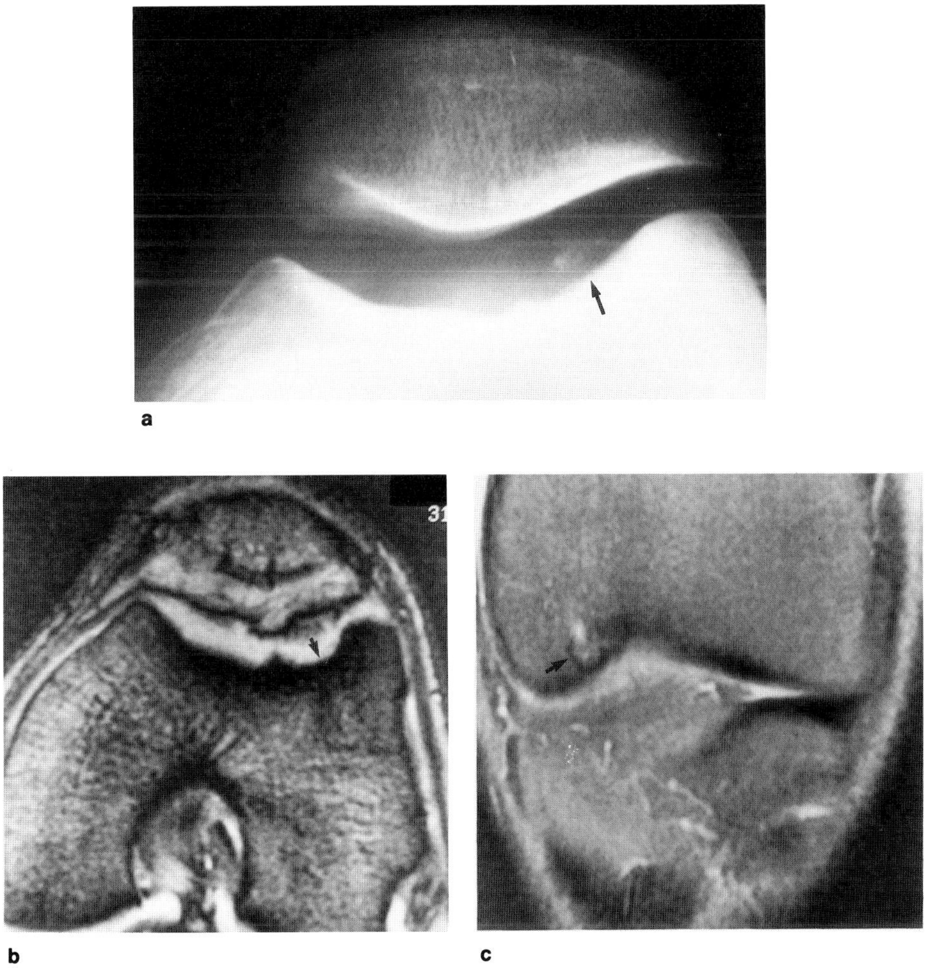

FIGURE 6.35. Osteochondritis dissecans—lateral femoral condyle. (a) Merchant view—there is chondral irregularity and abnormal calcification at the anterior aspect of the lateral femoral condyle within the trochlear sulcus (arrow). (b) Axial gradient echo (TR/TE 4000/16) and (c) coronal fast spin-echo proton density (TR/TE 5000/19) MRI with fat suppression demonstrates a chondral defect and subchondral cystic changes with slight separation of the osteochondral fragment (arrows).

in contour of the articular cartilage (Figure 6.23). Examination of the articular cartilage surface may be facilitated if a joint effusion is present, providing high contrast against the intermediate signal articular cartilage (Figure 6.24). Based on this principle, the utility of intra-articular injection of gadopentatate dimeglumine contrast prior to MRI (MRI arthrography) is being investigated in the shoulder and the knee.[83–85]

MRI is sensitive for the detection of advanced CMP (stages III and IV) with a high predictive value (Figures 6.25 and 6.26).[79,80,86] Stages I and II disease are not reliably evaluated,[68,79–81,86] as signal alterations and surface blistering may not be apparent on MRI and, when seen, these changes do not reliably correlate with cartilage disease. Interpretation of abnormal internal signal within articular cartilage is often subjective and is subject to interobserver variability, much as arthroscopic detection and diagnosis of early CMP is.

In summary, MRI detection and characterization of CMP based on morphologic criteria,

FIGURE 6.36. Osteochondritis dissecans (OCD)—medial femoral condyle. (a) Fast spin echo proton density (TR/TE 5000/17) sagittal MRI with fat suppression. There is an osteochondral defect at the weight-bearing surface of the medial femoral condyle. This represents OCD in situ, with surrounding joint fluid indicating that the fragment is unstable. (b) Coronal image (same parameters) demonstrates an additional loose intra-articular osteochondral fragment in the medial recess of the joint (arrow), from the same donor site.

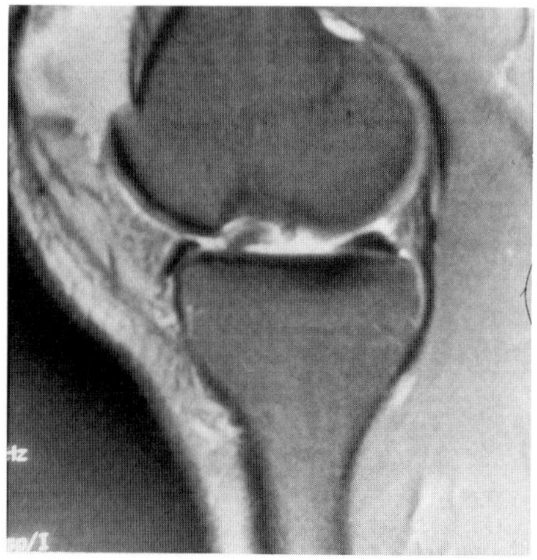

a

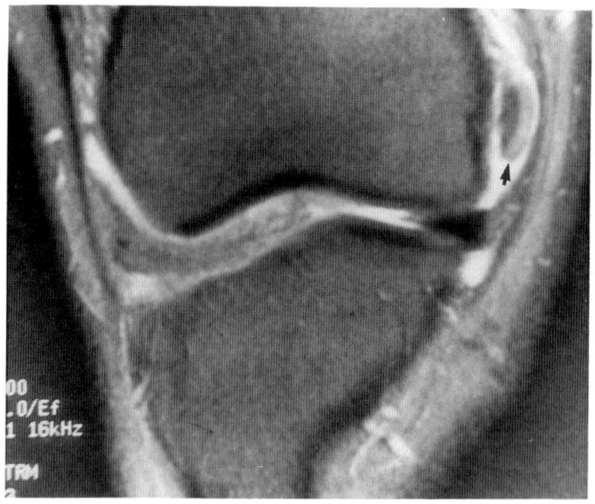

b

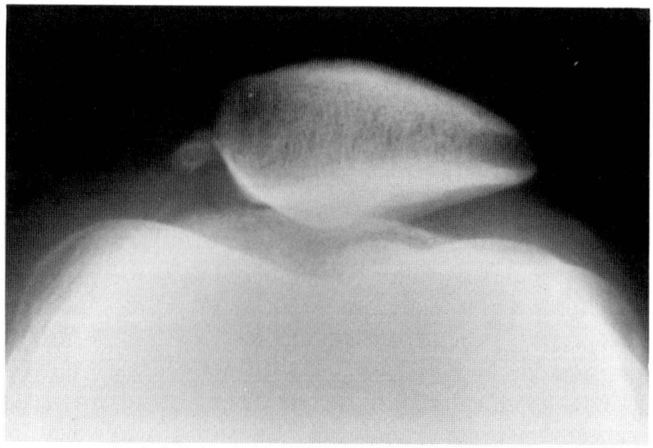

FIGURE 6.37. Traumatic lateral patellar dislocation. There is a well-corticated fracture fragment at the medial margin of the patella. The patella spontaneously reduced prior to presentation.

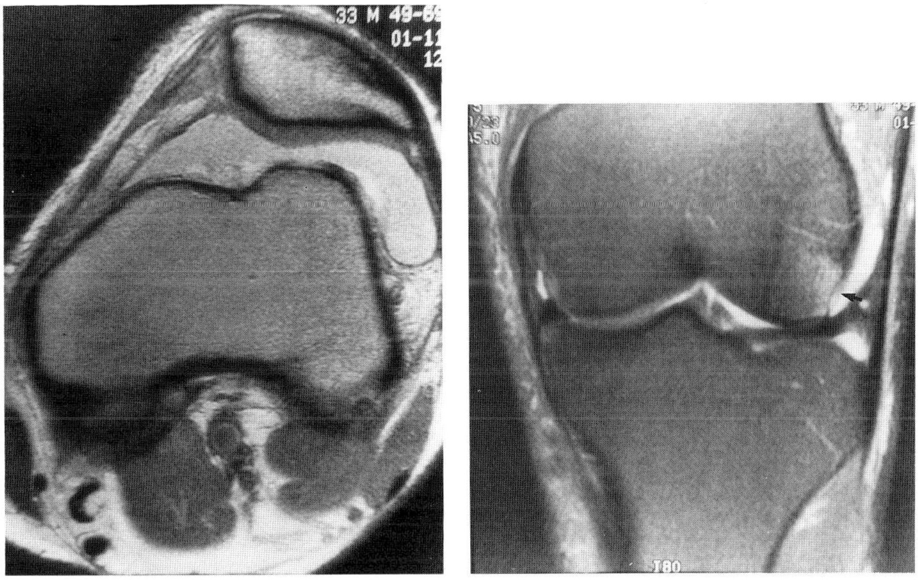

a b

FIGURE 6.38. Lateral patellar dislocation. (a) Axial fast spin echo proton density MRI. There is residual lateral patellar subluxation with disruption of the medial retinaculum (compare with the normal low-signal-intensity lateral retinaculum). (b) Coronal fast spin echo proton density (TR/TE 4500/18) MRI with fat suppression. Abnormal increased signal intensity in the lateral femoral condyle consistent with characteristic bone bruise (arrow).

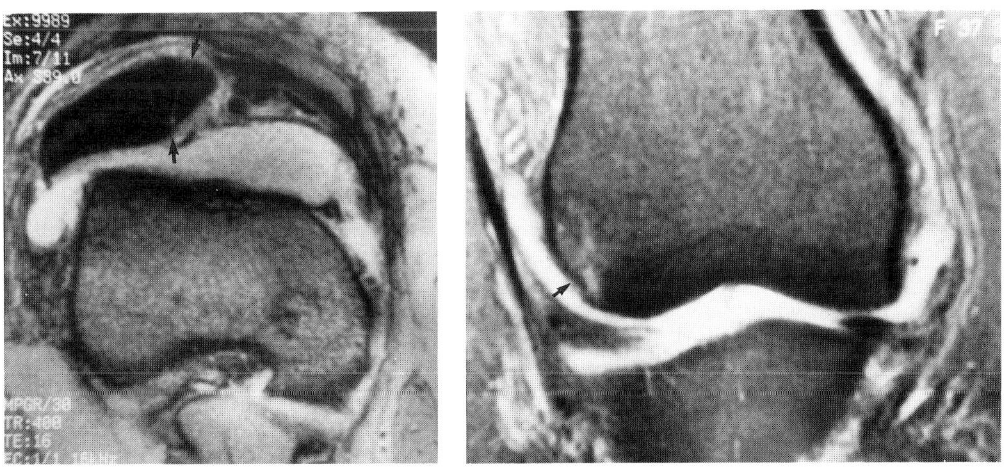

a b

FIGURE 6.39. Lateral patella dislocation. (a) Axial gradient echo (TR/TE 400/16) and (b) coronal fast spin echo proton density MRI with fat suppression. Strikingly similar findings to the patient in Figure 6.38 are seen, including medial retinacular disruption and bone contusion of the lateral femoral condyle (arrow in b). This patient also sustained a fracture of the medial patella, faintly seen as a line of increased signal intensity (arrows in a).

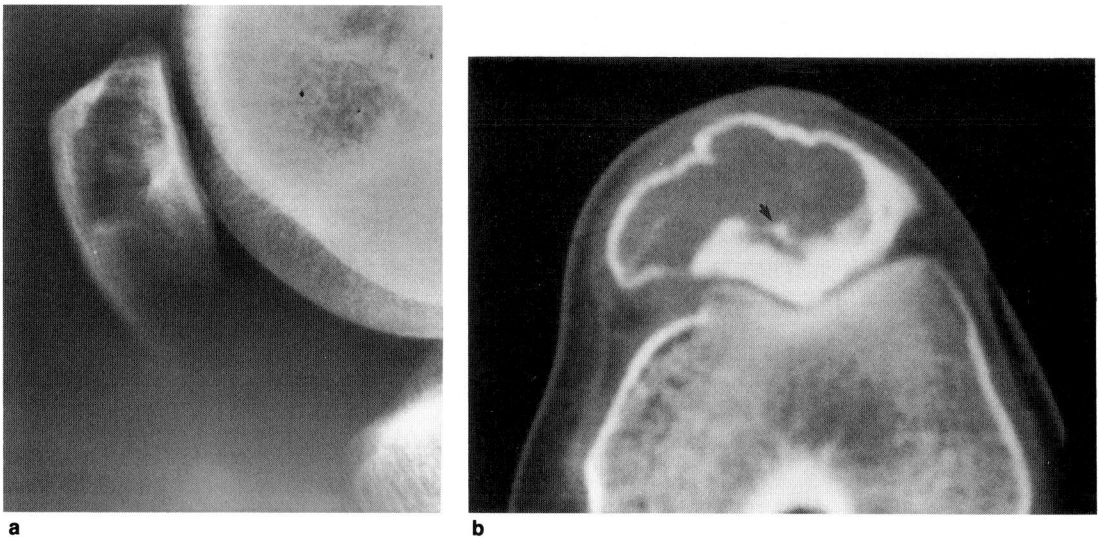

FIGURE 6.40. Chondroblastoma. (a) Lateral view of the patella. There is a lytic lesion involving the upper half of the patella, with a suggestion of central calcification. (b) Axial unenhanced CT scan. The tumor involves the majority of the cross section of the patella. Intralesional chondroid calcification is seen (arrow).

such as surface "blisters" and cartilage fibrillation, contour irregularity, and ulceration, have proved to be highly sensitive and reliable. However, diagnosis of early (stage I) disease based on internal signal changes cannot be made reliably because of limitations in specificity and a high incidence of false-positive examinations.[68] As reported in a correlative study by Handelberg et al.,[68] sensitivity for detection of CMP by MRI has been high (up to 100%), with an overall accuracy of over 80%. Specificity is limited to approximately 50%, largely owing to the inclusion of the less clinically significant stage I disease.

Synovial Disease

Synovial Plicae

Synovial plicae are embryologic remnants of synovial tissue that originally divided the knee into three compartments. Plicae normally exist as thin folds, which may be complete or incomplete, and are commonly asymptomatic. The three most commonly encountered plicae are (1) the infrapatellar, (2) the suprapatellar, and (3) the medial patellar, in decreasing order of frequency.[87,88] Plicae syndrome is characterized by abnormal thickening of these normally thin, pliable folds, resulting in nonspecific symptoms that often mimic meniscal or articular pathology. Of the three plicae, the medial patellar plica ("shelf") is the one classically implicated in this syndrome.

Plicae are readily demonstrated on double-contrast arthrography.[89–91] The suprapatellar plica is best seen on a lateral projection. Because of their orientation, the medial and infrapatellar plicae are more difficult to examine on conventional arthrography. CT arthrography is ideal for examination of patients with plica syndrome, as the medial patella plica, which is usually oriented in the coronal plane, is easily seen on axial CT images (Figure 6.27). In addition, the articular cartilage of the patella can be assessed for CMP, which is not uncommonly seen in patients with plicae syndrome. Indeed, Hodge et al. found that 29% of patients with plica syndrome had associated moderate to severe CMP.[92]

CT arthrography consistently demonstrates plicae whether or not there is associated joint effusion, unlike MRI, where evaluation of pli-

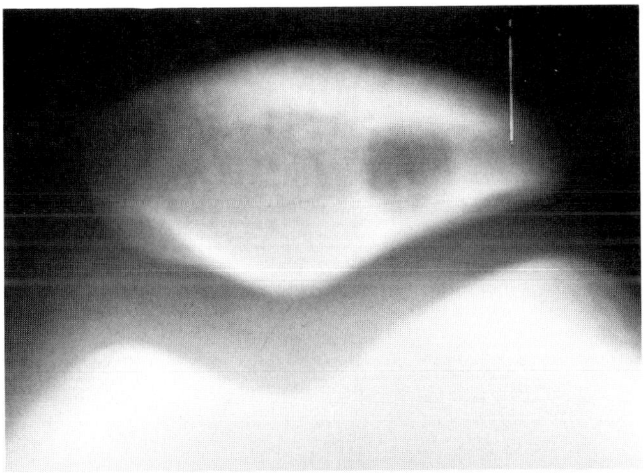

FIGURE 6.41. Hemangioma—Merchant view. There is a well-circumscribed, rounded lytic lesion in the lateral patella. The lesion was "hot" on the bone scan.

cae is limited if a joint effusion is not present. However, in the presence of joint fluid, excellent contrast resolution and anatomic definition of plicae are provided on MRI (Figure 6.28). Also, other pathologic processes in the knee that may be implicated in patients with symptoms of plica syndrome may be detected by this modality.

Pigmented Villonodular Synovitis

Pigmented villonodular synovitis (PVNS) most commonly occurs in the knee joint and can be suggested by conventional radiographic findings by virtue of its variable pressure erosive effect on the adjacent bones. In the knee, however, where the joint cavity is relatively capacious, pressure erosions are rarely seen. The infrequency of bony changes in the knee and the absence of calcifications in these lesions limits the utility of conventional radiographs in diagnosis. The nodular synovium can be demonstrated on arthrography as multiple lucent-filling defects with irregular nodular thickening of the synovium (Figure 6.29);[74,93] this, combined with a hemorrhagic joint aspirate, strongly suggests the correct diagnosis. While a presumptive diagnosis can be made on arthrography, MRI can definitively diagnose this condition by virtue of its signal characteristics. Specifically, the hemosiderin, which is typically contained in these hemorrhagic lesions, results in low signal intensity masses on both T_1- and T_2-weighted sequences (Figure 6.30).[93,94]

Injuries to the Extensor Mechanism of the Knee

The extensor mechanism of the knee is composed of the quadriceps muscle and the tendon, the patella, and the patella tendon. Injury to the extensor mechanism occurs by forced flexion of the knee against a contracted quadriceps mechanism, and results in loss of extensor function.

Quadriceps Tendon Tear

The quadriceps tendon is a multilayered structure composed of the following four muscles: (1) vastus intermedius, (2) vastus lateralis, (3) vastus medialis, and (4) rectus femoris, which all converge above the patella to form the quadriceps tendon and insert on the superior patella. The tendon has a trilaminar structure, with the rectus femoris most superficial and the vastus intermedius deepest. The MRI appearance of the normal quadriceps tendon reflects this laminated anatomy, with two to four layers visible 92% of the time.[95]

Quadriceps tendon tears may be partial or complete. The normal tendon does not usually rupture under stress.[96,97] Predisposing factors are often present, including advanced age, ste-

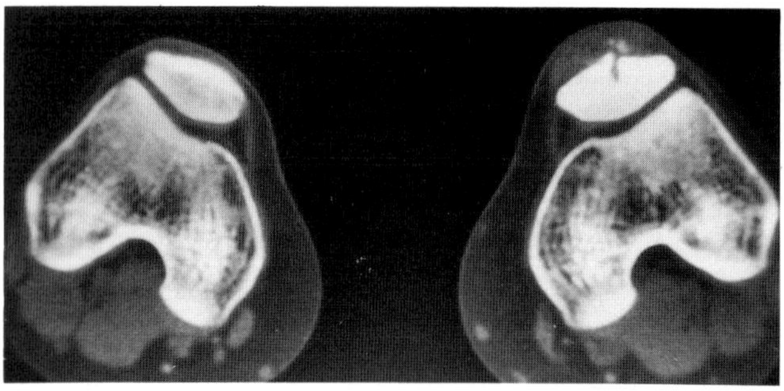

a

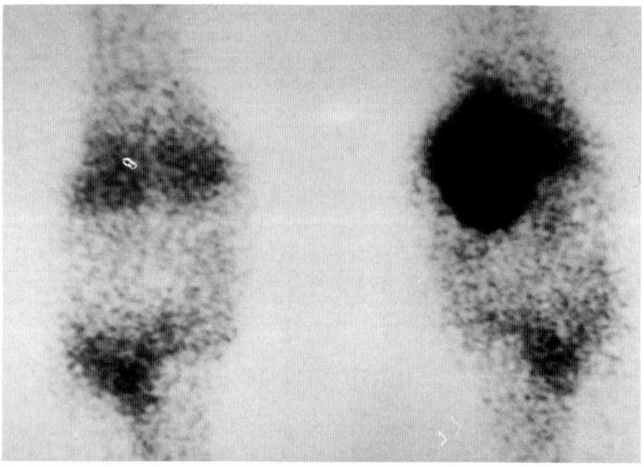

b

FIGURE 6.42. Osteosarcoma. (a) Axial unenhanced CT scan of both knees. The left patella is diffusely sclerotic secondary to extensive neoplastic involvement. The biopsy tract can be seen anteriorly in the patella with associated fragmentation. (b) Bone scan. Frontal view of both knees shows greatly increased activity in the left patella. The right knee is normal for a child.

roid therapy, obesity, systematic lupus erythematosus, diabetes mellitus, and chronic renal failure.[98-100] Rupture most commonly occurs at the teno-osseous junction at the superior patella. The diagnosis is usually suspected clinically and confirmed by conventional radiography. Plain film findings of quadriceps tendon rupture are best visualized on a lateral radiograph and include joint effusion (hemarthrosis), suprapatella soft-tissue mass (retracted tendon and muscle), punctate calcifications in the suprapatella region, poor definition of the distal tendon, tendinous discontinuity, and patella baja (Figure 6.31).[100,101] Arthrography has been used in the past to document tendinous disruption; contrast injected into the suprapatella bursa extends through the tear into the quadriceps tendon or anterior soft tissues.[102] MRI can exquisitely define the location and the extent of tendon tears, demonstrating discontinuity of the normally dark tendon, as well as tendinous retraction and degree of separation for complete tears.[81] The integrity of the patella retinaculum can also be depicted on axial images. Partial tendon tears result in intratendinous edema and/or hemorrhage, seen on T_2-weighted axial and sagittal images as a foci of increased signal intensity.

Patella Tendon Injury

Patella Tendinitis

The patella tendon, seen on a lateral conventional radiograph, normally appears fairly uniform in thickness with distinct margins. Patella tendinitis results in thickening of the tendon, with indistinct margins, and soft-tissue infiltration of the adjacent fat pads secondary to associated edema. Radiographic changes are usually absent or subtle early in the disease.[103] Expensive imaging techniques such as MRI are rarely needed, as the diag-

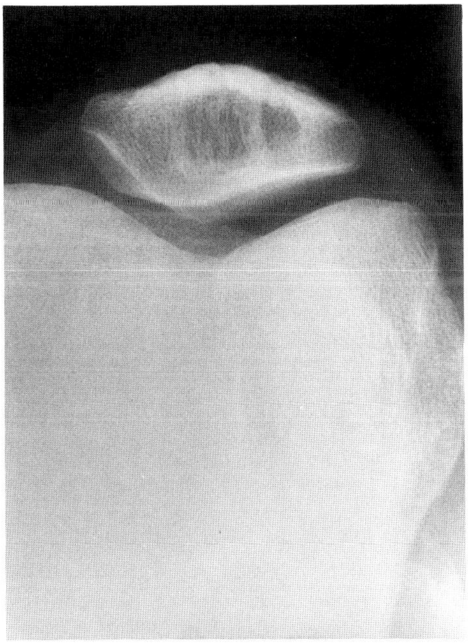

FIGURE 6.43. Gout: Merchant view shows a lytic lesion in the patella in a patient with gouty involvement at other sites in the skeleton.

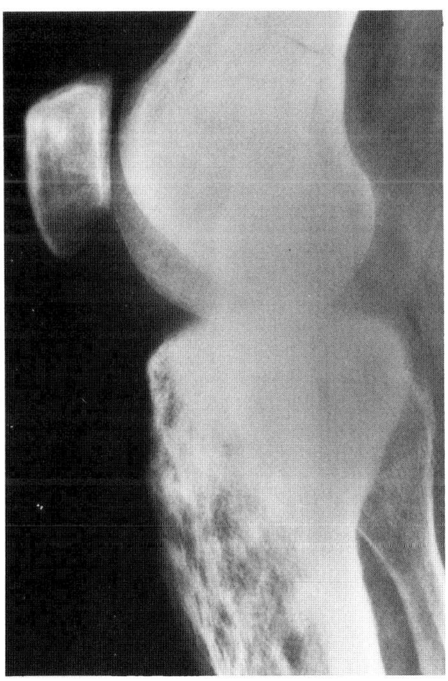

FIGURE 6.44. Paget disease. There is extensive Paget disease involving the proximal tibia manifested by increased density, and cortical and trabecular thickening. Similar findings involve the superior patella.

nosis is typically made clinically. However, in athletes who fail to respond to conservative therapy, or when the diagnosis remains in question, MRI can be used to confirm the presence of disease, assess therapeutic response on followup studies, and judge the severity and the extent of disease when considering surgical intervention.[104] The normal patella tendon appears straight and well defined with homogeneously low signal intensity on MRI. Patella tendinitis results in focal (most commonly proximal) or diffuse thickening of the tendon with abnormal internal signal.[104,105] Of note, normal variation in internal signal of the patella tendon has been described with a V-shaped area of increased intratendinous signal, sometimes seen at the posterior patella attachment of the tendon, and less frequently at its tibial insertion;[104] this should not be mistaken for tendinitis or tendon tear. Thickening of the patella tendon in patella tendinitis has also been described on ultrasound and CT.[106,107] Patella tendinitis may result in increased activity at the inferior pole of the patella on the radionuclide bone scan.[108]

Patella Tendon Tear

Unlike quadriceps tears, which typically occur in older persons or those with predisposing diseases, patella tendon tears are usually seen in younger, active, often athletic patients. This difference is clearly demonstrated by an extensive review of the literature, which found that 80% of quadriceps ruptures occurred in patients older than 40 years of age, while 80% of patella tendon ruptures occurred in those less than 40 years of age.[109] Patella tendon tears are the least common cause of disruption of the extensor mechanism,[101] most commonly seen at the junction of the lower patella with the patella tendon. As with quadriceps tears, patella tendon tears may be partial or complete. On plain films, complete tears result in traumatic patella alta, poor definition of the patella tendon, surrounding soft-tissue edema, and occasionally an avulsion fracture of the lower patella (Figure 6.32). MRI can define the location and extent of injury as a site of dis-

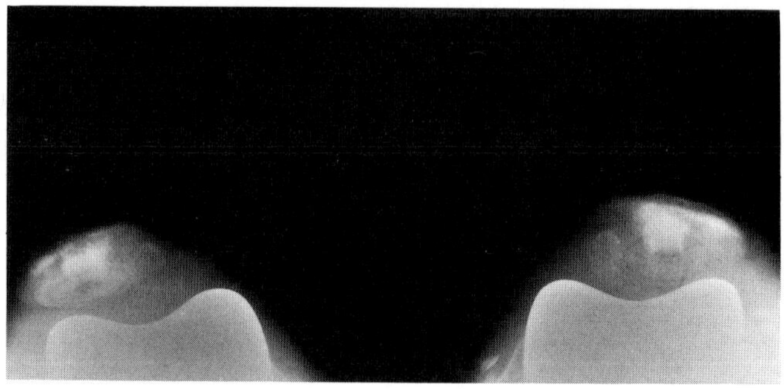

FIGURE 6.45. Bilateral lateral patellar subluxation following arthroplasty. Mild bilateral lateral patellar subluxation (right greater than left) is seen on this Merchant view.

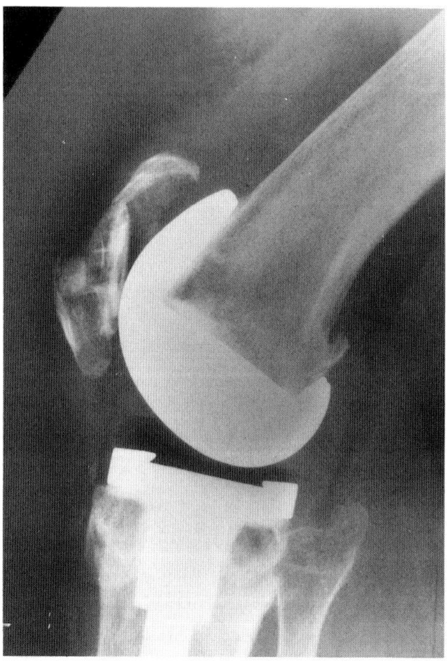

FIGURE 6.46. Patella fracture following arthroplasty. There is a comminuted fracture with superior displacement of the fragments.

continuity of the normally low signal bandlike tendon. Partial tears result in abnormal intratendinous signal, with or without surrounding soft-tissue changes (Figure 6.32).

Patella Fracture

Acute Fracture

Patella fractures comprise approximately 1% of all skeletal injuries[110] and can occur by either direct or indirect trauma.[111] AP and lateral views are usually sufficient in classifying the fracture orientation and degree of displacement (see Figure 6.4). Degree of fracture displacement is dependent on the presence and the extent of associated retinacular disruption; an intact retinaculum can provide continued extensor function and prevent displacement, despite patella fracture.

Stress Fracture

Stress fractures can be divided into the following two groups: (1) fatigue fractures, which occur in normal bone subjected to excessive repetitive activity; and (2) insufficiency fractures, which occur in abnormal bone subjected to the usual degree of physiologic stress. Although stress fractures in the lower extremities are seen most commonly in the metatarsals, tibia, calcaneus, and tarsal navicular, patella stress fractures with and without endoprostheses have been reported (Figure 6.33).[112,113] Conventional radiographs are notoriously insensitive in detecting these injuries.[114] Radionuclide bone scan and MRI are highly sensitive in reflecting the physiologic and anatomic alterations associated with stress fractures at an earlier stage than plain films.[115,116] Stress fractures appear hot on bone scans, owing to increased radionuclide uptake associated with the reparative process. On MRI, stress fractures typically appear as a band of low signal intensity on T_1-weighted images, which is usually perpendicular to the

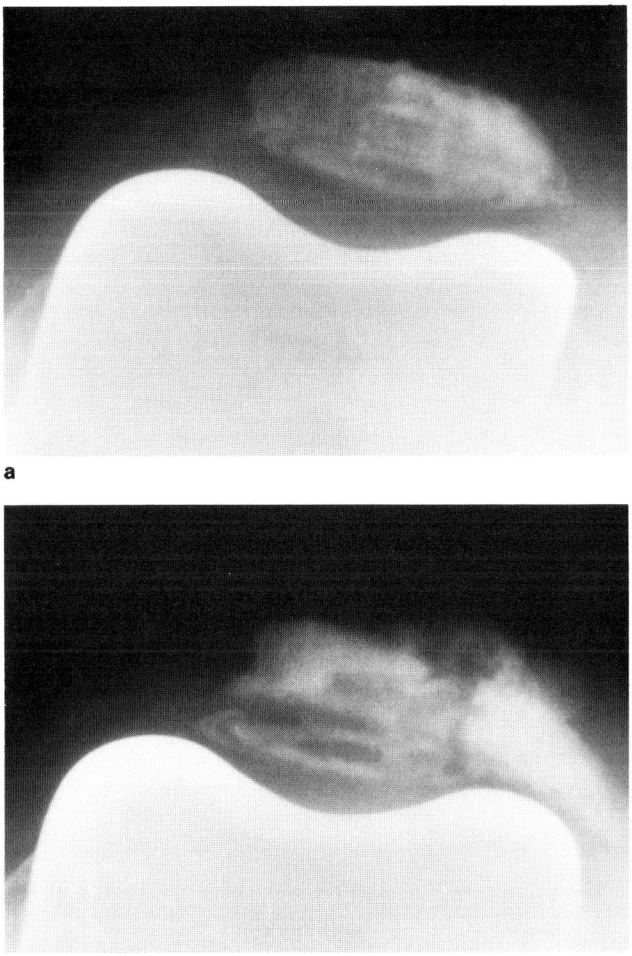

FIGURE 6.47. Patella fracture following arthroplasty. (a) Merchant view of the knee six months after arthroplasty with patella resurfacing shows mild sclerosis of the lateral patella, with the patella appearing intact on all views. (b) Eleven months later there is a fracture of the patella with sclerosis of the lateral fragment, likely secondary to necrosis.

cortex, and appears bright on T_2-weighted sequences.

Osteochondritis Dissecans

In osteochondritis dissecans (OCD), a portion of the articular surface becomes partially or completely separated from the underlying bone. Although the most common site in the knee for this osteochondral injury is the medial femoral condyle (about 85%),[117] the lesion is occasionally seen in the lateral femoral condyle and rarely in the patella (Figures 6.34 through 6.36). OCD has a propensity to affect the convexity of articular surfaces. As such, when the patella is involved, the lesion is often located near the median ridge, most commonly in the medial facet.[118-120] The upper half of the patella and the odd facet are typically spared.[118]

OCD can be readily diagnosed by conventional radiography; however, those lesions that primarily involve articular cartilage with early osseous involvement may be radiographic occult. MRI is valuable in detecting subtle chondral defects and defining the extent of bony involvement. In addition, MRI has also proved useful in determining stability of osteochondral lesions;[120] the sensitivity and specificity for predicting lesion stability is about 92% and 90%, respectively.[121,122]

The following imaging characteristics correlate with lesion instability: size greater than 1 cm, linear or diffuse increased signal intensity beneath the lesion at the donor site, and focal increased activity on radionuclide bone scan.[121,122] The high accuracy of MRI in defining the presence, extent, and stability of osteochondral lesions and the treatment implications of these findings make this the modality of choice for evaluation.

Patella Dislocation

In traumatic dislocation of the patella, the patella typically dislocates laterally and usually relocates prior to clinical presentation. Indeed, most patients are unaware they have had a lateral patellar dislocation[123] and 50% to 75% of patients will not be correctly diagnosed at initial presentation based on clinical and plain film examination.[124,125] Therefore, in a patient with the appropriate clinical history and mechanism of injury, further imaging is often warranted despite an apparently normally located patella on conventional radiographs. Conventional radiographs may demonstrate residual lateral patella tilt or subluxation, large joint effusion (hemarthrosis), or fracture of the medial margin of the patella. This latter sign, best seen on axial views, is an osteochondral injury thought to be pathognomonic of lateral dislocation of the patella (Figure 6.37).[126] It is due to impaction of the medial patella facet against the lateral femoral condyle during dislocation and relocation. MRI is ideal for detecting the soft-tissue and the osteochondral injuries that commonly accompany patella dislocation. Specifically, associated injuries such as medial retinacular and capsular disruption, bone contusion, occult osteochondral injury (medial patella and lateral femoral condyle), loose bodies, and hemarthrosis are well demonstrated (Figures 6.38 and 6.39).[123]

Neoplastic Disease

Although neoplastic involvement of the patella is rare, comprising less than 1% of all primary bone tumors,[127] these lesions typically present with acute or chronic anterior knee pain and should, at least, be considered in the differential diagnosis. Lytic lesions of the patella have a wide differential diagnosis, including neoplasms (primary and secondary) (Figures 6.40 through 6.42), osteomyelitis, brown tumor of hyperparathyroidism, subchondral cyst, and dorsal defect of the patella. The distinct majority of patella tumors are benign,[128] with chondroblastoma and giant cell tumor occurring most commonly;[128,129] followed by simple benign cyst; and aneurysmal bone cyst, osteoblastoma, and hemangioma.[130] The patella is a sesamoid bone and is therefore considered to be an epiphyseal equivalent, explaining the relative frequency of chondroblastoma and giant cell tumor. Unlike other bones, where classic epiphyseal lesions such as giant cell tumor and diametaphyseal lesions such as bone cyst are seen in predictable locations, the patella, by virtue of its embryologic development, has the unique characteristic of being a site where any of a variety of lesions can occur, regardless of their typical site propensity.

Malignant lesions of the patella include lymphoma, angiosarcoma, and metastases. Metastatic involvement of the patella is extremely uncommon, perhaps owing to the relatively poor blood supply to this sesamoid bone.[131] Only a handful of metastases to the patella have been reported,[132] usually in patients with known primary tumors. Patella tumors are typically seen as lytic lesions with well-defined, often sclerotic margins. Margins of malignant patella tumors may be well defined,[133] making this an unreliable sign for assessing malignancy or benignity. Metastatic lesions often demonstrate areas of sclerosis; rapid progression; and occasionally, soft-tissue mass. The radiographic appearance of patella tumors is nonspecific. Biopsies of the lesions are easily done percutaneously, owing to the relatively superficial location of the patella.

Miscellaneous Conditions

The patella can be affected by a variety of local and systemic disease states. In addition to those mentioned previously, infection or arthritis (most commonly osteoarthritis and CPPD) may involve the patella in addition to less commonly seen diseases such as gout (Figure 6.43) and Paget's disease (Figure 6.44).

Prosthesis Failure

Patellofemoral complications comprise a large percentage (up to 50%)[134] of total knee arthroplasty revisions and are seen in up to 9% of arthroplasties.[135] Complications include patella subluxation (Figure 6.45); fracture (Figures 6.46 and 6.47); infection; loosening of the patella component; and less commonly, polyethylene wear of metal-backed patella prosthesis and patella ligament avulsion.[136,137] The Merchant view is crucial in assessing patella position and integrity of the patella prosthesis after total knee arthroplasty. Polyethylene wear is manifested by diminished width of the lucency between the patella component and the adjacent condylar portion of the metallic femoral prosthesis.[138] Displacement of the polyethylene may be seen as a lucent shadow in the knee, usually into the fat pad. Conventional radiography is the most important tool in diagnosing patella prosthetic component failure, making the correct diagnosis about 90% of the time.[136] Clinical history and physical examination are limited in their detection and characterization of complications of patella prosthesis placement.

Conclusion

Several methods of diagnostic imaging techniques are available to the clinician to diagnose patellofemoral disorders, depict their extent, and detect associated abnormalities. Knowledge of the advantages and limitations of these imaging modalities for specific disorders, as well as a systematic approach tailored to the individual patient are important in prompt and accurate diagnosis.

References

1. Pavlov, H: *Radiographic Examination,* in Insall JN, Windsor RE, Scott WN, et al. (eds.): *Surgery of the Knee,* ed. 2. New York: Churchill Livingstone, 1993, pp. 83–110.
2. Altman RD, Fries JF, Bloch DA, et al.: Radiographic assessment of progression of osteoarthritis. *Arthritis Rheum* 1987;30:1214–1225.
3. Carson WG Jr., James SL, Larson RL, et al.: Patellofemoral disorders: Physical and radiographic evaluation. Part II: Radiographic examinations. *Clin Orthop* 1984;185:178–186
4. Macnab I: Recurrent dislocation of the patella. *J Bone Joint Surg Am* 1952:34A:957–967.
5. Brattstrom H: Patella alta in non-dislocating knee joints. *Acta Orthop Scand* 1970;41:578–586.
6. Freeman BL: Recurrent dislocations, in Crenshaw AH (ed.): *Campbell's Operative Orthopedics,* ed. 7. St. Louis, CV Mosby Co., 1987, pp. 2173–2218.
7. Insall J, Aglietti P, Tria AJ Jr.: Patellar pain and incongruence II. Clinical application. *Clin Orthop* 1983;176:225–232.
8. Osgood RB: Lesions of the tibial tubercle occurring during adolescence. *Boston Med Surg J* 1903;148:114–117.
9. Schlatter C: Verletzungen des schnabelörmigen fortsatzes der oberen tibiaepiphyse. *Bruns' Beitr Klin Chir* 1903;38:874–887.
10. Sinding-Larsen C: A hitherto unknown affection of the patella in children. *Acta Radiol* 1921;1:171–179.
11. Johansson S: Eine bisher nicht bescheriebene erkrankung der patella. *Hygica* 1922;84:161–167.
12. Cobby MJ, Schweitzer ME, Resnick D: The deep lateral femoral notch: An indirect sign of a torn anterior cruciate ligament. *J Radiol* 1992;184:855–858.
13. Warren RF, Kaplan N, Bach BR: The lateral notch sign of anterior cruciate ligament insufficiency. *Am J Knee Surg* 1988;1:119–124.
14. Jakob RP, von Gumpenberg S, Engelhardt P: Does Osgood Schlatter disease influence the position of the patella? *J Bone Joint Surg Br* 1981;63B:579–582.
15. Schmidt H, Freyschmidt J, Holthusen W. *Kohler/Zimmer's Borderlands of Normal and Early Pathologic Findings in Skeletal Radiography,* ed. 4. New York, Thieme Medical Publishers, 1993.
16. Newberg A, Wales L: Radiographic diagnosis of quadriceps tendon rupture. *Radiology* 1977;125:367–371.
17. Scuderi C: Ruptures of the quadriceps tendon: Study of 20 tendon ruptures. *Am J Surg* 1958;95:626–634.

18. Blumensaat C: Die lagaebweichungen und verrenkungen der kneischeibe. *Ergeb Chir Orthop* 1938;31:149–223.
19. Insall J, Salvati E: Patella position in the normal knee joint. *Radiology* 1971;101:101–104.
20. Norman O, Egund N, Ekelund L: The vertical position of the patella. *Acta Orthop Scand* 1983; 54:908–913.
21. Blackburne JS, Peel TE: A new method of measuring patellar height. *J Bone Joint Surg Am* 1977;59A:241–242.
22. Caton J, Deschamps G, Chambat P, et al.: Les rotules basses. A propos 128 observations. *Rev Chir Orthop* 1982;68:317.
23. Linclau L: Measuring patellar height. *Acta Orthop Belg* 1984;50:70.
24. Scuderi GR: Radiographic assessment of patellar length, thickness and height. Presented at the American Academy of Orthopaedic Surgeons meeting, Washington DC, 1992.
25. Merchant AC, Mercer RL, Jacobsen RH, et al.: Roentgenographic analysis of patellofemoral congruence. *J Bone Joint Surg Am* 1974;56A: 1391–1396.
26. Laurin CA, Dussault R, Levesque HP: The tangential x-ray investigation of the patellofemoral joint: X-ray technique, diagnostic criteria and their interpretation. *Clin Orthop* 1979;144:16–26.
27. Brattstrom H: Shape of the intercondylar groove normally and in recurrent dislocation of the patella. A clinical and x-ray anatomical investigation. *Acta Orthop Scand* 1964; 68(suppl.):1–138.
28. Aglietti P, Insall JN, Cerulli G: Patellar pain and incongruence. *Clin Orthop* 1983;176:217–223.
29. Shellock FG, Mink JH, Deutsch AL, et al.: Patellar tracking abnormalities: Clinical experience with kinematic MR imaging in 130 patients. *Radiology* 1989;172:799–804.
30. Kujala M, Kormano M, Kujala UM, et al.: Patellofemoral relationships in recurrent patellar dislocation. *J Bone Joint Surg Br* 1989;71B: 788–792.
31. Schutzer SF, Ramsby GR, Fulkerson JP: The evaluation of patellofemoral pain using computed tomography. *Clin Orthop* 1986;204:286–293.
32. Behrman RE, Vaughan VC: *Nelson Textbook of Pediatrics,* ed. 13. Philadelphia, WB Saunders Co., 1987.
33. Sillverman FN. The limbs, in Silverman FN, Kuhn JP (eds.): *Essentials of Caffey's Pediatric X-ray Diagnosis.* Chicago, Year Book Medical Publishers, 1990, pp. 737–1006.
34. Wiberg G: Roentgenographic and anatomic studies on the femoropatellar joint. *Acta Orthop Scand* 1941;12:319–410.
35. Hennsge J. Arthrosis deformans des patella gleitweges. *Zentralbl Chir* 1962;32:1381–1387.
36. Berquist TH: *Imaging of Orthopedic Trauma,* ed. 2. New York, Raven Press, 1991.
37. Ficat RP, Philippe J, Hungerford DS: Chondromalacia patellae: A system of classification. *Clin Orthop* 1979;144:55–62.
38. Goergen TG, Resnick D, Greenway G, et al.: Dorsal defect of the patella: A characteristic radiographic lesion. *Radiology* 1979;130:333–336.
39. Johnson JF, Brogdon BG: Dorsal defect of the patella;incidence and distribution. *AJR* 1982; 138:339–340.
40. van Holsbeeck M, Vandamme B, Marchal G, et al.: Dorsal defect of the patella: Concept of its origin and relationship with bipartite and multipartite patella. *Skeletal Radiol* 1987;16: 304–311.
41. Haswell DM, Berne AS, Graham CB: The dorsal defect of the patella. *Pediatr Radiol* 1976; 4:238–242.
42. Ho VB, Kransdorf MJ, Jelinek JS, et al.: Dorsal defect of the patella: MR features. *J Comput Assist Tomogr* 1991;15:474–476.
43. Duncan JG, Souter WA: Hereditary onycho-osteodysplasia. The nail-patella syndrome. *J Bone Joint Surg Br* 1963;45B:242–258.
44. Rutherford WJ: Hereditary knock-knee with recurrent dislocation of patella and aplasia of nails on fingers and toes. *Br J Children's Dis* 1933;30:34.
45. Kutz ER: Congenital absence of the patellae. *J Pediatr* 1949;34:760–762.
46. Bernhang AM, Levine SA: Familial absence of the patella. *J Bone Joint Surg Am* 1973;55A: 1088–1090.
47. Freiberger RH: Techniques of knee arthrography, in Freiberger RH, Kaye JJ (eds.): *Arthrography.* New York, Appleton-Century-Crofts, 1979, pp. 5–30.
48. Dye SF, Boll DA: Radionuclide imaging of the patellofemoral joint in young adults with anterior knee pain. *Orthop Clin North Am* 1986; 17:249–262.
49. Mink JH, Deutsch AL: Occult cartilage and bone injuries of the knee: Detection, classification and assessment with MR imaging. *Radiology* 1989;170:823–829.
50. Minkoff J, Fein L: The role of radiography in

evaluation and treatment of common anarthrotic disorders of the patellofemoral joint. *Clin Sports Med* 1989;8:203.
51. Fulkerson JP, Hungerford DS: *Disorders of the Patellofemoral Joint,* ed. 2. Baltimore: Williams & Wilkins Co., 1990.
52. Delgado-Martins H: A study of the position of the patella using computerized tomography. *J Bone Joint Surg Br* 1979;61B:442–444.
53. Boven F, Bellemans M, Geurts J, et al.: A comparative study of the patellofemoral joint on axial roentgenograms, axial arthrograms and computed tomography following arthrography. *Skeletal Radiol* 1982;8:183–185.
54. Stanford W, Phelan J, Kathol MH, et al.: Patellofemoral joint motion: Evaluation by ultrafast computed tomography. *Skeletal Radiol* 1988;17:487–492.
55. Shellock FG: Patellofemoral joint abnormalities in athletes: Evaluation by kinematic magnetic resonance imaging. *Top Magn Reson Imaging* 1991;3:71–95.
56. Shellock FG, Mink JH, Deutsch AL, et al.: Patellar tracking abnormalities: Clinical experience with kinematic MR imaging in 130 patients. *Radiology* 1989;172:799–804.
57. Shellock FG, Mink JH, Deutsch AL, et al.: Kinematic MR imaging of the patellofemoral joint: Comparison of passive positioning and active movement techniques. *Radiology* 1992; 184: 574–577.
58. Brossman J, Muhle C, Büll CC, et al.: Evaluation of patellar tracking in patients with suspected patellar malalignment: Cine MR imaging vs arthroscopy. *AJR* 1994;162:361–367.
59. Brossman J, Muhle C, Schröder C, et al.: Patellar tracking patterns during active and passive knee extension: Evaluation with motion-triggered cine MR imaging. *Radiology* 1993; 187:205–212.
60. Kujala VM, Osterman K, Kormano M, et al.: Patellar motion analyzed by magnetic resonance imaging. *Acta Orthop Scand* 1989;60:13–16.
61. Haas SB, Scuderi GR: Examination and radiographic assessment of the femoropatellar joint. *Semin Orthop* 1990;5:108–114.
62. Ghelman B, Hodge JC: Imaging of the patellofemoral joint. *Orthop Clin North Am* 1992; 23:523–543.
63. Hall FM, Wyshak G: Thickness of articular cartilage in the normal knee. *J Bone Joint Surg Am* 1980;62A:408–413.
64. Hayes CW, Conway WF: Evaluation of articular cartilage: Radiographic and cross-sectional imaging techniques. *Radiographics* 1992; 12: 409–428.
65. Conway WF, Hayes CU, Loughran T, et al.: Cross-sectional imaging of the patellofemoral joint and surrounding structures. *Radiographics* 1991;11:195–217.
66. Modl JM, Scth LA, Haughton VM, ct al.: Articular cartilage: Correlation of histologic zones with signal intensity at MR imaging. *Radiology* 1991;181:853–855.
67. Lehner KB, Rechl HP, Gmeinwieser JK, et al.: Structure, function and degeneration of bovine articular cartilage: Assessment with MR imaging in vitro. *Radiology* 1989;170:495–499.
68. Handelberg F, Shahabpour M, Castelyn PP: Chondral lesions of the patella evaluated with computed tomography, magnetic resonance imaging, and arthroscopy. *Arthroscopy* 1990;6: 24–29.
69. Wojtys E, Wilson M, Buchwalter K, et al.: Magnetic resonance imaging of knee hyaline cartilage and intraarticular pathology. *Am J Sports Med* 1987;15:455–463.
70. Hodler J, Bethiaume M, Schweitzer ME, et al.: Knee joint hyaline cartilage defects: A comparative study of MR and anatomic sections. *J Comput Assist Tomogr* 1992;16:597–603.
71. Ficat RP, Phillipe J, Hungerford DS: Chondromalacia patellae: A system of classification. *Clin Orthop* 1979;144:55–62.
72. Insall J, Falvo KA, Wise DW: Chondromalacia patellae: A prospective study. *J Bone Joint Surg Am* 1976;58A:1–8.
73. Goodfellow J, Hungerford DS, Woods C: Patello-femoral joint mechanics and pathology. II. Chondromalacia patella. *J Bone Joint Surg Br* 1976;58B:291–299.
74. Schneider R, Freiberger RH: Extrameniscal abnormalities, in Freiberger RH, Kaye JJ (eds.): *Arthrography.* New York, Appleton-Century-Crofts, 1979, pp. 109–135.
75. Ihara H: Double-contrast CT arthrography of the cartilage of the patellofemoral joint. *Clin Orthop* 1985;198:50–55.
76. Boven F, Bellemans M, Geurts J, et al.: The value of computed tomography scanning in chondromalacia patellae. *Skeletal Radiol* 1982; 8:183–185.
77. Weissman BNW, Sledge C: *Orthopedic Radiology.* Philadelphia, WB Saunders Co., 1986.
78. Shahriaree H: Chondromalacia. *Contemp Orthop* 1985;11:27–39.
79. Brown TR, Quinn SF. Evaluation of chondromalacia of the patellofemoral compartment

with axial magnetic resonance imaging. *Skeletal Radiol* 1993;22:325–328.
80. Yulish BS, Montanez J, Goodfellow DB, et al.: Chondromalacia patella: Assessment with MR imaging. *Radiology* 1987;164:763–766.
81. Deutsch AL, Shellock FG: The extensor mechanism and patellofemoral joint, in Mink JH, Reicher MA, Crues JV Jr III, Deutsch AL (eds.): *MRI of the Knee,* Ed. 2. New York: Raven Press, 1993, pp. 189–236.
82. Konig H, Sauter R, Deimling M, et al.: Cartilage disorders: Comparison of spin-echo, CHESS, and FLASH sequence MR images. *Radiology* 1987;164:753–758.
83. Winalski CS, Aliabadi P, Wright RJ, et al.: Enhancement of joint fluid with intravenously administered gadopentetate dimeglumine: Technique, rationale and implications. *Radiology* 1993;187:179.
84. Engel A. Magnetic resonance knee arthrography: Enhanced contrast by gadolinium complex in the rabbit and in humans. *Acta Orthop Scand* 1990;240(suppl):1–57.
85. Chardnani VP, Ho C, Chu P, et al.: Knee hyaline cartilage evaluated with MR imaging: A cadaveric study involving multiple imaging sequences and intraarticular injection of gadolinium and saline solution. *Radiology* 1991;178: 557–561.
86. Hayes C, Sawyer RW, Conway WF: Patellar cartilage lesions: In vitro detection and staging with MR imaging and pathologic correlation. *Radiology* 1990;176:479–483.
87. Hardaker WT, Whipple TL, Bassett FH III: Diagnosis and treatment of the plica syndrome of the knee. *J Bone Joint Surg Am* 1980;62A:221–225.
88. Patel D: Arthroscopy of the plicae—Synovial folds and their significance. *Am J Sports Med* 1978;6:217–225.
89. Apple JS, Martinez S, Hardaker WT, et al.: Synovial plicae of the knee. *Skeletal Radiol* 1982;7:251–254.
90. Deutsch AL, Resnick D, Dalinka MK: Synovial plicae of the knee. *Radiology* 1981;141:627–634.
91. Resnick D: Arthrography, in Resnick D (ed.): *Bone and Joint Imaging.* Philadelphia; WB Saunders Co., 1989, pp. 154–184.
92. Hodge JC, Ghelman B, O'Brien SJ, et al.: Synovial plicae and chondromalacia patellae: Correlation of results of CT-arthrography with results of arthroscopy. *Radiology* 1993;186:827–831.
93. Reicher, MA: The spectrum of knee joint disorders, in Mink JH, Reicher MA, Crues JV III, Deutsch AL (eds.): *MRI of the Knee,* ed. 2. New York, Raven Press, 1993, pp. 333–399.
94. Jelinek JS, Kransdorf MJ, Utz JA, et al.: Imaging of pigmented villonodular synovitis with emphasis on MR imaging. *AJR* 1989;152:337–342.
95. Zeiss J, Saddemi SR, Ebraheim NA: MR imaging of the quadriceps tendon: Normal layered configuration and its importance in cases of tendon rupture. *AJR* 1992;159:1031–1034.
96. Daffner RH, Riemer BL, Lupetin AR, et al.: Magnetic resonance imaging in acute tendon ruptures. *Skeletal Radiol* 1986;15:619–621.
97. McMaster PE: Tendon and muscle ruptures. Clinical and experimental studies on the causes and location of subcutaneous ruptures. *J Bone Joint Surg Am* 1933;15A:705–722.
98. Ramsey R, Muller GE: Quadriceps tendon rupture: A diagnostic trap. *Clin Orthop* 1970;70: 161–164.
99. Halpern AA, Horowitz BG, Nagel DA: Tendon ruptures associated with corticosteroid therapy. *West J Med* 1977;127:378–382.
100. Newberg A, Wales L: Radiographic diagnosis of quadriceps tendon rupture. *Radiology* 1977;125:367–371.
101. Nance EP Jr., Kaye JJ: Injuries of the quadriceps mechanism. *Radiology* 1982;142:301–307.
102. Jelaso DV, Morris GA: Rupture of the quadriceps tendon: Diagnosis by arthrography. *Radiology* 1975;116:621–622.
103. Roels J, Martens M, Mulier JC, et al.: Patellar tendinitis (jumper's knee). *Am J Sports Med* 1978;6:362–368.
104. El-Khoury GY, Wira RL, Berbaum KS, et al.: MR imaging of patellar tendinitis. *Radiology* 1992;184:849–854.
105. Bodne D, Quinn SF, Murray WT, et al.: Magnetic resonance imaging of chronic patellar tendinitis. *Skeletal Radiol* 1988;17:24–28.
106. Fritschy D, de Gantad R: Jumper's knee and ultrasonography. *Am J Sports Med* 1988;16: 637.
107. Davies SG, Baudouin CJ, King JB, et al.: Ultrasound, computed tomography and magnetic resonance imaging in patellar tendinitis. *Clin Radiol* 1991;43:52–56.
108. Kahn D, Wilson MA: Bone scintigraphic findings in patellar tendinitis. *J Nucl Med* 1987; 28:1768–1770.
109. Siwek KW, Rao JP: Ruptures of the extensor mechanism of the knee joint. *J Bone Joint Surg Am* 1981;63A:932–937.

110. Boström J: Fractures of the patella. *Acta Orthop Scand* 1972;143(suppl.):1–80.
111. Hohl M, Larson RL, Jones DC: Fractures and dislocations of the knee, in Rockwood CA Jr., Green DP (eds.): *Fractures in Adults.* Philadelphia: JB Lippincott Co., 1984, pp. 1429–1591.
112. Jerosch JG, Castro WHM, Jantea C: Stress fracture of the patella. *Am J Sports Med* 1989; 17:579–580.
113. Devas MB: Stress fractures of the patella. *J Bone Joint Surg Br* 1960;42B:71–74.
114. Breaney RB, Gerber FH, Laughlin RL, et al.: Distribution and natural history of stress fractures in U.S. Marine recruits. *Radiology* 1983; 146:339–346.
115. Lee JK, Yao L: Stress fractures: MR imaging. *Radiology* 1988;169:217–220.
116. Yao L, Lee JK: Occult intraosseous fracture: Detection with MR imaging. *Radiology* 1988; 167:749–751.
117. Resnick D, Goergen TG, Niwayama G: Physical trauma, in Resnick D (ed.): *Bone and Joint Imaging.* Philadelphia, WB Saunders Co., 1989, pp.801–898.
118. Edwards DH, Bentley G: Osteochondritis dissecans patellae. *J Bone Joint Surg Br* 1977; 59B:58–63.
119. Blum GM, Tirman PFJ, Crues JR III: Osseous and cartilaginous trauma, in Mink JH, Reicher MA, Crues JR III, Deutsch AL (eds.): *MRI of the Knee,* ed. 2. New York: Raven Press, 1993, pp. 295–332.
120. Nelson DW, DiPaola J, Colville M, Schmidgall J: Osteochondritis dissecans of the talus and knee: Prospective comparison of MR and arthroscopic classifications. *J Comput Assist Tomogr* 1990;14:804–808.
121. DeSmet A, Sapega AA, Banakdarpour A, et al.: Osteochondritis dissecans of the knee: Value of MR imaging in determining lesion stability and the presence of articular cartilage defects. *AJR* 1990;155:549–553.
122. Mesgarzadeh M, Sapega AA, Banakdarpour A, et al.: Osteochondritis dissecans: Analysis of mechanical stability with radiography, scintigraphy and MR imaging. *Radiology* 1987; 165:775–780.
123. Kirsch MD, Fitzgerald SW, Friedman H, et al.: Transient lateral patellar dislocation: Diagnosis with MR imaging. *AJR* 1993; 161: 109–113.
124. Casteleyn PP, Handelberg F: Arthroscopy in the diagnosis of occult dislocation of the patella. *Acta Orthop Belg* 1989;55:381–383.
125. Keene JS: Diagnosis of undetected knee injuries: Interpreting subtle clinical and radiologic findings. *Postgrad Med* 1989; 85: 153–163.
126. Freiberger RH, Kotzen LM: Fracture of the medial margin of the patella, a finding diagnostic of lateral dislocation. *Radiology* 1967; 88:902–904.
127. Dahlin DC, Unni KK: *Bone Tumors: General Aspects and Data on 8542 Cases,* ed. 4. Springfield, Ill., Charles C Thomas Publisher, 1986.
128. Kransdorf MJ, Moser RP Jr, Vinh TN, et al.: Primary tumors of the patella, a review of 42 cases. *Skeletal Radiol* 1989;18:365–371.
129. Wilson JS, Genant HK, Carlsson A, et al.: Patellar giant cell tumor. *AJR* 1976;127:856.
130. Bansal VP, Singh R, Grewal DS: Haemangioma of the patella: A report of two cases. *J Bone Joint Surg Br* 1974;56B:139–141.
131. Stoler B, Staple TW: Metastases to the patella. *Radiology* 1969;93:853–856.
132. Sur RK, Singh DP, Dhillon MS: Patellar metastasis: A rare presentation. *Br J Radiol* 1992; 65:722–724.
133. Ehara S, Khurana JS, Kattapuram SV: Osteolytic lesions of the patella. *AJR* 1989;153:103–106.
134. Thomas WH, Ewald FC, Poss R: Duopatellar total knee arthroplasty. *Orthop Trans* 1980;4: 329–335.
135. Clayton ML, Thirupathi R: Patellar complications after total condylar arthroplasty. *Clin Orthop* 1973;94:153–165.
136. Brick GW, Scott RD: The patellofemoral component of total knee arthroplasty. *Clin Orthop* 1988;231:163–178.
137. Ranawat CS: The patellofemoral joint in total condylar knee arthroplasty. *Clin Orthop* 1986; 205:93–99.
138. Bayley JC, Scott RD: Further observations on metal-backed patellar component failure. *Clin Orthop* 1988;236:82–87.

7

Conservative Care of Patellofemoral Pain

K. Donald Shelbourne and William S. Adsit

Anterior knee pain is a common complaint of patients presenting to a general orthopedic or orthopedic sports medicine practice. Appropriate treatment of this problem begins with a careful and complete initial evaluation, involving a thorough history, a physical examination, and proper radiologic examinations. After a correct and specific diagnosis is made,[1,2] conservative treatment with a patient active rehabilitation program may be prescribed. In this chapter, we will review our approach to patients with patellofemoral symptoms and discuss our philosophy of conservative treatment.

History

Listening about the patient's problem is the first step toward a specific diagnosis. Pain as a chief complaint can be pursued with questions about its onset, duration, intensity, and location. Other direct questions to ask the patient include: (1) What activities bring on or make your pain worse?; (2) How much do your symptoms limit you?; (3) Does your knee swell and, if so, what activities bring on your swelling?; (4) Do you have any giving way sensations?; and (5) Have you had any previous treatment or surgery on the knee? Answers to these questions will enable the physician to determine the magnitude of the patient's problem and will help in prescribing appropriate treatment.

One typical presentation is the gradual onset of knee pain in the adolescent girl. The pain is described as an ache, located in the anterior knee, worse with stair descent or prolonged flexion such as sitting in a car or at a theater. It is improved by changing to a position of knee extension. She has tried activity modifications, and though that helps some, the pain recurs when she is active again. She has not noted swelling. She is not sure about giving way, but the knee feels weak. This history, though suggestive of patellofemoral dysplasia, does not yet provide enough information for a specific diagnosis.

A history of patellar instability is slightly different. The patient may remember a specific episode of the knee giving way or an instant of sharp pain that rapidly resolved after a twisting activity such as cutting away from the planted foot on the affected side. There may be a feeling of a slipping or a clicking sensation in the knee. The patient may or may not remember indirect trauma (Figure 7.1) as an instigating factor.

Another presentation is the athlete who has started a preseason conditioning program, or who is training for a specific competition by a rapid or a significant increase in athletic activity. Athletes may also have pain with change in surfaces from the turf of a football field to the hardwood surface of a basketball court, and the transition from a running sport to a jumping sport. The onset of knee pain following one of these significant activity changes suggests overuse. The physical de-

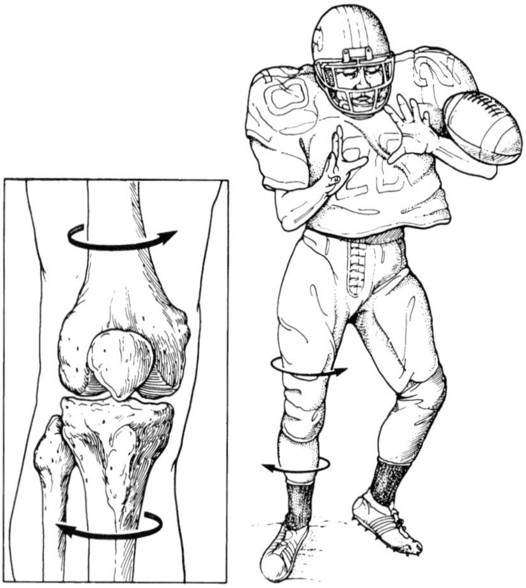

FIGURE 7.1. Indirect trauma. Internal rotation of the femur on a planted foot may cause patellar instability.

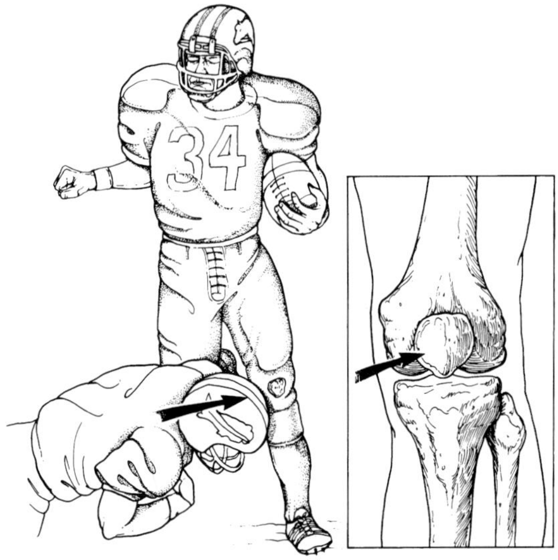

FIGURE 7.2. Direct trauma. A laterally directed force applied to the patella may cause patellar instability.

mands being placed on the knee extensor mechanism exceed its current level of fitness.

The balance of the extensor mechanism may be upset by direct blunt trauma to the anterior knee. This may vary from the knee striking the dashboard in a motor vehicle accident, to the knee striking the ground or an opponent in athletics (Figure 7.2). The trauma may be a cause of knee pain by itself, or it may unmask some underlying but previously silent cause of knee pain. Contusions can cause inflammation in a plica and, once inflamed, routine activities may be irritating enough to cause the persistent inflammation and symptoms.[3]

Previous surgery can directly cause anterior knee pain. Examples include painful scars, neuroma of surgical incisions, and arthroscopic portals. Failure to restore full motion equal to the contralateral normal knee after surgery can cause anterior knee pain when the patient attempts to return to full activity.[4]

If the patient complains of swelling, it is important to determine if the swelling is activity related or from a recent knee injury. Swelling should also be differentiated into an actual intra-articular knee effusion, or the appearance or feeling of swelling in some location around the knee. Knee effusion immediately following a knee injury is most commonly a hemarthrosis from a ligament tear, a retinacular tear, or an intra-articular fracture. Spontaneous or activity-related effusions suggest an articular cartilage lesion.[5]

Knee pain may be referred from the back, the hip, or other anatomic areas in the lower extremity. Other knee pathology such as ligamentous instability may lead to pain in the anterior knee, but the sensation is from the ligament deficiency rather than from the patellar instability. The distinction, however, may be difficult for the patient.

Physical Examination

The physical examination should begin with the observation of the patient dressed in loose-fitting athletic shorts and bare feet. The stance and gait should be observed, with attention to antalgia, quadriceps atrophy, limb alignment, genu varus or valgum, femoral anteversion, tibial torsion, and dynamic patellar positioning. Excessive foot pronation may contribute to patellofemoral pain.[5–7]

Flexibility should be observed and assessed in the lower back, quadriceps (Figure 7.3), hamstring (Figure 7.4), and gastrocnemius–soleus areas. Observations specific to the patella include a measurement of Q angle, both supine and with weight bearing. This angle is formed by the intersection of a line from the anterior superior iliac spine to the middle of the patella, and a line extending from the middle of the patella to the middle of the tibial tubercle[8,9] (Figure 7.5). Patellar tracking should be observed as the knee is flexed and extended. Does the patella slide smoothly into and out of the femoral trochlea, or does it slide laterally as it exits the trochlea in knee extension (the J sign)?[10] The positioning of the patella should also be observed as the knee is moved from full extension to full flexion.

The patellofemoral joint and its surrounding soft tissues are accessible to physical examination by palpation.[11,12] Some order should be used so no structures are missed. Starting proximally, palpation for tenderness proceeds across the distal quadriceps muscle

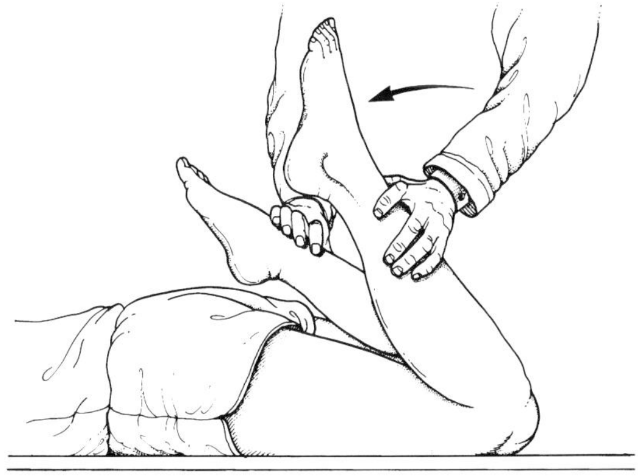

FIGURE 7.3. Quadriceps tightness. Quadriceps flexibility can be easily demonstrated with the patient in the prone position by flexing the knees and comparing the relative heel heights.

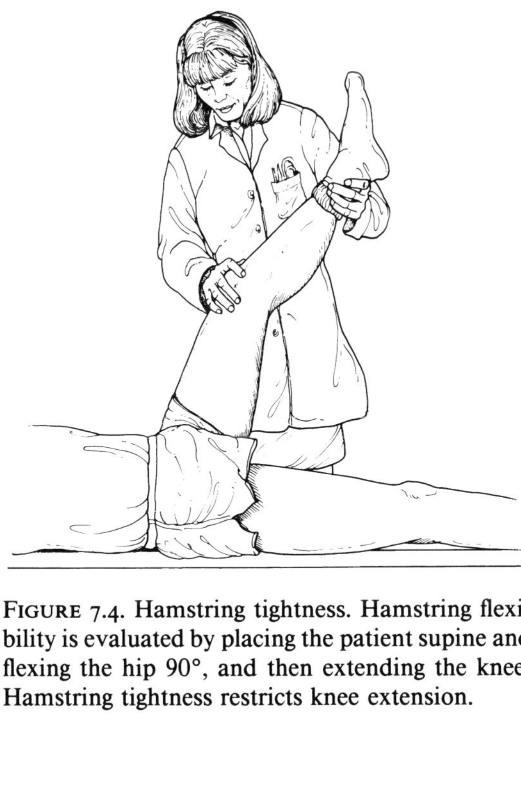

FIGURE 7.4. Hamstring tightness. Hamstring flexibility is evaluated by placing the patient supine and flexing the hip 90°, and then extending the knee. Hamstring tightness restricts knee extension.

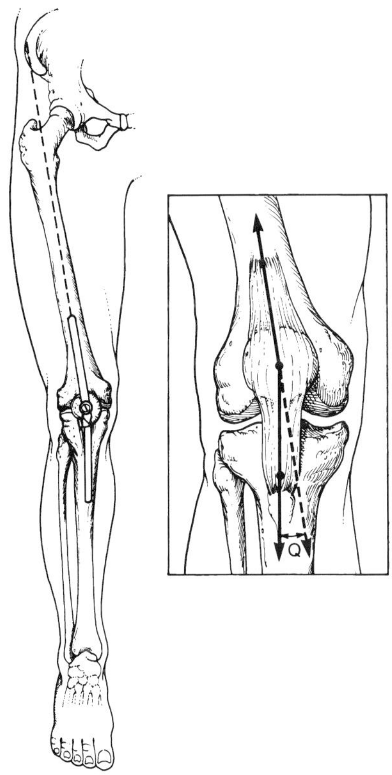

FIGURE 7.5. Q angle. The Q angle is formed by the intersection of a line from the anterior superior iliac spine to the center of the patella, and a line from the center of the patella to the middle of the tibial tubercle.

and tendon, and down onto the superior pole of the patella and the prepatellar bursa. The medial retinaculum, the plica and the medial facets, the lateral retinaculum, and the lateral facets are then examined. The examination is completed by palpating the distal pole of the patella, the patellar tendon, the tibial tubercle, and Hoffa's fat pad, along with the joint lines and the iliotibial band. The clinician should specifically observe and palpate for the presence of an effusion. All scars, both traumatic and surgical, should also be palpated for evidence of tenderness or neuroma formation.

Manipulation may help distinguish between patellar instability with retinacular laxity or retinacular tightness and knee pain.[13] The patella should be displaced laterally to assess the quantity of lateral glide and to observe for apprehension or the reproduction of symptoms. Medial glide should also be quantified (Figure 7.6). Lateral retinacular tightness can be assessed by observing patellar tilt and attempting to lift the lateral facet of the patella away from the femoral trochlea in addition to assessing how far medially the patella can be passively moved (Figure 7.7).

The physical examination is not completed until the knee, the lower back, and the remainder of the lower extremity has been examined sufficiently to exclude pain referred to the anterior knee from another source. The sitting patient is asked to flex and extend the knee. Initially, the movement of the patella is observed and smooth, graceful movements are differentiated from sudden, lateral or medial movements. Then the patella is palpated gently through the range of motion to assess the magnitude and the location of crepitus. Direct compression of the patellofemoral joint may also cause pain and this should be checked at various angles of knee flexion. If these maneuvers reproduce the patient's symptoms, that fact should be noted. The area of articulation in the patellofemoral joint shifts proximally on the patella and distally on the femur as the knee is flexed.[14] For example, pain and crepitus with greater knee flexion implies a more proximal location of an articular lesion on the patella.

The final manipulative test is the attempt to laterally sublux the patella and cause a response from the patient, the apprehension sign. This maneuver should be done at the end of the physical examination, as it may cause the patient sufficient discomfort to make relaxation difficult.

Radiographic Assessment

Routine radiographic assessment of the knee with suspected patellofemoral pathology consists of three views. A standing 45° posteroanterior weight-bearing radiograph[15] shows development variations, osteochondritis dissecans, fractures, and other knee joint pathology that may cause anterior knee pain.

Proper rotation to get good overlap of the femoral condyles is important for the lateral view. The knee is flexed 60° to be sure the patellar tendon is under tension. The method of Blackburne and Peel is used to calculate a

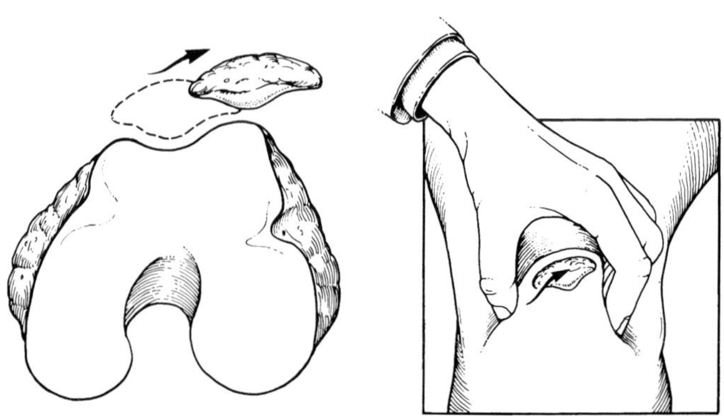

FIGURE 7.6. Patellar glide. The mobility of the patella is evaluated by manually attempting to shift it medially and laterally.

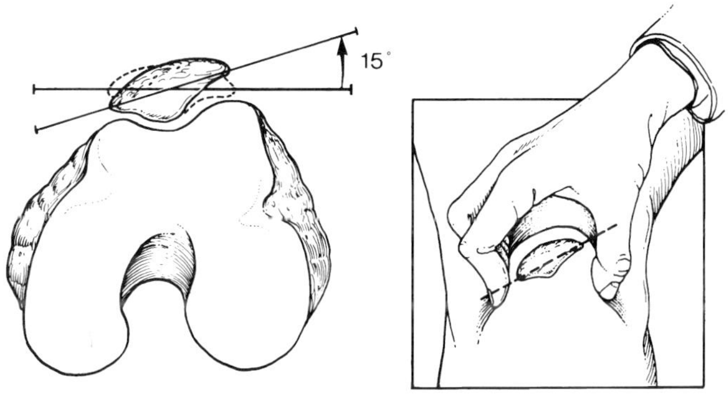

FIGURE 7.7. Patellar tilt. Manually rotating the lateral patellar facet away from the femoral trochlea assesses patellar tilt.

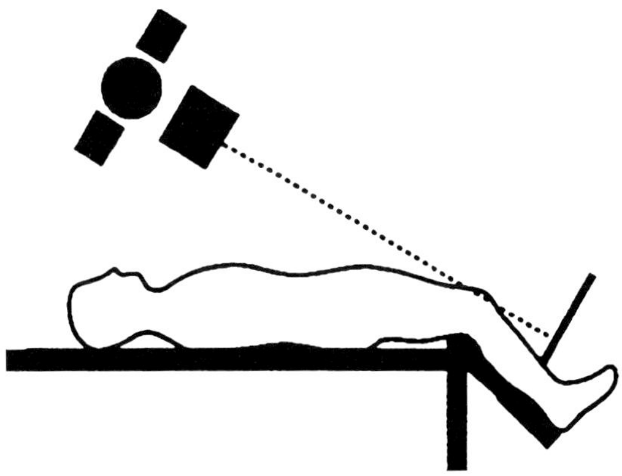

FIGURE 7.8. Axial patellofemoral radiographic technique. The patient lies supine, with knees supported on a board and quadriceps relaxed. (Reproduced by permission; Merchant AC. Patellofemoral Malalignment and Instabilities in *Articular Cartilage and Knee Joint Function: Basic Science and Arthroscopy,* J.W. Ewing, editor, Raven Press, Ltd, New York, 1990, pp 80.)

ratio of the height of the articular surface on the patella above the tibial articular surface to the length of the articular surface of the patella (patella baja versus patella alta).[16]

To specifically assess the patellofemoral joint, the Merchant axial view is added to these two routine radiographs.[17] A frame is used to hold the cassette, to maintain the standard 45° of knee flexion, and to allow the quadriceps muscle to relax (Figure 7.8). This frame improves the consistency of getting this view. The sulcus angle, the congruence angle, and the patellofemoral index are calculated from this axial view.[18,19]

Schutzer et al. note that plain axial views of the patellofemoral joint may not show lateral subluxation if the knee is flexed sufficiently for the patella to be engaged in the trochlea. The plain axial radiograph may also suffer from effects of overlap and the true position of the patella may not be appreciated.[20] A single midpatellar computed tomography (CT) scan cut with the knee flexed 20° and the quadriceps relaxed may best show the true position of the patella as it begins to enter the femoral trochlea (Post WR: Clinical and radiographic indications for successful surgical treatment of patellofemoral disorders, Instructional Course Lecture, American Orthopaedic Society for Sports Medicine Meeting, Sun Valley, Idaho July 1993). This CT scan is the basis for the classification system for subluxation and/or tilt, which, when correlated with an appropriate history and physical examination, may guide selection of appropriate treatment. Further radiographic assessment including multiple CT slices,[20] CT arthrography,[21] bone scan,[22] or magnetic resonance imaging (MRI)[23] are discussed in detail in Chapter 6 and have a role in more complex cases, including cases in which the symptoms and the signs do not correlate with routine radiographs, or as part of the preoperative evaluation. The triple-phase bone scan may assist in confirming reflex sympathetic dystrophy.

Determining a Diagnosis

With a careful history, a physical examination, and radiographs, the physician can then determine the appropriate diagnosis and recommend a treatment method for the patient. In our experience, most patellofemoral pain can be treated successfully with proper physical therapy and this should be the physician's first choice.[24] An understanding of the anatomy and biomechanics of the patellofemoral joint contributes to the design of any treatment program.

Arthroscopy has a limited role for diagnosis alone, but it can help to confirm clinical findings at the time of surgical intervention.[25–27] The arthroscopic appearance of the articular cartilage on the patella does not necessarily correlate with the patient's symptoms.[25,27] The best results of surgical treatment are attained when a specific and surgically correctable lesion is identified.[28,29]

Rehabilitation Program

Phase I

Conservative treatment of patellofemoral pain begins with aggressive attempts to control pain and restore some functional activity.[30] Pain control should be an early goal of conservative care to help gain the confidence of the patient and to allow rehabilitation to proceed. Pain, as a symptom, must be controlled to allow the patient to actively participate in the rehabilitation program and to allow functional activity. A strengthening program will be ineffective if sufficient pain with activity exists to reflexively shut down quadriceps activity.[31]

For patients with overuse, relative rest may be a part of the plan.[32] The treatment should be tailored to the individual patient. Rest, though helpful in controlling symptoms initially, may decondition the extremity to the point that the activities of daily living cause knee pain.[33] The patient transforms relative rest into complete rest with resultant quadriceps atrophy.[34] The history should be reviewed to determine a possible offending activity or overuse, and the restrictions on activity should be limited to only those necessary to decrease the pain.[35]

Anti-inflammatory medications may be useful during this phase.[36,37] The effectiveness of one over another or over placebo has not been proven by clinical trial, but some authors[30,32] recommend their use, at least in the short term.[30] Anti-inflammatory medications should be used with the understanding by the clinician and the patient that their role is to assist in initial pain control and the discomfort early in the rehabilitation process. These medications may also be useful in subsequent symptomatic flares. They all can have side effects and their long-term use is not recommended.

Physical modalities have a role in this phase. Cryotherapy in the form of ice massage, refreezable cold packs, or the Cryo/Cuff (Aircast, Inc., Summit, N.J.) may contribute significantly to pain control. Its judicious use may aid in returning the patient to functional activity more quickly. During a lunch break or after a day at work, a convenient method of icing the knee may help the patient get control of the pain and decrease knee swelling.

McConnell taping techniques may help some patients with pain control.[31,32] For those patient who do respond, the results can be dramatic. It is difficult to identify the specific patient who will respond, so a trial may be useful in patients who are severely symptomatic or who are early failures with other conservative modalities (Figure 7.9).

The second cornerstone in the early rehabilitation phase is rapidly returning the patient to some functional activity. Get the patient upright with the foot on the ground and functioning in a weight-bearing capacity. Walking, an exercise bike, aqua therapy, or some other activity to rapidly restore physiologic patterns of knee extensor mechanism function should be used.[30]

Other modalities that may help in the early phase include the use of cushion insoles or Vibram (Quabaug Corp., North Brookfield, Mass.) soles on the shoe to cushion impact forces, decrease peak ground reaction force, and improve comfort to the lower extremity with the return to functional activities. Some patients, noted to have excessive pronation of their feet during observed gait, may find sig-

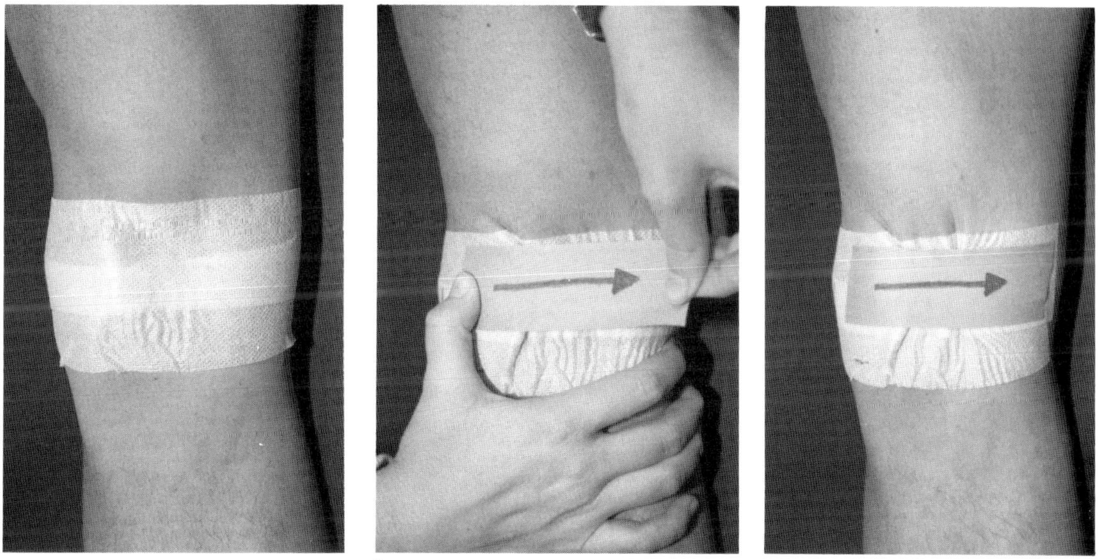

a b c

FIGURE 7.9. McConnell taping technique for patellar tilt. Two strips of tape are applied to the knee to fully cover the patella, the medial femoral condyle, and the lateral femoral condyle (a). A third piece of tape is applied from the center of the patella, pulling toward the medial side of the knee (b) and anchored behind the medial femoral condyle (c).

nificant relief with the use of off-the-shelf or custom orthotics for their shoes.[7,38]

Certain patients may also receive significant benefit from the use of patellar stabilizing braces, neoprene sleeves, or straps.[39–41] These devices should be individualized, with trials available for the patient.

Phase II

The next phase in the general rehabilitation program is the stretching and initial strengthening phase. Improved lower-extremity flexibility is emphasized at this time. Hamstring stretches include the Brady stretch (Figure 7.10), modified hurdler's stretch (Figure 7.11), step stretch (Figure 7.12), and contract/relax partner stretch (Figure 7.13). Quadriceps stretches include side lying (Figure 7.14) and standing quadriceps stretches (Figure 7.15). The lateral hip and iliotibial band areas are stretched with the pretzel (Figure 7.16) and standing iliotibial band stretch (Figure 7.17). Gastrocnemius–soleus flexibility is improved with wall leans (Figure 7.18) and inclined heel cord board (Figure 7.19).

The stretching technique is firm but gentle, with a static stretch held for 20 to 30 s with four to five repetitions per exercise. They should be part of the warm-up before strengthening or cool down after exercise. The goal is to restore balanced flexibility to the extremity and to decrease soft-tissue restraints to fluid motions of the extremity.

Selective strengthening of the vastus medialis obliquus (VMO) is possible by various techniques,[42–44] however the enhanced benefit of isolated VMO strengthening has not been proven by clinical trials.

Our preferred regiment uses closed kinetic chain techniques. Patients may put their feet on the floor, and walk and use crutches for assistance as necessary. The goal is to walk with a normal gait pattern without limping. The quadriceps muscle is exercised physiologically in the terminal short extensor arc with lower patellofemoral compression forces, which results in a more functional patient.

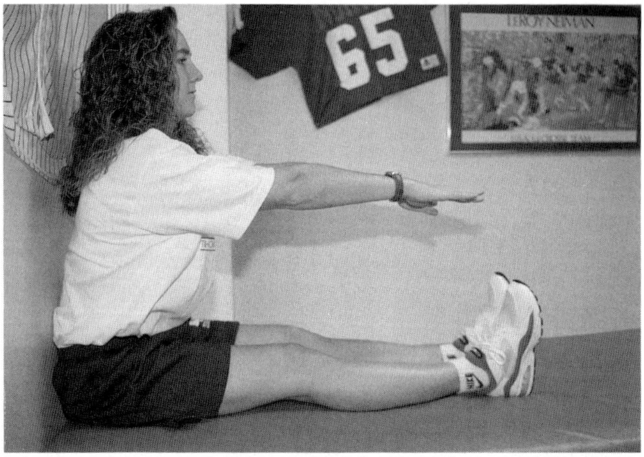

FIGURE 7.10. Brady stretch. Sit upright on the floor or against a wall. With knees straight and arms raised in front, lean forward, moving at the hips. Keep the back straight.

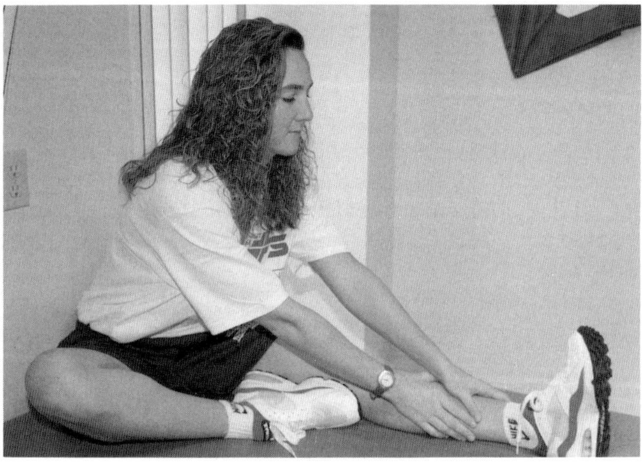

FIGURE 7.11. Modified hurdler's stretch. Sit on the mat as shown. While keeping the back and the knee straight, stretch toward the toes, pulling chest toward the thigh. Alternate legs.

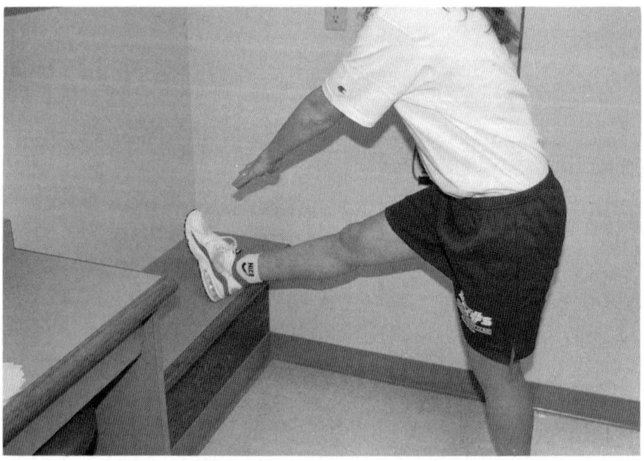

FIGURE 7.12. Step stretch. With one foot on a step (or a bleacher) approximately knee high, the ankle in a neutral position, and the knees straight, reach toward the ankle, bringing the chest toward the thigh. Keep the back straight. Repeat with the other leg.

The next step is literally that, a step of low height such as a brick, a book, a wooden block, or a step exercise machine with variable step height. The patient stands upon the platform with the affected leg as the support leg (Figure 7.20). The knee is flexed to allow the toe of

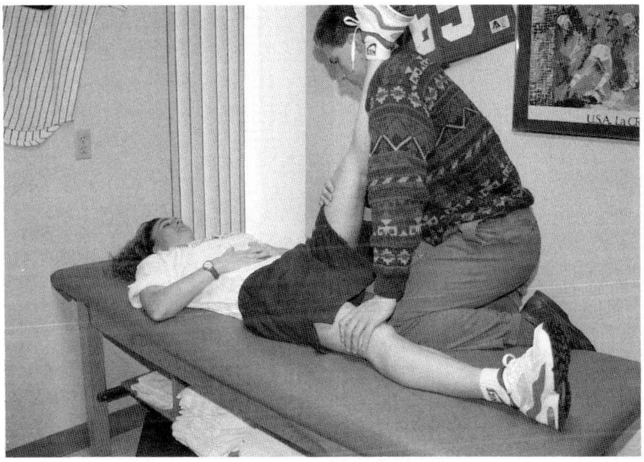

FIGURE 7.13. Contract/relax partner stretch. Patient is supine on the mat. Partner holds opposite leg on the mat and lifts the patient's calf with the partner's shoulder, holding the knees straight. Lift until tension develops in the patient's hamstring. Partner holds the position while the patient contracts the hamstring pushing the upper leg toward the floor for 10 to 15 s. Relax the muscle and the partner stretches the hamstring by lifting the leg farther from the floor.

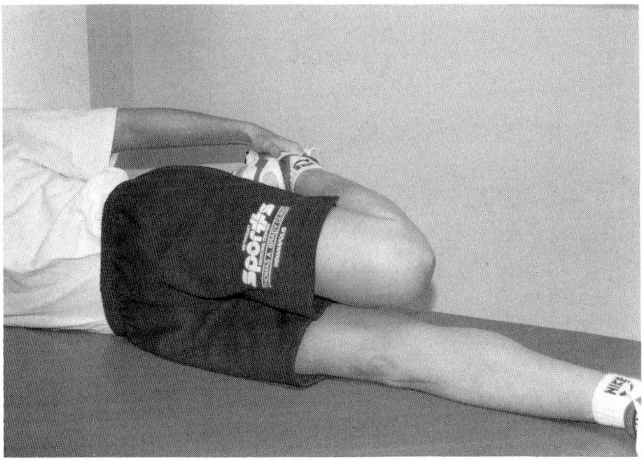

FIGURE 7.14. Side lying stretch. Lay on your side. With a belt, a towel, or your hand, pull the heel toward the buttock.

the free leg to touch the ground. The affected knee is then extended to return to the starting position. This again is a closed kinetic chain quadriceps strengthening exercise in the terminal extensor arc. The difficulty can be varied considerably by adjusting the height of the platform, or touching the free heel versus the toe of the non-weight-bearing foot.

The goal is to gradually progress the quadriceps strengthening exercises within the patient's tolerance while continuing pain modulation (e.g., ice, nonsteroidal anti-inflammatory drugs, braces, or other modalities). Progression takes the form of increased duration of exercise from 5 to 10 min and increased height of the platform. Access to a fitness center or physical therapy office with a step machine that allows variable step height such as a Stairmaster (Tri-tech, Inc., Tulsa, Okl.) is an extremely convenient way of achieving the same regiment. Initially, extremely small step heights for short durations can follow the functional walking program. Progression is again made in step height and duration of exercises. One complaint of this step regiment is boredom while doing the exercises. Once mastered, the exercises do not require much mental concentration and can be done while watching television, listening to music, talking on the phone, or reading a book.

Another closed kinetic chain exercise is the use of an exercise bicycle with the seat high to decrease knee flexion and with low resistance to decrease patellofemoral contact pressures.[45] Progressive load and duration of ex-

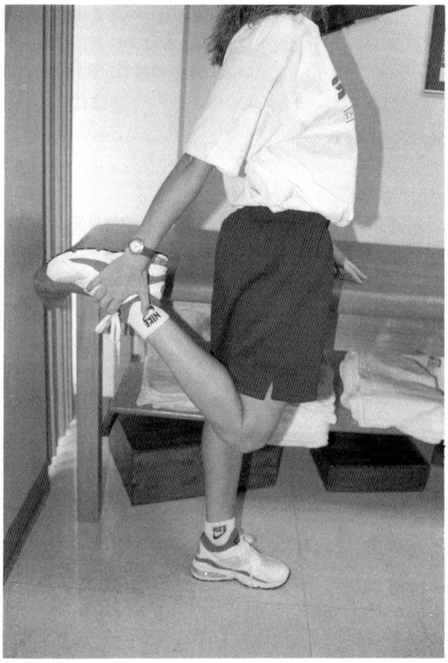

FIGURE 7.15. Standing quadriceps stretch. Standing and holding on support for balance, grab the ankle with the hand on the same side and pull the heel toward the buttock. Increase the stretch by extending at the hip. Keep the trunk vertical.

ercise improves quadriceps strength. These rehabilitation techniques share a philosophy of physiologic restrengthening through a pain-free arc of knee flexion. The exercises should be tailored to the individual patient to achieve that goal by adjustments in platform height, step height, or seat height.

While our preference is for the closed kinetic chain exercise program previously outlined, traditional quadriceps strengthening exercises are included in this discussion for completeness.[35] Many clinicians have used these regiments and have reported good results.[46–48]

Quadriceps strengthening exercises with the knee fully extended includes the quadriceps set. The patient is supine. The contralateral hip and the knee are flexed to stabilize the pelvis and to avoid lower back pain. The quadriceps musculature on the affected leg is voluntarily maximally contracted with the foot dorsiflexed for 8 to 10 s. Ten repetitions completes one set.

Straight leg raises begin in the same position as the quad set. The knee is held fully extended and the foot is lifted 12 in (30.5 cm) off the table for 8 to 10 s; the foot is then lowered. The patient should work up to three sets of ten repetitions. The final open chain exercise is the short arc knee extension. With the patient supine, a bolster supports the distal thigh, with the knee flexed approximately 30°. The foot is lifted from the table, extending the knee, but the thigh is still supported by the bolster. This position of knee extension is held for 8 to 10 s; the foot is lowered to the table completing the exercise.

The VMO can be strengthened by hip adduction with care to keep the knee extended to avoid adductor tendinitis.[35] Further strengthening is then generally done with closed chain techniques as previously outlined.[42]

Phase III

Phase III is the final phase in the conservative treatment program and encompasses the sports-specific functional progression needed to return to sport and a long-term maintenance plan for the individual. Therapy is directed at correcting any remaining deficits in strength, speed, flexibility, or agility that would preclude return to full and unrestricted sports activities. Additional strength techniques include the leg press, the hip sled, quarter squats, and lunges.

Patients may return to sports after completing the appropriate functional progression. Leg strength may be measured by a Cybex (a division of Lumex, Inc., Ronkonkoma, N.Y.) isokinetic dynamometer to monitor progress through rehabilitation. Care should be used early in the program and at slow speeds, as the testing may aggravate the knee pain in some patients. Improvements may plateau after return to sports. Athletes may concentrate on other parts of the game, and unconsciously develop bad habits by compensating for their weakness. Patients should be specifically encouraged to add some stretching and strength work to their workout and during off seasons

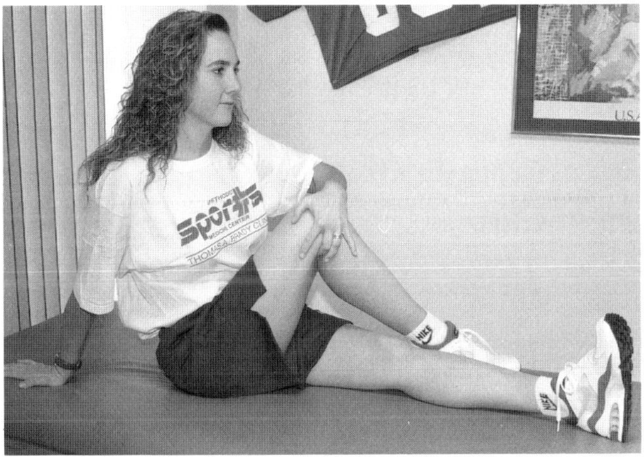

FIGURE 7.16. Pretzel stretch. Assume position as illustrated. Pull the knee of the bent leg across the body and toward the opposite shoulder.

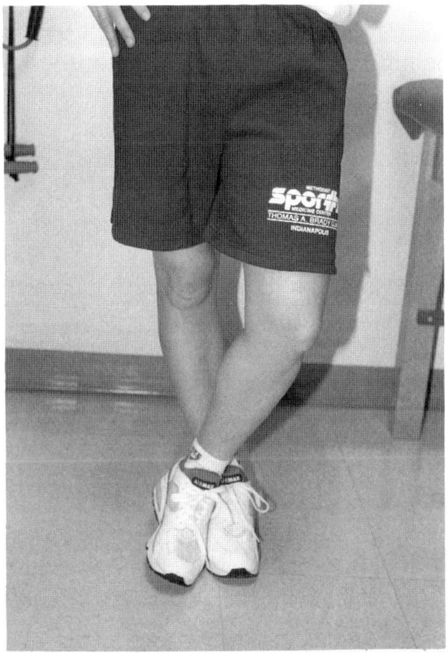

FIGURE 7.17. Standing iliotibial band stretch. Stand with knees straight. Cross the affected leg behind the noninvolved leg as far as possible. Lean the hips away from the involved leg. Maintain balance by holding a table or the wall. Repeat with the other leg.

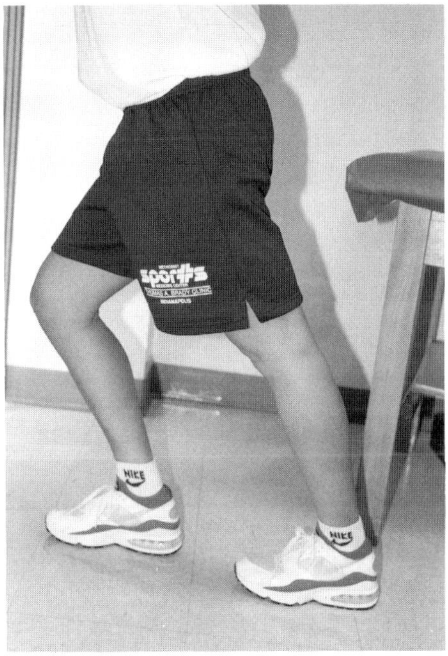

FIGURE 7.18. Wall lean, gastrocnemius stretch. Stand about 2 ft (60 cm) away, but face a wall. Feet should be straight ahead or slightly internally rotated. Step one foot toward the wall. Keeping both heels on the floor and the back knee straight, lean hips toward the wall by bending the knee of the front leg. Keep the heels on the floor.

as part of a maintenance program to prevent recurrent symptoms.

The patient should have a good understanding of the knee problem and, having worked through rehabilitation, the various techniques that then will help control the symptoms. The maintenance programs will be individualized. Some patients will have restored the balance to their extensor mechanism and will not need any formal, ongoing exercise programs. Others will need to continue the stretching and

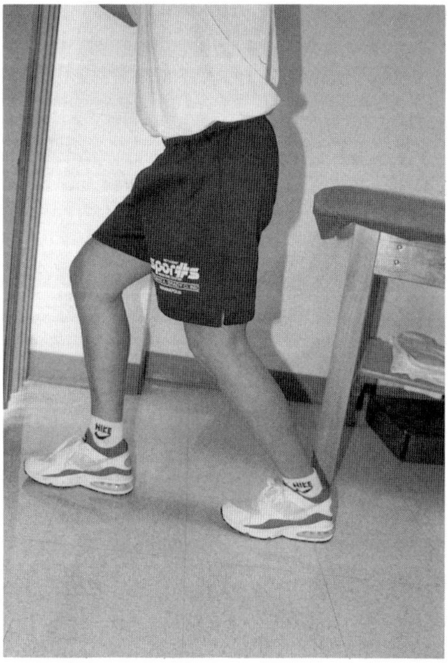

FIGURE 7.19. Wall lean, soleus stretch. From the starting position of the gastrocnemius stretch, bend the back knee, keeping the heels on the floor.

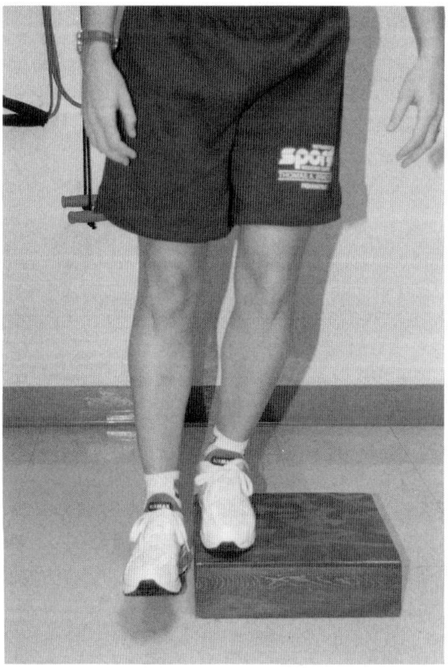

FIGURE 7.20. Lateral step. The affected leg is up on the step. The knee is flexed, lowering the foot of the well leg to the floor. The knee is then extended fully and the exercise is repeated.

strengthening on a regular basis, and may note a return of symptoms when they attempt to taper off their exercise program.

Complications of Conservative Care

Though complications are generally associated with operative management, conservative care also has potential problems. Absolute rest will make some patients absolutely miserable. The goal in phase I is to reduce the patients' symptoms to the point that they feel they are in control and can return to some function. Greater rest than necessary may lead to greater muscle atrophy and even patella osteopenia. These patients can become so deconditioned that they have significant pain even with activities of daily living. The absolute rest approach is best avoided.

Another potential cause of problems with conservative treatment is misdiagnosis. The literature reports success in 70% to 90% of these patients with conservative care.[31,46–48] Treatment failure in a specific patient should lead to careful reassessment before operative intervention is considered.

Operative techniques can yield good results in the properly selected patient.[28,29] Again, the key to success is doing the right surgery for the right diagnosis. Though "failure of conservative treatment" is one indication for surgery, it should not be the first. Some patients remain symptomatic despite conservative care, but there may not be a good surgical solution to their problems. Presently, for example, there is not a reliable surgical technique for a symptomatic patient with a hypermobile patella and a shallow trochlear groove. Physicians should realize the limits of success with surgical procedures for patellofemoral problems in order to prevent compounding problems that can result.

Summary

The conservative care of patellofemoral pain begins with a careful clinical assessment, with a goal of determining a specific diagnosis for the patient. The importance of a complete history and a careful physical examination cannot be overemphasized. Appropriate radiographic studies may confirm the suspected clinical diagnosis. Conservative care begins in phase I, with the goals of rapidly controlling the symptoms of pain and instability with activity modification, cryotherapy, medications, and other modalities as necessary to allow a rapid return to daily functional activities. Phase II is the stretching and strengthening phase in which, after receiving education in a physical therapy department, the patient can do the great majority of work at home or at a fitness center. The goal is to restore balance to the extensor mechanism and the affected extremity. Phase III is the final phase in which any remaining deficits in strength, endurance, speed, flexibility, or agility are specifically addressed to allow the patient to return to sports activity through a functional progression program. Patients are also instructed in maintenance stretching and strengthening programs to decrease the recurrence of symptoms. Patient education and participation are requirements for success with conservative care of patellofemoral pain.

References

1. Merchant A: Classification of patellofemoral disorders. *Arthroscopy* 1988;4:235–240.
2. Jacobson K, Flandry F: Diagnosis of anterior knee pain. *Clin Sports Med* 1989;8:179–195.
3. Tindel N, Nisonson B: The plica syndrome. *Orthop Clin North Am* 1992;23:613–618.
4. Aglietti P, Buzzi R, D'Andria S, et al.: Patellofemoral problems after intra-articular anterior cruciate reconstruction. *Clin Orthop* 1993; 288:195–204.
5. Fulkerson J, Shea K: Current concepts review. Disorders of patellofemoral alignment. *J Bone Joint Surg Am* 1990;72A:1424–1429.
6. Beckman M, Craig R, Lehman R: Rehabilitation of patellofemoral disfunction in the athlete. *Clin Sports Med* 1989;8:841–860.
7. Cox J: Patellofemoral problems in runners. *Clin Sports Med* 1985;4:699–715.
8. Aglietti P, Insall J, Cerulli G: Patellar pain and incongruence. I: Measurements of incongruence. *Clin Orthop* 1983;176:217–224.
9. Horton M, Hall T: Quadriceps femoris muscle angle: Normal values and relationships with gender and selected skeletal measures. *Phys Ther* 1989;69:897–901.
10. Kettlekamp D: Current concepts review. Management of patellar malalignment. *J Bone Joint Surg Am* 1981;63A:1344–1348.
11. Fulkerson J: Awareness of the retinaculum in evaluating patellofemoral pain. *Am J Sports Med* 1982;10:147–149.
12. Fulkerson J: Evaluation of the peripatellar soft tissues and retinaculum in patients with patellofemoral pain. *Clin Sports Med* 1989;8:197–202.
13. Kolowich P, Paulos L, Rosenberg T, et al.: Lateral release of the patella: Indications and contraindications. *Am J Sports Med* 1990;18:359–365.
14. Hungerford D, Barry M: Biomechanics of the patellofemoral joint. *Clin Orthop* 1979;144:9–15.
15. Rosenberg T, Paulos L, Parker R, et al.: The 45° posteroanterior flexion weight-bearing radiograph of the knee. *J Bone Joint Surg Am* 1988;70A:1479–1483.
16. Blackburne J, Peel T: A new method of measuring patellar height. *J Bone Joint Surg Br* 1977;59B:241–242.
17. Merchant A, Mercer R, Jacobsen R, et al.: Roentgenographic analysis of patellofemoral congruence. *J Bone Joint Surg Am* 1974;56A: 1391–1396.
18. Laurin C, Dussault R, Levesque H: The tangential x-ray investigation of the patellofemoral joint. *Clin Orthop* 1979;144:16–26.
19. Dowd G, Bentley G: Radiographic assessment in patellar instability and chondromalacia patellae. *J Bone Joint Surg Br* 1986;68B:297–300.
20. Schutzer S, Ramsby G, Fulkerson J: Computed tomographic classification of patellofemoral pain patients. *Orthop Clin North Am* 1986;17: 235–248.
21. Ghelman B, Hodge J: Imaging of the patellofemoral joint. *Orthop Clin North Am* 1992;23: 532–543.
22. Dye S, Boll D: Radionuclide imaging of the patellofemoral joint in young adults with anterior knee pain. *Orthop Clin North Am* 1986; 17:249–261.
23. McCauley T, Kier R, Lynch K, et al.: Chondromalacia patellae: Diagnosis with MR imaging. *AJR* 1992;158:101–105.
24. Sandow M, Goodfellow J: The natural history of anterior knee pain in adolescents. *J Bone Joint Surg Br* 1985;67B:36–38.

25. Casscells S: The arthroscope in the diagnosis of disorders of the patellofemoral joint. *Clin Orthop* 1979;144:45–50.
26. Fu F, Maday M: Arthroscopic lateral release and the lateral patellar compression syndrome. *Orthop Clin North Am* 1992;23:601–612.
27. Greenfield M, Scott W: Arthroscopic evaluation and treatment of the patellofemoral joint. *Orthop Clin North Am* 1992;23:587–600.
28. Ceder L, Larson R: Z-plasty lateral retinacular release for the treatment of patellar compression syndrome. *Clin Orthop* 1979;144:110–113.
29. Dandy D, Griffiths D: Lateral release for recurrent dislocation of the patella. *J Bone Joint Surg Br* 1989;71B:121–125.
30. Zappala F, Taffel C, Scuderi G: Rehabilitation of patellofemoral joint disorders. *Orthop Clin North Am* 1992;23:555–566.
31. McConnell J: The management of chondromalacia patella: A long term solution. *Aust J Physiother* 1986;32:215–223.
32. Shelton G: Conservative management of patellofemoral dysfunction. *Prim Care* 1992;19: 331–350.
33. Insall J: "Chondromalacia patellae": Patellar malalignment syndrome. *Orthop Clin North Am* 1979;10:117–127.
34. Muller E: Influence of training and of inactivity on muscle strength. *Arch Phys Med Rehabil* 1970;51:449–462.
35. Henry J: Conservative treatment of patellofemoral subluxation. *Clin Sports Med* 1989;8:261–278.
36. Chrisman D: The role of articular cartilage in patellofemoral pain. *Orthop Clin North Am* 1986;17:231–234.
37. Chrisman D, Snook G, Wilson T: The protective effect of aspirin against degeneration of human articular cartilage. *Clin Orthop* 1972;84: 193–196.
38. Steadman J: Nonoperative measures for patellofemoral problems. *Am J Sports Med* 1979;7: 374–375.
39. Cherf J, Paulos L: Bracing for patellar instability. *Clin Sports Med* 1990;9:813–821.
40. Palumbo P: Dynamic patellar brace: A new orthosis in the management of patellofemoral disorders. *Am J Sports Med* 1981;9:45–49.
41. Villar R: Patellofemoral pain and the infrapatellar brace. *Am J Sports Med* 1985;13:313–315.
42. Hanten W, Schulthies S: Exercise effect on electromyographic activity of the vastus medialis oblique and vastus lateralis muscles. *Phys Ther* 1990;70:561–565.
43. Ingersoll C, Knight K: Patellar location changes following EMG biofeedback of progressive resistive exercises. *Med Sci Sports Exerc* 1991; 23:1122–1127.
44. Soderberg G, Minor S, Arnold K, et al.: Electromyographic analysis of knee exercises in healthy subjects and in patients with knee pathologies. *Phys Ther* 1987;67:1691–1696.
45. Ericson M, Nisell R: Patellofemoral joint forces during ergometric cycling. *Phys Ther* 1987;67: 1365–1369.
46. DeHaven K, Dolan W, Mayer P: Chondromalacia patellae in athletes: Clinical presentation and conservative management. *Am J Sports Med* 1979;7:5–11.
47. Fulkerson J: The etiology of patellofemoral pain in young, active patients. *Clin Orthop* 1983;179:129–133.
48. Malek M, Mangine R: Patellofemoral pain syndromes: A comprehensive and conservative approach. *J Orthop Sports Phys Ther* 1981;2: 108–116.

Suggested Readings

Bentley G, Dowd G: Current concepts of etiology and treatment of chondromalacia patellae. *Clin Orthop* 1984;189:209–228.

Bigos S, McBride G: The isolated lateral retinacular release in the treatment of patellofemoral disorders. *Clin Orthop* 1984;186:75–80.

Bose K, Kanagasuntheram R, Osman M: Vastus medialis oblique: An anatomic and physiologic study. *Orthopedics* 1980;3:880–883.

Brattstrom H: Patella alta in non-dislocating knee joints. *Acta Orthop Scand* 1970;41:578–588.

Broom M, Fulkerson J: The plica syndrome: A new prospective. *Orthop Clin North Am* 1986; 17: 279–281.

Chen S, Ramanathan E: The treatment of patellar instability by lateral release. *J Bone Joint Surg Br* 1984;66B:344–348.

Crosby E, Insall J: Recurrent dislocation of the patella. *J Bone Joint Surg Am* 1976;58A:9–13.

Dandy D: Arthroscopy in the treatment of young patients with anterior knee pain. *Orthop Clin North Am* 1986;17:221–229.

Dzioba R: Diagnostic arthroscopy and longitudinal open lateral release. *Am J Sports Med* 1990;18: 343–348.

Carson W, James S, Larson R, et al.: Patellofemoral disorders: Physical and radiographic evaluation, part I physical examination. *Clin Orthop* 1984; 185:165–177.

Carson W, James S, Larson R, et al.: Patellofemoral disorders: Physical and radiographic evaluation, part II radiographic examination. *Clin Orthop* 1984;185:178–186.

Fisher R: Conservative treatment of patellofemoral pain. *Orthop Clin North Am* 1986;17:269–272.

Fulkerson JP, Hungerford DS: *Disorders of the Patello-Femoral Joint, ed. 2.* Baltimore, Williams & Wilkiens Co., 1990.

Goodfellow J, Hungerford D, Zindel M: Patellofemoral joint mechanics and pathology. Functional anatomy of the patellofemoral joint. *J Bone Joint Surg Br* 1976;58B:287–290.

Goodfellow J, Hungerford D, Woods C: Patellofemoral joint mechanics and pathology. Chondromalacia patellae. *J Bone Joint Surg Br* 1976; 58B:291–299.

Grana W, Kriegshauser L: Scientific basis of extensor mechanism disorders. *Clin Sports Med* 1985; 4:247–257.

Grood E, Suntay W, Noyes F, et al.: Biomechanics of the knee-extension exercise. *J Bone Joint Surg Am* 1984;66A:725–734.

Hallisey M, Doherty N, Bennett W, et al.: Anatomy of the junction of the vastus lateralis tendon and the patella. *J Bone Joint Surg Am* 1987;69A: 545–549.

Hardaker W, Whipple T, Bassett F: Diagnosis and treatment of the plica syndrome of the knee. *J Bone Joint Surg Am* 1980;62A:221–225.

Hayes C, Sawyer R, Conway W: Patellar cartilage lesions: In vitro detection and staging with MR imaging and pathologic correlation. *Radiology* 1990;176:479–483.

Henry J, Goletz T, Williamson B: Lateral retinacular release in patellofemoral subluxation. *Am J Sports Med* 1986;14:121–129.

Hungerford D, Lennox D: Rehabilitation of the knee and disorders of the patellofemoral joint: Relevant biomechanics. *Orthop Clin North Am* 1983;14:397–402.

Hughston J: Subluxation of the patella. *J Bone Joint Surg Am* 1968;50A:1003–1026.

Insall J: Patellar pain. *J Bone Joint Surg Am* 1982; 64A:147–151.

Insall J, Aglietti P, Tria A: Patellar pain and incongruence. II. Clinical application. *Clin Orthop* 1983;176:225–232.

Insall J, Salvati E: Patella position in the normal knee joint. *Radiology* 1971;101:101–104.

Kaufer H: Patellar biomechanics. *Clin Orthop* 1979; 144:51–54.

Lancourt J, Cristini J: Patella alta and patella infera. *J Bone Joint Surg Am* 1975;57A:1112–1115.

Larsen E, Lauridsen F: Conservative treatment of patellar dislocations. *Clin Orthop* 1982;171:131–136.

Lieb F, Perry J: Quadriceps function. *J Bone Joint Surg Am* 1968;50A:1535–1548.

Macdonald D, Hutton J, Kelly I: Maximal isometric patellofemoral contact force in patients with anterior knee pain. *J Bone Joint Surg Br* 1989; 71B:296–299.

Maquet P: Mechanics and osteoarthritis of the patellofemoral joint. *Clin Orthop* 1979;144:70–73.

Mariani P, Caruso I: An electromyographic investigation of subluxation of the patella. *J Bone Joint Surg Br* 1979;61B:169–171.

Micheli L: Overuse injuries in children's sports: The growth factor. *Orthop Clin North Am* 1983; 14:337–360.

Paulos L, Rusch K, Johnson C, et al.: Patellar malalignment. A treatment rationale. *Phys Ther* 1980;60:1624–1632.

Patel D: Plica as a cause of anterior knee pain. *Orthop Clin North Am* 1986;17:273–277.

Reider B, Marshall J, Koslin B, et al.: The anterior aspect of the knee joint. An anatomical study. *J Bone Joint Surg Am* 1981;63A:351–356.

Reider B, Marshall J, Ring B: Patellar tracking. *Clin Orthop* 1981;157:143–148.

Reider B, Marshall J, Warren R: Clinical characteristics of patellar disorders in young athletes. *Am J Sports Med* 1981;9:270–274.

Reynolds L, Levin T, Medeiros J, et al.: EMG activity of the vastus medialis oblique and the vastus lateralis in their role in patellar alignment. *Am J Phys Med* 1983;62:61–70.

Seedhom B, Takeda T, Tsubuku M, et al.: Mechanical factors and patellofemoral osteoarthrosis. *Ann Rheum Dis* 1979;38:307–316.

Terry G: The anatomy of the extensor mechanism. *Clin Sports Med* 1989;8:163–177.

Tria A, Palumbo R, Alicea J: Conservative care for patellofemoral pain. *Orthop Clin North Am* 1992;23:545–554.

Walsh W, Helzer-Julin M: Patellar tracking problems in athletes. *Prim Care* 1992;19:303–330.

Woodall W, Welsh J: A biomechanical basis for rehabilitation programs involving the patellofemoral joint. *J Orthop Sports Phys Ther* 1990; 11:535–542.

Yates C: Patellofemoral pain—A prospective study. *Orthopedics* 1986;9:663–667.

Yulish B, Montanez J, Goodfellow D, et al.: Chondromalacia patellae: Assessment with MR imaging. *Radiology* 1987:164:763–766.

8

Rehabilitation of the Patellofemoral Joint

Suanne S. Maurer, Glenn Carlin, Robert Butters, and Giles R. Scuderi

The incidence of anterior knee pain within the general population is reported to be as high as one in four, with the proportion increasing in the athletic population.[1] This is the most encountered knee problem seen today.[2]

Anterior knee pain that results from abnormal tracking of or pressure on the patellofemoral articulation without disruption of the patella's articular cartilage may be referred to as *patellofemoral pain syndrome* (PFPS).[3] Most commonly PFPS is a result of extensor mechanism malalignment that is caused by three main factors: (1) abnormalities of patellofemoral configuration, (2) deficiency of supporting musculature or guiding mechanics, and (3) malalignment of the extremity relating to the knee mechanics.[4] All these can be treated conservatively as well as surgically.

The conservative approach is usually exhausted before surgical intervention is attempted. Many PFPS patients will respond well if conservative treatment focuses on controlling inflammation, releasing tight lateral structures, quadriceps strengthening, and avoidance of harmful activities. The various causes of PFPS gives rise to several rehabilitative techniques shown to be effective. To date, there has not been one protocol that has proven to be universally effective. The purpose of this chapter is to explore varied approaches in dealing with those patients suffering from PFPS. The assorted techniques described have been shown to be an effective means of decreasing patellofemoral pain.

The cause of the PFPS must be identified through a thorough lower-extremity evaluation to effectively treat the patient. Patient individuality must be ensured; therefore, a "cookbook" approach should not be used when dealing with patients who have PFPS. It is important, however, that the clinician knows the appropriate progression and integration of therapeutic techniques.

Stretching and Mobilization

The unrestricted movement of the entire lower kinetic chain is vital for proper functioning of the patellofemoral joint. The PFPS patient should be examined thoroughly for comparative passive and active motions. Restrictions, contractures, neural inhibitions, or spasms in relation to the patient's particular pain pattern will need to be evaluated.

Travell and Simons describe trigger point pain patterns associated with anterior knee pain.[5] Travell and Simons define a *trigger point* as a focal area of hypersensitivity in a tissue that may be locally tender or painful, and may give rise to referred pain and tenderness, referred autonomic phenomena, and proprioceptive distortion.[5] The restrictions are most readily observed in the rectus femoris, while restricted vastus medialis obliquus (VMO) or vastus lateralis (VL) will result in disruption of patella alignment. Figures 8.1 and 8.2 show the common locations of trigger points of the VMO and the VL, respectively.

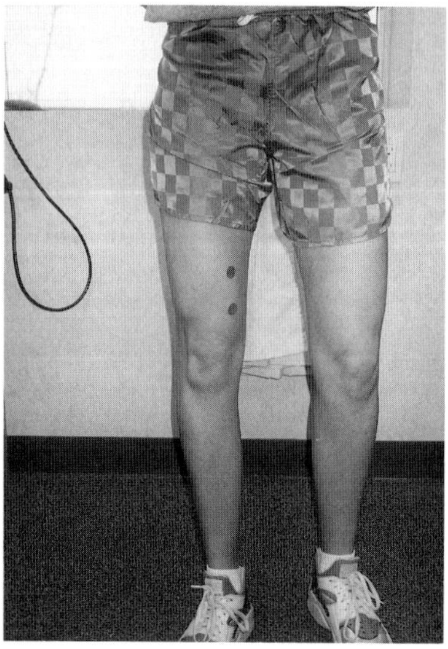

FIGURE 8.1. Common trigger point locations of the VMO.

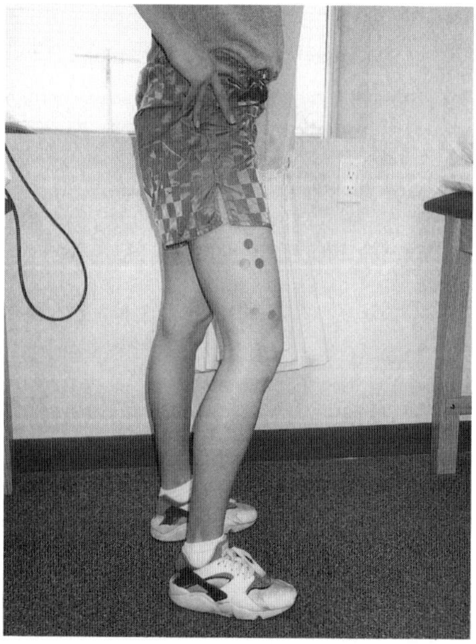

FIGURE 8.2. Common trigger point locations of the VL.

Trigger points in the rectus femoris and the VMO may refer pain to the anterior knee.[5]

Antich et al. showed that hamstring and quadriceps tightness was found in involved extremities relative to the opposite limb.[6] They suggest that this increases the potential of extensor mechanism overload. Kramer and others have implemented tight lateral retinaculum as a cause of PFPS.[7–9] When restricted, the iliotibial band and the tensor fasciae latae have also been shown as contributing factors in lateral patellar tracking.[8,5] Travell and Simons attribute anterior lateral knee pain to trigger points in the tensor fasciae latae and the VL. They describe this condition as the "stuck patella."[5] Additionally, tight hip flexors, hip external rotators, and gastrocnemius muscles should be considered when checking for pathologic restrictions.

The use of therapeutic exercises are vital in the attempt to correct the lower-limb biomechanics by releasing restrictions. Modalities may be used to enhance this process. Ultrasound, electric muscle stimulation (EMS), thermotherapy, and cryotherapy are excellent complementary modalities. Several techniques are available to correct abnormal range of motion (ROM). Cryostretch, propioceptive neuromuscular fascilitation (PNF) stretches, contract–relax, reciprocal inhibition, myofacial release, soft-tissue mobilization, CPM,[10] and stationary bike are techniques that can be used to reestablish normal ROM.[11,5] Figure 8.3 shows assisted passive stretching of tight lateral structures.

Stretching and soft-tissue mobilization techniques should be taught to the patient and updated periodically. Figure 8.4 shows self-stretches for the lateral structures, quadriceps femoris, and the hamstrings, respectively. The patient should be instructed to perform static stretches that are held between 20 and 40 s at the point of mild tension of the stretched muscle, stopping short of pain, and then relaxing for 5 to 10 s. This should be repeated a minimum of five times bilaterally for each exercise.

Tennis ball exercises can be used to release trigger points in the VL. The patient will lay on the affected side and place the tennis ball under the tender points in the lateral thigh (Figure 8.5). The patient should control the pressure so that mild to moderate discomfort is experienced and pain is avoided. This can be performed for 1 or 2 min for each trigger point once each day, or every other day.[5]

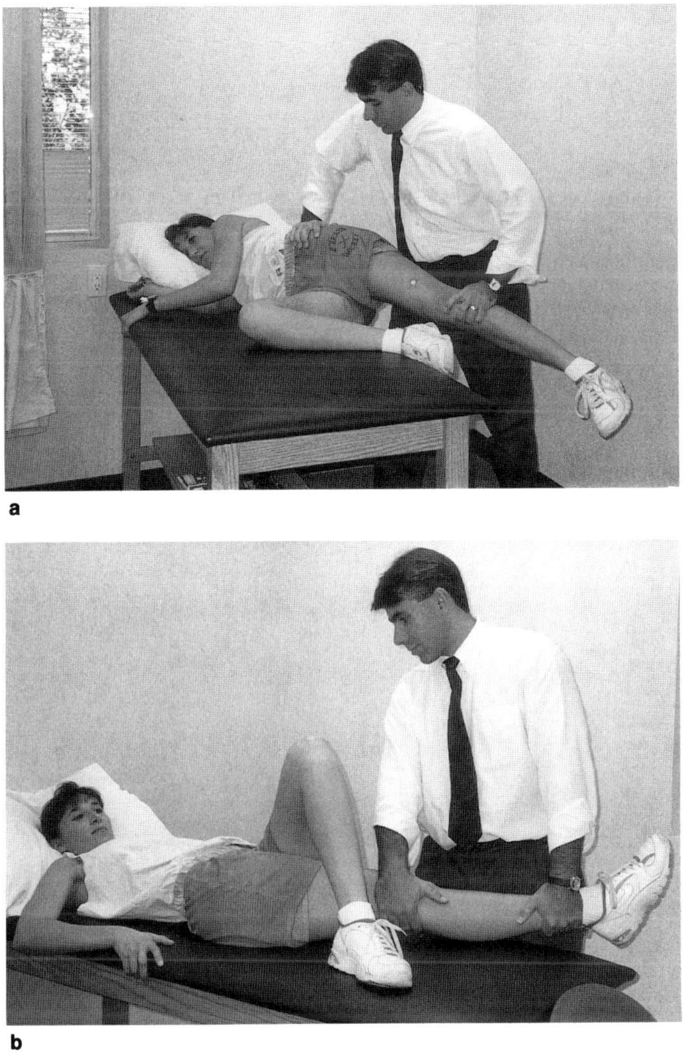

FIGURE 8.3. Assistive passive stretching for tight lateral structures. (a) Lateral decubitus position and (b) supine position.

Kramer also discusses two techniques in soft-tissue mobilization designed to decrease lateral pressure and enhance cartilage metabolism.[7] Maitland and others have suggested the potential for healing articular cartilage.[10,12,13] These authors suggest that controlled forces applied to collagen increases articular nutrition and metabolism, while decreasing capsular contractures, joint stiffness, and the effects of disuse.

As Kramer described, the first technique involves a medial glide of the patella.[7] Begin with the thumb pads on the lateral border of the patella and mobilize the patella medially (Figure 8.6). The amplitudes are progressively increased, and are held initially for no more than 30 s and progressed up to 1 min for larger amplitudes. This can be taught to patients for self-mobilizations.

This technique can be combined with longitudinal movements and with a compression movement as healing dictates.[14] After pain and effusion have subsided, patella compression tracking can be attempted in order to facilitate cartilage metabolism. Figure 8.7 depicts this second technique. The patient begins seated with the knee bent up to 90° of flexion. The patient actively extends the knee while the patella is compressed and tracked medially by the rehabilitation specialist.[7,14] The degree of

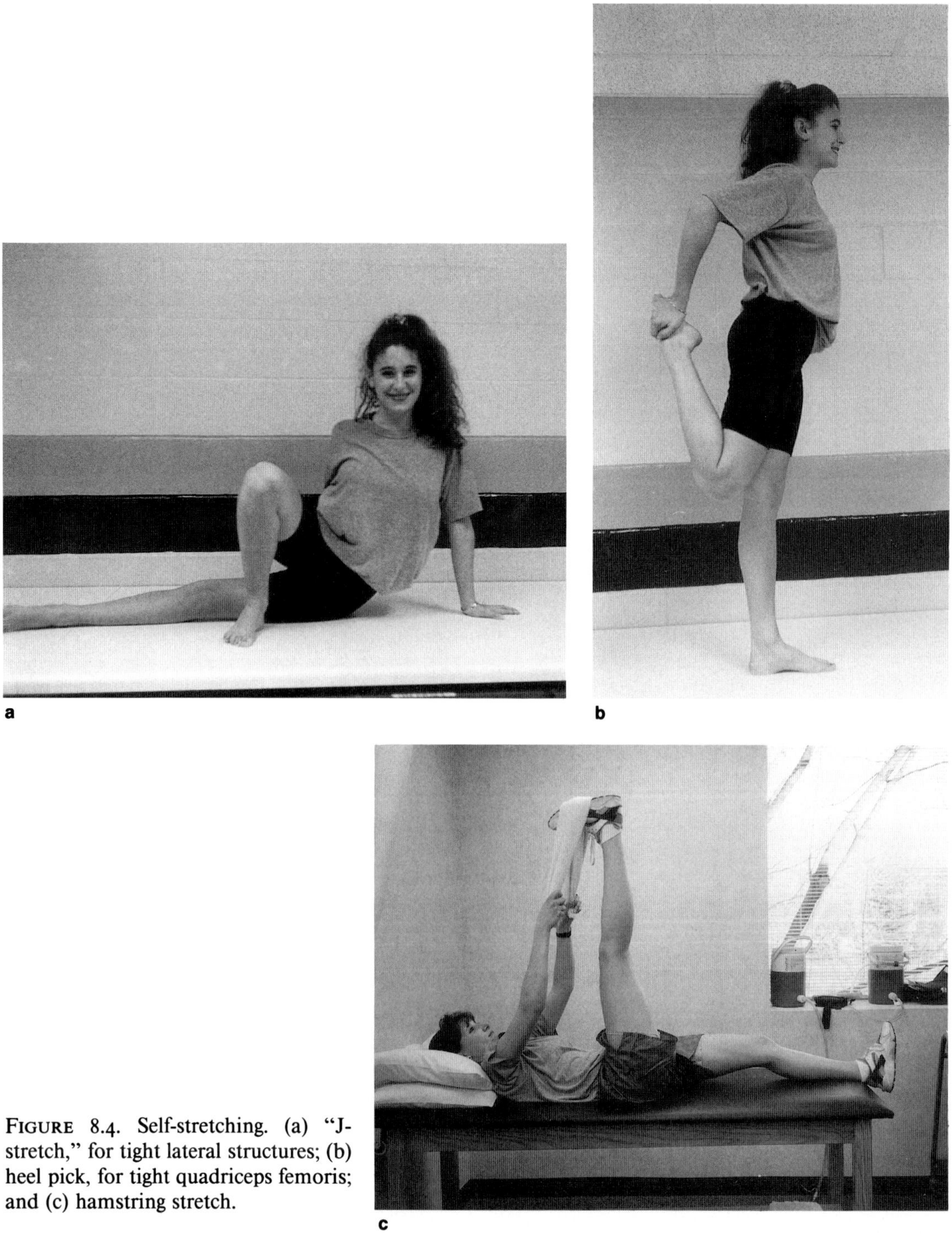

FIGURE 8.4. Self-stretching. (a) "J-stretch," for tight lateral structures; (b) heel pick, for tight quadriceps femoris; and (c) hamstring stretch.

flexion and the amount of compression should be carefully graded to avoid increasing pain and effusion.

These techniques must be initiated carefully and gently with the patient's particular level of pain and tissue damage kept in mind. As pain decreases, the mobilization can increase until maximum amplitude can be achieved with a strong compressive component.[14]

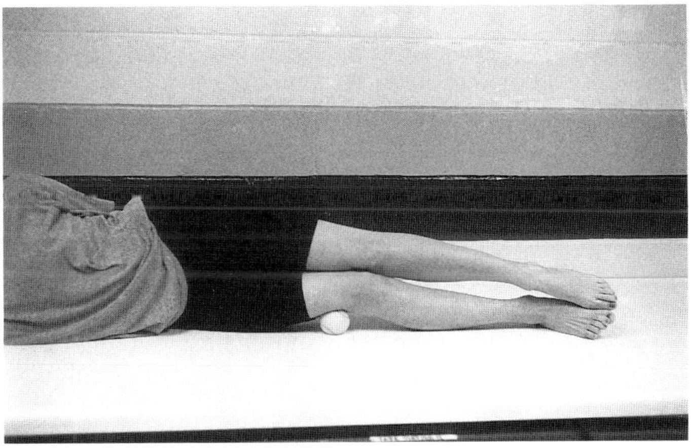

a

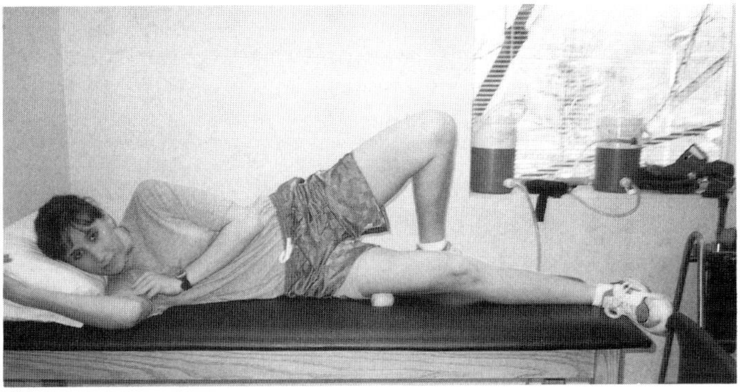

b

FIGURE 8.5. Tennis ball exercises (a) for common distal VL trigger points and (b) for common proximal VL trigger points.

Neuromotor Control

Neuromotor control is fundamental for proper functioning of the knee. After an injury, immobilization, or a period of non-weight bearing, there is a deterioration of proprioception and kinesthesis.[11] The reestablishment of proper functioning of the mechanoreceptors of the lower extremities is crucial in regaining proper functioning.[15] This neuromotor retraining should occur early in the rehabilitation program and should emphasize closed kinetic chain (CKC) exercises that simulate near-normal functioning.

Closed kinetic chain may be defined as a series of connecting joints that creates an intricate motor system in which the distal segment is fixed. This is in contrast to open kinetic chain (OKC), where the distal segment is free.[11,16] CKC exercises aid in neuromuscular reeducation and restore lower-extremity joint integration.

Pain and swelling in the knee will result in neural inhibition of the quadriceps. Spencer et al. found that the VMO was inhibited after only 20 mL being present in the joint, as apposed to 50 to 60 mL of saline being required before inhibition of the rectus femoris and VL muscles.[17] If left unchecked, these inhibitions and subsequent neuromuscular deficits can cause mechanical alterations of the extensor mechanism, which may potentially lead to the onset of PFPS.

Bennett and Stauber have suggested that PFPS may be a result of improper neuromotor control of the quadriceps muscle, specifically during the eccentric phase of control.[18] McConnell also suggests that timing of the VMO contraction should be stressed during rehabilitation rather than just increasing activity.[8]

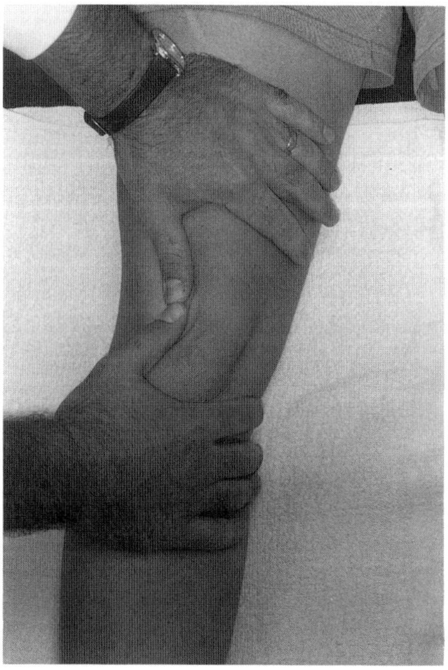

FIGURE 8.6. Medial patella mobilizations.

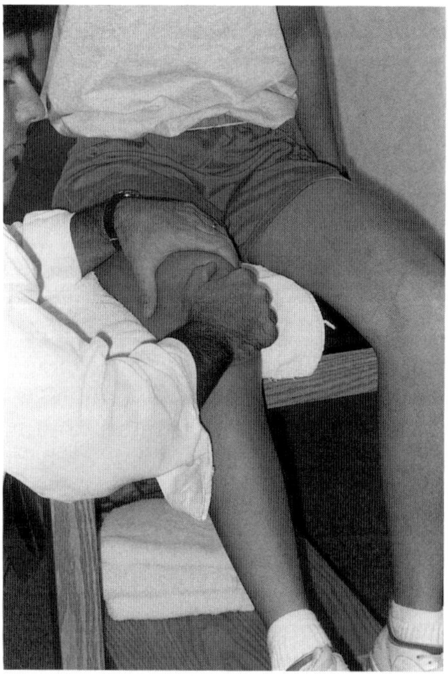

FIGURE 8.7. Patella compression tracking. The clinician provides compression of the patella against the articular surfaces while maintaining a medial tracking as the knee is extended.

Neuromotor control should be the main emphasis in PFPS rehabilitation.

Affected knees have demonstrated a greater concentric muscle contraction (CMC) quadriceps torque than eccentric muscle contraction (EMC).[18] EMC in the normal quadriceps muscle should produce greater tension for the same motor unit activation, support more weight, and have greater torque than CMC.[9,19,20] Eccentric peak torque has also been shown to increase or remain constant with increases in movement velocities when compared with CMC, which decreases.[19,21]

Upon specific training, the reversal of the EMC/CMC deficit and of the PFPS symptoms occurred in such a brief period of time that the change was presumed to have occurred because of changes in neurologic functioning.[18] The same effect did not occur for patients with knee pain from other causes such as meniscal tears. These neural adaptations are similar to those that Knight[15,22] described in explaining the quick effects of the DAPRE (daily adjustable progressive resistive exercise) program explained in Table 8.1.

Using the following protocol, Bennett and Stauber were able to facilitate neuromuscular control.[18] These exercises were performed eccentrically in a range between 0° and 50° flexion that was pain-free and subjectively adjusted daily according to the patient's tolerance. Three sets of ten repetitions at speeds of 30°, 60°, and 90°/s were performed isokinetically for a total of 90 repetitions per session. The strengthening was continued until the patient's pain was relieved.

Neurologic control can also be facilitated with the use of CKC activities such as minisquats, lunges, steps, leg press, balancing boards (Figure 8.8), and sliding boards. Proprioceptive balancing activities should also be a focus and can include stork standing (Figure 8.9), BAPS board (Figure 8.10) (CAMP, Jackson, Mich.), Plyo Rebounder (Figure 8.11) (EFI/Total Gym, San Diego), and unilateral balancing. Various movements of the contralateral hip can be used to alter the neuromotor input such as using static and dynamic actions in abduction, extension, and flexion, and then adding resistance to the contralateral hip. The

TABLE 8.1. DAPRE technique

	Set 1	Set 2	Set 3	Set 4
Percentage of working weight	50	75	100	Adjusted*
No. of repetitions	10	6	Max	Max†

Working weight adjustment		
A	B	C
No. of repetitions performed during the set	Adjusted working weight for set 4	Working weight for the next day
0–2	Decrease 5–10 lb (2.3–4.5 kg)	Decrease 5–10 lb (2.3–4.5 kg)
3–4	Decrease 0–5 lb (0–2.3 kg)	Keep the same
5–7	Keep the same	Increase 2.5–7.5 lb (1.1–3.4 kg)
8–10	Increase 2.5–5 lb (1.1–2.3 kg)	Increase 5–10 lb (2.3–4.5 kg)
More than 10	Increase 5–10 lb (2.3–4.5 kg)	Increase 10–15 lb (4.5–6.8 kg)

*The adjusted working weight for set 4 is determined by the number of repetitions performed during set 3. Use columns A and B as a guide.
†The number of repetitions performed during set 4 determines the working weight for the next day. Use columns A and C as a guide.
Source: Knight. Reprinted with permission of Waverly and Knight, K.: Quadriceps Strengthening with the DAPRE Technique Med Science Sports Exercise 17:647. 1985.

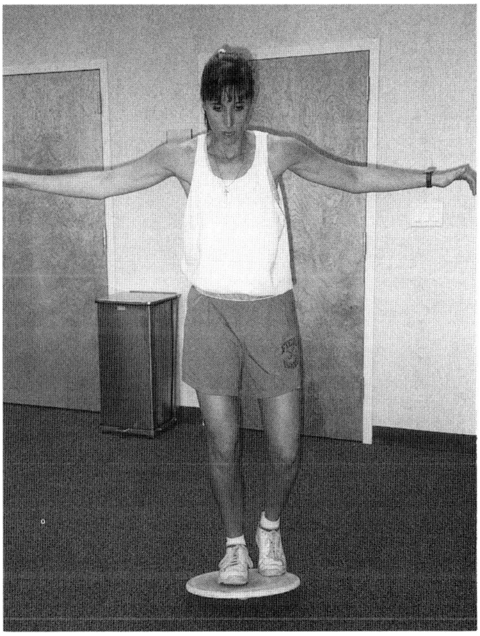

FIGURE 8.8. Balance board exercises in an unsupported position.

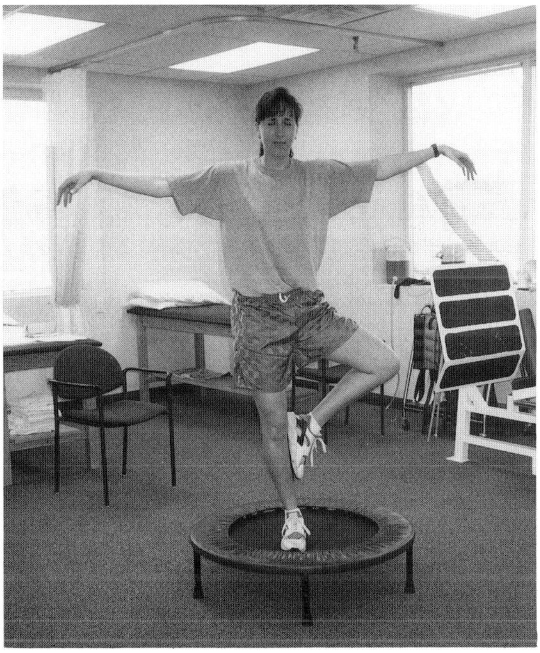

FIGURE 8.9. Stork stance on the trampoline with eyes closed.

BAPS board can also be used in several ways and can be facilitated by the use of biofeedback. Progressions involve manipulating such variables as supported to unsupported; two feet to one; eyes open and looking down, straight ahead, and eyes closed; and adding the use of the Plyo Rebounder.

Tubing exercises, both high-speed straight

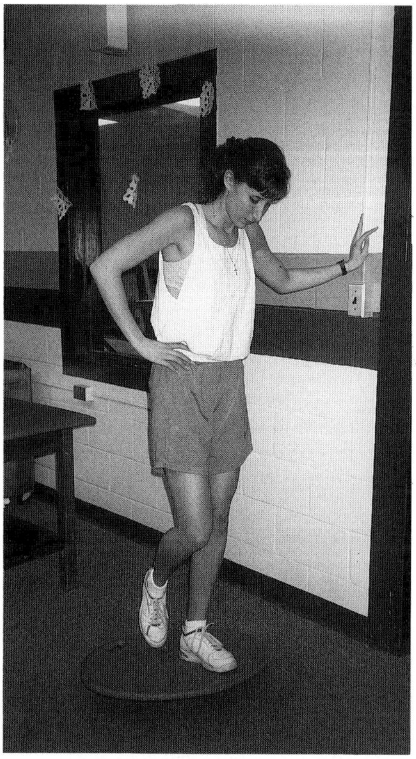

FIGURE 8.10. BAPS board unilateral with support.

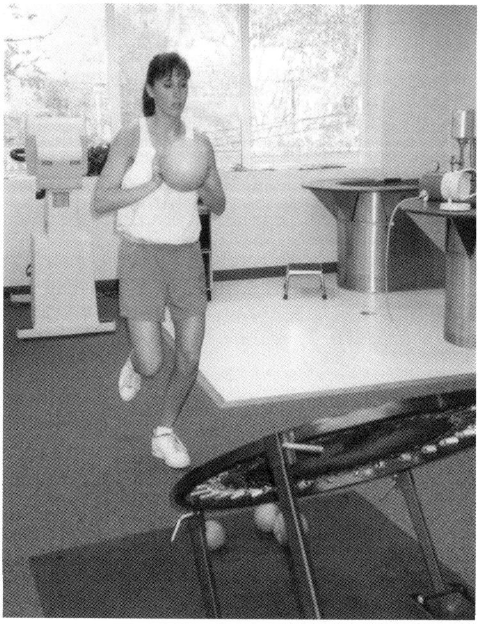

FIGURE 8.11. Plyo Rebounder. The patient balances unilaterally while dynamically stabilizing against the force of decelerating and accelerating a weighted ball.

leg and eccentric yo-yo exercises, can also be used to enhance neuromotor redevelopment. High-speed tubing exercises may be performed with the involved leg completing a straight leg adduction exercise with a strong VMO contraction (Figure 8.12), and with hip flexion and extension again using the tubing to create resisted adduction. The patient should perform these at predetermined ROM and at progressive speeds. The yo-yo exercises are an excellent facilitator of neuromuscular control because they require the patient to actively control the force produced by the quadriceps in an eccentric submaximal load.[23] The yo-yo exercise involves attaching a length of rubber tubing with a hanging weight to the patient's lower leg and then having the patient rhythmically contract the quadriceps. Figure 8.13 illustrates this technique. The object is to perform a series of smooth, controlled bounces with the weight. This exercise emphasizes neuromuscular control and not force.

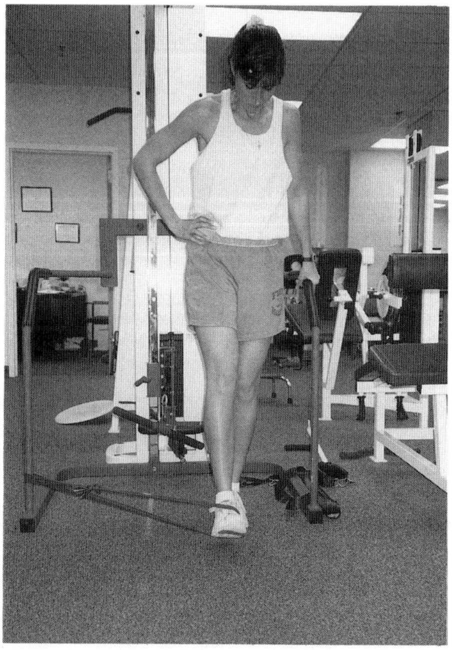

FIGURE 8.12. Tubing adduction with hip flexed slightly and knee extended.

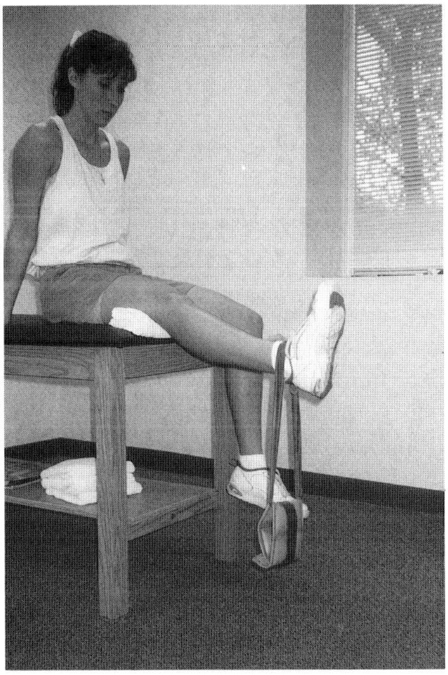

FIGURE 8.13. Yo-yo exercise. Eccentric loading of the knee extensors in the terminal range. Maintaining a smooth, even bounce should be emphasized.

Strengthening Techniques

Traditionally, the strength of the musculature surrounding the knee, especially the quadriceps, has been the main focus in rehabilitating patients with PFPS. Research has led clinicians to believe that increasing quadriceps strength is directly correlated to decreasing patellofemoral pain.[15,24] Recently, however, much focus has been placed on redeveloping functional strength, especially through CKC exercises. The lower compressive and shearing forces in the patellofemoral joint associated with CKC exercises have made them the mainstay of the PFPS rehabilitation process, yet the appropriate use of OKC exercises can also enhance this process.

The use of OKC exercises must be incorporated when CKC exercise is contraindicated or too difficult for the patient to perform. A progressive integration of strengthening exercises is necessary to accomplish the patient's desired goals through the PFPS rehabilitation program.

Specific VMO strengthening techniques need to be incorporated into the program. The function of the VMO is to realign the patella during extension.[25] This is the only medial stabilizer and any insufficiency will cause the patella to drift laterally.[26,27] The goal of the rehabilitation is to achieve a dynamic balance between the VMO and the VL.[2,27,28] The prescribed exercises should attempt to selectively activate and strengthen the VMO to reduce muscle imbalance.[29] Travell and Simons describe the VMO as the "quitter muscle" because this muscle will become inhibited and unexpectedly weak as a response to injury or pain.[5] The VL is the bulk of the quadriceps femoris group and, according to the law of valgus, will naturally pull the patella laterally.[5] When this is associated with other factors such as VMO inhibition or weakness, tight lateral structures, or biomechanical abnormalities, patellofemoral dysfunction results.

Perhaps the two most common exercises described for PFPS rehabilitation include the isometric quadriceps set and the straight leg raise (SLR).[30–32] Justification for use of these exercises includes decreased joint compression, graded tension, and little or no joint movement. O'Neil believes that SLRs are an effective means of increasing quadriceps strength early in the rehabilitation program, while ROM is limited.[31] These often are initiated while the patient is still in the immobilizer.

Knight suggests that isometric quadriceps sets can be performed with increasing resistance using the DAPRE program.[15] The resistance will be adjusted according to the patient's neuromuscular redevelopment. The advantage of this program is that it is graded and progressive. This exercise protocol is outlined in Table 8.1. Antich and Brewster suggest that ankle dorsiflexion can be incorporated with quadriceps isometrics to decrease pain.[33] Heckman suggests that isometric quadriceps are performed with as strong a contraction as possible below the pain threshold.[30] Ten-second contractions can be used and should be completed in sets of ten, ten times per day. When a strong active contraction is not possible because of pain, swelling, etc., the use of electric stimulation and/or biofeedback (Figure 8.14) may be incorporated, with concentration on the VMO.[30]

As ROM and pain permits, the isometrics may be performed at various degrees of flexion, usually a carry-over effect of 15° to 20° will allow strengthening through the range.[30,34]

Once a strong active contraction can be performed, patients may begin SLRs in all four planes. If lateral compression syndrome exists, abduction should be omitted. The SLRs can be completed with the patient laying down or standing on the uninvolved leg. Active isometric contraction of the VMO should be maintained throughout the entire exercise, completing three to five sets of ten to 15 repetitions with no weight initially and progressing to 20 lb (9 kg) or 10% of the patient's body weight.[30] The VMO activity may be enhanced with electric muscle stimulators and/or biofeedback.

McConnell states that initial training should include an adduction component to facilitate VMO contraction while eliminating as much as possible the VL and the rectus femoris from

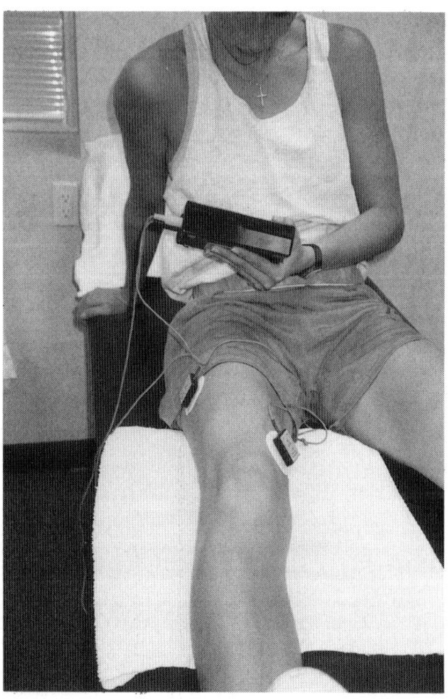

FIGURE 8.14. Quadriceps set using biofeedback to enhance VMO redevelopment.

initiating the contraction.[33,35] These exercises could include medicine ball squeezing both in non-weight bearing (Figure 8.15) and weight bearing (Figure 8.16), rubber tubing exercises, and use of low-pulley exercises. Later, adduction exercise can be decreased and isolated VMO work should be emphasized.

With the continued improvement of ROM and muscular control short arc quadriceps (SAQ) exercises can be initiated. A short arc quadriceps (SAQ) is a dynamic strengthening exercise that is completed in a small segment relative to the full ROM. Recommendations on safe angles vary. Malek and Mangine, and Heckman suggest exercising around crepitus using a range of 90° to 45° or the flexion arc.[3,30] Sczepanski et al. define this arc as 60° to 85°.[29] The rationale is that patellofemoral joint surface contact is the highest for dispersal of forces between the patella and the femoral condyles.[3,30] Other authors recommend the use of SAQ at the terminal ranges, although the cited boundaries vary.[36,37,38] The rationale for this is that patellofemoral joint contact surfaces are the lowest and the quadriceps tension is the highest. The correct prescription of exercises will focus on pain-free ROM while avoiding the suspected contact pressure ranges and the patient's ability to alter muscular imbalances. Pain-free ROM should be the primary guideline and needs to be evaluated daily, avoiding the area of crepitation because this is usually associated with patellofemoral chondrosis. These exercises should be performed with emphasis on the VMO and progressive weights can be used as symptoms allow.

The DAPRE program, as referred to previously, is an excellent technique that allows for maximal strength increases by accommodating to the patient's neuromuscular redevelopment. These exercises should include both limbs, exercising the injured limb first.

SAQ may also be performed in the CKC. The patient may perform short arc leg press (Figure 8.17), minisquats (Fig 8.18), and Don Tigney exercises (Figure 8.19) in an effort to increase the functional nature of the rehabilitation and to further decrease patellofemoral joint forces.[11,24] Steinkamp et al. suggested that

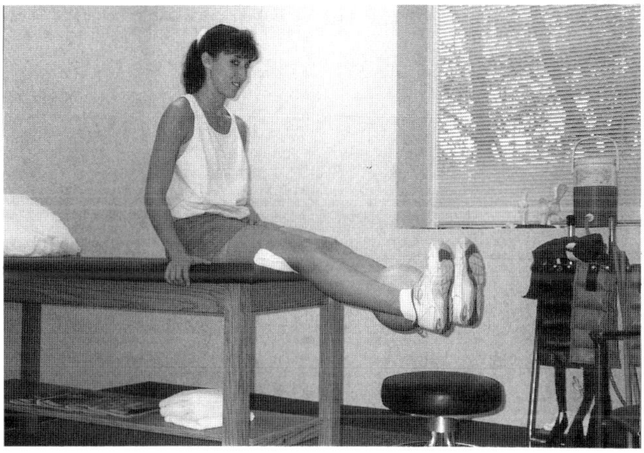

FIGURE 8.15. Adduction squeeze exercise incorporating knee extension. These can be completed both isometrically or in short arc quadriceps (SAQ) to enhance VMO recruitment.

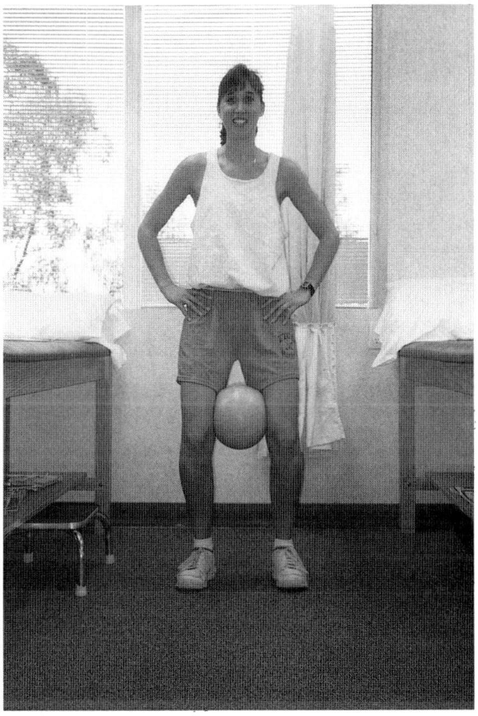

FIGURE 8.16. Adduction squeeze exercise combined with minisquats unsupported to enhance VMO strengthening.

PFPS patients respond better to leg press exercises than to leg extension exercises in the functional range of 0° to 30°.[24]

The muscle stress should be progressive, beginning with no more than 25% of the patient's body weight for the leg press and increasing as symptoms permit. Minisquats can be progressed using various combinations of the following: bilaterally to unilaterally, supported to unsupported, wall slides to free-standing position, and by increasing external resistance as with the use of hand-held weights or rubber tubing (Figure 8.18).[11]

Another useful CKC exercise is the step-up. This can be progressed by increasing the height of the step, which, in turn, will increase the flexion arc. However, patellofemoral joint reactivity should be closely monitored with increases in step height as higher angles of flexion are correlated to higher patellofemoral compressive forces.[24,39] The addition of adduction tubing will further increase strength development of the VMO.

Care must be taken to ensure good technique, especially to avoid flexion into pain and remembering to keep the feet hip width apart while keeping the knees in line with the laces. McConnell states that knee extension with internal femoral rotation will increase the pull of the tensor fasciae latae, and thereby increase the lateral tracking of the patella and decrease the VMO effectiveness.[35]

Isokinetics may also be incorporated in SAQ exercises using faster velocities (120°/s).[34] The patellofemoral joint contact force is decreased because of a decrease in surface pressure at synovial fluid interfaces, but Sczepanski et al. also suggest that there is an in-

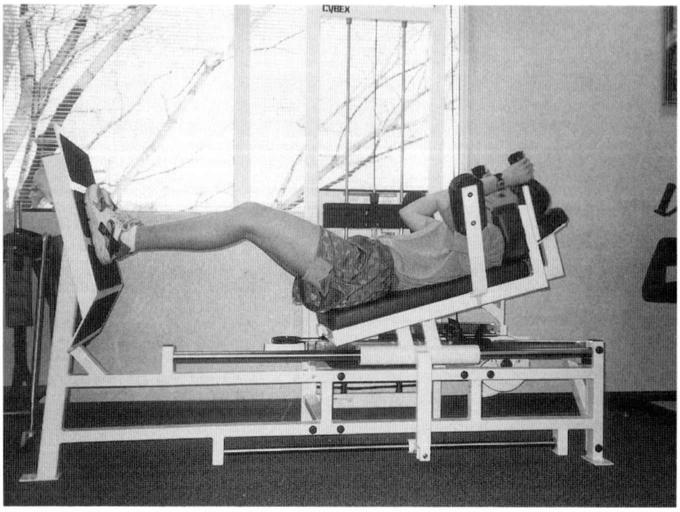

FIGURE 8.17. Leg press. The CKC SAQ exercises are performed in the 0° to 30° of flexion range.

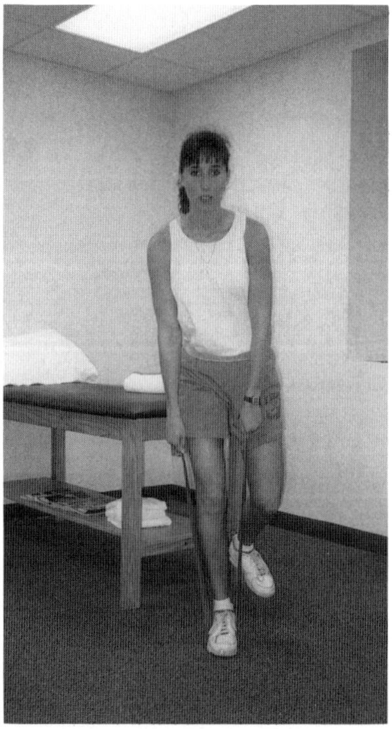

FIGURE 8.18. Minisquats unsupported unilaterally with tubing to increase intensity.

crease in VMO activity relative to the VL at higher speeds (120°) of concentric isokinetics.[29] The patient should begin at 50% intensity and progress to 100% as symptoms permit. These exercises can also be performed in a CKC manner as in the Don Tigney exercise shown in Figure 13.19b.

Once leg strength has increased and has tested at 70% to 80% of the uninvolved side, advanced functional strengthening exercises (i.e., jog–run progressions) can be initiated.[11,30] The leg press and partial squats can be progressions for plyometric-type exercises. The preplyometrics can begin on the leg press (Figure 8.20) and gradually can be progressed to full weight-bearing plyometrics as the patient's specific goals dictate to ensure a safe return to activity. Strength and endurance training for uninvolved musculature and the contralateral limb should also be addressed in a comprehensive program, which should include ankles, knees, hips, buttocks, and lower back.

McConnell Taping and Biofeedback

McConnell suggests that a decrease in patellofemoral pain can be achieved with proper patellar orientation.[35] She believes that by gaining a base as to patellar orientation, one can physically alter the position of the patella by taping it (Figure 8.21). This could then bring the patella into proper positioning, decrease patellofemoral pain, and thereby facilitate the rehabilitation process.

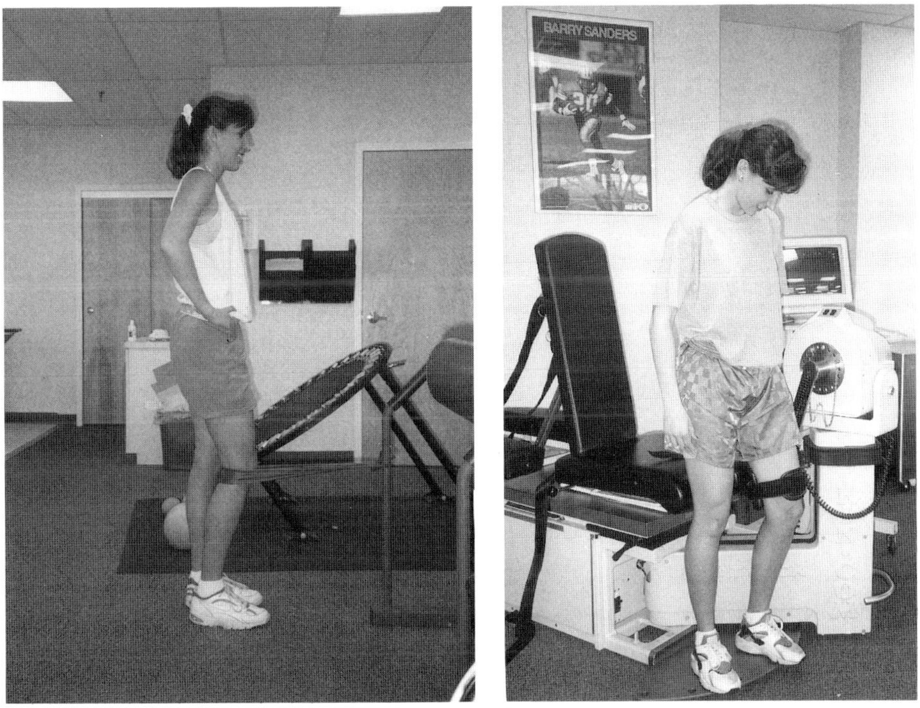

a b

FIGURE 8.19. Don Tigney exercises using (a) tubing and (b) isokinetics.

FIGURE 8.20. Preplyometrics using the leg press bilaterally. The toes are released from the footpad by only a few centimeters.

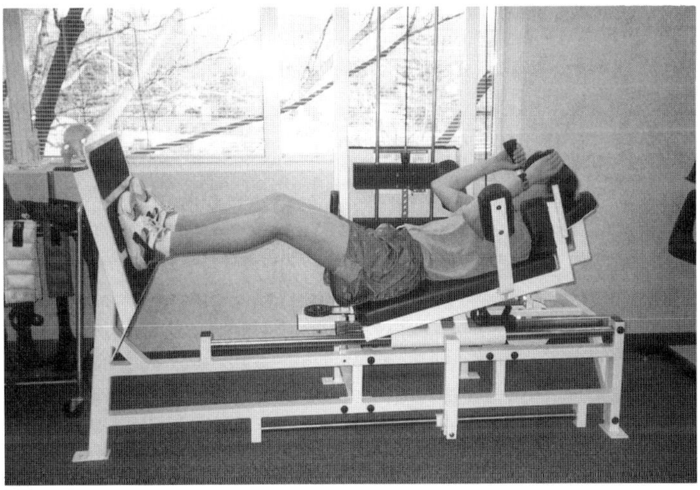

McConnell feels that the following three components must be evaluated with each patient: (1) tilt, (2) glide, and (3) rotation.

The *tilt* is detected by using the thumb and index finger on the lateral and the medial borders. Both fingers should be level. If the medial border sits higher that the lateral, the lateral structures are tight, as most commonly seen in PFPS patients.[35] Correction of the lateral tilt can be made by "firm taping of the midline of the patella medially."[8] This lifts the lateral border and provides a passive stretch to the lateral structures.

The *glide* component determines the

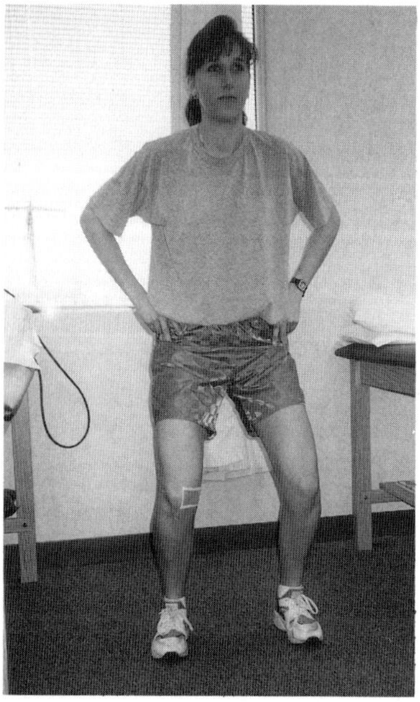

FIGURE 8.21. McConnell knee taping to control patella alignment while performing an unsupported minisquat.

amount of lateral deviation of the patella in the frontal plane. Almost all patients will require a medial glide of their patella. The amount of glide will vary, depending on the tightness of the lateral structures and on the relative amount of activity in the VMO as compared with the VL.[8]

In normal patellar alignment, the longitudinal axis of the patella (the superior and the inferior poles) should be in line with the longitudinal axis of the femur. Deviations from this are termed *rotation.* To correct abnormal patellar rotation, "firm taping from either the middle superior pole downwards and medially (to correct internal rotation of the inferior pole) is applied" or vise versa.[8] This taping technique can be used to assist in the rehabilitation process and should be combined with a VMO strengthening program to achieve lasting results. When attempting to assist the patient in training the VMO, an important factor is in the instruction to the patient to concentrate on a more specific VMO contraction.

The focus in VMO training is to achieve a 1:1 VMO/VL ratio throughout weight-bearing range of motion with simultaneous activation of the two muscles.[40] Biofeedback may be used to assist in initial VMO training. The following is taken from a protocol developed for the Pathway MR-100 (Prometheus Group, Portsmouth, N.H.). This is a set of preprogrammed parameters conforming to the McConnell approach of VMO insufficiency.[40] The following six different positions are used: (1) sitting, (2) standing, (3) minisquat, (4) walk stance, (5) step-down, and (6) wall slide. Modification and addition to these to meet the needs of specific patients is encouraged.

The protocol calls for six repetitions at each position with a 6-s contraction and a 10-s relaxation time. More advanced training may consist of a 2-s contraction and a 2-s relaxation.[40] The quality of the contraction is more important than the quantity of contractions. For those patients who perform too many contractions, the VMO will fatigue, and the VL will dominate. This, in turn, will lead to lateral tracking of the patella.

This protocol was designed to keep daily living activities in mind. Therefore, the patient will use the following functional CKC activities:

1. *Sitting.* The patient is sitting near the end of a chair and is weight bearing with the involved leg. The knees position can range from neutral to 90° of flexion (Figure 8.22). The patient attempts to perform an isolated VMO contraction. Be sure the patient does not internally rotate the hip, curl the toes, or shift weight. Multiple angles of flexion may be performed. For those patients who are having a difficult time, adduction thigh squeezes may facilitate contraction of the VMO.
2. *Standing.* The patient is standing with the feet hip width apart and equal weight bearing on each foot. The knee is in a neutral or slightly flexed position. The patient attempts to contract the VMO while maintaining a good alignment of the lower extremity.
3. *Minisquat.* The patient begins in the same position as in the standing exercise (Figure 8.23). The patient keeps both knees in line

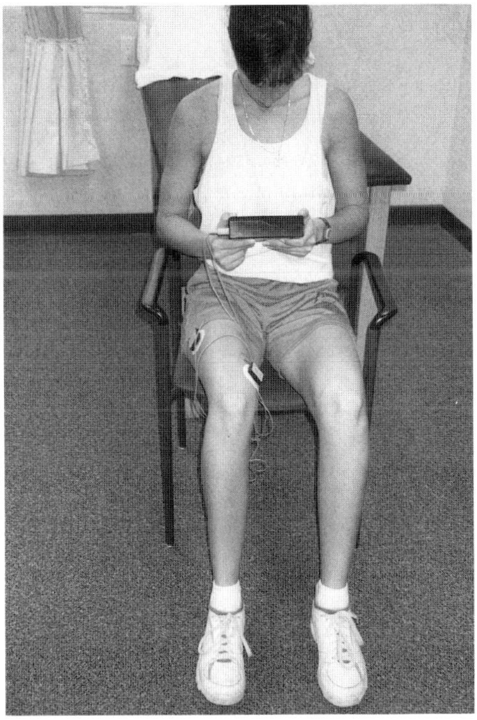

FIGURE 8.22. Biofeedback isometric quadriceps sets in the sitting position.

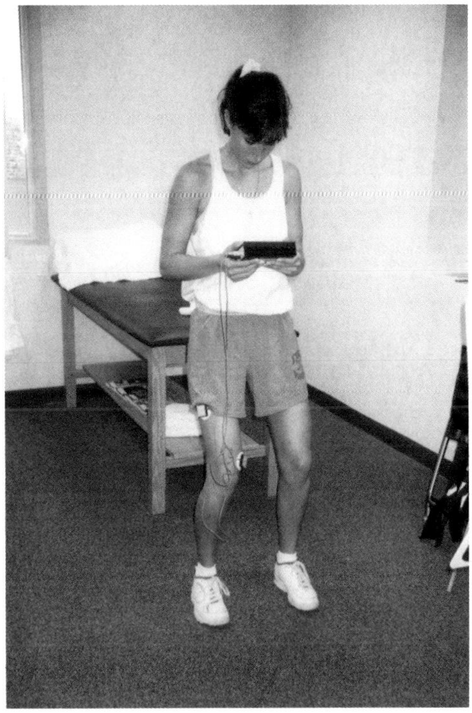

FIGURE 8.23. Biofeedback dynamic quadriceps exercise while performing a minisquat.

over the shoe laces as the partial squat is performed.

4. *Walk stance.* This position mimics the stage of gait in which weight bearing occurs. The patient steps forward with full weight bearing on the involved leg. The back foot should be positioned with the heel lifted as in the push-off phase in gait. The back foot is used for balance only (Figure 8.24).
5. *Step-down.* A proper step height should be selected based upon the patient's condition and irritation to the patellofemoral joint. The patient stands with the involved leg remaining on the step, preparing to lower the opposite leg to the floor. The patient slowly lowers the leg, making sure there is correct alignment of the lower leg (Figure 8.25). As the patient improves, the step height can be raised.
6. *Wall slide.* The patient will keep equal weight bilaterally and keep the back flat on the wall (Figure 8.26). The patient will then perform a wall slide in any position, however, one-quarter and one-half squats are most commonly used. Adduction exercises may also be used with the wall slide. The patient could squeeze a medicine ball between the knees and perform a wall slide. The patient needs to be sure they are not training through pain. Pain will inhibit the VMO and enhance patellar problems. In addition, biofeedback training can be used in conjunction with the McConnell taping techniques already discussed.

Bracing and Orthotics

Aside from surgical intervention or physical therapy, bracing and orthotic applications have proved beneficial in treating patients with anterior knee pain. There are many braces available whose manufacturers claim will treat multiple knee ailments. There are braces claiming to treat extensor mechanism problems, including such diagnosis as chon-

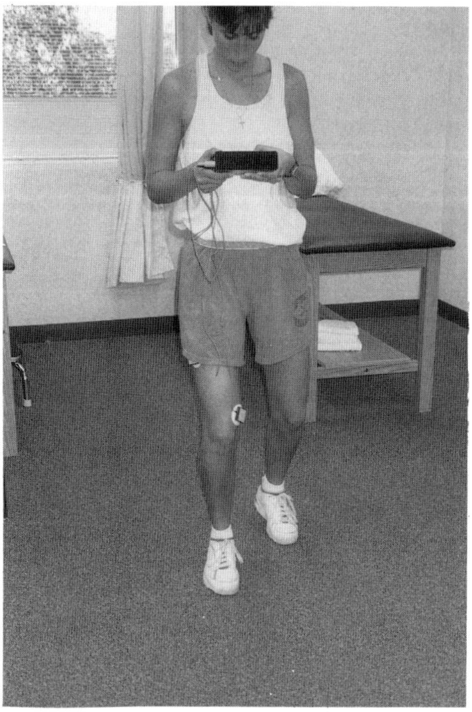

FIGURE 8.24. Biofeedback isometric quadriceps set in the walking stance position.

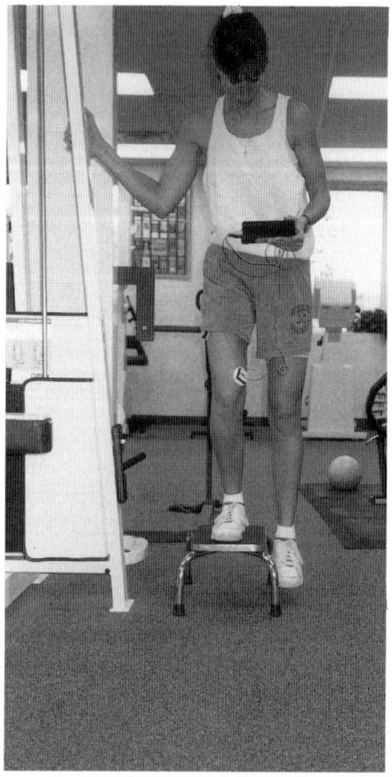

FIGURE 8.25. Biofeedback dynamic quadriceps exercise while performing a step-down.

dromalacia, PFPS, patellar tendinitis, and patellar instability.[41] Reported functions of test braces include dissipation of force, maintenance of alignment, improved patellar tracking, and prevention of patellar subluxation and dislocation.[42] In 1979, Levine and Splain looked at the use of an infrapatellar strap with patients diagnosed with anterior knee pain.[43] Seventy-seven percent of the patients received enough relief to resume normal activity.

In 1976, Palumbo reported that his dynamic patellar brace was found to reduce symptoms in 93% of 62 patients with patellofemoral dysfunction.[44] Lysholm et al. studied quadriceps muscle strength isokinetically in patients with patellofemoral arthralgia.[45] Patients performed exercise with and without patellar bracing. Eighty-eight percent of those patients tested showed improvements in their strength test with the brace. These data are not conclusive because other investigators have refuted the benefits of bracing. Villar[46] was unable to produce Levine and Splain's success rate because he found only 24% of his patients improved following brace application.

The mechanical function of these devices seems limited to applying a medially directed force to the lateral aspect of the patella. This is the one function of patellar bracing that is based on sound principal, and to assume that this principal might be applicable in treating other causes of anterior knee pain is speculative.[41] The senior author, G.R. Scuderi, prefers a patellar cutout sleeve with a lateral buttress pad. In some patients, several braces should be tried in order to find one that provides symptomatic relief. Bracing used in combination with other therapeutic techniques is beneficial but should not be the sole means of treating patellofemoral problems.

Reduction of patellofemoral symptoms through the use of foot orthoses has been widely reported, especially in those patients with abnormalities of the foot and the ankle.[47–49] Based on the theory of linkage and synchronicity between joints in the gait cycle, ab-

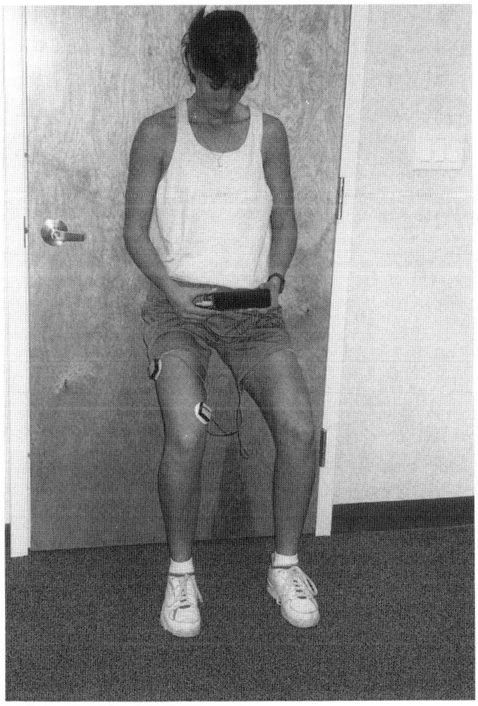

FIGURE 8.26. Biofeedback isometric quadriceps set in the wall slide position.

normal joint motion of the foot and the ankle affects knee biomechanics.[48] Therefore, if abnormal subtalar joint motion is noted in a patient with anterior knee pain, orthotic application has been helpful to correct this deforming force. Correction of any subtalar joint malalignment should reduce the tibiofemoral stress and the resultant patellofemoral pain. Similar to bracing, orthotics are an adjunct to a sound rehabilitation program.

Rehabilitation Phases

The most successful rehabilitation program customizes and individualizes the specific application of the program to each patient, avoiding a universal, cookbook approach.[50] The focus presented draws from various techniques in order to gain the most beneficial protocol for each patient. The program has been divided into three therapeutic phases and one maintenance phase. These phases are not rigid but, rather, flexible, depending on the patient's progress.

Phase I

Phase I is the acute injury or immediate postoperative phase. The main goals of this phase are to modulate pain, reduce swelling, and decrease the effects of disuse atrophy.[11,30,51] Several modalities are beneficial, including ice, ultrasound, electric stimulation, transcutaneous electrical nerve stimulation (TENS), occasional medication, patellar mobilizations, quadriceps sets, and gentle range of motion exercises. It is important in this phase to control and reduce swelling, as swelling inhibits recovery. Cryotherapy has been the most successful modality to reduce pain and inflammation.[6,52] Rest and avoidance of aggravating activities such as deep squatting, stairs, or sitting with the knee bent for long periods should be stressed, and bracing can also be useful in this phase. Paramount to a successful recovery is patient education and a clear understanding of the goals of therapy. It is also at this time that a therapist develops a relationship with the patient.

The next goal of phase I is to restore normal range of motion and to gain neuromuscular control of the quadriceps. This phase combines active and passive range of motion exercises, and includes a home stretching program that addresses each patient's specific needs.

Initially, neuromuscular redevelopment includes isometric quadriceps contractions that can be coupled with an EMS unit to aid in recruitment of more quadriceps muscle units. Quadriceps sets and SLRs can be performed in an immobilizer when tissue healing constraints dictate. The patient should be able to perform a tight isometric contraction before advancing to SLRs out of an immobilizer. This will further redevelop muscular control. Isometric adduction with VMO activation is also important at early stages of patellofemoral rehabilitation. The introduction of CKC is pivotal at this stage in the form of progressive weight-bearing exercises, leading up to Don Tigney exercises.

Exercising the contralateral limb should be included in this phase. Care should also be taken to avoid aggravating preexisting injuries such as lower back pain. Initially, the exercises are performed from one to three times per day and should last 15 to 30 min.[15,30] Exacerbation of pain must be avoided, so the program is modified according to symptoms. All exercises should end with the application of ice to reduce swelling.

Phase II

Advancement to phase II of rehabilitation is dependent upon the improvement in the patient's symptoms, including patient's diminution of pain and swelling, as well as an increase in range of motion and muscle control.[7,30,41] The main goal of this phase is to regain full pain-free range of motion, to restore normal gait, and to increase muscle strength and flexibility along with improved joint proprioception. At the end of phase II the clinician would like to see 70% to 80% quadriceps peak torque isokinetically as compared with the uninjured side. More advanced biofeedback training can also be incorporated within this phase.

To facilitate restoration of muscle control, graded isometric exercises at varying angles are used with progression to isotonic exercises, including the SLR with weights. Concentric and eccentric exercises are introduced in the available SAQ range, while isokinetics and rubber tubing can be used to retrain neuromuscular deficits.[18] Continued strengthening of the adductor muscles with CKC exercises such as one-quarter squats while squeezing a ball between the knees as well as OKC activities need to be continued.

Patellar mobilization and the stretching of tight soft-tissue structures should be continued at this time. Patellar compression tracking can also be carefully initiated.[7]

During this phase the patient can begin cycling exercise for increasing muscular strength and cardiovascular endurance. When presenting cycling exercises it is important to take into account the seat height and wheel tension in order to reduce patellofemoral forces. Initially, the seat should be set high so that the down leg comes to near full extension. A helpful adjunct at this time is hydrotherapy and pool exercises. This allows a comfortable environment for exercise.

Phase III

The criteria for progression into phase III is for the ROM, pain, and swelling to be within the normal range. The goal of phase III is to reach maximum strength while concentrating on developing muscular endurance, power, and functional activities.[30] The guidelines during this stage are based upon the patient's progression, goals, and desired outcome. The continuation of stretching and self-mobilization with compression tracking should still be utilized. Strengthening is continued with the introduction of advanced closed chain activities, preplyometrics, and specific functional activities according to the patient's goals (Table 8.2).

Once adequate muscular strength and power have been redeveloped, usually around 70% to 80% contralateral (or uninvolved side), advanced functionally specific rehabilitation

TABLE 8.2. Functional progressions.*

Protective immobilization/active rest
ROM exercises
Strengthening in OKC exercises
Progressive weight-bearing exercises (i.e., weight shifts)
Strengthening in CKC exercises (i.e., Don Tigney exercises)
Neuromuscular redevelopment (i.e., BAPS board, balancing)
Strengthening the VMO (biofeedback)
Minisquat progression
Retrowalking
Step-up progression
Walk–jog
Jog–run
Sprints
Agility drills (figure eights, right angle cuts)
Specific functional activities
Return to function

*The activities listed are a general order of exercise progressions. These often are overlapping with adaptable sequences and multiple applications in accordance with the patient's needs.

Source: Adapted from Kegerises et al.[53]

may begin.[30] The goal of rehabilitation programs is to return the patient to a preinjury activity level without the threat of aggravation or reinjury. Specific functional exercises (Table 8.3) allow the patient to resume the specific sport- or activities of daily living (ADL)-related activity. Initially, these functional exercises are broken down into individual components—running, jumping, and twisting—and then they are combined together in order to re-create the sport-specific movements. It is this interplay of functional exercise that brings the patient closer to resumption of preinjury activity.[15,30,53]

CKC exercises are incorporated with endurance activities and are directed towards the

TABLE 8.3. Rehabilitation phases.

Goals	Treatment strategies
Phase I: Acute/postoperative stage	
1. Decrease pain, swelling, and atrophy	1. (a) Cryotherapy, ultrasound, electric stimulation, TENS, non steroidal anti-inflammatory medications, immobilizers/brace (b) Quadriceps sets, ankle pumps, SLRs
2. Increase ROM and neuromotor control	2. (a) AROM, PROM, hamstring stretch, patella mob.s, stationary cycling (b) Progressive weight bearing, proprioception, Don Tigney exercises, minisquats
3. Issue home program	3. Self-stretches, self-mob.s, tennis ball, quadriceps sets, SLRs, proprioception
Criteria for progression:	1. Decreased pain 2. Strong isometric contraction 3. SLRs with weight 4. Good ambulation
Phase II: Intermediate/strengthening stage	
1. Full ROM	1. PROM, AROM, stationary cycling
2. Increase strength—especially VMO, power, and endurance—as tolerated	2. Continue SLR with weight, progressive resistance exercises (PREs) with SAQs, leg press, minisquats, isokinetics submaximal (180–300), closed chain activities
3. Increase proprioception and eccentric extensor lag	3. Balancing, BAPS board, Plyo rebounder, tubing–yo yo, hip flexion/extension with increasing speed as tolerated
4. Functional activities	4. Specific components
5. Strengthen hamstrings, ankles, and hips bilaterally	
Criteria for progression:	1. No pain or minimal intermittent pain 2. Strength 70% to 80% uninvolved side
Phase III: Functional activities stage	
1. Maximize strength, endurance, and power	1. Continue PREs progressing as tolerated, advanced CKC, preplyometrics, full body weight leg press, step-ups, maximal isokinetics, cycling for speed and endurance
2. Specific functional activity	2. Functional progressions
Criteria for progression:	1. No pain 2. Full ROM isokinetics 90% uninvolved 3. Full body weight leg press
Phase IV: Maintenance stage	
1. Maintain ROM, strength, functioning, etc.	1. Continue self-stretches, advanced home program, specific activities, brace and orthotics

patient's specific goals. Creative use of these components can greatly enhance recovery. The overlapping nature of this phase must be kept in mind, as progressions from simple to complex movement skills and from half-speed to full-speed activities need to be integrated properly.

Combining functional exercises from simple to complex movement skills enhances agility and recovery. The exercises are integrated into the workout program and progressed from half-speed to full-speed activity. The full speed of complex movements should correlate closely with the specific sport or activity. This phase is complete when the desired goals have been reached at functional speeds, frequencies, and durations without the reoccurrence of pain, swelling, or limitations of motion.[53] Delayed onset muscle soreness or residual pain may be experienced the next day. As with all rehabilitation exercises, ice, in conjunction with other modalities of choice, should be used at the conclusion of each session.

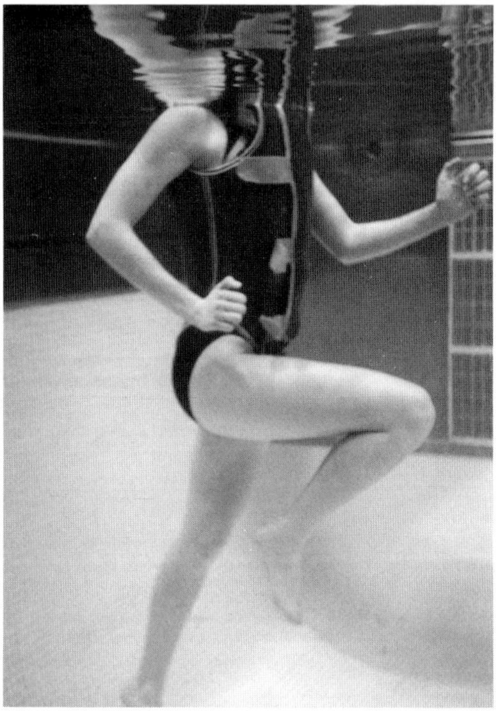

FIGURE 8.27. Pool exercises in a non-weight-bearing mode using the Wet Vest (Sports Support, Dallas) for flotation during running.

Phase IV

Once the patient has successfully returned to the activity, the acquisitions in the rehabilitation program will deteriorate if a maintenance program is overlooked. Maintenance includes the flexibility exercises, used as a warm-up as well as a cool down, progressive resistance exercises (PREs), and functional exercises for specific muscle groups. These exercises should be continued two to three times per week as dictated by the needs of the patient while endurance exercise can be performed on alternated days.[30]

Finally, the patient's education should be directed towards instructing the individual as to why the problem developed and rationale for prevention of future and further injury. The use of bracing, patella support, or orthotics during this final phase can help ensure proper patellar alignment and safeguard against reinjury.

Pool Exercises

Pool therapy can be an excellent compliment to the rehabilitation of PFPS. Early exercise has been promoted as a means of decreasing the effects of injury while stimulating the redevelopment of mechanoreceptors in the lower extremities. The buoyancy and assistive qualities of water aid in decreasing the potential harm of early exercise on healing tissue while the resistive and supportive qualities serve to promote earlier neuromuscular recovery. McNeil has found that patients undergoing pool exercise programs reestablish their normal gait patterns and dynamic stability in less time than patients undergoing traditional programs.[54]

The benefits of pool exercises include decreasing pain while increasing strength, ROM, flexibility, balance, coordination, muscle endurance, and general conditioning. One additional advantage is that hydrotherapy allows for earlier progressive weight bearing and functional skill redevelopment.[54] Patients with little or no water skills can easily be instructed in pool exercises using flotation devices.

The patient should be progressively and

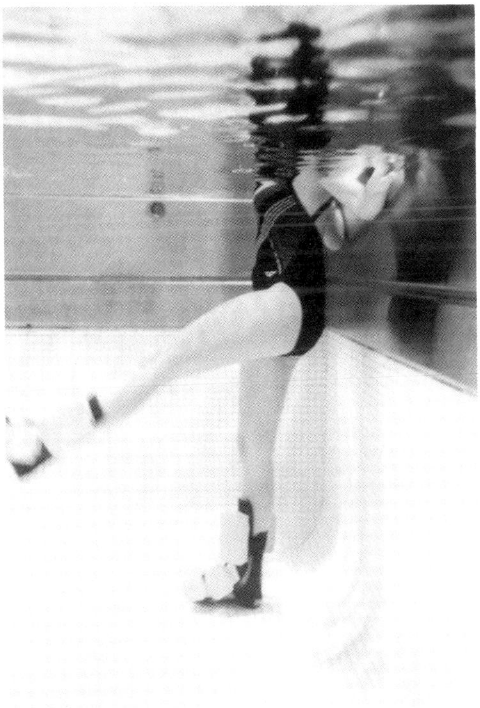

FIGURE 8.28. Pool exercises in a weight-bearing mode performing hip flexion exercises with resistive boots.

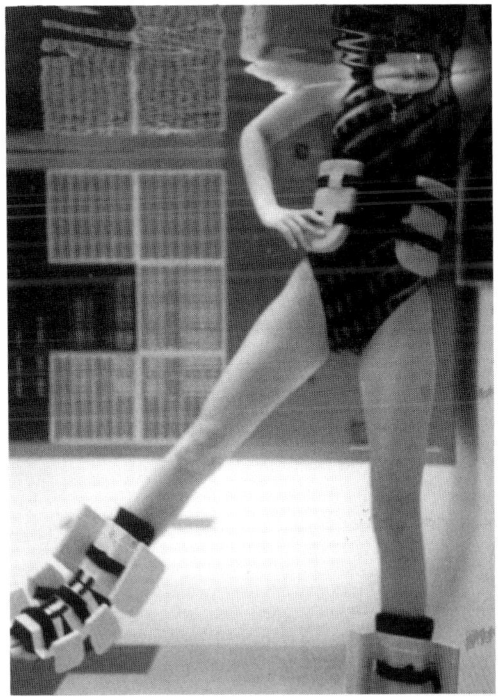

FIGURE 8.29. Pool exercises in the non-weight-bearing mode using the flotation belt and boots to perform adduction exercises. Care must be taken to avoid forceful return to the abducted position if tight lateral structures are present.

carefully introduced to the program. Initially, treatments should serve only as an orientation and exploration. During phase I, most exercises are modifications of those used out of the water, which easily permits a transition through familiarity. The exercises are performed slowly in a controlled fashion through a pain-free ROM while maintaining a quadriceps contraction or cocontraction for stability. Exercises that cause greater amounts of flexion or forceful abduction should be avoided until a decrease in symptoms occur. The speed and the ROM are gradually increased as exercises are added in accordance with the patient's needs and symptoms. The smooth resistance of the water over the entire limb provides the patient with feedback in redeveloping neuromuscular control. Change of direction exercises that progress from slow to fast, with an emphasis on positioning and technique, are excellent.

In cases in which weight bearing is restricted or patellar loading is contraindicated, the patient may perform exercises in the deep end of the pool where the bottom is not contacted (Figure 8.27). When flotation devices are not available, the patient may use a kickboard, a buoy, or simply hold on to the wall.

Once progressive weight bearing is allowed, the patient should begin a functional progression in the pool by varying the effects of water buoyancy. This can be accomplished by altering the depth of the water: neck-deep submersion correlates to the patient supporting about 10% of the body weight, chest-deep water is about 25% body weight, and waist-deep water is about 50%.[54] This technique can be used to modify the intensity of weight-bearing exercises while focusing on correct function, posture, and technique.

Phase II exercises include the SLR into hip flexion and hip extension. Figure 8.28 shows this in a weight-bearing mode. Adduction ex-

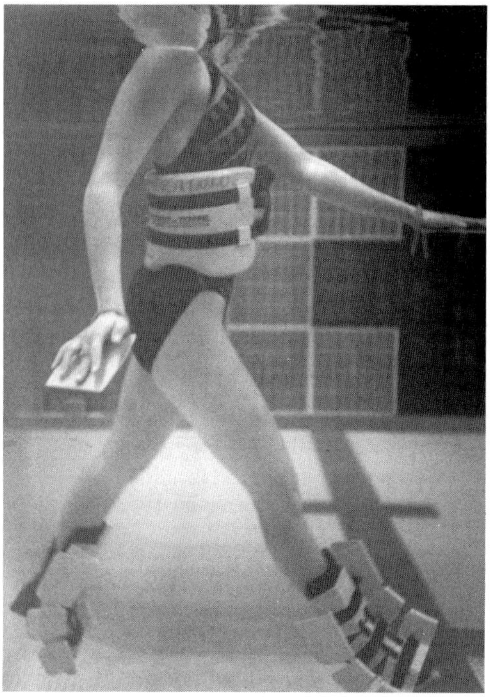

FIGURE 8.30. Pool exercises in the non-weight-bearing mode performing the scissors kick using the belt for flotation, and hand paddles and boots for resistance.

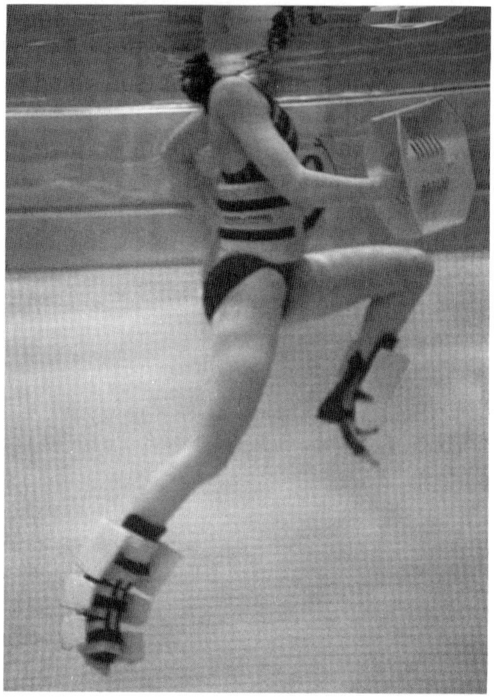

FIGURE 8.31. Pool exercises in the non-weight-bearing mode using Hydro-Tone Jogger Belt (Hydro-Tone International, Oklahoma City) for flotation with resistive boots and hand bells.

ercises are important (Figure 8.29), however, the return to the abducted position should be completed slowly to avoid tightening lateral structures. Scissors kicks can be used in the sagittal plane, concentrating on keeping the legs straight. These exercises can be performed in the corner using only the legs, or they can be used in deeper water with both arms and legs moving in opposition as to simulate functional gait (Figure 8.30). Toe raises and calf stretches can be completed in the shallow end, along with single leg standing, minisquats, forward walking, and retrowalking. McNeil also points out that lap work may be added if the legs are not used for forceful kicking.[54]

In phase III, the previously mentioned exercises are used with an increase in speed and ROM. Also diagonal leg exercises, SLRs with external hip rotation, and sideways walking are added. Scissors kicks are progressed to stationary running by adding slight knee flexion (Figures 8.27 and 8.31). Flutter kicks are also initiated at this stage. The use of resistive devices such as boots, wings, or bells (Figure 8.31) can be added. Running is also progressed to laps with or without weight bearing and the flutter kick is advanced to laps with a kickboard and a flipper on the involved limb. Functional skill development is progressed to return to activity out of the pool.

In phase IV, the pool is used only for maintenance and general fitness.

Surgical Intervention

The conservative approach outlined previously for the PFPS patient is attempted first and usually is exhausted prior to the initiation of more aggressive intervention. For persistent symptoms, several surgical techniques can be used that range from the release of tight structures to realignment of the extensor mechanism. Later chapters will review common techniques shown to be effective in the surgical management of PFPS patients.

Regardless of the surgical techniques the physician performs, the goals of rehabilitation are the same—to return to normal pain-free activity as soon as possible. The various surgical techniques will require specialized rehabilitative approaches. Precaution, contraindications, and time frames will vary, depending on the complexity of the surgery and the individual patient's goals.

Summary

This chapter has attempted to give the framework in which one may develop a sound rehabilitation protocol for PFPS. This approach is multifaceted and requires constant interaction between the practitioner and the patient. The comprehensive treatment approach will address all the applicable components—decreasing pain and swelling, and increasing strength, neuromotor control, and healing parameters—in an effort to meet the patient's particular goals.

The rehabilitation of the PFPS patient is initially conservative, with an emphasis on CKC activities, restoring neuromuscular function, and retraining the VMO. Additionally, rehabilitation should decrease lateral compressive forces and protect the joint from compressive stress that may occur during rehabilitation. Taping, bracing, and orthotics have also shown to be effective adjuncts to this program. Pool exercises may help hasten restoration of normal function.

When the rehabilitation program has not alleviated PFPS, surgical intervention may be prompted. As previously stated, various techniques can be used when dealing with PFPS. The clinician must keep in mind that surgical intervention alone will not relieve the patient from PFPS. The clinician must also prescribe a sound rehabilitation program.

References

1. Outerbridge RE: Further studies on the etiology on chondromalacia patellae. *J Bone Joint Surg Br* 1964;46B:179–190.
2. Souza DR: Anatomy and pathomechanichics of patellafemoral pain syndrome, in *Postgrad Stud Sport Phys Ther Cont Ed Course I–IX.* Forum Medicum, 1991.
3. Malek M, Mangine R: Patellofemoral pain syndromes: A comprehensive and conservative approach. *J Orthop Sports Phys Ther* 1981;2:108–116.
4. Outerbridge RE, Dunlop J: The problem of chondromalacia patellae. *Clin Orthop* 1975;110: 177–196.
5. Travell J, Simons D: *Myofacial Pain and Dysfunction: The Trigger Point Manual: Lower Extremity,* ed. 1. Baltimore, Williams & Wilkins Co., 1992.
6. Antich TJ, Randall CC, Westbrook RA, et al.: Evaluation of knee extensor mechanism disorders: Clinical presentation of 112 patients. *J Orthop Sports Phys Ther* 1986;8:248–254.
7. Kramer PG: Patella malalignment syndrome: Rationale to reduce excessive lateral pressure. *J Orthop Sports Phys Ther* 1986;8:301–309.
8. McConnell J: The management of chondromalacia patellae: A long-term solution. *Aust J Physiother* 1986;32:215–223.
9. Grana WA, Kreisshauser LA: Scientific basis of extensor mechanism disorder. *Clin Sports Med* 1980;4:247–257.
10. Salter R, Simmons D, Malcom B, et al.: The biological effects of continuous passive motion on the healing of full-thickness defects in articular cartilage. *J Bone Joint Surg Am* 1980;62A: 1232–1251.
11. Andrews J, Harrolson G: *Physical Rehabilitation of the Injured Athlete,* ed. 1. Philadelphia: WB Saunders Co., 1991.
12. Maitland G: The hypothesis of adding compression when examining and treating synovial joints. *J Orthop Sports Phys Ther* 1980; 2:7–14.
13. McCarthy M, O'Donoghue P, Yates C, et al.: The clinical use of continuous passive motion in physical therapy. *J Orthop Sports Phys Ther* 1992;15:132–140.
14. Maitland G: *Peripheral Manipulation,* ed. 2. Boston, Butterworth, 1977.
15. Knight K: Quadriceps strengthening with DAPRE technique: Case studies with neurological implications. *Med Sci Sports Exerc* 1985;17:646–650.
16. Stendler A: *Kinesiology of the Human Body Under Normal and Pathological Conditions.* Springfield, Ill., Charles C Thomas Publisher, 1970.
17. Spencer JD, Hayes KC, Alexander IL: Knee

joint effusion and quadriceps reflex inhibition in man. *Arch Phys Med Rehabil* 1984;65:171–177.

18. Bennett JG, Stauber WT: Evaluation and treatment of anterior knee pain using eccentric exercise. *Med Sci Sport Exerc* 1986;18:526–530.
19. Komi P: Measurement of the force velocity relationship in muscle under concentric and eccentric contractions. *Med Sports* 1973;8:224–229.
20. Doss WS, Karpovich PV: A comparison of concentric, eccentric and isometric strength of elbow flexors. *J Appl Physiol* 1965;20:351–353.
21. Cress N, Peters K, Chandler JM: Eccentric and concentric force-velocity relationship of the quadriceps femoris muscle. *J Orthop Sports Phys Ther* 1992;16:82–85.
22. Knight K: Rehabilitating chondromalacia patellae. *Physician Sportsmed* 1979;7:147–148.
23. Hisamoto J: Evaluation and treatment of shoulder impingement and anterior knee pain, in *Sportworks' Seminar.* Uniondale, N.Y. June 1993.
24. Steinkamp L, Dillingham M, Markel M, et al.: Biomechanical considerations in patellofemoral joint rehabilitation. *Am J Sports Med* 1993;21:438–444.
25. Lieb F, Perry J: Quadriceps function: An anatomical and mechanical study using amputated limbs. *J Bone Joint Surg Am* 1968;59A:1535–1548.
26. Gruber MA: The conservative treatment of chondromalacia patellae. *Orthop Clin North Am* 1979;10:105–115.
27. LeVeau B, Rogers C: Selective training of the vastus medialis muscle using emg biofeedback. *Phys Ther* 1980;60:1410–1415.
28. Wise HH, Fiebert IM, Kates JL: EMG biofeedback as treatment for patellafemoral pain syndrome. *J Orthop Sports Phys Ther* 1984;6:95–103.
29. Sczepanski LT, Gross MT, Duncan PW, et al.: Effects of contraction type, angular velocity and arc of motion on vmo:vl emg ratio. *J Orthop Sports Phys Ther* 1991;14:256–262.
30. Heckman TP: Conservative vs postsurgical patella rehabilitation, in Mangine R (ed.): *Physical Therapy of the Knee.* New York: Churchill Livingstone, 1988, pp. 127–143.
31. O'Neil DB, Micheli LJ, Warner JP: Patellofemoral stress: A prospective analysis of exercise treatment in adolescents and adults. *Am J Sports Med* 1992;20:151–156.
32. Amusa LO, Obajuluwa VA: Static vs dynamic training programs. *J Orthop Sports Phys Ther* 1986;8:243–247.
33. Antich TJ, Brewster CE: Modification of quadriceps femoris muscle exercises during knee rehabilitation. *Phys Ther* 1986;66:1246–1251.
34. Davies G: *A Compendium of Isokinetics in Clinical Usage and Rehabilitation Techniques,* ed. 2. LaCrosse, Wis., S&S Publisher's, 1985.
35. McConnell, J: Patella alignment and quadriceps strength, in *Proceedings of the MTAA Conference.* Manipulative Therapist Association of Australia, Melbourne, Victoria, Australia, November 1987.
36. Case WS: Minimizing patellofemoral joint compression during knee rehab. *Phys Ther Forum* 1985;4:1–4.
37. Brunet ME, Stewart GW: Patellofemoral rehabilitation. *Clin Sports Med* 1989;8:319–329.
38. Dehaven KE, Dolan WA, Mayer PJ: Chondromalacia in athletes: Clinical presentation and conservative management. *Am J Sports Med* 1979;7:5–14.
39. Reynolds N, Worrel T, Perrin D: Effects of a lateral step up exercise protocol on quadriceps isokinetic peak torque values and thigh girth. *J Orthop Sports Phys Ther* 1992;15:151–155.
40. Tremain L: Vastus Medialis Obliquus (VMO) Protocol, in *Operator's Guide to the Pathway MR-100 Muscle Rehabilitation System.* Portsmouth, N.H., Prometheus Group, 1993.
41. Paulos L, Rusche K, Johnson C, et al.: Patella malalignment: A treatment rationale. *Phys Ther* 1980;60:1624–1632.
42. Cherf J, Paulos L: Bracing for patella instability. *Clin Sports Med* 1990;9:813–821.
43. Levine J, Splain S: Use of the infrapatellar strap in the treatment of patellofemoral pain. *Clin Orthop* 1979;139:179–181.
44. Palumbo P: Dynamic patellar brace: A new orthosis in the management of patellofemoral disorders. *Am J Sports Med* 1976;1:45–49.
45. Lysholm J, Nordin M, Ekstrand J, et al.: The effect of patella brace on performance in a knee extension strength test in patients with patellar pain. *Am J Sports Med* 1977;2:110–112.
46. Villar R: Patellofemoral pain and the infrapatellar brace. *Am J Sports Med* 1980;5:313–315.
47. Bogan R, Jenkins D, Hyland T: The runner's knee syndrome. *Sports Med* 1978;78:159–177.
48. Tibero D: The effects of subtalar joint pronation on patellofemoral mechanics: A theoretical model. *J Orthop Sports Phys Ther* 1987;9:160–165.
49. Buchbinder M, Napora N, Biggs E: The relationship of abnormal pronation to chondro-

malacia of the patella in distance runners. *J Am Podiatr Med Assoc* 1979;69:159–162.
50. Beckman M, Craig R, Lehman RC: Rehabilitation of patellofemoral dysfunction in the athlete. *Clin Sports Med* 1989;8:841–860.
51. Knight K: Guidelines for rehabilitation of sports injuries. *Clin Sports Med* 1985;4:405–416.
52. Sheldon GL, Thigpen LK: Rehabilitation of patellofemoral dysfunction: A review of the literature. *J Orthop Sports Phys Ther* 1991;14:243–249.
53. Kegereis S, Malone T, McCaroll J: Functional progressions: An aid to athletic rehabilitation. *Physician Sportsmed* 1984;12:67–71.
54. McNeil R: *Aquatic Therapy,* ed. 2. Abingdon, Md., Aquatic Therapy Services, 1988.

9

Patellar Problems in the Young Patient

Joseph M. Stefko and Freddie Fu

Patellofemoral joint pathology is a frequent cause of disabling knee pain in the young patient. Prior to our recent understanding of patellofemoral disorders, chondromalacia patellae was diagnosed in all patients with knee pain attributed to the patellofemoral joint. In 1924, Konig[1] first described this all-inclusive term. Since then, other authors have used the term *chondromalacia patellae* to describe the associated patellar surface changes consisting of fissuring and softening. Confusion over diagnosis occurred in those young patients with anterior knee pain and no demonstrable lesions of the articular cartilage. By categorizing all anterior knee pain as chondromalacia patellae, the clinician fails to recognize the numerous causes of patellofemoral pain and fails to establish a meaningful treatment plan. Because patellar surface fissuring and softening is universally present in the older population, chondromalacia may actually describe the early pathologic findings noted with articular cartilage degeneration (Figure 9.1).

In 1977, Ficat and Hungerford[2] elucidated the differential diagnosis for painful conditions of the patellofemoral joint. With an expanded focus toward patellofemoral pathology, the term *chondromalacia patellae* has since been restricted to the clinical observation of articular cartilage discontinuity. Recently, Merchant[3] devised a detailed classification of patellofemoral disorders (Table 9.1) that allows uniformity in the medical literature concerning the patellofemoral joint and the development of diagnosis-specific treatment protocols. This classification system catalogs patellofemoral disorders by their reported etiology: acute trauma, dysplasia, idiopathic chondromalacia patellae, osteochondritis dissecans, and synovial plicae syndrome. Although this classification provides a useful framework for understanding patellofemoral disorders, it fails to recognize congenital and genetic conditions that are peculiar to the pediatric knee.

This chapter will review the multifactorial etiologies of anterior knee pain in the young patient. Because the concepts of patellofemoral instability and arthritis are discussed elsewhere in this book, this chapter will focus on patellofemoral disorders caused by acute or chronic trauma and other idiopathic conditions. It is our hope that the reader will ostracize the term *chondromalacia patellae* as a specific cause of anterior knee pain in young people. This is typified by the title of a recent article from Radin,[4] "Anterior Knee Pain: The Need for a Specific Diagnosis, Stop Calling It Chondromalacia!"

Lateral Retinacular Pain and the Excessive Lateral Pressure Syndrome

Young patients with anterior knee pain may or may not show evidence of patellofemoral malalignment. Historically, soft cartilage or chondromalacia was assumed to cause ante-

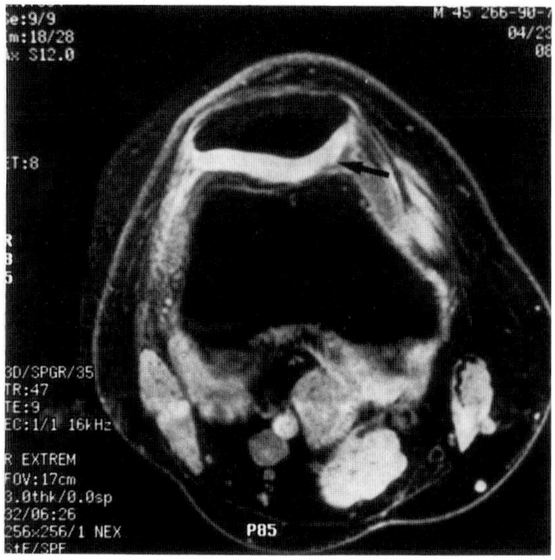

FIGURE 9.1. Magnetic resonance imaging (MRI) of the patellofemoral joint. This axial-spoiled fat-saturated image of the patellofemoral joint demonstrates chondromalacia of the medial facet and odd facet characterized by low signal intensity within the articular cartilage along with surface irregularity (arrow).

TABLE 9.1. Classification of patellofemoral disorders.

- I. Trauma (conditions caused by trauma in the otherwise normal knee)
  - A. Acute trauma
    - 1. Contusion
    - 2. Fracture
      - a. Patella
      - b. Femoral trochlea
      - c. Proximal tibial epiphysis (tubercle)
    - 3. Dislocation (rare in the normal knee)
    - 4. Rupture
      - a. Quadriceps tendon
      - b. Patellar tendon
  - B. Repetitive trauma (overuse syndromes)
    - 1. Patellar tendinitis ("jumper's knee")
    - 2. Quadriceps tendinitis
    - 3. Peripatellar tendinitis (e.g., anterior knee pain of the adolescent owing to hamstring contracture)
    - 4. Prepatellar bursitis ("housemaid's knee")
    - 5. Apophysitis
      - a. Osgood–Schlatter disease
      - b. Sinding–Larsen–Johansson disease
  - C. Late effects of trauma
    - 1. Posttraumatic chondromalacia patellae
    - 2. Posttraumatic patellofemoral arthritis
    - 3. Anterior fat pad syndrome (posttraumatic fibrosis)
    - 4. Reflex sympathetic dystrophy of the patella
    - 5. Patellar osseous dystrophy
    - 6. Acquired quadriceps fibrosis
- II. Patellofemoral dysplasia
  - A. Lateral patellar compression syndrome
    - 1. Secondary chondromalacia patellae
    - 2. Secondary patellofemoral arthritis
  - B. Chronic subluxation of the patella
    - 1. Secondary chondromalacia patellae
    - 2. Secondary patellofemoral arthritis
  - C. Recurrent dislocation of the patella
    - 1. Associated fractures
      - a. Osteochondral (intra-articular)
      - b. Avulsion (extra-articular)
    - 2. Secondary chondromalacia patellae
    - 3. Secondary patellofemoral arthritis
  - D. Chronic dislocation of the patella
    - 1. Congenital
    - 2. Acquired
- III. Idiopathic chondromalacia patellae
- IV. Osteochondritis dissecans
  - A. Patella
  - B. Femoral trochlea
- V. Synovial plicae (anatomic variant made symptomatic by acute or repetitive trauma)
  - A. Medial patellar ("shelf")
  - B. Suprapatellar
  - C. Lateral patellar

Source: Merchant AC: Classification of patellofemoral disorders. Arthroscopy 4(4):236, 1988. Reprinted with permission of Raven Press.

rior knee pain in patients with or without instability. Recently, many reports have shown a weak association between anterior knee pain and morphologic evidence of articular cartilage softening.[5–8] Fulkerson,[9] along with Ficat and Hungerford,[2] stress the importance of not only a detailed patella examination, but also adequate examination of the peripatellar soft tissue in patients who exhibit anterior knee pain. Certain patellofemoral painful disorders have been attributed to the peripatellar soft tissue. Fulkerson[10] described a group of patients with anterior knee pain who exhibited a focal area of discomfort over the lateral retinaculum. A subsequent study demonstrated small nerve injuries in the lateral retinaculum of patients with chronic anterior knee pain.[11] Larson et al.[12] and Johnson[5] have further substantiated the role of the lateral retinaculum in anterior knee pain and occasionally they recommend surgery before adaptive changes occur.

Lateral retinacular pain typically presents in the second decade of life with anterior knee pain that is aggravated by physical activity. A consistent pathologic finding is shortening of the lateral patellar retinaculum. The cause of this adaptive contracture is speculative. We postulate either an occult injury to the extensor mechanism with resulting fibrosis, or shortening in response to some form of extremity malalignment (i.e., torsional deformity or malunion). The net effect is anterior knee pain, with knee flexion secondary to excessive stress placed on the shortened lateral retinaculum as the patella is drawn into the trochlear groove and the iliotibial band pulls posteriorly.

A patient with a symptomatic lateral retinaculum commonly exhibits pain where the lateral retinaculum interdigitates with the vastus lateralis tendon and in the inferomedial peripatellar area. Patellar tilt may or may not be noted at this time. By manually displacing the patella in the medial direction, the lateral retinaculum is placed under stress and specific painful bands may be palpated. Pain relief with the injection of local anesthetic over this area may confirm the diagnosis. Deficient medial patellar glide compared with the contralateral side may suggest excessive lateral patellar tethering. With further shortening of the retinaculum, patellar tilt becomes clinically evident (Figure 9.2). Increasing degrees of tilt, along with further contracture of the lateral retinaculum, results in structural findings consistent with the diagnosis of lateral patellar compression syndrome.

Ficat and Hungerford[2] developed the concept of excessive lateral pressure syndrome (ELPS). The characteristic findings in these patients are patellar arthrosis caused by stress overload on the lateral patellar facet and altered pressure distribution on the medial facet. Chronic patellar tilt (Figure 9.3) is routinely noted and is felt to contribute to the pressure overload on the lateral facet. The syndrome probably originates with adaptive contracture of the lateral retinaculum. The tightened lateral structures establish a lateral and posterior vector on the patella. With the presence of a normal Q angle and medial restraints, patellar tilt develops without evidence of overt subluxation. A chronic imbalance in pressure distribution results in the characteristic morphologic findings. It is uncertain whether the pathology of ELPS initiates from a congenitally tilted patella[13] or from one of the many factures that may lead to an adaptively shortened lateral retinaculum (Figure 9.4). Neverless, the end result is premature arthrosis of the patellar facets.

Our preferred radiographic study to examine the patellofemoral joint is the Merchant view.[14] Patients with isolated retinacular pain and no evidence of patellar tilt rarely show radiographic abnormalities. The lateral patellofemoral angle and the patellar angle that Laurin et al.[15] described are good indicators of abnormal patellar tilt. According to Laurin et al., 97% of normal subjects have a lateral opening of their patellofemoral angle. Parallel lines or a medial facing patellofemoral angle are associated with abnormal patellar tilt or subluxation. Patellar tilt angles are believed to be more reliable when measured on computerized tomographic (CT) scans and referenced with the posterior condyles.[16] Significant loss of articular cartilage can occur with excessive lateral compression syndrome. Early arthrosis

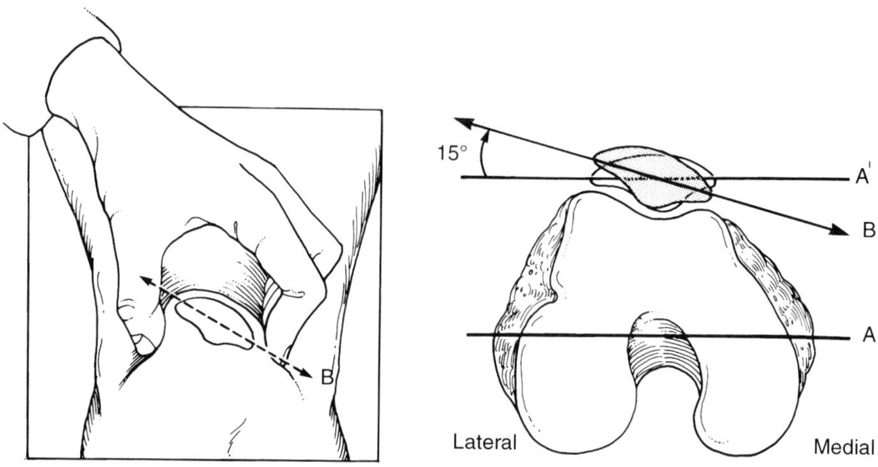

FIGURE 9.2. The clinical determination of normal passive patella tilt.

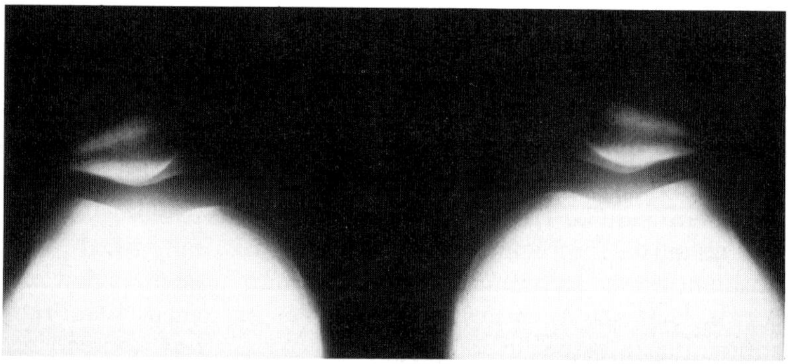

FIGURE 9.3. Merchant view radiograph of a 16-year-old girl with ELPS, demonstrating bilateral patellar tilt.

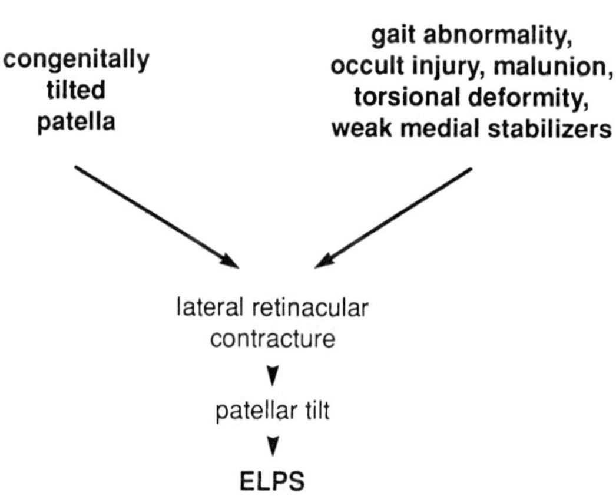

FIGURE 9.4. Proposed etiology of ELPS.

occurs at the intersection of the medial ridge and the transverse ridge on the lateral one half of the patella. Figure 9.5 illustrates common radiographic findings seen on axial view radiography in patients with ELPS.

A patient who presents with lateral retinacular pain and evidence of lateral soft-tissue contracture is not destined to develop ELPS. This early stage is most responsive to a nonoperative treatment approach, which includes activity restriction. The goal of treatment is to mobilize the tight lateral retinacular structures, iliotibial band, and hamstring stretching, along with vastus medialis strengthening. By stretching the tight lateral structures, pa-

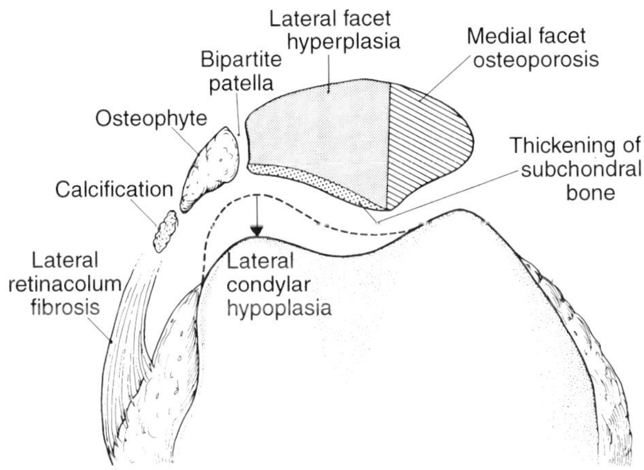

FIGURE 9.5. Common radiographic findings seen on axial view radiographs of patients with ELPS.

tellar tilt is reduced, which alters the pathologic articular load distribution. Doucette and Goble[17] recently reported that 84% of their patients with significant lateral compression were pain-free after eight weeks of rehabilitation. O'Neill et al.[18] notes good results with an isometric quadriceps strengthening program, even when lower-extremity alignment is normal. Patellar bracing and taping techniques also have been shown to be efficacious.[19,20] Lysholm et al.[21] report that 88% of their patients with patellofemoral arthralgia treated with a patellar brace significantly improved quadriceps peak strength with a Cybex-II isokinetic dynamometer. Selective use of an orthotic, along with appropriate footwear, may be beneficial to the patient with anterior knee pain.[22,23] When early arthrosis occurs, it initially may be managed with nonsteroidal anti-inflammatory medication.

Patients who have not responded to conservative measures may benefit from surgical release of the tight lateral structures. Many studies have documented the efficacy of lateral retinacula release in patients with patellofemoral pain.[6,7,24–31] Intractable lateral retinacular pain without other patellofemoral pathology may respond beneficially to lateral retinacular release.[7] Lateral retinacular release apparently decreases the lateral and the posterior force vector placed on the patella during knee flexion, thus reducing the articular load on the lateral facet. It currently is believed that lateral release is most efficacious when treating patellofemoral pain associated with patellar tilt.[13] Kolowich et al.[32] report that 74% and 76% of their good or excellent results after lateral release had preoperative examination findings, suggestive of patellar tilt and lateral patellar compression syndrome, respectively. A cadaver study using pressure-sensitive film[33] demonstrates no specific change in patellar contact pressure after a lateral release is performed on specimens without patellar tilt. Using lateral patellofemoral angles and CT, Fulkerson et al.[16] illustrate a reduction in abnormal patellar tilt after lateral release. If ELPS causes significant arthrosis and collapse of the lateral facet, lateral release was shown to be less effective in reducing patellar tilt. If radiographs are suspicious of lateral facet arthrosis, we routinely perform arthroscopy before lateral release in order to further document the extent of disease. In the presence of significant articular disease (Outerbridge 3–4), some believe that anterior displacement of the tibial tubercle is indicated[34] in skeletally mature persons.

Patellar Tendinitis (Jumper's Knee)

Jumper's knee, also known as patellar tendinitis or partial rupture of the patellar ligament, is a painful tendinitis caused by repetitive stress overload of the bone–ligament junction at the lower patellar pole. This term–also has been used to describe less common painful conditions of the quadriceps mechanism at the upper pole of the patella or the the tibial tuberosity. Jumper's knee is especially evident in persons who participate in repetitive activity (microrupture), such as running, or explosive activity (macrorupture), such as jumping and kicking. These activities require repetitive eccentric quadriceps muscle contractions that overcome the tendon's strength. Complete patellar ligament rupture is rare,[35,36] and usually is seen in young athletes or patients with systemic diseases.[37–40]

The patient typically presents in the second or third decade of life, with aching in the knee centered over the infrapatellar or the suprapatellar region after activity. Complaints of giving way, weakness, or locking are common. Symptoms usually resolve with a brief period of rest. Unlike other painful patellofemoral conditions, patellar tendinitis patients can train intensively if excessive eccentric quadriceps contractions can be avoided.[41] The classification scheme that Blazina et al.[42] devised outlines the natural history of the disease (Table 9.2). The majority of patients present with either stage 1 or stage 2 disease, which can be easily arrested with activity restriction. Early examination usually reveals a focal area of sharp pain to palpation at the inferior pole of the patella. Other signs may include quadriceps wasting and crepitus. Kujala et al.[43] recognized the common association of patellar tendinitis with patella alta, patellofemoral laxity, and leg length inequalities. End-stage jumper's knee, or patellar tendon rupture, occurs in patients with chronic patellar tendinitis because of primary structural weakening of the degenerative tendon.

TABLE 9.2. Blazina classification of patellar tendinitis.

Stage	Classification
1	Pain after sports activity
2	Pain at the beginning of sporting activity, disappearing with warm-up, and sometimes reappearing with fatigue
3	Pain at rest and during activity; inability to participate in sports
4	Rupture of the patellar tendon

Source: Blazina ME, Kerlan RK, Jobe FW, et al.: Jumper's knee. Orthop Clin North Am 4:655, 1973

Blazina ME, et al. (42)

The histopathology of patellar tendinitis has been well described.[35,41,44] The abnormality is located within the osteotendinous junction where Ferretti et al.[45] noted pseudocystic cavities with myxomatous and hyaline metaplasia at the border between mineralized fibrocartilage and bone. Fibrocartilage ossification and mineralization also are observed distal to the "blue line" (Figure 9.6). The tendon substance far from the bone–tendon junction is normal but may exhibit mucoid degeneration, fibrinoid necrosis, and neovascularization if prior cortisone injections were administered.

Histologic findings also have correlated with ultrasound, CT imaging, and magnetic resonance imaging (MRI). All three procedures appear to be equally efficacious.[46] Ultrasound is recommended as the initial diagnostic investigation because it is the least expensive, the quickest, and the easiest means of confirming the diagnosis (Figure 9.7). A 7.5-mHz probe shows sagittal or coronal plane images, demonstrating thickening of the tendon at its insertion (when compared with the normal opposite side). More confluent areas of hypoechogenicity represent small partial tears.[47] CT scans and MRI should be reserved for difficult cases in which uncertainty exists after ultrasound. CT detects central tendinous expansion at the insertion to the lower border of the patella and progressing for a variable length down the tendon.[46] The drawback to the use of CT is the use of ionizing radiation. MRI demonstrates signal intensity changes owing to necrosis, inflammation, and synovial proliferation.[48] The most common MRI finding in patients with patella tendinitis is tendon thickening, along with focal signal changes.[46] Partial saturation and short tau inversion recovery (STIR) sequences enhance the detection of focal signal changes compared with the spin echo protocol.

Jumper's knee may be prevented by proper training that focuses on conditioning and strengthening tissues to withstand stress. Emphasis should be placed on exercises that build eccentric quadriceps strength. All patients

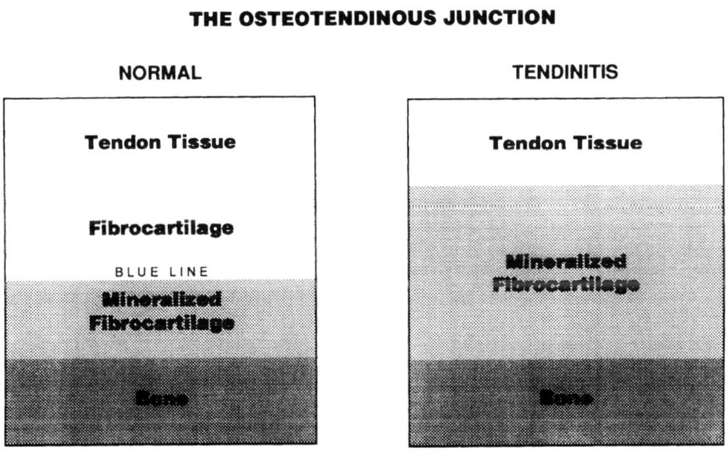

FIGURE 9.6. A graphic representation of the normal histology seen at the osteotendinous junction (left). With chronic tendon inflammation (right), the fibrocartilage distal to the "blue line" becomes mineralized.

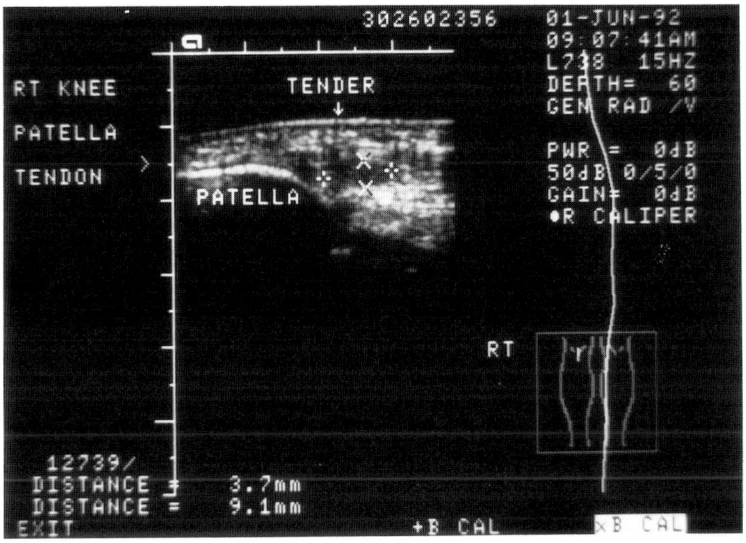

FIGURE 9.7. A 22-year-old athlete with chronic patellar tendinitis. Sagittal plane ultrasound study demonstrates hypoechogenicity over the proximal one third of the patellar tendon. This area corresponds to the location of maximal tenderness.

with patellar tendinitis should initially be treated conservatively. Early intervention could avoid progression to a chronic pathologic state. Rest, ice, ultrasound therapy, and nonsteroidal anti-inflammatory drugs are effective treatment modalities. Stanish et al.[49] documented 90% good or excellent results with a therapy program that focuses on eccentric loading in patients with chronic inflammation. The athlete may continue to exercise with activities that do not bring on any symptoms. Patients with refractory cases should not be injected with cortisone because of the resulting change in the tendon morphology and the increased incidence of patellar tendon rupture.[35,45,50,51] If all conservative measures fail in a patient with severe patellar tendinitis, surgery may be indicated.

Several surgical procedures have been described. These include excision of devitalized tendinous tissue along resection of the lower pole of the patella and tendon reattachment[52], excision of the degenerated portion of the patellar tendon alone,[53–55] and patellar distal pole drilling.[56] Our preferred treatment is surgical excision of only the diseased tissue. Its margins are adequately defined by preoperative physical examination and adjunctive ultrasound study. This area commonly represents the central one third of the patellar tendon at its bone insertion site. Karlsson et al.[55] reported excellent or good functional results and complete resumption of sporting activities in 71 of 78 patients after simple removal of the diseased tissue from the ligament.

Synovial Plica Syndrome

A *plica* is a normal embryonic synovial septum that can persist into adult life.[57] The vast majority of plicae are asymptomatic but occasionally the medial patellar plica can produce knee symptoms when it becomes inflamed, thickened, and less elastic. A symptomatic plica can mimic a torn meniscus, a loose body, osteochondritis dissecans of the patella or trochlea, and patellofemoral syndromes. The plica syndrome is a diagnosis of exclusion that is based mainly on a careful history and a physical examination. Radiography rarely provides assistance in establishing this diagnosis.

Embryologically, the knee develops from three pouches separated by a thin synovial membrane. Absorption of the dividing membrane leads to the formation of a single-cavity knee joint. Incomplete absorption of the septa leads to persistent synovial folds known as *plicae*.[57,58] Three major types of plicae have been identified[59,60] (Figure 9.8). They are named according to their relationship to the patella. The anterior plica, or ligamentum mucosum, is the most commonly seen. It is present, to some extent, in most persons as a thin redundant membrane that originates from the intercondylar notch and extends to the inferior fat pad. The anterior plica has not been associated with any pathologic conditions. The suprapatellar plica can demonstrate much anatomic variation.[57,61] Commonly, it bridges the medial wall of the suprapatellar pouch to the inferior surface of the quadriceps tendon. Rarely, a prominent suprapatellar plica can isolate the suprapatellar pouch from the rest of the joint. When this occurs, a small opening or *porta* across this dividing membrane may allow loose bodies to be concealed within the suprapatellar pouch.[59,62]

The medial patellar plica is clinically the most significant because it has been implicated with the plica syndrome. It originates from the synovium adjacent to the medial patella and extends to the synovial lining of the infrapatellar fat pad. Sakakibara[63] separates medial patellar plica into four groups, depending on the thickness of the synovial fold and whether the synovial fold covers the anterior surface of the medial femoral condyle. Only the large shelf-like plica that covers the medial femoral condyle is felt to be potentially symptomatic.[60] With the knee flexion, the large shelf-like plica impinges on the medial femoral condyle. This stretches pain receptors in the plica itself and potentially can lead to medial femoral condyle chondrosis.

The vast majority of plicae are innocuous. The *plica syndrome* refers to a constellation of nonspecific symptoms that are attributed to a thickened and inflamed medial patellar plica. Of the 730 arthroscopies that Broom and Fulkerson performed,[64] only 29 knees had clinical and arthroscopic findings consistent with this diagnosis. Nottage et al.[65] reported a 5.2% incidence of plica syndrome in patients undergoing arthroscopy for knee pain. Nearly all patients with the plica syndrome initially present with nonspecific anterior knee pain.[62,64–66] Pain may not be localized over the pathologic medial patellar plica. Other symptoms include snapping or clicking, weakness, a sense of instability, pseudolocking, or swelling. The most common clinical examination finding is tenderness over the femoral condyle.[62,65–67] Effusion, joint line tenderness, quadriceps atrophy, and patellofemoral crepitus also may be present. The most common misdiagnoses in patients with the plica syndrome are medial meniscal tear and patellofemoral syndrome.[62,64]

The preoperative diagnosis of the plica syndrome is dependent upon the history and the physical examination. Routine radiography provides no assistance in establishing the diagnosis but is necessary to eliminate other pathologic causes of knee pain. Other techniques available to document the presence of a prominent medial patellar plica include double-contrast arthrography, CT, ultrasonography, and MRI.[68–72] The utility of these studies is limited because of the difficulty in diagnosing a pathologic plica.

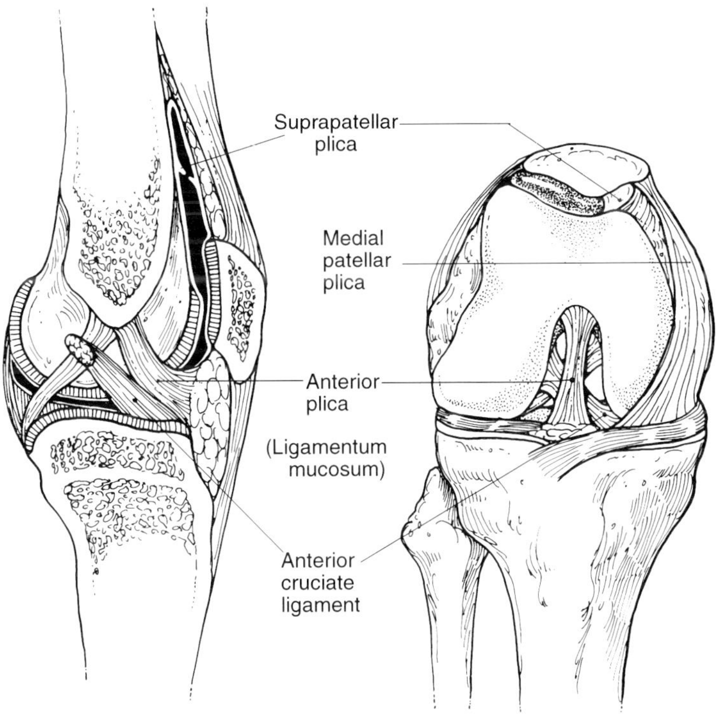

FIGURE 9.8. Anatomy of the knee synovial plicae.

Most plica are incidental arthroscopic findings unrelated to the true knee pathology. According to Jackson et al.,[73] a thick, rounded, fibrotic plica, and plica with a white inner border should be considered pathologic. Observing impingement of the plica on the underlying medial femoral condyle, along with evidence of articular cartilage wear, supports the diagnosis of the plica syndrome.

All patients diagnosed with the plica syndrome should initially enroll in a conservative treatment program.[74] This should include rest, nonsteroidal anti-inflammatory medication, quadriceps strengthening, and stretching. Older patients with chronic symptoms unresponsive to conservative measures may be candidates for surgical intervention. A detailed arthroscopic examination should be performed to rule out the presence of other pathologic conditions. If the patient's complaint is clearly related to the pathologic plica, it may be easily excised arthroscopically. Surgical excision of the medial patellar plica is not an innocuous procedure and should not be performed in nonpathologic states.

Patellar Bursitis

Bursae surrounding the knee are synovial-lined cavities that function to reduce friction between tendons and dermal tissue or bone. Acute trauma or chronic irritation of the bursa may lead to a symptomatic inflammatory response. Because of the anatomic proximity to the patella, knee bursal pathology may mimic patellofemoral disease. Normally, bursae are thin-walled cavities that are hardly noticeable between tissue planes (Figure 9.9). However, when affected by inflammation, trauma, or a pyogenic process, the bursal tissue becomes distinct.

Prepatellar Bursitis

The superficial prepatellar bursa is located subcutaneously at the level of the midportion of the patella. Repetitive irritation from prolonged kneeling may lead to a symptomatic inflammatory response of the prepatellar bursa. This has been commonly referred to as

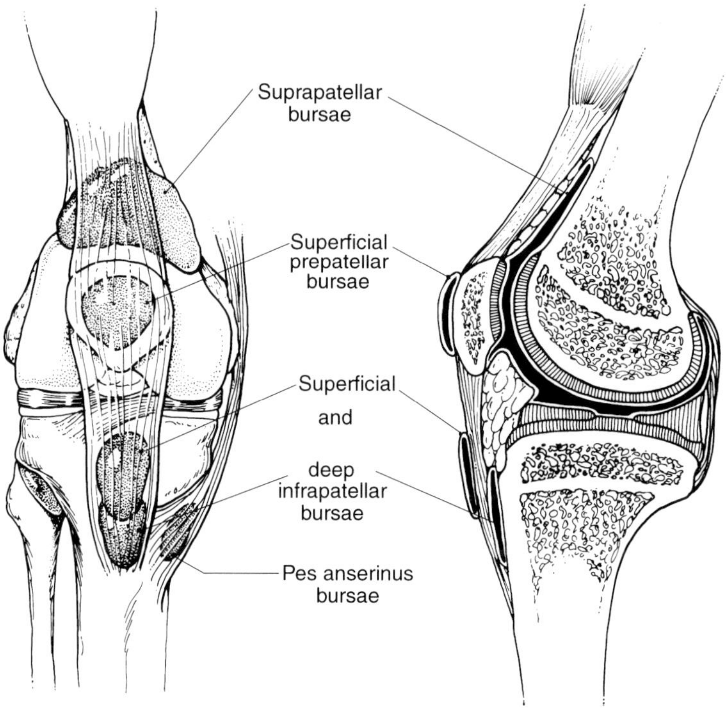

FIGURE 9.9. The bursae surrounding the knee.

a housemaid's knee. Other reported etiologies of prepatellar bursitis include a direct blow to the anterior knee and a significant abrasion-type injury to the skin above the patella. Wrestlers and athletes performing on artificial turf are particularly at risk.[75,76] Janecki and Hechtman[77] reported on a patient who developed an acute prepatellar bursitis from a lost meniscal fragment after arthroscopic meniscectomy. In acute cases of bursitis, the prepatellar bursa is fluctuant, swollen, and focally tender. Subacute and chronic cases are less evident on physical examination and an index of suspicion should be maintained in order to differentiate prepatellar bursitis from a more serious patellofemoral disease.

Septic prepatellar bursitis probably results from bacterial inoculation of the bursa after anterior knee trauma. The most common organisms are *Staphylococcus* and *Streptococcus* species.[78,79] Gram stain and bacterial culture results from the bursal aspirate differentiates between aseptic inflammation and an infectious process.

Infrapatellar Bursitis

The superficial and the deep infrapatellar bursae protect the distal patellar tendon from the adjacent dermal tissue and bone, respectively. Like prepatellar bursitis, chronic irritation, trauma, and bacterial infection can cause the infrapatellar bursa to become inflamed, swollen, and painful. It may be difficult on physical examination to differentiate infrapatellar bursitis from tendinitis, meniscal pathology, fat pad syndrome, and Osgood–Schlatter disease. Palpation of the infrapatellar region with the knee fully extended and the quadriceps muscle relaxed isolates the infrapatellar bursa and elicits tenderness.

Pes Anserinus Bursitis

The pes anserinus bursa underlies the combined insertion of the sartorius, semitendinosus, and gracilis tendons into the anteromedial aspect of the proximal tibia. Pes anserinus bursitis occurs classically in both distance runners and intermediate distance sprinters. Overuse of the medial hamstring secondary to inadequate rest periods, running on uneven terrain, and inadequate stretching can result in chronic pes anserinus bursal inflammation. Pain is located on the medial aspect of the knee approximately 6 cm below the joint line in the area of the pes anserinus bursa. With the knee held in extension, the patient may note palpable discomfort near the joint line, but if the knee is flexed, the tenderness will be detected over the pes anserinus bursa, a fact that differentiates between pes anserinus bursitis and medial joint pathology. Differential diagnosis includes medial meniscus tears, medial knee compartment degenerative disease, stress fractures, bone tumors, and hamstring tendinitis.[80]

Treatment

Initial treatment of inflammatory conditions of the knee bursae is conservative and includes rest, ice, compression, and immobilization. Oral anti-inflammatory agents are especially effective. Not only does bursal aspiration differentiate between a septic and an aseptic process, it also may relieve much of the pain associated with bursal distention. Because of the potential of causing infection, intrabursal injection of corticosteroids is not recommended.[79] Surgical excision of the entire bursa is indicated in those cases of chronic bursitis unresponsive to conservative measures. Kerr[81] described a three portal arthroscopic technique for resection of the prepatellar bursa.

Pyogenic bursitis first may be treated with bursal aspiration and initiation of anti-staphylococcal antibiotics. The final bacterial culture report may dictate the most appropriate antibiotic coverage. Initial intravenous antibiotics followed by a seven- to ten-day course of oral antibiotics are usually sufficient. If no clinical response is noted after 24 hours, formal incision and drainage may be required.

Fat Pad Syndrome

Hoffa[82] originally described a specific inflammatory condition involving the infrapatellar fat pad that appears to be distinct from generalized synovitis of the knee. Isolated trauma to the infrapatellar fat pad, either by a direct blow or by being caught between the femoral condyles and the tibial plateaus on extension, may initiate an inflammatory reaction accompanied by tenderness to direct palpation and occasionally by signs of swelling.[83] Diagnosis of fat pad syndrome is based on the location of the tenderness and by comparing the adipose tissue consistency with that of the contralateral knee. Symptoms usually abate with conservative measures and rarely is surgical debridement required.

Bipartite Patella

Since the original description of a bipartite patella by Gruber[84] in 1883, this anatomic variation has raised much debate. Prior to 1970, the orthopedic community believed that a bipartite patella was a normal variant of patellar development and was incapable of being symptomatic (Figure 9.10). Later observations

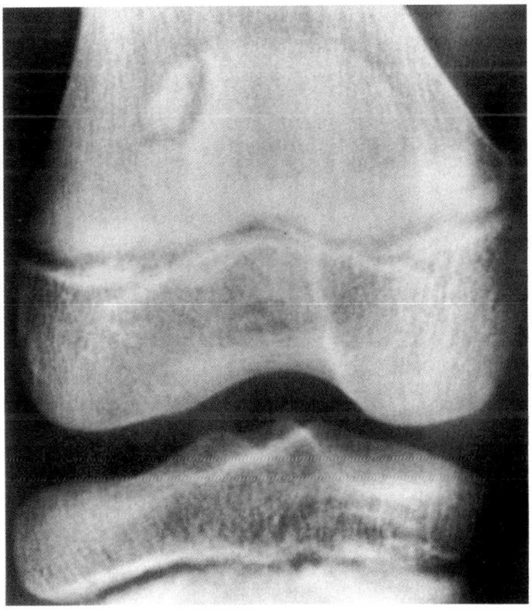

FIGURE 9.10. The typical superior lateral location of a secondary ossification center of the patella (bipartite patella). The finding was incidentally found on this 11-year-old boy.

by Green[85] and Weaver[86] recognized this accessory ossific nucleus as a potentially painful foci in atheletic persons. Its anatomic appearance is often indistinguishable from a fracture or pseudoarthrosis, which has caused difficulty in differentiating a bipartite patella from acute trauma.[87] Some authors fail to recognize this normal anatomic variation and believe that a bipartite patella actually represents a stress fracture.[88,89]

The rudimentary patella is known to develop in the ninth week of embryonic life as a cartilaginous mass lying deep to the extensor mechanism. Ossification of this cartilaginous analog occurs between 3 and 6 years of age. Ossification occurs in many irregular centers, which gradually coalesce by the second decade of life. Accessory ossification centers usually appear in early adolescence and occasionally persist into adulthood. There appears to be a male predilection.

The overall incidence of bipartite patellae has been reported to be as low as 0.05% by Stucke[90] to as high as 1.66% by Blumensaat.[91] Approximately one half of the occurrences are bilateral.[85,92] Weaver[86] estimates that only 2% to 3% of patients with bipartite patellae eventually require medical intervention.

Saupe[93] devised a classification of bipartite patellae based on the location of the accessory ossification center: inferior (type 1), lateral margin (type 2), and superolateral (type 3). The vast majority of symptomatic bipartite patellae occur with Saupe type 3 deformity.[86] With the experience of other authors, Saupe type 1 patellae are also capable of producing painful symptoms.[94,95] Pain is thought to result from excessive tension at the chondro-osseous junction, which leads to the accretion of fibrous tissue and fibrocartilage.[96] The histologic findings are similar to those found in Osgood–Schlatter disease and Sinding–Larsen–Johansson syndrome. Actually, Saupe type 1 lesion is thought to represent the end result of Sinding–Larsen–Johansson syndrome because no true secondary ossification center exists at the inferior patellar pole.[94] Type 2 patellae are most likely the result of traumatic patellar subluxation or dislocation.[97]

A bipartite patella may become spontaneously symptomatic but more frequently a history of trauma antedates symptoms. At times it can be difficult to differentiate a Saupe type 3 bipartite patella from a fracture of the superolateral margin. The following assist in making the diagnosis of a fracture: a history of significant trauma to the superolateral patella, localized point tenderness, hematoma, crepitation, and a radiograph demonstrating an irregular outline at the site of concern. If examination occurs weeks after the injury, diagnosis may be difficult because a pseudoarthrosis will have the same radiographic appearance as a bipartite patella. A radiograph of the patella prior to the accident may substantiate the diagnosis.

Cylinder cast immobilization usually differentiates a symptomatic bipartite patella from a fracture. A fracture is noted to heal after four to six weeks of cast treatment, whereas a bipartite patella continues to reveal a separation between the primary and the accessory ossification centers. A painful bipartite patella may be initially managed with immobilization, anti-inflammatory therapy, and injection of steroids into the area of localized tenderness. Excision of the accessory ossification center is usually effective when conservative therapy fails to resolve symptoms. Weaver[86] reviewed 21 athletes with symptomatic bipartite patellae. Surgical excision was curative in 13 out of 16 patients. Those who did not completely respond had mild residual symptoms.

Osteochondritis Dissecans of the Patella

Osteochondritis dissecans (OCD) of the patella is defined as partial of total separation of a portion of articular cartilage from the underlying patellar bone. To date, approximately 100 cases of OCD of the patella have been reported in the world literature. The exact incidence of this disease is unknown, but Schwarz et al.[98] estimates an operative incidence of 0.15% from a surgical knee registry of more than 30,000 operations. The osteochondral fragment may remain nondisplaced, become partially detached, or form a loose body (Figure 9.11).

OCD of the patella primarily involves the middle and lower thirds of the medial facet and the medial ridge of the patella.[98,99] The lesion occurs less frequently on the lateral facet and the superior aspect of the patella. The margins of the patella and the medial "odd facet" appear to be spared. The preferential involvement of the lower and middle thirds of the articular surface may be explained by the patellofemoral force transmission during knee flexion. At 10° to 15° of knee flexion, the lower third of the patella contacts the trochlear groove. With increasing degrees of flexion, patellar contact moves proximally. Not until 90° of flexion does the upper third of the patella establish contact. Because normal gait and most sporting activities only require 65° of flexion,[100] the lower two thirds of the patella appears to be exposed to the majority of the high shear and contact pressures of the patellofemoral articulation. Cumulative microtrauma eventually leads to separation of an osteochondral fragment. Other possible etiologies for OCD of the patella include ischemia,[101] endocrine factors,[102] genetic predisposition,[103] and anomalies of ossification.[104] Most likely, OCD of the patella has a multifactorial etiology and there may be factors not yet appreciated that interplay with microtrauma in its development.

The majority of patients with OCD of the patella present in the second decade of life with clinical features similar to the patellofemoral pain syndrome.[105] The average age at presentation has been reported to be 17 years old and the number of male patients significantly outnumber females (2.5–9 to 1).[106–108] Common complaints are anterior knee pain, swelling, locking, and giving way. Pain is usually aggravated by activities such as ascending and descending stairs, and is relieved by rest. One third of patients may recall a history of trauma.[98] The most common physical examination finding is patellofemoral crepitation.[98,99] Other findings include subpatellar pain with compression, quadriceps wasting, and effusion. It is unusual to have restricted knee motion or evidence of patellofemoral instability.

The diagnosis of OCD of the patella is confirmed with anteroposterior, lateral, and Merchant view radiographs. The lesion is most clearly seen in the lateral view. The Merchant view helps to localize the defect to the medial or the lateral patellar facets. Radiographs should be inspected carefully for intra-articular loose bodies. Nondisplaced, healing OCD lesions are readily appreciated on routine radiographs. Pfeiffer et al.[109] believe that MRI can assess the viability and attachment of the OCD fragment to the underlying cancellous bone, which may have implications for prognosis and guide treatment.

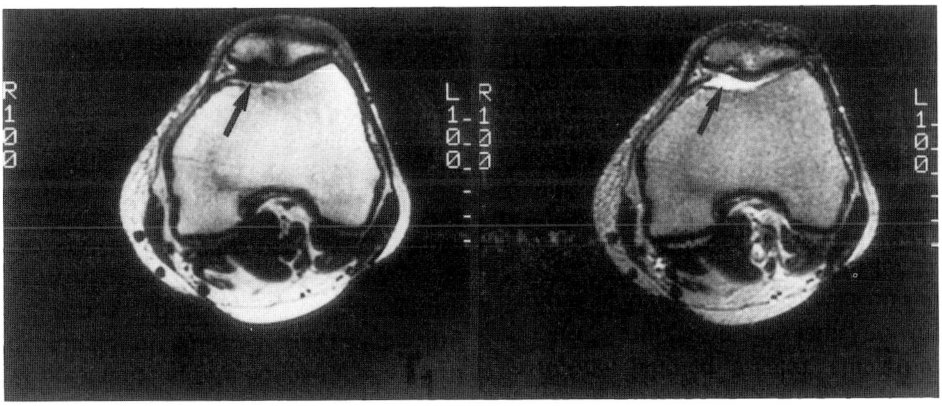

FIGURE 9.11. OCD of the patella. T_1 (left) and T_2 (right) MRI of the patellofemoral joint. Note the decreased subchondral signal of the medial facet on T_1 and the internal high signal on T_2. An osteochondral flap is evident on the T_2 image.

Patients with OCD of the patella have a guarded prognosis. Best results are obtained in those patients with minimally displaced lesions that show no sclerosis at their margins. These patients may be managed with activity restriction and immobilization. The high shear and contact pressures of the patellofemoral articulation prohibits healing of displaced OCD lesions. Most authors agree that surgical excision of the osteochondral fragment is indicated if there is subchondral sclerosis or separation of the fragment from its underlying cancellous bone bed.[98,99,110,111] The anatomic location of the OCD lesion may have some prognostic significance. Schwarz et al.[98] notes better long-term results with superior or inferior lesions. An equatorial position is associated with a poor result. Also, lesions greater than 2 cm in diameter demonstrate poor healing and persistent discomfort after operative debridement.[99,108,111]

Displaced OCD lesions of the patella may be treated with excision of the fragment combined with curettage or drilling of the bone crater.[98,99,107,111] Bone curettage or drilling is thought to open new channels for vascular ingrowth, stimulating healing and reconstitution of the articular surface through metaplasia of the underlying bone to fibrocartilage.[112] The OCD lesion may be addressed with the arthroscope or through a standard midline arthrotomy. Published operative treatment results of patellar OCD have been variable. Desai et al.[99] report good or excellent results in ten out of 11 patients treated with fragment excision and crater curettage. Similar good results are reported by other authors.[108,110,111] A larger study by Schwarz et al.[98] reports less optimism, with as many as 62% of their patients having fair or poor results. Persistent pain with restricted function and residual patellofemoral crepitation were noted on followup. Stougaard[107] also documented poor followup results in more than one half of his patients treated surgically. To date, there are few reports of surgical fixation of the osteochondral fragment with either bone pegs or pins and no outcome assumptions can be made.[110,113] Given the reported residual complaints after debridement and curettage, internal fixation of the fragment may be a reasonable option for larger fragments. The role of patching the bone crater with an osteochondral allograft has yet to be defined.

Patellar Fracture

Patellar fractures in skeletally immature patients are relatively rare. It has been estimated that less than 1% of patellar fractures occur in patients younger than 15 years of age.[114–116] The infrequent occurrence of these fractures in children may be explained by the patella's large cartilaginous content, increased mobility, and association with a resilient periarticular soft tissue.[117–120] The immature patella exhibits both adult fracture patterns and a unique avulsion-type injury.

Houghton and Ackroyd popularized the sleeve fracture of the patella in children.[121] This fracture represents an avulsion of the lower pole of the patella with wide separation

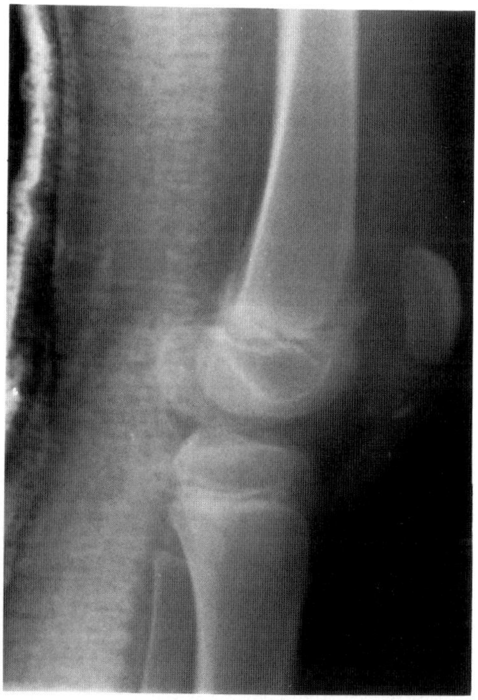

FIGURE 9.12. Classic patellar sleeve fracture in a 13-year-old girl. Note the avulsed inferior patellar pole and the resulting patellar alta.

of the fracture fragments (Figure 9.12). Along with a segment of bone, a large sleeve of articular cartilage is pulled off the main body of the bony patella. A later report by Grogan et al.[122] illustrates that avulsion fractures may involve any segment of the patellar periphery. Avulsion and transverse fractures constitute the vast majority of pediatric patellar fractures. The unique occurrence of patellar avulsion fractures in the pediatric population may be explained developmentally. Patellar chondro-osseous transformation proceeds as separate small foci of ossification progressively incorporating into the main patellar ossified body. The marginal bone is the least mature and is most susceptible to the varying amounts of tensile pull through the quadriceps mechanism and the retinacular tissue.[123]

Patellar fractures result from a direct or indirect blow to the knee, or from a twisting motion to the knee, causing subluxation or dislocation of the patella.[117,118,124,125] It is not uncommon for the diagnosis of patellar fracture in a child to be missed or significantly delayed.[117,126] Because of the relatively large cartilaginous bulk of the developing patella, the size of the fracture fragments may be underestimated radiographically. Also, a symptomatic bipartite patella may be confused with an acute fracture, making accurate clinical and radiographic diagnosis difficult.

Patients universally present after an acute injury to the anterior aspect of the knee. This may be caused by a direct blow, a sudden and violent quadriceps contraction, or by high tensile forces created by the quadriceps muscle and the patellar ligaments. An active patient with a history of chronic anterior knee pain prior to the acute event should raise suspicion of a patellar stress fracture.[127–129] Acute fractures demonstrate considerable swelling, ecchymosis, and limited knee extension against gravity. A palpable defect within the substance of the patella is a clinical tip-off. If extensor mechanism disruption has occurred, patella alta may be present. Standard radiographs always should be obtained and should include contralateral extremity views in order to differentiate acute fracture from variations in normal patellar ossification. A bone scan may assist in diagnosing a patellar stress fracture.[127] CT and MRI also are useful adjuncts in defining the exact location and extent of the injury. Table 9.3 lists the common patella fracture patterns in young people. The fracture geometry varies according to the mechanism of injury.

Transverse, Stellate, and Longitudinal Fractures

A violent blow to the flexed anterior knee can produce a transverse, stellate, or longitudinal fracture pattern. Ray and Hendrix[130] noted these fracture patterns to occur in half of all pediatric patellar fractures over a 12-year period at their institution. Other authors also have recognized these common fracture patterns in childhood and adolescence, and remark on their similarity to the adult injury.[97,117,119,120,131,132] A transverse fracture may result from acute displacement of a chronic stress insult.[129] A history of chronic anterior knee pain in a running or a jumping athlete, along with proof of insignificant trauma antedating the displaced patella fracture, is suggestive of a previous stress fracture.

Indications for surgery with transverse, stellate, or longitudinal fracture patterns in children and adolescents are the same as those for adults. If the fracture is nondisplaced and active knee extension is maintained, nonoperative treatment is recommended.[118,119,130] Open reduction and internal fixation is advisable if separation between the fragments of the patella is greater than 4 mm and if the step-off is greater than 3 mm.[117,120,121,124,133] Retinacular repair should follow bone fixation. Open frac-

TABLE 9.3. Patella fracture patterns.

Stage	Pattern
1	Transverse
2	Stellate
3	Longitudinal
4	Avulsion (marginal)
	a. Inferior (classic sleeve fracture)
	b. Medial
	c. Superior
	d. Lateral (? bipartite patella)
5	Stress (tensile injury)

tures, regardless of displacement, should undergo irrigation and debridement plus fixation as indicated.[118,119,134]

Avulsion (Marginal) Fracture

Grogan et al.[122] classify avulsion fractures by their anatomic location: inferior, medial, superior, and lateral. All have been associated with trauma and may be caused by chronic stress weakening of the pediatric bone. Lateral marginal fractures are not discussed here because of their infrequent occurrence and may possibly represent a bipartite patella.

Inferior Avulsion Fractures

Inferior avulsion injuries represent the classic sleeve fracture that Houghton and Ackroyd[121] described. This fracture exclusively occurs in children and adolescents who participate in jumping activities.[121,135] Some authors believe the inferior sleeve fracture could be a variant of the Sinding–Larsen–Johansson disease.[135–137] Inherent weakness of the lower patellar pole during adolescence, along with strain on the patellar tendon during vigorous activity, can result in distal pole weakening.[138,139] With jumping activity, the knee is forcefully extending against resistance, causing the extensor mechanism to fail at the osteochondral junction of the inferior pole. At the time of fracture, the distal avulsed fragment retains a large sleeve of articular cartilage. With further pull of the quadriceps musculature, the denuded patella is separated from its inferior pole. The patella is commonly high riding and a palpable gap is noted between the displaced fragments. The majority of sleeve fractures are significantly displaced and require anatomic restoration of the articular surface through open reduction and internal fixation[94,121,122,130,135] (Figure 9.13).

Medial Avulsion Fractures

Medial avulsion fractures represent an osteochondral injury associated with acute lateral dislocation of the patella. Osteochondral fractures are reported to occur in approximately 5% of all patellar dislocations in children.[137,140] The patella is forced laterally over the ridge of the lateral trochlea. Because of the continued pull of the medial stabilizers, an osteochondral portion of the medial patella is avulsed (Figure 9.14). The fracture also may result from spontaneous or manual reduction of the dislocation. With reduction, a segment of the medial patella may be sheared from the main body of the patella. This injury is commonly associated with longitudinal disruption of the medial retinaculum and quadriceps fascia. Like sleeve fractures, articular incongruity and displacement are usually present and anatomic reduction, along with fracture stabilization, is indicated with larger bone fragments.[122,141,142]

Superior Avulsion Fractures

Superior pole avulsion fractures are the least common fracture pattern. Grogan et al.[122] reports on seven patients with variable degrees of superior pole separation. Five out of seven patients were treated with cast immobilization in extension for three to eight weeks. By three months after immobilization, all patients had adequate return of quadriceps strength and function. None of the patients demonstrated radiographic deformity of the patella. Of those patients in the literature that are treated with open reduction, a large cartilaginous fragment is consistently found and considerable separation exists between fracture fragments.[122,143] The small osseous fragment seen on a radiograph fails to quantitate the size of the articular segment. Although short-term results appear to be acceptable with immobilization alone, we believe that restoration of the articular surface in significantly displaced fractures through open reduction will lessen the chance of later posttraumatic arthrosis and extensor mechanism dysfunction.

Stress Fracture

Adolescent stress fractures most commonly occur in the tibia and the fibula. The first description of patellar stress fracture in the English literature was by Devas in 1960.[144] Since then, many reports have been published de-

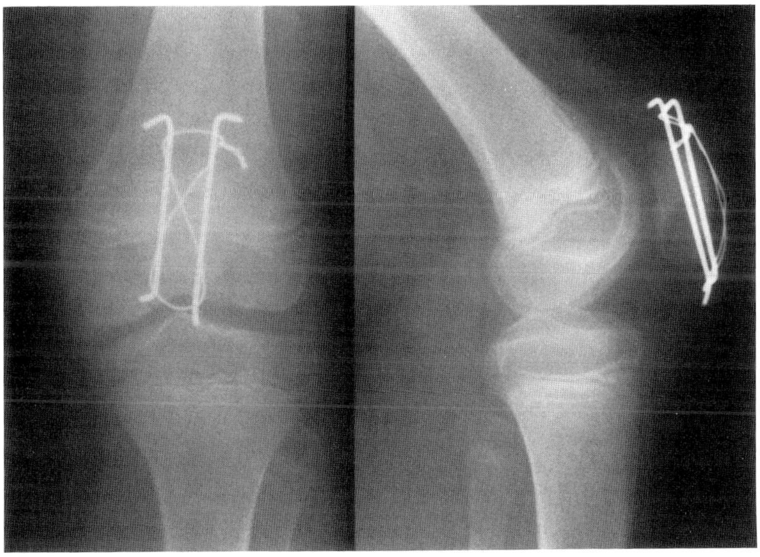

FIGURE 9.13. Anatomic reduction of a patellar sleeve fracture and stabilization with the AO tension band technique.

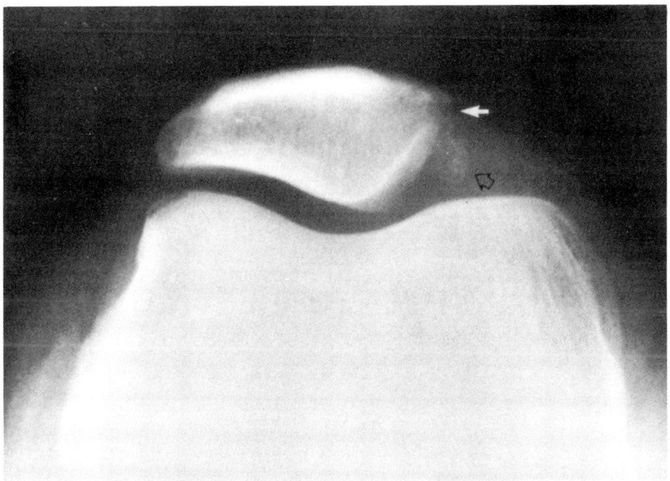

FIGURE 9.14. Osteochondral fracture of the medial facet of the patella in a 27-year-old man whose knee "gave out" while playing racquetball. The osteochondral fragment (open arrow) and its source of origin from the medial facet of the patella (white arrow) are demonstrated. (Reprinted with permission: Rogers LF, Hendrix RW: Radiology of skeletal trauma. Churchill Livingstone, New York, 1992)

scribing this injury in patients with cerebral palsy[145–147] and adolescent athletes.[148–152] In the athletic group, patellar stress fractures have occurred exclusively in patients participating in running and jumping activities.[144,149,150,152,153] Most stress fractures of the patella are the transverse type. Stress fractures in the longitudinal plane also have been reported.[148,153] Some authors believe that a painful bipartite patella actually may represent a stress fracture.[88,89,154]

With knee flexion, tensile forces are applied to the anterior surface of the patella through the quadriceps tendon and the patellar tendon. Perry et al.[155] found quadriceps force to be 210% of the body weight at 30° of flexion. This quadriceps force equaled 50% of the average maximal quadriceps strength and is capable of producing stress-induced failure of the patella initiated in tension. Cyclic loading of the extensor mechanism below the yield strength of the bone initiates stress fracturing. A fatigue fracture results when the frequency of loading overshadows the remodeling necessary to prevent failure.

Cerebral palsy patients with knee flexion contractures are known to develop patellar stress fractures.[145–147] The tonically active extensor mechanism provides a constant tensile load, which is believed to disrupt bone maturation. Stanitski et al.[156] argue that bone integrity can be compromised by the mechanical insult from concentrated muscle forces. The common link between cerebral palsy patients and athletic persons who suffer patellar stress fractures is the frequent tensile overload on the patella caused by the overcontracting quadriceps musculature.

A high index of suspicion must be maintained when examining any adolescent athlete with patellar pain. The vast majority of stress fractures occur in adolescents participating in activities such as basketball, volleyball, and other sports involving jumping. The athlete usually presents with the insidious onset of dull patellar pain. Examination reveals tenderness directly over the bone. These patients rarely have swelling, effusion, or patellofemoral crepitation. Radiographic examination should include anteroposterior, lateral, and sunrise views of the patella. Increased uptake on a lateral technetium bone scan may support the diagnosis (Figure 9.15).

Any athlete who presents with a chronic history of anterior knee pain and localized tenderness directly over the patella, suggestive of a patellar stress fracture, should be treated conservatively. Four to six weeks of immobilization and activity restriction allows remodeling of the compromised bone. A symptomatic bipartite patella also is likely to respond to this treatment regime. Patients with patellar pain who present acutely with fracture fragment displacement after insignificant trauma probably experienced acute failure of a stressed, weakened patella (Figure 9.16). Displaced fractures should be managed with open reduction and internal fixation. Patellar stress fractures heal more slowly than a normal patella fracture and avascular changes of the patellar substance may occur.

Avulsion Fractures of the Tibial Tuberosity

Avulsion fractures of the tibial tuberosity are infrequent, acute traumatic injuries that occur during adolescence. Forceful quadriceps contracture during sporting activity can cause the developing tibial tuberosity to fail in tension (Figure 9.17). Because of the unique anatomic relationship between the immature proximal tibial physis and tibial tuberosity, combined injuries with intra-articular involvement are not uncommon. To date, many authors have noted the association between preexisting Osgood–Schlatter disease and tibial tuberosity avulsion injuries.[157–160] It is believed that Osgood–Schlatter disease causes structural modifications in the physeal cartilage of the developing tibial tubercle, predisposing it to an altered biomechanical response when exposed

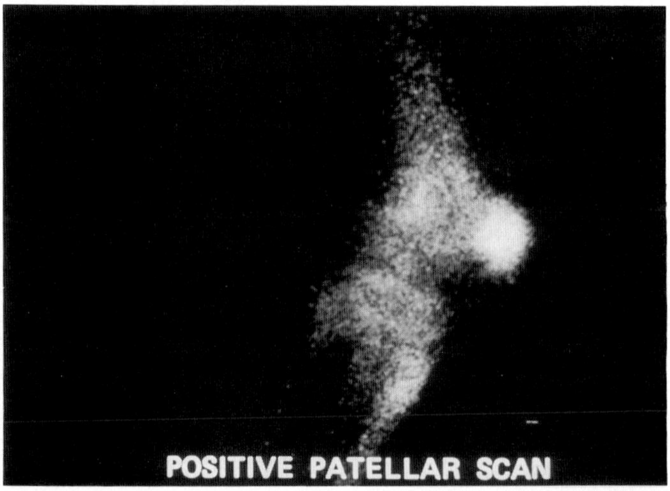

FIGURE 9.15. A 21-year-old man with a 6-week history of activity-induced anterior knee pain. A greatly positive technetium bone scan over the patella supported the diagnosis of a patellar stress fracture.

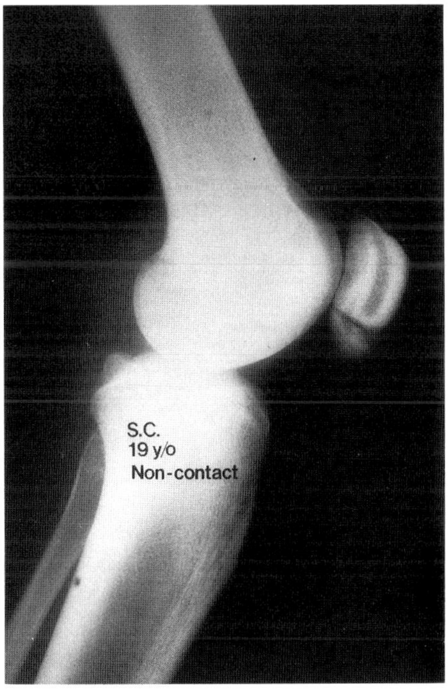

FIGURE 9.16. Acute lower-pole patellar fracture after insignificant trauma in a patient known to have a patellar stress fracture.

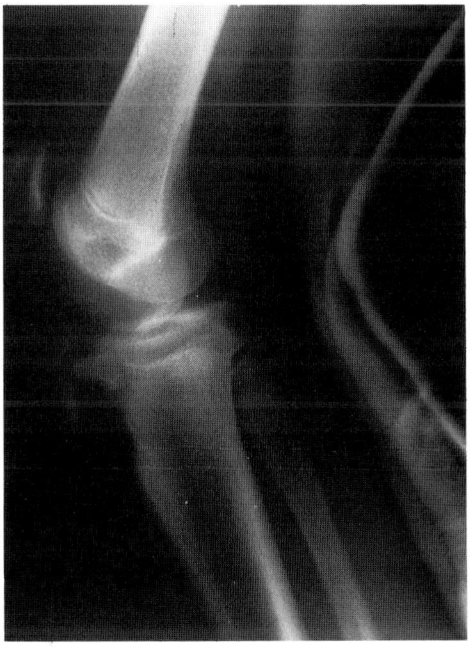

FIGURE 9.17. This 15-year-old boy basketball player sustained an Ogden type 2B tibial tubercle fracture while jumping off the ground.

to the strain transmitted by the patellar tendon.

Tibial tubercle avulsion fractures occur predominantly in adolescent boys between 12 and 17 years of age. Sports that require jumping are responsible for more than 50% of the cases. Other sports such as football, track, and gymnastics are less contributory. The patient usually presents with complete functional disability because of severe acute anterior knee pain. Physical examination always reveals swelling on the proximal anterior surface of the tibia and a knee hemarthrosis. Less consistent findings include patella alta or a prominent bone spike palpated subcutaneously. Lateral radiographs confirm the diagnosis. The radiographic classification system that Ogden et al.[161] defined considers both the different fracture patterns and the degree of displacement of the avulsed fragment (Figure 9.18).

The fracture pattern does not relate to the age at which it occurs, but it is dependent upon the vector pull of the patellar tendon at the time of injury.[158] When the tensile force exerted by the extensor mechanism is greater than the inherent strength of the apophyseal cartilage, an avulsion fracture results. At full extension, the patellar tendon force is concentrated solely on the tibial tubercle. Forceful quadriceps contracture in a nearly extended knee can occur while springing off the ground, while jumping, or during the landing phase of a jump. This mechanism has been associated with isolated anterior tibial tuberosity injuries (Ogden type 1 and 2). With progressive knee flexion, the patellar tendon vector pull is redirected through the anterior tibial epiphysis, resulting in the more complex fracture patterns as Ogden described (Ogden type 3).

Nondisplaced and minimally displaced tibial tubercle avulsion fractures can be treated by closed means.[158,161,162] Minimally displaced injuries may be reduced with gentle digital pressure applied over the tuberosity. After reduction is obtained, one month of cylinder cast immobilization usually is sufficient. Displaced injuries (Ogden type 1B, 2B, and 3) require open reduction and internal fixation.[158,159,163] A parapatellar surgical approach

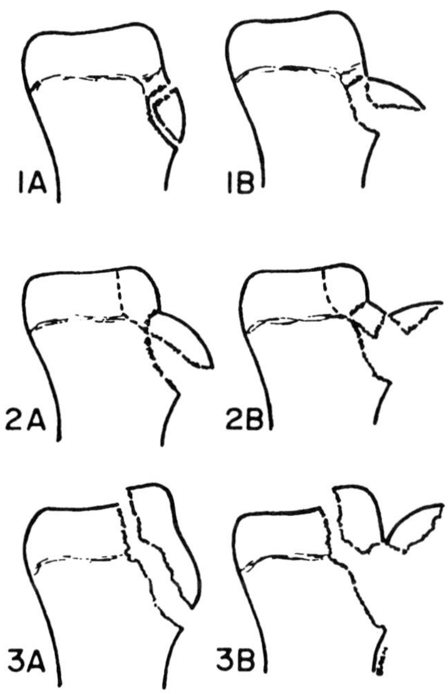

FIGURE 9.18. Types of injury to the tibial tuberosity. Type 1A: The fracture is distal to the normal junction of the ossification centers of the proximal end of the tibia and tuberosity. Displacement is minimal. Type 1B: The fragment is hinged (displaced) anteriorly and proximally. Type 2: In type 2A, the primary fracture failure is at the junction of the ossification of the proximal end of the tibia and tuberosity, essentially in line with a transverse continuation of the proximal tibial epiphysis. In type 2B, the tuberosity fragment is comminuted and the more distal fragment may end up being more proximally displaced. Type 3: The fracture extends into the joint and is associated with displacement of the anterior fragment of fragments, leading to discontinuity of the joint surface. In type 3A, the tuberosity and anterior aspect of the proximal tibial epiphysis are a composite unit. In type 3B, the unit is comminuted, with the major site of fragmentation being the juncture of the ossification centers of the tuberosity and proximal end of the tibia. (Reprinted with permission: Ogden JA, Tross RB, Murphy MJ. Fracture of the tibial tuberosity in adolescents. J Bone Joint Surg 62A:206, 1980)

allows sufficient exposure of the fracture fragments. After fracture reduction, one or two cancellous bone screws with washers adequately stabilizes the tuberosity. Following rigid operative fixation, the extremity may be mobilized as early as three weeks. Reported complications associated with this injury include anterior compartment syndrome, refracture, painful nonunion, and metal irritation after surgical fixation.[159]

Quadriceps and Patellar Tendon Rupture

The knee extensor mechanism is analogous to a chain link and may be disrupted at any portion. The location of the disruption is dependent upon the mechanism of knee trauma or the presence of a predisposing condition structurally weakening the bone or the tendon tissue. Quadriceps and patellar tendon disruptions usually occur after maximal contracture of the quadriceps musculature with the knee held in flexion. Other mechanisms of tendon rupture include lacerations or a direct blow. The extensor mechanism is more likely to fail at the musculotendinous junction, the muscle belly, or the bone–tendon interface. A local tendinitis may structurally weaken the midsubstance of the tendon, causing it to fail prematurely. The tendon may be affected by systemic inflammatory conditions such as rheumatoid arthritis and gout, overuse tendinitis, degenerative joint disease, diabetes tenosynovitis, metabolic diseases, tumor, or infection. Steroid injections may cause microscopic damage to the tendon's vascular supply, predisposing it to rupture.[35,45,50,51]

Patellar tendon ruptures seem to occur in a younger population than quadriceps tendon tears. In 1981, Siwek and Rao[164] described 117 cases of knee tendon rupture over a three-year period. Eighty percent of patellar tendon ruptures were in patients less than 40 years old. In contrast, 88% of quadriceps ruptures were in patients older than 40 years. The earlier occurrence of patellar tendon ruptures may be explained by the increased involvement of the younger age group in sporting activities that place chronic tensile stress on the extensor mechanism, leading to tendinous degeneration and jumper's knee.[42] The majority of patients with quadriceps tendon ruptures have systemic diseases affecting the quality of the tendinous tissues or significant degenerative diseases of the patellofemoral joints.

Early diagnosis and treatment is the key to a successful outcome. Recognizing the diagnosis after a two-week delay affects the results of treatment. The majority of patients present with acute pain and loss of knee extensor function. The younger patient suffering a patellar tendon disruption may describe an audible "pop" while landing on a semiflexed knee. Physical examination usually reveals a tense knee hemarthrosis, palpable step-off, and varying degrees of active knee extension. The degree of injury determines the amount of patellar retinacular disruption. Intact retinacular tissue may allow compensatory knee extensor function. With extensive patellar tendon disruption, patella alta may be evident on plain radiographs. MRI may be helpful in diagnosing subtle tendon tears in the presence of a functioning extensor mechanism. Although rare, bilateral quadriceps tendon ruptures have been reported more often than bilateral patellar tendon injuries.[165–167]

Early in the 20th century, surgical repair of the disrupted extensor mechanism became the treatment of choice.[168,169] Primary surgical repair within two weeks from the time of rupture consistently yields the best results.[164] The rupture frequently occurs at the bone–tendon junction. After debridement of the frayed tendon margins, both ruptured quadriceps and patellar tendons should be repaired primarily to the patella using no. 2 nonabsorbable suture. The suture must pass through healthy tendinous tissue and through bone tunnels created along the periphery of the patella. A cancellous bony trough should be created adjacent to the repair site. This trough provides a bleeding bone bed that may stimulate tendon-to-bone healing. The ruptured retinaculum should be repaired with absorbable suture using a figure-eight-type stitch. One must avoid shortening the tendon when performing the repair. This may disrupt the relationship between the patella and the trochlear groove, leading to a patellar alta or baja deformity. Patellar tilt may be created if the surgical repair is not adjacent to the articular surface of the patella. Postoperatively, the patient should be immobilized in extension for six weeks. Afterwards, an aggressive physical therapy program should concentrate on quadriceps strengthening and knee range of motion.

If the tendon margins are not easily approximated without excessive tension across the repair site, reinforcement of the repair may be indicated. Many reinforcement techniques have been described. These include the use of circular stainless steel wire, Mersilene tape, fascial grafts, Dacron vascular grafts, and semitendinous tendon transposition.[168,170–173] Specifically for quadriceps tendon ruptures, Scuderi[174] described an anterior quadriceps turn-down flap. All of these reinforcement procedures function to share the load across the surgical repair site until sufficient healing has occurred.

Delayed surgical repair presents a particular problem. By as little as two weeks after the injury, significant quadriceps contracture has occurred, prohibiting tendon approximation. The Codivilla V to Y quadriceps tendon lengthening technique is useful for delayed quadriceps tendon repairs.[175] Preoperative patellar traction may be required for delayed repairs of the patellar tendon.[164] All delayed repairs of the quadriceps or patellar tendon should be reinforced with any of the surgical means described previously.

Osgood–Schlatter Disease

Tibial tubercle apophysitis, or Osgood–Schlatter disease (OSD), was originally described by Osgood[176] and Schlatter[177] at the beginning of the 20th century. It represents a benign lesion of the tibial tubercle affecting rapidly growing and active adolescents. A history of activity-related discomfort over the tibial tubercle, along with signs of swelling and tenderness, implies the diagnosis of OSD. The patient's presentation may resemble other more serious conditions, such as malignant disease or local infection, and a misdiagnosis can delay early institution of appropriate treatment.[178–180]

Prior reports suggest that OSD is more common in the adolescent boy population. However, the disease prevalence appears to be increasing in adolescent girls because of their increased participation in competitive sports, in particular gymnastics and soccer. Boys commonly present at 12 to 15 years of age compared with girls, who present one to two years earlier. Because of the age differences between sexes, this disorder appears to be related to the degree of skeletal maturity rather than gender. The majority of patients with OSD participate in regular athletic activities, particularly those requiring running, climbing, or jumping. Athletic adolescents were noted to have a 21% prevalence of OSD and only 4.5% of similar age nonathletic persons were symptomatic.[181] Bilateral knee involvement has been documented in 20% to 30% of patients.[178,182] Kujala et al.[181] noted siblings of affected persons to be more likely to develop OSD when compared with a control population.

The maturing tibial apophysis appears to be susceptible to chronic tensile strain. Repetitive microtrauma acting on the immature junction of the patellar ligament and the tibial tubercle causes an avulsion injury, which leads to attempted osseous repair.[157,183] Histologic studies note chronic inflammation or an apophysitis of the tibial tubercle.[182] Commonly, an adjacent bony ossicle and fibrous bursal tissue are present. Chronic inflammation leads to the proliferation of cartilage and bone, resulting in a tender and prominent tibial tubercle, which characterizes this condition.

Physical examination demonstrates distal extensor mechanism swelling and intense local discomfort. Resisted knee extension usually reproduces the symptoms, which leads to a functional extensor lag. The remainder of the examination is typically normal. Some authors have reported an unclear association between OSD and patellofemoral malalignment and instability.[181,184–186]

Radiographic examination to the knee differentiates OSD from other more serious conditions affecting adolescents, most notably infections and tumors (Figure 9.19). Findings on plain radiographs in OSD include swelling of soft tissues and an ill-defined margin between the patellar tendon and its bony insertion. The tibial tubercle may demonstrate a separate, discrete ossicle in 10% to 50% of cases.[182,187] Although CT and MRI reveal distal patellar tendinitis and ossicle formation, clinical examination and plain radiographs provide the same information, therefore not necessitating these costly studies. Lanning and Heikkinen[188] have proposed ultrasound as a simple, fast, and reliable method for the diagnosis of OSD. Specific ultrasound findings include an echogenic tendon with an anechoic zone of edema seen anterior to the tibial tubercle. Bone scan does not appear to be helpful in establishing the diagnosis.[189]

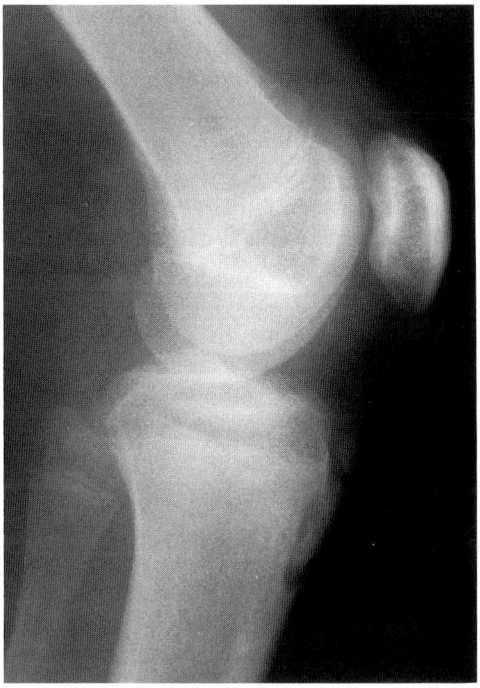

FIGURE 9.19. OSD. Note the irregular outline of the tibial tubercle and the presence of a discrete ossicle within the substance of the patellar tendon.

The preponderance of patients with OSD should be treated nonoperatively. Spontaneous resolution of symptoms occur with normal tibial tubercle apophyseodesis. By adulthood, most patients are noted to be asymptomatic.[187] If initial symptoms are neglected and protracted, morbidity occurs, as many as 30% of patients may eventually require surgical intervention.[181] Early treatment consists of activity restriction, ice, anti-inflammatory medication, and flexibility exercises. If symptoms persist, a trial of formal extremity immobilization may be indicated. Once the patient is capable of returning to the sporting activity, the level of participation should be based on symptom severity. Cushioned knee and foot orthoses may provide symptomatic relief to the young athlete. Steroid injections into the tibial tubercle are not recommended because they may result in patellar tendon rupture or skin problems.[50,190]

Surgical intervention has shown good results in those patients who do not respond to conservative measures and demonstrate a symptomatic ossicle or ossicles.[182,191] Removal of all loose intratendinous ossicles and overlying bursal tissue is the procedure of choice, both from a functional and a cosmetic point of view.[192]

Sinding–Larsen–Johansson Disease

Sinding–Larsen–Johansson disease (SLJ), also called patellar epiphysitis, represents a form of jumper's knee that is exclusive to the adolescent population. Its association with OSD has been well described.[193,194] Both conditions represent a traction phenomenon in which repeated strain at the patellar tendon causes chondro-osseous tensile failure of the immature skeleton.[96,145] SLJ is self-limited, like OSD, although it is shorter in duration and is seen in a younger group of patients (a range of 10 to 13 years old).[193]

The involved child elicits a history of chronic anterior knee pain with running, jumping, prolonged sitting, and ascending stairs. These repetitive loaded knee flexion activities lead to a traction tendinitis with partial tendon avulsion and de novo calcification of the proximal patellar tendon. Using radiographic findings, Medlar and Lyne[193] devised a classification scheme that also outlines the natural progression of the disease (Table 9.4).

TABLE 9.4. Radiographic stages of Sinding–Larsen–Johansson disease.

Stage	Classification
1	Normal findings
2	Irregular calcification at the inferior patellar pole
3	Coalescence of the calcification
4A	Incorporation of the calcification into the patella to yield a normal roentgenographic configuration of the area
4B	Coalesced calcification mass separate from the patella

Source: Medlar RC, Lyne ED: Sinding–Larsen–Johansson Disease: Its etiology and natural history. J Bone Joint Surg 60A(8):1113, 1978

Like jumper's knee in the adult skeleton, treatment centers on conservative measures. Nearly all patients are disease-free and have returned to a full level of activity by 13 months after symptom onset.[193] Surgery is only indicated in "catastrophic" jumper's knee when there is acute avulsion of the patellar or the quadriceps tendon.

Congenital and Genetic Disorders

Congenital Dislocation of the Patella

Congenital dislocation of the patella is a result of lateral displacement of the extensor mechanism that could be permanent and irreducible, or unstable and capable of being manually reduced.[195] Genetic factors or in utero distress may lead to failure of normal medial rotation of the skeletal myotome that contains the quadriceps and the development of fibrotic muscular and fascial attachments to the patella. The derangement appears to occur both unilaterally and bilaterally, and has been postulated to have a familial association.[196,197] Even though the majority of cases are seen in children with genetic abnormalities, this condition may be observed in otherwise normal children.[198]

Dislocation is present at birth but the diagnosis is often delayed until the parents note disability or secondary deformity. Early in infancy the child may show good knee extensor function with no cosmetic abnormalities. Walking is not prohibited even though there is documented extensor weakness and inability to completely straighten the knee. With further growth of the child, genu valgum, external tibial torsion, lateral tibial subluxation, and a fixed knee flexion deformity results. The lateral femoral condyle is prominent on physical examination and the hypoplastic patella is displaced posteriorly to the region of the fibular head. Pain is rarely present but may signify early arthrosis.

Radiographic diagnosis is difficult until age 3 to 4 years, at which time patellar ossification is noted to occur. Preossification findings include loss of the normal anterior knee soft-tissue shadow on lateral projection. Once ossification occurs, radiographs reveal lateral patellar displacement along with significant patellofemoral hypoplasia. We have found MRI to be useful in establishing the diagnosis in young children. MRI defines the anatomic location of the extensor mechanism along with associated dysplasia.

The goal of treatment is to restore the extensor mechanism alignment before secondary arthrosis results. Closed patellar reduction is not possible and surgical realignment is required. A combination of medial plication, lateral retinacular release, patellar tendon realignment, or Galeazzi's procedure[199] may be required. Bony realignment should be avoided until skeletal maturity.

Duplication of the Extensor Mechanism

Duplication of the extensor mechanism is a rare congenital abnormality noted to occur more commonly in patients with multiple epiphyseal dysplasia (MED) syndrome. Along with the finding of irregular ossification of multiple epiphyses, patellofemoral abnormalities are noted in approximately 50% of MED patients.[200] Both coronal and sagittal plane duplications have been reported.[201] Successful results have been obtained by resecting the more hypoplastic structures along with centralization of the remaining patella.[202]

Down Syndrome

Down syndrome has been classically associated with mental retardation, muscle hypotonia, and soft-tissue laxity. Dugdale and Renshaw studied 361 Down syndrome patients and noted an 83% incidence of patellar instability.[203] A fewer percentage of patients possess clinically significant instability that warrants a surgical procedure.[204] We have not observed an association between instability and functional status. Operative treatment should be reserved for those patients who exhibit significant instability along with pain, frequent falls, and lack secondary deformities related to Down syndrome.[204] The preferred treatment is medial soft-tissue plication along with lateral retinacular release. The reoccurrence rate of patellar subluxation or dislocation is high.

Nail–Patella Syndrome

Nail–patella syndrome or onycho-osteodysplasia is an autosomal dominant disorder associated with nail abnormalities, radial head dysplasia, "iliac horns," and patellar hypoplasia or complete absence.[205] Clinical examination reveals an anterior knee sulcus with flexion. The hypoplastic patella may be ovoid or triangular in shape and patellar baja is sometimes observed. Despite the significant anatomic abnormality, disability rarely occurs and reconstruction is infrequently indicated.[206]

Patellar Lesions

Dorsal Defect of the Patella

Dorsal defect of the patella (DDP) is a rare benign patellar tumor that may present with symptoms of swelling, pain, and giving way. In 1972, Caffey[207] first reported this condition, which probably represents a developmental abnormality. Since its original description, 32 cases have been documented in the English literature.[207–213]

DDP is a sharply marginated, round, radiolucent lesion that borders on the dorsal subchondral bone of the superolateral aspect of the patella (Figure 9.20). The histology of DDP is similar to a fibrous cortical defect in that bone spicules are noted in a bed of fibrous tissue. It is currently believed that fibrous cortical defects arise from an alteration in the periosteum. Because the patella is devoid of true periosteum, most pathologists are reluctant to equate a DDP with a fibrous cortical defect. A common pathologic diagnosis is a "nonspecific, benign lesion." Because the superolateral corner of the patella is a common location of secondary ossification centers, it has been postulated that DDP represents a cartilaginous abnormality that inhibits the patellar ossification process.[211]

Not all patients with DDP are symptomatic.[209,210] This lesion is commonly a spurious finding during radiographic examination of other knee pathologies. Symptomatic patients with DDP universally have increased uptake on technetium bone scanning.[208-210] Unlike OCD, the articular surface does not appear to be violated on either a knee arthrogram or an MRI study. The majority of symptomatic patients respond to conservative measures including activity restriction and anti-inflammatory medications. Followup radiographic studies may demonstrate spontaneous resolution of the lesion.[211] If a symptomatic DDP is not responsive to a long course of conservative treatment, surgical excision of the lesion along with bone grafting of the bone crater can provide rapid and successful resolution of the problem.[208,209]

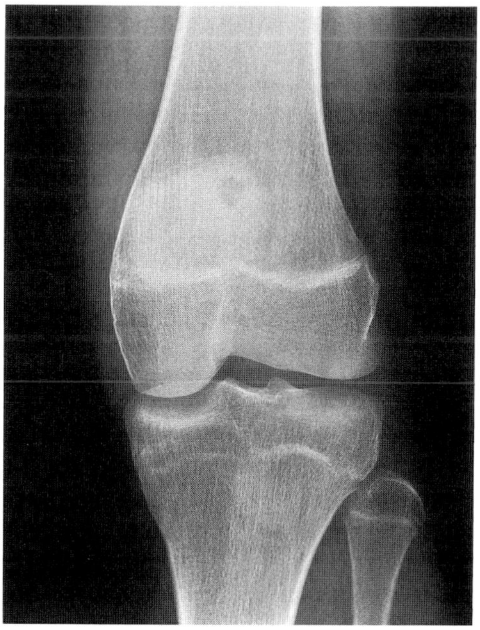

FIGURE 9.20. Dorsal defect of the patella.

Patellar Tumors

Primary and metastatic bone tumors are known to occur within the patella. The majority of patients with patellar tumors present with nonspecific anterior knee pain resembling other pathologic patellar conditions. Diagnostic studies include plain radiographs, technetium bone scanning, CT, and MRI. The diagnosis is confirmed with surgical biopsy. The most common primary patellar tumors reported in the literature are giant cell tumors[214,215] followed by osteosarcoma.[216] Less common primary tumors include chondroblastoma, hemangioma, osteoblastoma, enchondroma, reticulum cell sarcoma, myeloma, eosinophilic granuloma, brown tumor of hyperparathyroidism, and Paget's disease. Patellar metastases are even more rare. If present they commonly originate from the esophagus and the breast.[217-219] Osteomyelitis of the patella can resemble a bone tumor (Figure 9.21) and must be included in the differential diagnosis.[220,221]

Conclusions

It is important to establish a differential diagnosis when examining a patient with patellofemoral complaints. By classifying all painful patellar conditions as chondromalacia patella, the clinician fails to recognize the disease etiology and fails to establish a successful treatment plan. A detailed history and physical examination supplemented by plain radiographs of the patellofemoral joint should provide enough information to establish a definitive diagnosis in the majority of cases. Almost all nontraumatic afflictions of the patella initially should be treated in a conservative

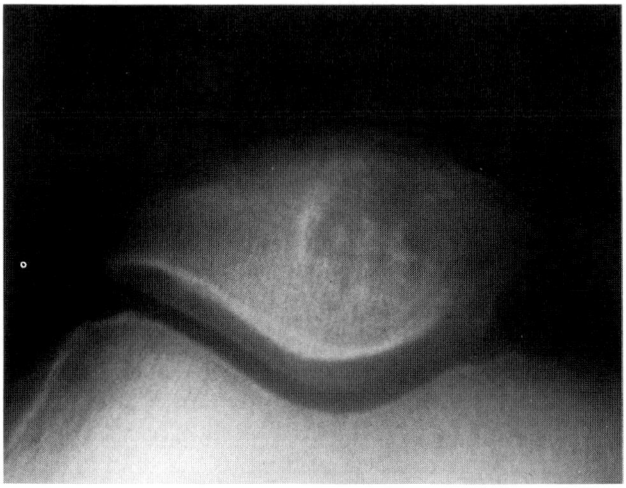

FIGURE 9.21. A 22-year-old woman dialysis patient with a chronic fungal infection of the patella. Although patellar bone lesions are rare, it is difficult to distinguish osteomyelitis from a neoplastic lesion.

manner. By understanding the pathophysiology of the patellofemoral joint, surgical options can be recommended to those patients resistant to nonoperative methods of treatment.

References

1. Owre A: Chondromalacia patellae. *Acta Chir Scand* 1936;77(suppl. 41).
2. Ficat RP, Hungerford DS: *Disorders of the Patellofemoral Joint.* Baltimore, Williams & Wilkins Co., 1977.
3. Merchant AC: *Classification of patellofemoral disorders. Arthroscopy* 1988;4(4):235.
4. Radin FL: Anterior knee pain: The need for a specific diagnosis, stop calling it chondromalacia! *Orthop Rev* 1985;14:123.
5. Johnson R: Lateral facet syndrome of the patella. *Clin Orthop* 1989;238:148–158.
6. McGinty JB, McCarthy JC: Endoscopic lateral retinacular release: A preliminary report. *Clin Orthop* 1981;158:120.
7. Krompinger WJ, Fulkerson JP: Lateral retinacular release for intractable lateral retinacular pain. *Clin Orthop* 1983;179:191–192.
8. Grana WA, Kriegshauser LA: Scientific basis of extensor mechanism disorders. *Clin Sports Med* 1985;4:247–257.
9. Fulkerson JP: Evaluation of the peripatellar soft tissues and retinaculum in patients with patellofemoral pain. *Clin Sports Med* 1989;8: 197–202.
10. Fulkerson JP: Awareness of the retinaculum in evaluating patellofemoral pain. *Am J Sports Med* 1982;10:147–149.
11. Fulkerson JP, Tennant R, Jaivin JS, Grunnet M: Histologic evidence of retinacular nerve injury associated with patellofemoral malalignment. *Clin Orthop* 1985;197:196–205.
12. Larson RL, Cabaud HE, Slocum DB, et al.: The patellar compression syndrome: Surgical treatment by lateral retinacular release. *Clin Orthop* 1978;134:158–167.
13. Fulkerson JP, Hungerford DS: *Disorders of the Patellofemoral Joint* ed. 2. Baltimore, Williams & Wilkins Co., 1990.
14. Merchant AC, Mercer RL, Jacobsen RH, Cool CR: Roentgenographic analysis of patello-femoral congruence. *J Bone Joint Surg Am* 1974; 56A:1391–1396.
15. Laurin CA, Dussault R, Levesque HP: The tangential x-ray investigation of the patellofemoral joint: X-ray technique, diagnostic criteria and their interpretation. *Clin Orthop* 1979;144:16–26.
16. Fulkerson JP, Schutzer SF, Ramsby GR, Bernstein RA: Computerized tomography of the patellofemoral joint before and after lateral release or realignment. *Arthroscopy* 1987; 3(1): 19–24.
17. Doucette SA, Goble EM: The effect of exercise on patellar tracking in lateral patellar compression syndrome. *Am J Sports Med* 1992;20(4): 434–440.
18. O'Neill DB, Micheli LJ, Warner JP: Patellofemoral stress, A prospective analysis of exercise treatment in adolescents and adults. *Am J Sports Med* 1992;20:151–156.
19. Moller RN, Krebs B: Dynamic knee brace in the treatment of patellofemoral disorders. *Arch Orthop Trauma Surg* 1986;104:377–379.
20. McConnel J: The management of chondro-

malacia patellae: A long-term solution. *Austr J Physiother* 1986;32:215–223.
21. Lysholm J, Nordin M, Ekstrand J, Gillquist J: The effect of a patella brace on the performance in a knee extension strength test in patients with patellar pain. *Am J Sports Med* 1984;12: 110–112.
22. James S, Bates G, Osternig L: Injuries to runners. *Am J Sports Med* 1978;6:40.
23. McKenzie DC, Clement DB, Taunton JE: Running shoes, orthotics, and injuries. *Sports Med* 1985;2:334–347.
24. Schonholtz G: Lateral retinacular release of the patella. *Arthroscopy* 1987;3:269–272.
25. Metcalf R: An arthroscopic method for lateral release of the subluxating of dislocating patella. *Clin Orthop* 1982;167:9–18.
26. Grana W, Hinkley B, Hollingsworth S: Arthroscopic evaluation and treatment of patellar malalignment. *Clin Orthop* 1984;186:122–128.
27. Schonholtz GJ, Zahn MG, Magee CM: Lateral retinacular release of the patella. *Arthroscopy* 1987;3:269–272.
28. Aglietti P, Pisaneschi A, Buzzi R, Gaudenzi A, Allegra M: Arthroscopic lateral release for patellar pain of instability. *Arthroscopy* 1989; 5: 176–183.
29. Christensen F, Soballe K, Snerum L: Treatment of chondromalacia patella by lateral retinacular release of the patella. *Clin Orthop* 1988;234:145–147.
30. Betz R, Magill JT, Lonergan RP: The percutaneous lateral retinacular release. *Am J Sports Med* 1987;15(5):477–482.
31. Dzioba RB, Strokon A, Mulbry L: Diagnostic arthroscopy and longitudinal open lateral release: A safe and effective treatment for "chondromalacia patellae." *Arthroscopy* 1985; 1(2): 131–135.
32. Kolowich PA, Paulos LE, Rosenberg TD, Farnsworth S: Lateral release of the patella: Indications and contraindications. *Am J Sports Med* 1990;18(4):359–365.
33. Huberti HH, Hayes WC: Contact pressures in chondromalacia patellae and effects of capsular reconstructive procedures. *J Orthop Res* 1988; 6(4):499–508.
34. Fulkerson JP, Schutzer SF: After failure of conservative treatment for painful patellofemoral malalignment: Lateral release or realignment? *Orthop Clin North Am* 1986;17(2):283–288.
35. Kelly DW, Carter VS, Jobe FW, et al.: Patellar and quadriceps tendon ruptures—Jumper's knee. *Am J Sports Med* 1984;12:375.
36. Rosenberg JM, Whitaker JH: Bilateral infrapatellar tendon rupture in a patient with jumper's knee. *Am J Sports Med* 1991;19:94.
37. Maddox PA, Garth WP: Tendinitis of the patellar ligament and quadriceps (jumper's knee) as an initial presentation of hyperthyroidism. *J Bone Joint Surg Am* 1986;68A:288.
38. Kricun R, Kricun ME, Arangio GA, et al.: Patellar tendon ruptures with underlying systemic diseases. *Am J Radiol* 1980;135:803.
39. Martin JR, Wilson CL, Mathews WH: Bilateral rupture of the ligamenta patellae in a case of disseminated systemic lupus erythematosus. *Arthritis Rheum* 1958;1:548.
40. Sulivan RL: Traumatic bilateral patellar tendon rupture with chronic renal disease. *Wis Med J* 1986;85:12.
41. Feretti A: Epidemiology of jumper's knee. *Sports Med* 1986;3:289.
42. Blazina ME, Kerlan RK, Jobe FW, et al.: Jumper's knee. *Orthop Clin North Am* 1973;4:665.
43. Kujala UM, Kvist M, Osterman K: Factors predisposing to patellar chondropathy and patellar apicitis in athletes. *Int Orthop* 1986;10: 195.
44. Molnar TJ, Fox JM: Overuse injuries of the knee in basketball. *Clin Sports Med* 1993;12(2): 349.
45. Ferretti A, Ippolito E, Mariani P, et al.: Jumper's knee. *Am J Sports Med* 1983;11:58.
46. Davies SG, Baudouin CJ, King JB, Perry JD: Ultrasound, computed tomography and magnetic resonance imaging in patellar tendonitis. *Clin Radiol* 1991;43:52.
47. Harke HT, Grissom LE, Finklestein MS: Evaluation of the muscularskeletal system with sonography. *AJR* 1988;150:1253.
48. Bodne D, Quinn SF, Murray WT, et al.: Magnetic resonance images of chronic patellar tendonitis. *Skeletal Radiol* 1988;17:24.
49. Stanish WD, Curwin S, Rubinovich RM: Tendonitis: The analysis and treatment for running. *Clin Sports Med* 1985;4:21.
50. Ismail AM, Balakrishmann R, Rajakamur MK: Rupture of the patellar ligament after steroid infiltration. *J Bone Joint Surg Br* 1969; 51B: 503.
51. Kennedy JC, Willes RB: The effect of local steroid injections on tendons. *Am J Sports Med* 1991;4:11.
52. Van der Ent A, de Baere AJ: Jumper's knee; results of operative therapy. *Acta Orthop Scand* 1985;55:450.
53. Martens M: Tendonitis of the patellar tendon. *Acta Orthop Belg* 1982;48:453.
54. Martens M, Wooters P, Burssens A, et al.: Pa-

tellar tendonitis: Pathology and results of treatment. *Acta Orthop Scand* 1982;53:445.
55. Karlsson J, Lundin O, Lossing IW, Peterson L: Partial rupture of the patellar ligament: Results after operative treatment. *Am J Sports Med* 1991;19(4):403.
56. Smillie IS: *Injuries of the Knee Joint,* ed. 3 Edinburgh, Churchill Livingstone, 1962.
57. Pipkin G: Knee injuries. The role of suprapatellar plica and suprapatellar bursa in simulating internal derangements. *Clin Orthop* 1971; 74:161.
58. O'Conner RL: *Arthroscopy.* Philadelphia, JB Lippincott Co., 1977.
59. Patel D: Arthroscopy of the plicae-synovial folds and their significance. *Am J Sports Med* 1978;6:217.
60. Munzinger U, Ruckstuhl J, Scherrer H, et al.: Internal derangement of the knee due to pathologic synovial folds: The mediopatellar plica syndrome. *Clin Orthop* 1981;155:59.
61. Pipkin G: Lesions of the suprapatellar plica. *J Bone Joint Surg Am* 1950;32A:363.
62. Hardaker WT, Whipple TL, Bassett FH: Diagnosis and treatment of the plica syndrome of the knee. *J Bone Joint Surg Am* 1980;62A:211.
63. Sakakibara J: Arthroscopic study on lino's band. *Nippon Seikeigeka Gakkai Zasshi* 1976; 50:513.
64. Broom MJ, Fulkerson JP: The plica syndrome: A new perspective. *Orthop Clin North Am* 1986;17(2):279.
65. Nottage WM, Sprague NF, Auerbach BJ, et al.: The medial patellar plica syndrome. *Am J Sports Med* 1983;11:211.
66. Muse GL, Grana WA, Mollingsworth S: Arthroscopic treatment of medial shelf. *Arthroscopy, J Arthroscopic Rel Surg* 1983;102:67.
67. O'Dwyer KJ, Peace PK: The plica syndrome. *Injury* 1988;19:350.
68. Kinnard P, Levesque RY: The plica syndrome: A syndrome of controversy. *Clin Orthop* 1984; 183:141.
69. Nicholas JA: Double contrast arthrography of the knee. *J Bone Joint Surg Am* 1970;52A:203.
70. Boven R, DeBoeck M, Protliege R: Synovial plicae of the knee on computed tomography. *Radiology* 1983;147:805.
71. Derks WMJ, De Mooge P, Van Linge B: Ultrasonographic detection of the patellar plica in the knee. *J Clin Ultrasound* 1986;14:355.
72. Pianka G, Combs J: Arthroscopic diagnosis and treatment of symptomatic plicae, in Scott WN (ed.): *Arthroscopy of the Knee: Diagnosis and Treatment.* Philadelphia, WB Saunders Co., 1990, p. 83.
73. Jackson RW, Marshall DJ, Fujisawa Y: The pathologic medial shelf. *Orthop Clin North Am* 1982;13:307.
74. Amatuzzi MM, Fazzi A, Varella MH: Pathologic synovial plica of the knee: Results of conservative treatment. *Am J Sports Med* 1990;18: 466.
75. Mysnyk MD, Wroble RR, Foster DT, et al: Prepatellar bursitis in wrestlers. *Am J Sports Med* 1986;14:46.
76. Larson RL, Osternig LR: Traumatic bursitis and artificial turf. *Am J Sports Med* 1974;2:183.
77. Janecki CJ, Hechtman KS: Prepatellar bursitis: A complication of arthroscopic surgery of the knee due to a lost meniscal fragment. *Arthroscopy* 1989;5:343.
78. Canoso JJ, Yood RD: Reaction of the superficial bursae in response to specific disease stimuli. *Arthritis Rheum* 1979;22:1361.
79. Canoso CJ, Sheckman PR: Septic subcutaneous bursitis: Report of 16 cases. *J Rheumatol* 1979;6:196.
80. Boland A: Soft tissue injuries of the knee, in Nicholas JA, Hershman EB (eds.): *The Lower Extremity and Spine in Sports Medicine,* St. Louis, CV Mosby Co., 1986, pp. 983–1012.
81. Kerr DR: Prepatellar and olecranon arthroscopic bursectomy. *Clin Sports Med* 1993; 12(1):137.
82. Hoffa A: The influence of the adipose tissue with regards to the pathology of the knee joint. *JAMA* 1904;43:795.
83. Smillie IS: *Injuries of the Knee Joint.* Baltimore, Williams & Wilkins Co., 1962.
84. Gruber W: In bildungsanomalie mit bildunghemmung begrundete bipartition beider patellae eines jungen subjektes. *Wirchows Arch Pathol Anag* 1883;94:358.
85. Green WT: Painful bipartite patella: A report of three cases. *Clin Orthop* 1975;110:197.
86. Weaver JK: Bipartite patella as a cause of disability in the athlete. *Am J Sports Med* 1977; 5:137.
87. Adams JD, Leonard RD: A developmental anomaly of the patella frequently diagnosed as a fracture. *Surg Gynecol Obstet* 1925;41:601.
88. Echeverria TS, Bersane FA: Acute fracture simulating a symptomatic bipartite patella. *Am J Sports Med* 1980;8:48–50.
89. Roels J, Martens M, Mulier JC, et al.: Patellar tendinitis (jumper's knee). *Am J Sports Med* 1978;6:362–368.
90. Stucke K: Die Patella partita in ihren Bezie-

hungen zum Unfall und zer Wehrdienstbeschadignung. *Monatsschr Unfallheilk* 1950;53: 238.
91. Blumensaat C: Patella partitia traumatische spaltpatella. *Patellarfraktur Arch Orthop Unfallchir* 1932;32:263.
92. Tos L, Salvi V: La patologia non traumatico della rotule. *Minerva Med* 1968;60:79.
93. Saupe H: Primaire knochenmark seilerung die kneischeibe. *Dtsch Z Chir* 1943;258:386.
94. Thabit G, Micheli LJ: Patellofemora pain in the pediatric patient. *Orthop Clin North Am* 1992;23(4):567–585.
95. Schmidt DR, Henry JH: Stress injuries of the adolescent extensor mechanism. *Clin Sports Med* 1989;8:343.
96. Ogden JA, McCarthy S, Jokl P: The painful bipartite patella. *J Pediatr Orthop* 1982;2:263.
97. Ogden JA: *Skeletal Injury in the Child.* Philadelphia, WB Saunders Co., 1990.
98. Schwarz C, Blazina ME, Sisto DJ, Hirsh LC: The results of operative treatment of osteochondritis dissecans of the patella. *Am J Sports Med* 1988;16(5):522.
99. Desai SS, Patel MR, Mitchelli LJ, Silver JW, Lidge RT: Osteochondritis dissecans of the patella. *J Bone Joint Surg Br* 1987;69B:320.
100. Kettelkamp DB, Johnson RJ, Smidt GL, Chao EYS, Walker M: An electrogoniometric study of knee motion in normal gait. *J Bone Joint Surg Am* 1970;50A:775.
101. Campbell CJ, Ranawat CS: Osteochondritis dissecans: The question of etiology. *J Trauma* 1966;6:201.
102. Smillie IS: Osteochondritis dissecans: Loose bodies in joints: Etiology, pathology, treatment. Edinburgh Churchill Livingstone, 1960.
103. Fraser WNC: Familial osteochondritis dissecans. *J Bone Joint Surg Br* 1966;48B:598.
104. Sontag LW, Pyle SI: Variations in the calcification pattern in epiphyses: Their nature and significance. *AJR* 1941;45:50.
105. Goodfellow J, Hungerford DS, Woods C: Patello-femoral joint mechanics and pathology. *J Bone Joint Surg Br* 1976;58B:291.
106. Rideout DF, Davis S, Navani SV: Osteochondritis dissecans patellae. *Br J Radiol* 1966;39:673.
107. Stougaard J: Osteochondritis dissecans of the patella. *Acta Orthop Scand* 1974;45:111.
108. Pantazopoulos T, Exarchou E: Osteochondritis dissecans of the patella. Report of four cases. *J Bone Joint Surg Am* 1971;53A:1205.
109. Pfeiffer WH, Gross ML, Seeger LL: Osteochondritis dissecans of the patella: MRI evaluation and a case report. *Clin Orthop* 1991; 271:207.
110. Smillie IS: in *Diseases of the Knee Joint.* London, Churchill Livingstone, 1980. p. 387.
111. Edwards DH, Bentley G: Osteochondritis dissecans patellae. *J Bone Joint Surg Br* 1977; 59B:58.
112. DePalma AF, McKeever CD, Subin DK: Process of repair of articular cartilage demonstrated by histology and autoradiography with tritiated thymidine. *Clin Orthop* 1966;48:229.
113. Herzberger M, Schuler P, Rossak K: Osteochondritis dissecans of the patella. *Z Orthop Ihre Grenzgeb* 1982;120:268.
114. Schoenbauer HR: Bruche der kniescheibe. *Ergeb Chir Orthop* 1959;42:56–79.
115. Brostrom A: Fracture of the patella. *Acta Orthop Scand* 1972;43:1–80.
116. Diebold O: Uber kniescheibenbruche im kindesalter. *Arch Klin Chir* 1927;147:664–681.
117. Belman DA, Neviaser RJ: Transverse fracture of the patella in a child. *J Trauma* 1973;13: 917.
118. Pollen AG: in *Fractures and Dislocations in Children.* Edinburgh, Churchill Livingstone, 1973, p. 173.
119. Rang MC: *Children's Fractures,* ed. 2. Philadelphia, JB Lippincott Co., 1983.
120. Crawford AH: Fractures about the knee in children. *Orthop Clin North Am* 1976;7:639.
121. Houghton GR, Ackroyd CE: Sleeve fractures of the patella in children. *J Bone Joint Surg Br* 1979;61B:165.
122. Grogan DP, Carey TP, Leffers D, Ogden JA: Avulsion fractures of the patella. *J Pediatr Orthop* 1990;10(6):721.
123. Ogden JA, McCarthy SM, Jokl P. Fractures of the tibial tuberosity in adolescents. *J Bone Joint Surg Am* 1980;62A:205.
124. Blount WP: Fractures of the patella, in Blount WP (ed.). *Fractures in Children.* Baltimore, Williams & Wilkins Co., 1954, pp. 171–172.
125. Nummi J: Fractures of the patella: A clinical study of 707 patellar fractures. *Ann Chir Gynaecol Fenn* 1971;179(suppl.):1–85.
126. Hallopeau P: De certaines fractures de la rotule chez l'enfant. *J Med Paris* 1923;42:927–929.
127. Schmidt DR, Henry JH: Stress injuries of the adolescent extensor mechanism. *Clin Sports Med* 1989;8(2):343.
128. Jerosch JG, Castro WH, Jantea C: Stress fracture of the patella. *Am J Sports Med* 1989; 17(4):579.

129. Teitz CC, Harrington RM: Patellar stress fracture. *Am J Sports Med* 1992;20(6):761.
130. Ray JM, Hendrix J: Incidence, mechanism of injury, and treatment of fractures of the patella in children. *J Trauma* 1992;32(2):464.
131. Ogden JA: *Pocket Guide to Pediatric Fractures.* Baltimore, Williams & Wilkins Co., 1987.
132. Rockwood CA, Wilkins KE, King RE: Fractures: Children and adolescents, vol. 3. Philadelphia, JB Lippincott Co., 1985.
133. Andrews JR, Hughston JC: Treatment of patellar fractures by partial patellectomy. *South Med J* 1977;70:809.
134. Weber MJ, Janecki CJ, McLeod P, et al.: Efficacy of various forms of fixation of transverse fractures of the patella. *J Bone Joint Surg Am* 1980;62A:215.
135. Wu C, Huang S, Liu T: Sleeve fracture of the patella in children. *Am J Sports Med* 1991;19: 525.
136. Gardiner JS, McInerney VK, Avella DG, Valdez NA: Injuries to the inferior pole of the patella in children. *Orthop Rev* 1990; 19(7): 643.
137. Heckman JD, Alkire CC: Distal patellar pole fractures, a proposed common mechanism of injury. *Am J Sports Med* 1984;12:424.
138. Hawley GW, Griswold AS: Larsen-Johansson's disease of the patella. *Surg Gynecol Obstet* 1928;47:68.
139. Medlar RC, Lyne ED: Sinding-Larsen-Johansson's disease. *J Bone Joint Surg Am* 1978; 60A:1113.
140. Rorabeck CH, Bobechko WP: Acute dislocation of the patella with osteochondral fracture: A review of 18 cases. *J Bone Joint Surg Br* 1976;58B:237.
141. Griswold AS: Fractures of the patella. *Clin Orthop* 1954;4:44.
142. Peterson L, Stener B: Distal disinsertion of the patellar ligament combined with avulsion fracture at the medial and lateral margins of the patella. *Acta Orthop Scand* 1976;47:680.
143. Bishay M: Sleeve fracture of upper pole of patella. *J Bone Joint Surg* 1991;73B:339.
144. Devas MB: Stress fracture of the patella. *J Bone Joint Surg Br* 1960;42B:71.
145. Rosenthal RK, Levine DB: Fragmentation of the distal pole of the patella in spastic cerebral palsy. *J Bone Joint Surg Am* 1977;59A:934.
146. Mann M: Fatique fracture of the lower patellar pole in adolescents with cerebral movement disorders. *Z Orthop* 1984;122:167.
147. Kaye JJ, Freiberger RH: Fragmentation of the lower pole of the patella in spastic lower extremities. *Radiology* 1971;101:97.
148. Devas M: Stress fractures of the patella, in Devas M (ed.). *Stress Fractures.* Edinburgh, Churchill Livingstone, 1975, pp. 130–137.
149. Hanel DP, Burdge RE: Consecutive indirect patellar fractures in an adolescent basketball player. *Am J Sports Med* 1981;9:327.
150. Dickason JM, Fox JM: Fracture of the patella due to overuse syndrome in a child: A case report. *Am J Sports Med* 1982;10:248.
151. Sugiura Y, Ikuta Y, Muroh Y: Stress fractures of the patella in athletes. *Nippon Seikeigeka Gakkai Zasshi* 1977;51:1421.
152. Hensal F, Nelson T, Pavlov, et al.: Bilateral patellar fractures from indirect trauma. A case report. *Clin Orthop* 1983;178:207.
153. Iwaya T, Tukatori Y: Lateral longitudinal stress fracture of the patella. Report of three cases. *J Pediatr Orthop* 1985;5:73.
154. Tarsney FF: Catastrophic jumper's knee: A case report. *Am J Sports Med* 1981;9:60.
155. Perry J, Antonelli D, Ford W: Analysis of knee-joint forces during flexed knee stance. *J Bone Joint Surg Am* 1975;57A:961.
156. Stanitski CL, McMaster JH, Scranton PE: On the nature of stress fractures. *Am J Sports Med* 1978;6:391.
157. Ogden JA, Southwick W: Osgood-Schlatter's disease and tibial tuberosity development. *Clin Orthop* 1976;116:180.
158. Balmat P, Vichard P, Pem R: The treatment of avulsion fractures of the tibial tuberosity in adolescent athletes. *Sports Med* 1990; 9(5): 311.
159. Wiss DA, Schilz JL, Zionts L: Type III fractures of the tibial tubercle in adolescents. *J Orthop Trauma* 1991;5(4):475.
160. Bowers KD: Patellar tendon avulsion as a complication of Osgood-Schlatter disease. *Am J Sports Med* 1981;9(6):356.
161. Ogden JA, Tross RB, Murphy MS: Fracture of the tibial tuberosity in adolescents. *J Bone Joint Surg Am* 1980;62A:205.
162. Christie MJ Ovonch VM: Tibial tuberosity avulsion fractures in adolescents. *J Pediatr Orthop* 1981;1(4):391.
163. Nimityongskul P, Montague WL, Anderson LD: Avulsion fracture of the tibial tuberosity in late adolescence. *J Trauma* 1988;28:505.
164. Siwek CW, Rao JP: Ruptures of the extensor mechanism of the knee joint. *J Bone Joint Surg Am* 1981;63A:932.
165. Kamali M: Bilateral traumatic rupture of the

infrapatellar tendon. *Clin Orthop* 1979;142: 131.
166. MacEachern AG, Plews JL: Bilateral simultaneous spontaneous rupture of the quadriceps tendons: Five case reports and a review of the literature. *J Bone Joint Surg Br* 1984; 66B:81.
167. Stern RE, Harwin SF: Spontaneous and simultaneous rupture of the quadriceps tendons. *Clin Orthop* 1980;147:188.
168. Gallie WE, LeMesurier AB: The late repair of fractures of the patella and of rupture of the ligamentum patellae and quadriceps tendon. *J Bone Joint Surg Am* 1927;9A:47.
169. Quenu E, Duval P: Traitement operatoire des ruptures sousrotuliennes du quadriceps. *Rev Chir* 1905;31:169.
170. McLaughlin HL, Francis KC: Operative repair of injuries to the quadriceps extensor mechanism. *Am J Surg* 1956;91:651.
171. Miskew WBW, Pearson RL, Pankovich AM: Mersilene strip suture in repair of disruptions of the quadriceps and patellar tendons. *J Trauma* 1980;20:867.
172. Frazier CH, Clark EM: Major tendon repairs with Dacron vascular graft suture. *Orthopedics* 1980;3:323.
173. Ecker ML, Lotke PA, Glazer RM: Late reconstruction of the patellar tendon. *J Bone Joint Surg Am* 1979;61A:884.
174. Scuderi C: Ruptures of the quadriceps tendon: Study of 20 tendon ruptures. *Am J Surg* 1958; 95:626.
175. Hass SB, Callaway H: Disruption of the extensor mechanism. *Orthop Clin North Am* 1992;23(4):687.
176. Osgood RB: Lesions of the Tibial Tubercle Occuring during adolescence. *Boston Med J* 1903;148:114.
177. Schlatter C: Verletzungen des schnabelformigen fortsatzes der oberen tibiaepiphyse. *Beitr Klin Chir* 1903;38:874.
178. Mital MA, Matza RA: Osgood-Schlatter disease: The painful puzzler. *Physician Sportsmed* 1977;5:60.
179. Season EH, Miller PR: Primary subacute pyogenic osteomyelitis in long bones of children. *J Pediatr Surg* 1976;11:347.
180. Knutsson, F: Two synovial fibrosarcomas. *Acta Radiol* 1948;29:4.
181. Kujala UM, Kvist M, Heinonen O: Osgood-Schlatter's disease in adolescent athletes. Retrospective study of incidence and duration. *Am J Sports Med* 1985;13:236.
182. Mital MA, Matza RA, Cohen J: The so-called unresolved Osgood-Schlatter lesion. *J Bone Joint Surg Am* 1980;62A:732.
183. Ogden JA: Radiology of postnatal skeletal development. Patella and tibial tuberosity. *Skeletal Radiol* 1984;11:246.
184. Lancourt JE, Christini JA: Patella alta and patella infera: Their etiological role in patella dislocation, chondromalacia, and apophysitis of the tibial tubercle. *J Bone Joint Surg Am* 1975;57A:1112.
185. Jakob RP, Gumppenberg S, Engelhardt P: Does Osgood-Schlatter disease influence the position of the patella? *J Bone Joint Surg Br* 1981;63B:579.
186. Blackburne JS, Peel TE: A new method of measuring patellar height. *J Bone Joint Surg Br* 1977;59B:241.
187. Krause BL, Williams JP, Catterall A: Natural history of Osgood-Schlatter disease. *J Pediatr Orthop* 1990;10:65.
188. Lanning P, Heikkinen E: Ultrasonic features of the Osgood-Schlatter lesion. *J Pediatr Orthop* 1991;11:538.
189. Rosenberg ZS, Kawelblum M, Cheung YY, et al.: Osgood-Schlatter lesion: Fracture of tendinitis? Scintigraphic, CT, and MRI imaging features. *Radiology* 1992;185(3):853.
190. Rostron PKM, Calver RF: Subcutaneous atrophy following methylprednisolone injection in Osgood-Schlatter epiphysitis. *J Bone Joint Surg Am* 1979;61A:627.
191. Glynn MK, Regan BF: Surgical treatment of Osgood-Schlatter disease. *J Pediatr Orthop* 1983;3:216.
192. Binazzi R, Felli L, Vaccari V, Borelli P: Surgical treatment of unresolved Osgood-Schlatter lesion. *Clin Orthop* 1993;289:202.
193. Medlar RC, Lyne ED: Sinding-Larsen-Johansson disease: Its etiology and natural history. *J Bone Joint Surg Am* 1978;60A:1113.
194. Wolf J: Larsen-Johansson disease of the patella. Seven new case reports. Its relationship to other forms of osteochondritis. Use of male sex hormones as a new form of treatment. *Br J Radiol* 1950;23:335.
195. Stanisavljevic S, Zemenick G, Miller D: Congenital irreducible, permanent lateral dislocation of the patella. *Clin Orthop* 1976;116: 190.
196. Green JP, Waugh W: Congenital lateral dislocation of the patella. *J Bone Joint Surg Br* 1968;50B:285.
197. Lanny L: Le traitement de la luxation congenitale de la rotule. *Bull Soc Chir* 1936;27: 419.

198. McCall RE, Lessenberry H: Bilateral congenital dislocation of the patella. *J Pediatr Orthop* 1987;7:100.
199. Hall JE, Micheli LJ, McManama GB Jr.: Semitendinosus tenodesis for recurrent subluxation or dislocation of the patella. *Clin Orthop* 1979;144:31.
200. Mansoor IA: Dysplasia epiphysealis multiplex. *Clin Orthop* 1970;72:287.
201. Gasco J, DelPino J, Gomar-Sancho F: Double patella: A case of duplication in the coronal plane. *J Bone Joint Surg Br* 1987;69B:602.
202. Dahners LE, Francisco WD, Halleran WJ: Findings at arthrotomy in a case of double layered patellae associated with multiple epiphyseal dysplasia. *J Pediatr Orthop* 1982;2:67.
203. Dugdale T, Renshaw T: Instability of the patellofemoral joint in Down's syndrome. *J Bone Joint Surg Am* 1986;68A:405.
204. Mendez A, Keret D, MacEwen G: Treatment of patellofemoral instability in Down's syndrome. *Clin Orthop* 1988;234:148.
205. Letts M: Hereditary onycho-osteodysplasia. *Orthop Rev* 1991;20:267.
206. Duthie RB, Hect F: The inheritance and development of the nail-patella syndrome. *J Bone Joint Surg Br* 1963;45B:259.
207. Caffey J: *Pediatric X-Ray Diagnosis,* ed. 6. Chicago, Yearbook Medical Publishers, 1972, p. 943.
208. Gamble JG: Symptomatic dorsal defect of the patella in a runner. *Am J Sports Med* 1986;14(5):425.
209. Denham RH: Dorsal defect of the patella. *J Bone Joint Surg Am* 1984;66A:116.
210. Goergen TG, Resnick D, Greenway G, et al.: Dorsal defect of the patella (DDP): A characteristic radiographic lesion. *Radiology* 1979;130:333.
211. Haswell DM, Berne AS, Graham CB: The dorsal defect of the patella. *Pediatr Radiol* 1976;4:238.
212. Keats TE: *An Atlas of Normal Roentgen Variants.* Chicago, Yearbook Medical Publishers, 1975, p. 200.
213. Hunter LY, Hensinger RN: Dorsal defect of the patella with cartilaginous involvement. A case report. *Clin Orthop* 1979;143:131.
214. Kelikjan H, Layton J: Giant cell tumor of the patella. *J Bone Joint Surg Am* 1957;39A:414.
215. Linscheid RL, Dahlin DC: Unusual lesions of the patella. *J Bone Joint Surg Am* 1966;48A:1359.
216. Goodwin MA: Primary osteosarcoma of the patella. *J Bone Joint Surg Br* 1961;43B:338.
217. Stoler B, Staple TW: Metastases to the patella. *Radiology* 1969;93:853.
218. Keeley CD: Bilateral patellar metastases from carcinoma of the male breast. *Can J Surg* 1973;16:328.
219. Taylor GH: Pathologic fracture of the patella caused by metastatic carcinoma. *NY State J Med* 1964;64:430.
220. Evans DK: Osteomyelitis of the patella. *J Bone Joint Surg Br* 1962;44B:319.
221. Vaninbroukx J, Martens M, Verhelst M, et al.: Haematogenous osteomyelitis of the patella. Report of three cases. *Acta Orthop Scand* 1976;47:566.

10

Arthroscopic Examination and Treatment of the Patellofemoral Joint

Fred D. Cushner and W. Norman Scott

The patella is the largest sesamoid bone in the body and serves the following six basic functions[1]:

1. Increases the moment arm of the quadriceps mechanism, improving the force of extension 25% to 30%.
2. By cartilage-to-cartilage articulation, a low coefficient of friction is established, improving quadriceps efficiency.
3. The divergent forces of the four heads of the quadriceps are centralized and therefore are transmitted to the patellar tendon.
4. Protects the quadriceps and patellar tendon from friction.
5. Shields the articular cartilage on the anterior tibia as well as the anterior femur.
6. Serves a cosmetic function.

Pain associated with the patellofemoral joint is a common malady seen in the orthopedic office. Other chapters of this book will review anatomy, physical examination, and imaging of the patellofemoral joint. This chapter will focus on the arthroscopic examination and treatment of the patellofemoral joint. Attention will be given to our technique of arthroscopic examination as well as the treatment of chondromalacia, arthroscopic lateral release, and arthroscopic management of the dislocated patella. Results of these procedures will also be reviewed.

Diagnostic Arthroscopy and Examination of Patellar Tracking

The setup for arthroscopic examination of the patellofemoral joint is the same as for diagnostic arthroscopy. The patient is placed on the operative table in the supine position. A tourniquet is placed on the proximal thigh of the involved extremity and inflated at the initiation of the case. We prefer not to use a leg holder in order to have free control of the leg, but this is only an individual preference. The anesthetic choices include epidural, local, or general anesthesia.

The extremity is then examined for proper portal placement (Figure 10.1). A marking pen can be used to outline the appropriate portals. Both superior and inferior portals are used in the examination of the patellofemoral joint. The proximal portals are approximately three fingerbreadths from the superior pole of the patella along the patellofemoral joint line. The portal location is determined with the limb in full extension. Standard anteroinferomedial and anteroinferolateral portals are also used with care to keep the anterolateral portal just superior to the fat pad. These portals should be just above the inferior pole of the patella just adjacent to the patellar tendon. Our preference is to run the inflow through the scope on the anterolateral portal, although we have a low threshold to use a superomedial portal when additional inflow is needed. Currently,

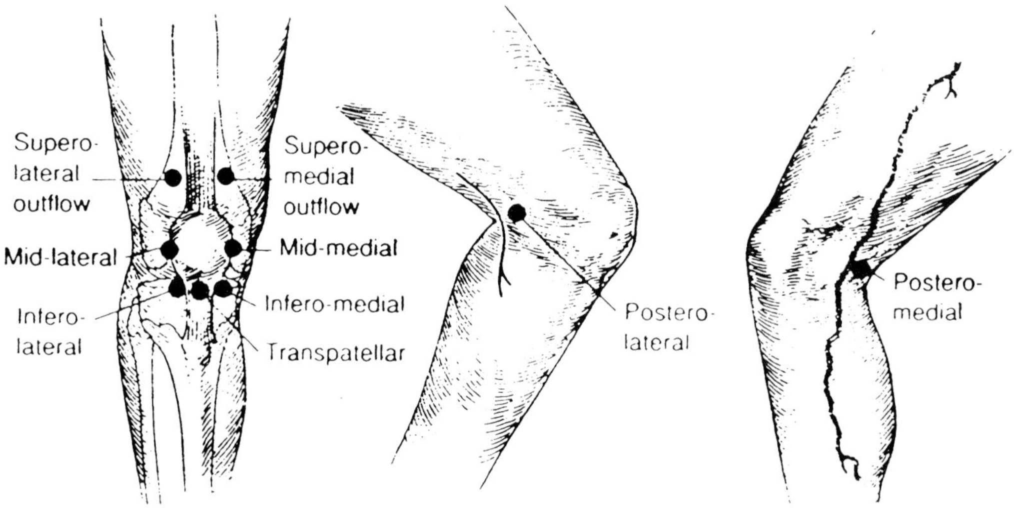

FIGURE 10.1. Standard portals for knee arthroscopy. From Tria and Klein, An Illustrated Guide to the Knee. Churchill Livingstone New York © 1992 with permission.

an arthroscopic pump is not used at the Insall Scott Kelly Institute, as we have found it to be unnecessary.

Prior to examination of patellar tracking, a comprehensive systematic inspection of the knee joint is performed. After the tourniquet is inflated, the arthroscope is placed in the anterolateral portal. Inspection begins with an examination of the articular surface of the patella and the femoral sulcus. The position of the patella in the femoral sulcus is also noted. A probe is used to palpate the articular cartilage and determine areas of softness. The lateral and the medial gutters are also examined for evidence of loose bodies, plicae, or synovitis. Attention is then turned to the medial and the lateral tibiofemoral joint spaces, as well as the femoral notch. Any articular abnormality, meniscal pathology, or ligament injury is noted and treated appropriately.

Once the diagnostic arthroscopy is completed, patellar tracking can be evaluated via both the diagnostic portals and/or a superolateral portal. An inflow cannula is then placed in the already-made inferolateral portal. A superolateral portal is then made for placement of the camera-equipped arthroscope. A 30° arthroscope is then placed to visualize patellofemoral tracking. A 70° arthroscope can be used if adequate examination of the patellofemoral joint cannot be obtained with a 30° arthroscope, but usually this is not necessary. Should there be difficulty, a 70° arthroscope can be obtained. There is flexibility in the position of the superomedial portal. If a superomedial portal was used for inflow, then this portal can be used for surgical instruments. Otherwise, a second superomedial portal can be placed at the desired location with the aid of a spinal needle.

To evaluate patellar tracking, the anteromedial portal is used and the patella is viewed through a complete range of flexion to full extension. The patella is examined in full extension and any medial offset or lateral overhang is noted (Figure 10.2).

There is no agreement on what constitutes normal anatomy of the patellofemoral joint. Casscells[2] performed anatomic measurements on several cadaver knees and found that the average depth of the patellar groove was 5.2 mm, while the mean height of the lateral femoral condyle above the medial femoral condyle is 4.5 mm. These numbers represent the mean and a wide variety of normal variations can be seen (Figure 10.3).

In extension, only the lateral facets should be engaging the lateral femur, but as the knee flexes, both the medial and the lateral patellar facets engage the femoral sulcus. During the

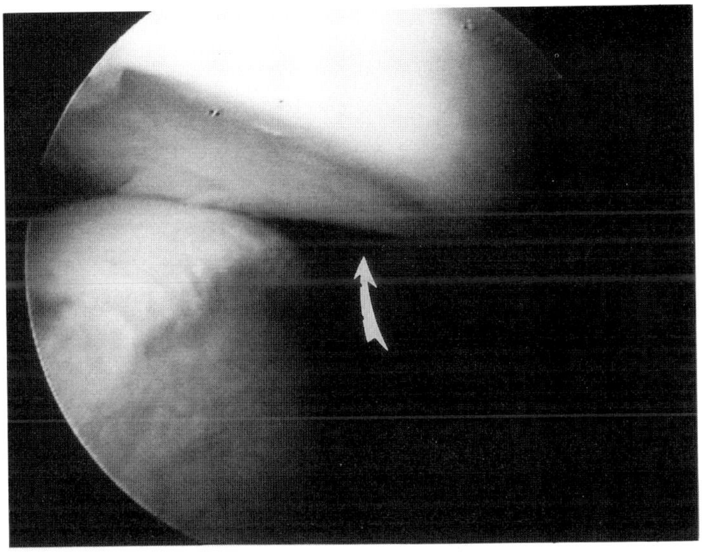

FIGURE 10.2. Arthroscopic examination demonstrating greater than 50% lateral overhang.

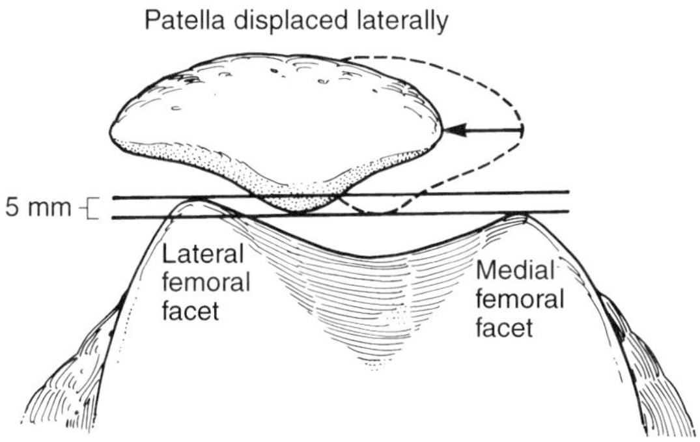

FIGURE 10.3. Tangential view of the patellofemoral joint.

first 45°, the midpatellar ridge should seat in the femoral sulcus. Casscells[2] and Metcalf[3] have defined *malalignment* as the failure of the midpatellar ridge to seat in the femoral sulcus during the first 45° of flexion (Figure 10.4). Sojbjerg et al.[4] examined 17 patients with a normal patellofemoral joint. They found that the lateral facet aligned at a knee flexion of 20°, the patellar ridge at 35°, and the medial facet at 50°. Compared with 12 patients that demonstrated patellar subluxation, there is no difference in alignment of the lateral facet. A difference, however, was noted in the alignment of the patellar ridge and the medial facet at a mean flexion of 55° and 85°, respectively.

Aside from patellar tracking, patellar stability can be evaluated with the knee in full extension. Stability is dependent not only on the sulcus height and condyle height, but also on the tightness of the lateral and the medial capsule. The patella can be visually examined for the potential to sublux or dislocate. Under direct vision, the patella can be manipulated medially and laterally, and the amount of displacement noted. This should be performed both in flexion and extension, and the amount of overall displacement and overhang should be noted.

Plicae

In 1918, Mayeda[5] described the anatomic presence of a plica after cadaveric examination of 100 knees. He reported the presence of plicae in 21% of the knees. Subsequently, the overall anatomic incidence of plica is estimated at 20% to 60% in all populations, with a higher incidence noted in the Japanese population.[6,7]

Synovial plicae are classified by their location, with the first and most common being the infrapatellar plica (Figure 10.5). Recently, its presence has been found to be 85% in normal knees.[8] The infrapatellar plica, synonymous with ligamentum mucosum, is visual-

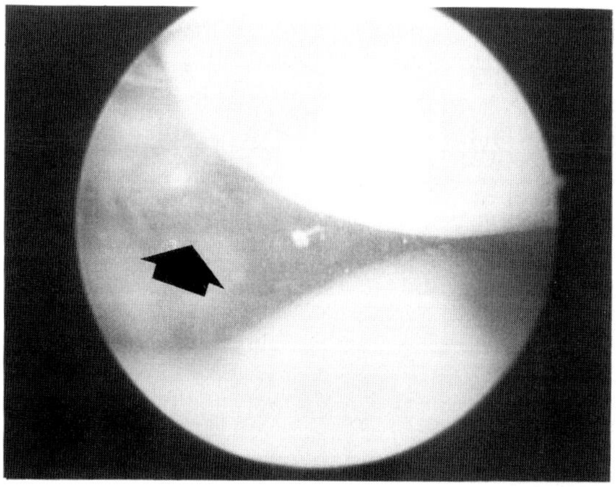

a

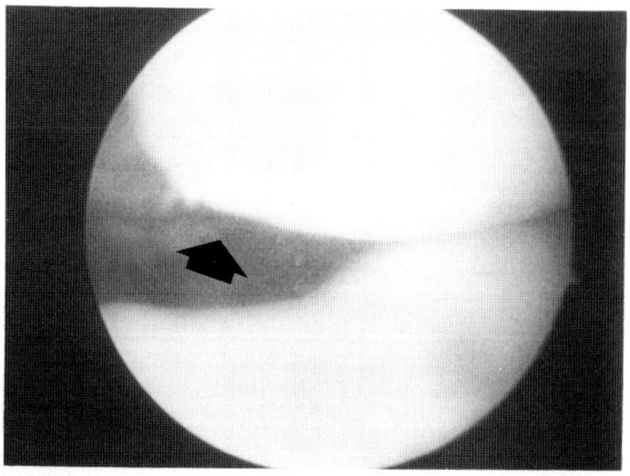

b

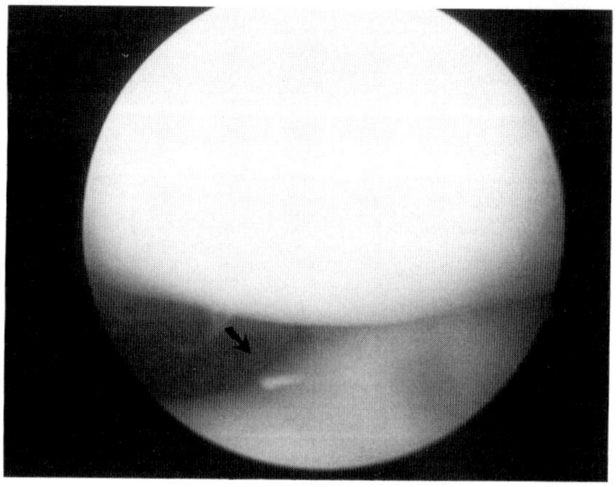

c

FIGURE 10.4. Abnormal patellar tracking with increased lateral overhang at full extension (a), 30° flexion (b), and 60° flexion (c).

ized as connecting the fat pad to the superior portion of the femoral notch. It parallels the anterior cruciate ligament and, to the novice, it can be mistaken for the anterior cruciate ligament. This infrapatellar plica inserts on the inferior fat pad and, although it may be troublesome when one attempts to examine the anterior cruciate ligament, no symptoms are noted with the presence of this plica.

A second commonly encountered plica is the suprapatellar plica (plica synovialis). This plica runs in a transverse fashion across the suprapatellar pouch. Often this plica is complete, but in some instances, a communication of variable size, a "porta," may be present. With flexion, this plica runs parallel to the femur, while in extension it runs transverse. On arthroscopic examination, the plica does not appear to contact the femoral condyle with flexion. On placement of a superomedial or a superolateral inflow cannula, resistance may be felt secondary to this plica.

A third variation of a plica is known as a medial patellar plica. The origin of this plica is the medial wall of the knee joint. This plica then runs obliquely in the direction of the medial inferopatellar fat pad (areolar ligament). This plica can arise or be separate from the suprapatellar plica. A variation of this plica can also be found on the lateral side but is much less common.

Debate remains as to the symptoms that occur with the presence of a plica. Is the plica itself symptomatic or is it the development of plica "syndrome," which causes the anterior knee pain? Jackson et al.[7] have outlined criteria for the diagnosis of a plica syndrome. The patient must give a history of typical plica

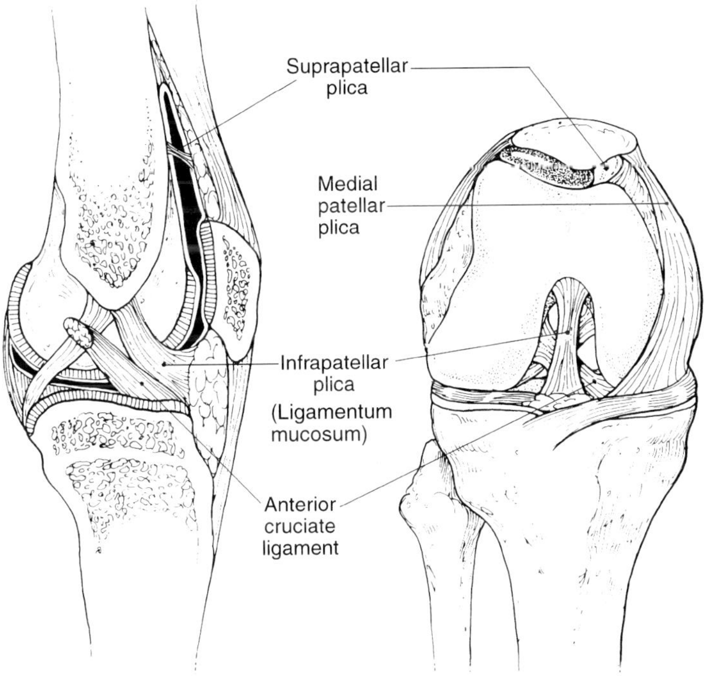

FIGURE 10.5. Anterior, posterior, and lateral views demonstrating plica locations.

symptoms; failed nonoperative treatment; and, at arthroscopy, have findings significant only for a plica with a fibrotic avascular edge that can be seen impinging on the femoral condyle with flexion. No other intra-articular abnormality should be found.

Typically, the symptoms of a symptomatic plica are vague. Often the pain is described as anterior and superior in location, and is common in children and adolescents. Pain is most severe if resultant articular damage is present. Symptoms include clicking, catching, locking, and pseudolocking. Often the symptomatic plica is palpable and can be felt "bowstringing" on the femoral condyle with flexion (Figure 10.6). Broom and Fulkerson[9] reported 64% of patients with symptoms of clicking, 59% giving way of the knee, and 45% with pseudolocking.

The majority of synovial plicae are normal, asymptomatic, anatomic variants. These plicae consist largely of elastic areolar tissue that are capable of changing in shape with flexion and extension of the knee. Etiologic factors

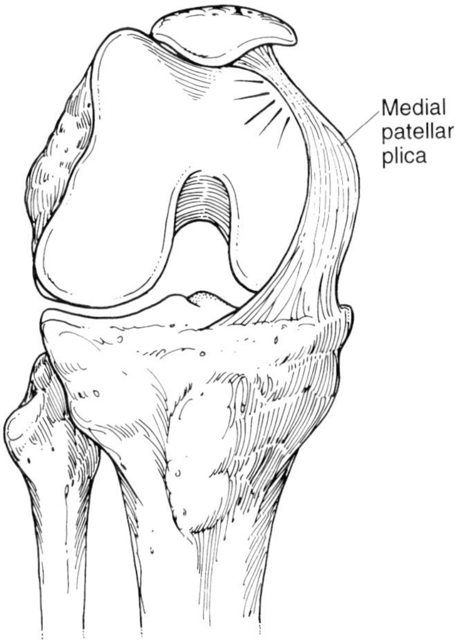

FIGURE 10.6. Pathologic plica demonstrating impingement on the medial femoral condyle.

then occur that stimulate an inflammatory response in this once-elastic tissue. Direct and indirect trauma are the most common factors, but other etiologies include strenuous activity, osteochondritis dissecans, meniscal injuries, or other injuries of the knee.[6,10,11]

Inflammation and edema result in a thickening of the previous elastic plica. The plica then loses some flexibility and snaps over the femoral condyle rather than gliding. With time, these changes become chronic with the elastic plica tissue replaced with the fibrous tissue. Rarely, hyalination and calcification occur. As a result, the thin, previously flexible residual synovial membrane is transformed into a thickened fibrotic pathologic structure. With repeated snapping of this fibrotic plica, recurring abrasions develop, which could lead to articular cartilage erosions. This usually involves the medial femoral condyle. Localized chondromalacia changes can also be found in areas such as the medial femoral condyle and the patellar facets.[11,12] Patel[13] noted medial patellar plica with chondromalacia of the medial femoral condyle in 40% of patients, while 60% had chondromalacia of the medial facet of the patella.

Regarding the history taken from the patient, further questioning reveals that activity exacerbates the symptoms. Pain is often noted as the knee flexes in the 45° to 90° range. Prolonged sitting can increase the symptoms as the plica is stretched over the femoral condyle. Patients may also give a history of pain when they stand after a prolonged period of sitting such as at a movie theater. Unfortunately, these symptoms are consistent with almost all types of patellofemoral pain. Patients are often young, athletic, and female, and may give a history of an increase in exercise or a change in footwear. Exercise-related swelling can also be noted.

Diagnosis of plica syndrome is not easy and thus imaging studies have played a small role in detection of plica. Plain films are of little help unless a loose body or osteochondritis dissecans lesion is noted. Arthrography has been shown to be of some value if anterior and posterior tangential views are obtained.[10] Ultrasound has also been shown to be successful in detecting plica, with a 92% sensitivity and a 73% specificity noted.[14] Technetium bone scans may show increased uptake for the impingement that occurs on the involved femoral condyle. Magnetic resonance imaging (MRI) clearly delineates any plica present and also gives details to the size and location of the plica.[15] This may be the best diagnostic test available today.[15]

The differential diagnosis of a symptomatic plica includes chondromalacia of the patella, or trochlea, lateral retinacular pain, injury to lateral retinacular nerves, patellar compression syndrome, Hoffa's disease, or intra-articular pathology such as articular cartilage damage or meniscal pathology. Physical examination may give some clue to the diagnosis of plica syndrome. A relative constant finding is a localized pain over the medial femoral condyle and the medial patellar plica sometimes can be palpated as it parallels the medial border of the patella. With rapid flexion and extension, an audible snap may be heard that can be confused with a positive "McMurray's" sign if joint line pain is also present.[11,16]

Confusion is common when differentiating medial plica syndrome from a medial meniscal tear. Broom and Fulkerson[9] diagnosed pathologic plica in 22 of 730 arthroscopes, with an initial diagnosis preoperatively to be a meniscal tear in more than one half of these patients. Nottage et al.[17] reviewed 1,304 arthroscopies, with 78 knees thought to be symptomatic for medial plica syndrome. In only 57% was the correct diagnosis made preoperatively.

Treatment begins with nonoperative modalities. Hardaker et al.[18] reviewed the results of rest, nonsteroidal anti-inflammatory drugs, localized heat, hamstring stretching, and progressive resistive exercises. This protocol was more successful in a population with a mean age of 21.5 years and symptoms of less than three-months duration. Repetitive trauma was the most common etiologic factor in this group. In those patients with a history of trauma, mean age of 28.5, and symptoms for six months or longer, conservative treatment was not as successful.[18] In a prospective study, Rovere and Adair[19] injected a long-acting anesthetic agent and steroid into the medial patellar plica region. Seventy-three percent of these patients reported lasting effects and were able to return to full activity. It appears that control of the inflammatory process limits long-term disability from a symptomatic plica.

If nonoperative treatment fails, arthroscopy can be not only a diagnostic tool, but it also can be a treatment modality. Arthroscopy can be used to rule out other internal derangements of the knee. Success rates for arthroscopy and arthroscopic resection of symptomatic plica range from 70% to 92%.[16,18,20–22] Hardaker et al.[18] treated 53 patients with arthroscopy and excision of the synovial plica with a reported 87% excellent result. Jackson et al.[7] reported arthroscopy with arthroscopic sectioning in 69 patients, with 70% stating significant improvement or complete relief. Muse et al.[23] showed similar results with 66% of patients with unrestricted activity and 26% with only mild pain with strenuous activity. The remaining 8% showed significant activity restriction secondary to pain.

Technique—Plicae Examination and Resection

Regarding the specific techniques for arthroscopic treatment of a symptomatic plica, the procedure begins with a systematic arthroscopic examination. Other intra-articular modalities such as meniscal injuries and loose bodies are ruled out.

Once completed, attention is turned to the diagnosis of a synovial plica and its subsequent treatment. The suprapatellar pouch is examined and the presence of a plica may be noted. Should a porta be present, the scope should be advanced through the porta to rule out loose bodies trapped in the suprapatellar pouch. The medial and the lateral gutters are examined, and the presence or absence of a plica is noted. If present, the plica should also be examined for fibrotic changes or any evidence of femoral condyle impingement. Chondromalacia may be noted on the medial patella on the corresponding femoral condyle.

The presence of a plica does not constitute the diagnosis of plica syndrome. Jackson et al.[7] reviewed 69 cases of pathologic medial plica. They differentiated between normal plicae, which are soft, wavy, vascularized, and with synovial covered edges, to pathologic plicae, which are thick, rounded, and fibrotic. According to Tindel and Nisonson,[15] the following three arthroscopic findings assist in making the diagnosis of plica syndrome: (1) plica appearance, (2) plica impingement on the femoral condyle or patella, and (3) articular wear in the area of impingement.

When the decision is made to resect a pathologic plica, certain maneuvers are helpful. When attempting to resect a suprapatellar plica, a standard anteroinferolateral portal can be used. Resistance may be felt on insertion of the trochar and occasionally a gentle pressure is needed to pop through the residual membrane. This allows an entrance into the suprapatellar pouch. Through the superolateral portal, arthroscopic instruments can be used to resect the septum. Resection can be completed with a high-speed shaver.

The infrapatellar plica has not been implicated as a cause of anterior knee symptoms. Care must be taken to visualize the complete anterior cruciate ligament (ACL) on arthroscopic examination. Should this plica inhibit adequate ACL visualization, then a shaver can be used to carefully remove the ligamentum mucosum as needed.

For the medial patellar plica, the anteroinferolateral portal is first used to visualize the pathology. The arthroscope is then inserted in the superolateral portal and often the insertion of the plica onto the infrapatellar fat pad can be seen. Not all plicae are symptomatic and need to be resected. Emphasis should be placed on resecting those that truly appear pathologic.

Many reviews of plica resection have been retrospective in nature. However, as described in a recent article, Johnson et al.[24] performed a prospective, randomize, controlled study of the benefits of plica resection. Forty-five knees (30 patients) were given the diagnosis of synovial plica syndrome based on the history of injury and pain, painful clicking, giving way, and a palpable tender plica. All patients received three months of physical therapy with emphasis on vastus medialis obliquus (VMO) and quadriceps training exercises. At arthroscopy, no other pathology except for a plica was noted, and this study group was randomized as to which would have the plica divided. The decision to excise the plica was based only on randomization and was not dependent on size, thickness, degree of fibrosis, or inflammation of the plica or impingement found. Results showed 83% overall success rate in those in the plica resection group compared with 29% of those with the plica left intact. Seventy percent of the resected plica group showed improvement once the plica was resected as a second procedure.

In closing, synovial plicae can be both a symptomatic or an asymptomatic finding in a knee undergoing arthroscopy. Often the source of anterior knee pain can be relieved by resection of this plica. Further information is needed to evaluate whether all plicae or just fibrotic nonelastic plicae are the source of pain and therefore demand resection.

Chondromalacia

Chondromalacia is a generalized term for the anatomic and histologic changes seen in articular cartilage. Aleman[25] first described chondromalacia in 1928 and the etiology is often unclear. It should be noted that chondromalacia is no longer synonymous with anterior knee pain of unknown etiology but rather as a distinct pathologic entity. Numerous studies have described the efficacy of arthroscopy for the diagnosis as well as the treatment of this condition.[2,4,5,26,27]

In 1961, Outerbridge[28] described the anatomic changes noted with chondromalacia. These findings were based on observations seen at 196 open meniscectomies. The Outerbridge classification is as follows:

- *Grade I.* Softening and swelling of the cartilage.
- *Grade II.* A 0.5-in (1.3 cm) or less fragmentation or fissuring.
- *Grade III.* Similar to grade II but larger than 0.5 in (1.3 cm) involved.
- *Grade IV.* Erosion to the bone.

At the Insall Scott Kelly Institute, we use the following modification of the Outerbridge classification:

- *Grade 0.* Normal cartilage.
- *Grade I.* The cartilage is light brown and yellow in color, and allows approximately 1 mm to pressure when probed. Commonly small blistering can be noted but fissuring and fragmentation are absent.
- *Grade II.* Fissuring is noted. Depression from 1 to 2 mm is present to probing.
- *Grade III.* Fissuring with fasciculations are present, although the subchondral bone is spared. This is often referred to as a "crab meat" appearance. Greater than one half of the articular thickness is involved.
- *Grade IV.* Erosion down to the subchondral bone is present. This stage is not distinguishable from osteoarthritis.

As noted in previous chapters, the differential diagnosis of anterior knee pain is multifocal. We prefer to use the classification system of Insall[29] based on the appearance of the articular cartilage (Table 10.1). Since extra-articular conditions have been discussed in other chapters, our scope will be towards intra-articular lesions of the patella that can be handled arthroscopically. When normal cartilage is noted on arthroscopic examination, extra-articular etiologies such as bursitis should be considered (Figure 10.7).

Conditions with variable cartilage involvement would include malalignment and syn-

TABLE 10.1. Insall's classification of patellofemoral disorders.

Articular damage
Chondromalacia
Osteoarthritis
Osteochondritis dissecans
Osteochondral fractures
Variable cartilage damage
Malalignment
Plicae
Normal cartilage
Peripatellar (bursitis tendinitis)
Overuse syndrome
Reflex sympathetic dystrophy (RSD)

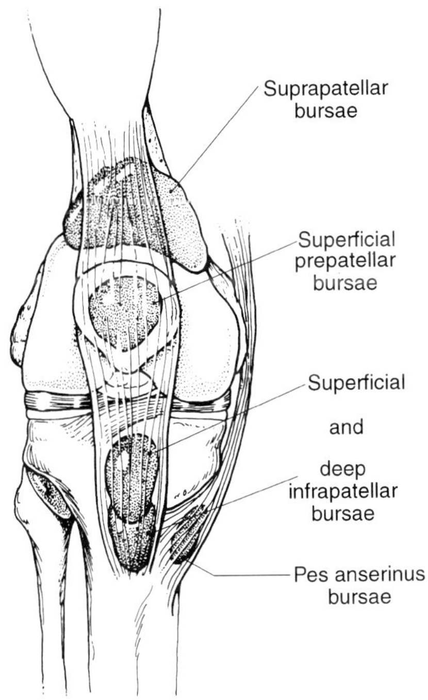

FIGURE 10.7. Bursae of the knee. All are possible sources of extra-articular knee pain.

ovial plica. Both patellar malalignment and synovial plica syndromes will be discussed elsewhere in this chapter.

Causes of anterior pain with significant cartilage damage would include chondromalacia, osteoarthritis, osteochondritis dissecans, and osteochondral fractures.

Several risk factors have been noted in the development of chondromalacia. This would include a poorly developed VMO, malalignment, patellar alta, trauma, and tight hamstrings. Chondromalacia is common in adolescents and has an increased incidence in females.

DeHaven et al.[30] has divided the etiology of chondromalacia into five groups. Recurrent subluxation was the most common with an estimated incidence of 51% in all chondromalacia cases. Other groups include idiopathic (30%), posttraumatic (10%), and recurrent dislocation (4%). Chondromalacia was also noted to develop secondary to rehabilitation of the knee with nonpatellar lesions (5%).

Although chondromalacia patellae is a common diagnosis made in the office, often the diagnosis is not accurate. Leslie and Bentley[31] performed arthroscopy on 78 patients with the clinical diagnosis of chondromalacia patellae. In only 51% was the diagnosis confirmed at arthroscopy. These investigators concluded that physical examination is unreliable ın predicting chondromalacia. They found that the most reliable physical finding was greater than 2-cm thigh atrophy compared with the uninvolved side effusion and retropatellar crepitus. Of these, 49% with no correlation with 58% were asymptomatic at one year.

Treatment

Treatment of chondromalacia of the patella begins with nonoperative treatment, which numerous authors have stressed.[3,29,32–35] According to Insall,[29] "In most patients, pain does not become progressively worse and in time a certain level becomes acceptable in their daily lives." Treatment begins with a well-supervised rehabilitation program. Lombardo and Bradley[25] described a three-phase program that is used at the Kerlan Jobe Clinic in Inglewood, Calif.

Phase I involves control of symptoms as well as isometric exercises. Modalities for this phase include electrostimulation to the VMO, quadriceps sets, straight leg raises, Achilles stretching, ice, compression, and nonsteroidal anti-inflammatory medication.

For phase II, phase I exercises continue but electrostimulation is stopped. Quadriceps sets, Cybex, and stationary bike are also added. Hamstring exercises were also begun at this phase.

As progress continues, phase III is initiated. Resistance on the stationary bike is increased and light jogging is begun. When the patient is able to jog 1.5 to 2 mi (2.4 to 3.2 km), agility drills are added. Ice is continued during this phase.

Although the patient's symptoms may improve, it is important that exercise therapy continues. DeHaven et al.[30] emphasize the importance of continuing a resistance exercise program even after normal activities have been reinitiated.

If no progress is made with nonoperative treatment, then arthroscopy should be considered. Indications for surgery include the following:

1. Failure of six to 12 months of a supervised rehabilitation program.
2. Progressive pain localized to the patella.
3. Inability to perform normal daily activities.
4. Expected associated pathology such as an osteochondral fracture or a meniscal injury.
5. Recurring instability.

Once arthroscopy is performed, a poor correlation exists between pain preoperatively and the appearance of the articular cartilage seen during arthroscopy.[2,31,36–40]

Technique

The arthroscopic approach to chondromalacia patellae is similar to the technique described previously. A complete examination of the knee is performed to rule out any associated pathology. The arthroscope is placed in the anteroinferior lateral portal, while the anteroinferior medial portal is used for placement of the arthroscope probe. The probe can be used not only to delineate the involved cartilage, but it can be used to measure the size of the cartilage defect. The degree of softening of the surrounding articular cartilage is also measured.

The areas of articular damage are noted not only on the patellar surface, but any corresponding lesions on the femoral trochlea are also recorded. Debate exists as to the most commonly involved patellar surface. Outerbridge[28] felt that the medial facet was the most common, while Insall et al.[41] felt that the medial part of the medial ridge was involved most commonly as well as in equal areas of softening on either side of the ridge medially and laterally.

Once the patellofemoral joint is completely examined, the attention then turns toward treatment. Using the anteroinferior medial portal, the power shaver or basket forceps is inserted. The damaged articular cartilage is then excised and smooth edges are obtained. Care is taken to leave the subchondral bone intact. Obviously, care is taken to avoid contact with the normal surrounding articular cartilage. The joint is then copiously irrigated to remove any loose fragments as well as collagenases. Although the shedding of debris in these joints is decreased, the biomechanical defects remain.

With respect to the grades of chondromalacia, the treatment is predicated by the degree of involvement. Grade 0 chondromalacia is usually left alone, but there is some debate as to how aggressive to be with grades II, III, and IV lesions.

Ogilvie-Harris and Jackson[42] reviewed 319 patients for chondromalacia patellae. Patients were treated by either of the following three methods: (1) lavage; (2) lavage and shaving; or (3) lavage, shaving, and lateral release. These patients were then observed at one- to five-year followup. For grade I lesions, lavage only was indicated. Satisfactory results were obtained both at the one- and five-year followup appointments.

For grade II lesions, the patients were treated by all three methods. No difference was noted at one-year followup between all three treatment groups. At five-year followup, there was a decrease in the satisfactory results for lavage only as well as lavage and shaving, but no decrease was noted in the lateral release, lavage and shaving group. For grade III lesions, again there was no difference noted between the three treatment modalities. For either of the treatments, a decrease in satisfactory results was noted at both the one- and five-year followup.

Wissinger[28] prospectively reviewed 100 patients that also included grade I lesions best treated with lavage only. For grade II lesions, treatment was carried out for lesions in the area of the center ridge, while grade III lesions were debrided with fissuring and flaps were present. For grade IV lesions, minimal debridement and lavage are done. It has been our experience with larger, aggressive debridement that the symptoms increase postoperatively. Unfortunately, this stage is similar to osteoarthritis, and no ideal procedure exists for this condition. Therefore, we consider patients with severe grade IV chondromalacia or degenerative joint disease as candidates for patellectomy or total knee arthroplasty, depending on the patient's age.

Considerable results have been reported successful with the treatment of chondromalacia. Henry and Crosland[43] looked at 145 patients with minor subluxating patellae. A 76% success rate was noted with conservative treatment. Sandow and Goodfellow[44] looked at the natural history in 54 adolescent girls with 52-months followup. Although 94.4% still have pain, the symptoms diminished in 46.3%. Fifty percent of these girls returned to sports and 60.7% had limited sports participation.

Results from arthroscopic lavage and debridement are mixed. DeHaven et al.[30] reviewed 100 patients with chondromalacia patellae. Eighty-two percent were judged to be successful. Sixty-six percent were able to return to unrestricted activities, while only 23% had some restriction of activities. Eleven percent were not able to return to their previous activity levels and 18% were considered as failures. Eight percent later required a second surgical procedure.

McCarroll et al.[45] looked at 184 knees with varying chondromalacia patellae. These patients were treated with a variety of open techniques and 3.9-years followup was obtained. In grades II and III lesions, shaving procedures had less satisfactory results in comparison with resection and drilling. The results were dependent on sex, age, and activity level of the patients. Better results were noted in patients greater than 45 years of age compared with those less than 25 years old. As expected, sedentary patients had better results than laborers.

Collagen healing has been a problem since the early days of medicine. In 1743, Hunter[46] stated "from Hippocrates to the present age, it is universally allowed that ulcerated cartilage is a troublesome problem and once destroyed is not repaired." In 1849, Leidy[47] stated "articular cartilage lacks regenerate power." Attempts were made to stimulate reparative cartilage formation. In 1959, Pridie[48] described joint debridement in which fibrous-like regenerative cartilage was formed. Although Pridie[48] recommended preservation of the patella, shaving of fissures and restoration of the cartilage were recommended. This concept of chondroplasty or abrasion arthroplasty has been refined with the modern arthroscopic equipment. The procedure consists of removal of the cartilage to the subchondral plate. This is followed by drilling of the subchondral plate to expose the cancellous patella. Copious irrigation is performed at the completion of this drilling.

Childers and Elwood[49] performed open chondrectomy and subchondral bone drilling in 29 knees. This procedure involved local arthroscopic chondrectomy and subchondral bone plate drilling. Good to excellent results were noted in patients less than 30 years of age. Less favorable results were achieved in the greater-than-30-years-of-age group.

Schonholtz and Ling[26] performed limited chondroplasty on various grades of chondromalacia patellae to remove loose fibrillations. At 40-months followup, 94% good to excellent results were noted. Ninety-two percent showed some improvement. No correlation was noted with the grade of chondromalacia present.

Although chondroplasty and abrasion arthroplasty have been shown to lead to the formation of reparative fibrocartilage tissue, it has been our experience that benefits are short lived. In part, this is due to the inability to relieve contact forces on this newly formed tissue while range of motion is maintained.

Lateral Release

Arthroscopic lateral release has gained popularity over recent years. Although the procedure for lateral release has been around since Roux's[50] description in 1888, when lateral release was just part of other procedures performed, it was Willner[51] who popularized this approach in the 1970s and Metcalf[3] who popularized the arthroscopic technique in the early 1980s. This procedure has become popular because of its low morbidity, small incision, and successful results, as well as the fact that "no bridges are burned." Often this procedure is used indiscriminately for a multitude of patellofemoral pain etiologies. Therefore, this section will not only outline the techniques of arthroscopic lateral release, but the indications and results will also be reviewed.

The offending structure for anterior patellofemoral pain is often a tight lateral retinaculum. This retinaculum consists of two separate layers: (1) the superior oblique retinaculum and (2) the deep transverse retinaculum. It is these structures that are released. With the knee in flexion, the lateral band is drawn posteriorly with the iliotibial band and displaces the patella laterally. The lateral force is counteracted by the medial stabilizers. If these medial stabilizers are stretched or the lateral structures are pathologically tight, the patella displaces and lateral tilt develops. Regarding the vascular anatomy, the lateral superior genicular artery is often cut as a lateral release is performed. This artery passes through the insertion of the lateral intramuscular septum and gives a superior lateral branch to the patella. This branch anastomoses with the superior genicular and the medial superior genicular artery approaching the superior medial aspect of the patella. The medial inferior genicular artery surrounds the patella and has branches that parallel the medial border of the patella as well as laterally to join the lateral inferior genicular artery.[52] By understanding the vascular anatomy, the primary complication of hemarthrosis can be avoided.

As with all medical conditions, a thorough history must be obtained prior to evaluating patellofemoral pain. The patient should be asked specifically concerning a history of a subluxation or dislocation of the patella, and whether spontaneous or manual reduction was needed. Patients will also give a history of catching, giving way, and anterior medial knee pain. Physical findings include apprehension, medial retinacular discomfort, and abnormal patellar tracking on flexion and extension of the knee. The amount of patellar glide, quadriceps angle, and overall joint laxity should also be evaluated.

Radiographic examination should also be performed. Standard anterior/posterior and lateral projections should be obtained to evaluate the degree of arthritic changes as well as to rule out any other bony lesion. A Merchant view will evaluate the amount of medial or lateral overhang. The tubercle sulcus angle can also be noted in this view. The strict indications for lateral release have yet to be decided. Initially, this procedure was advocated for subluxation and dislocation, and gradually the indications were stretched to all patellofemoral pain not resolving with conservative treatment. The absolute of indications for lateral release still remains debatable.

At the Insall Scott Kelly Institute, we do not perform lateral releases for isolated patellofemoral pain. Our surgical candidates can be divided into three groups. The first group is a patient with a tight lateral retinaculum, abnormal patellar tilt, and minimal chondromalacia (grades I or II). This group would include the so-called lateral pressure syndrome that Ficat and Hungerford[53] described (Figure

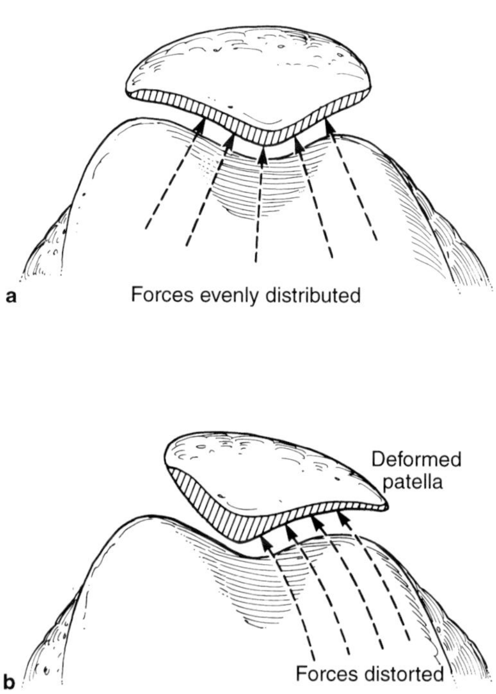

FIGURE 10.8. Evenly distributed patellofemoral contact forces (a) and uneven distribution of contact forces seen with abnormal patellar tilt (b).

10.8). This results in increased pressure on the lateral facet of the patella and with decreased pressure on the medial facet. With time, this leads to lateral scarring and shortening of the lateral retinaculum structures with resultant abnormal patellar tracking. Those patients with evidence of subluxation and a normal quadriceps angle constitute the second group, while malalignment and painful subluxation, and dislocation and minimal arthritis constitute the third group.

Contraindications for lateral release are multifold. These would include deficient medial restraints, patella alta, small hypermobile patella, severe malalignment, and an abnormal tubercle sulcus angle. With physical examination, other contraindications would include a positive patellar tilt as well as greater than three quadrant medial lateral glide. Severe patellofemoral pain without lateral tilt and patellofemoral arthritis are other contraindications.

Scuderi[54] noticed the presence of a hypermobile patella or a severe malalignment with patellar subluxation and dislocation may require additional proximal or distal procedures to increase the efficacy of a lateral release.

Technique

At the Insall Scott Kelly Institute, the attending surgeon's preference dictates the method of lateral release with subcutaneous arthroscopic assisted, and intra-articular arthroscopic release performed. The technique of both will be discussed as follows.

Subcutaneous Lateral Release with Arthroscopic Assistance

The setup is similar to methods already discussed. The case is performed under general or regional technique but local anesthesia is not advocated. Prior to the start of the case, the tourniquet is placed on the proximal thigh, and the leg is prepped and draped in the standard fashion. A routine arthroscopy is then performed and a complete examination done utilizing standard anteromedial and anterolateral portals. Any intra-articular pathology is treated prior to performing the lateral release to prevent lateral extravasation of the irrigant.

Once completed, attention then turns to the lateral release. A Mayo scissors is placed into the anterolateral portal and blunt dissection is performed between the subcutaneous and the lateral retinaculum. The lateral release is performed 1 cm from the lateral patellar border and, as a result, the retinaculum, capsule, and synovium are released. The release is performed from the musculotendinous junction of the vastus lateralis and goes distal to the joint line just lateral to the patellar tendon (Figure 10.9). To evaluate the release, inspection of the lateral aspect shows a mild bulge as the arthroscopic fluid extravasates through the lateral release. The patella is then grasped and attempts to evert the patella medially should show 60° to 90° of rotation. Henry et al.[55] referred to this as a "turn up" sign or a "flip" sign (Figure 10.10). Once completed, an electrocautery can be used to coagulate any bleeding vessels. As noted in previous studies, with the new insulated electrocautery tips,

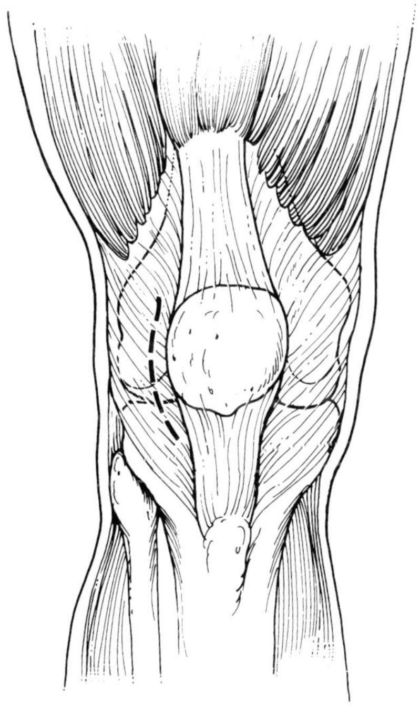

FIGURE 10.9. Site of surgical lateral release.

there is no need to change the irrigant to saline water or glycine.[37] It is the surgeon's preference whether to perform a lateral release with the tourniquet inflated or deflated, although we find that the initial arthroscopy examination is better resolved with a medial tourniquet inflation. If the surgeon prefers, the tourniquet is deflated upon completion of the lateral release to obtain hemostasis. The question does remain as to what effect joint distension has on patellar tracking. Muscle paralysis from the anesthesia and the tourniquet inflation may also have an effect on patellar tracking.

Technique of Electrocautery Lateral Release

Although good results can be obtained with the subcutaneous method of lateral release, other authors[56] advocate intra-articular release using electrocautery. The stated advantages of this method would include direct visualization; decreased postoperative pain, allowing earlier rehabilitation; and decreased cost secondary to the ability to perform this procedure on an ambulatory basis.

Technique of Intra-articular Release Using Electrocautery

Prior to the start of the case, the surgeon preferentially selects the electrocautery tips. A variety of hooks are available that concentrate the energy to a small area. These hooks vary as to the bend of the tip. A large inflow superior medial portal is used at the start of the case. As with most arthroscopic procedures, the anterior lateral portal is made for placement of the arthroscope, while the anteromedial portal is used for placement of the instruments (Figure 10.11).

Once the diagnostic examination and any intra-articular work are performed, attention is then turned to performing the lateral release. The coagulation and cut settings are set at 10 W, respectively, and are increased as needed. With the arthroscope in the anteromedial portal, the electrocautery tip is placed through a nonconducting short cannula into the anter-

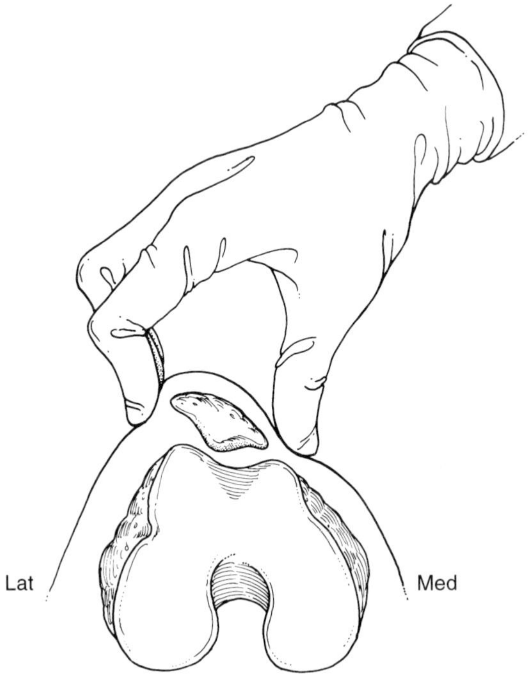

FIGURE 10.10. Adequate lateral release has been performed once a rotation of 70° to 90° is achieved.

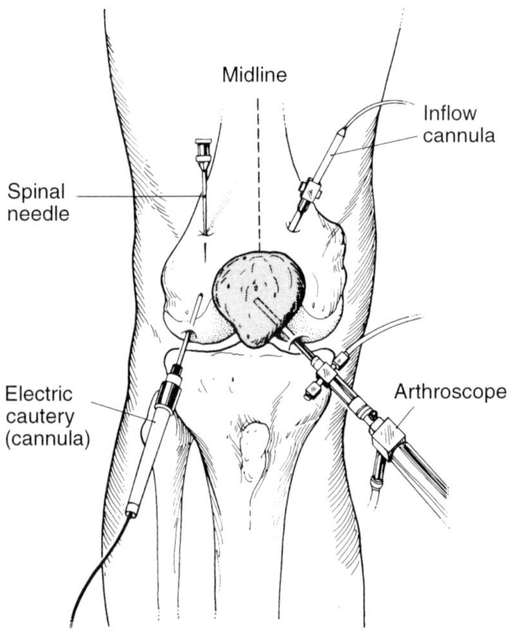

FIGURE 10.11. Surgical setup for arthroscopic lateral release.

olateral portal. The release is then performed 5 mm from the lateral patellar border and covers the distance from the superior patellar border to the bottom of the inferior portal (Figure 10.12). If the release is not adequate, it may need to be extended slightly into the vastus lateralis but extensive resection should be avoided. As the retinaculum is released, the subcutaneous fat is noted, especially at the anterior lateral portal. Care should be taken to avoid cutting into the fat because of its close proximity to the overlying skin to avoid a thermal burn. An 11-blade scalpel can be placed into the anterior lateral portal and angled distally to cut any remaining bands. At the close of the procedure, once again the passive patellar tilt should be from 60° to 90°. The arthroscope can be placed into the superomedial portal, and postoperative patellar tracking can be evaluated and the adequacy of the release judged. Once again cautery can be used to coagulate any bleeding vessels.

Postoperative rehabilitation is as important as the surgery itself. Initially, emphasis is

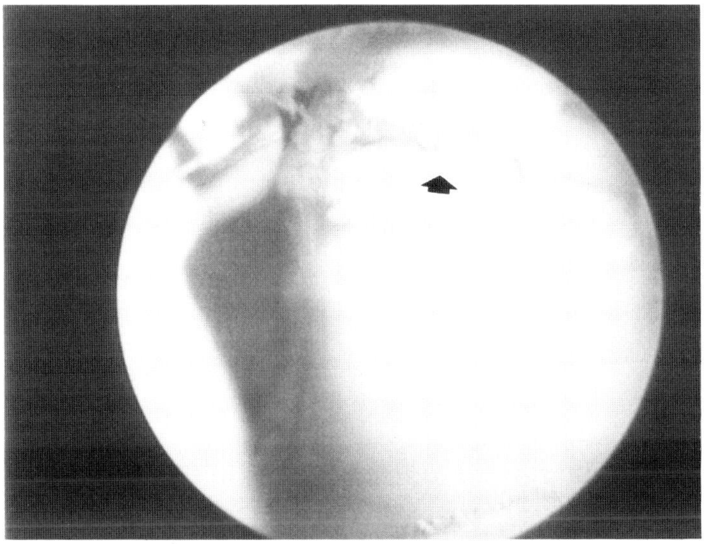

a

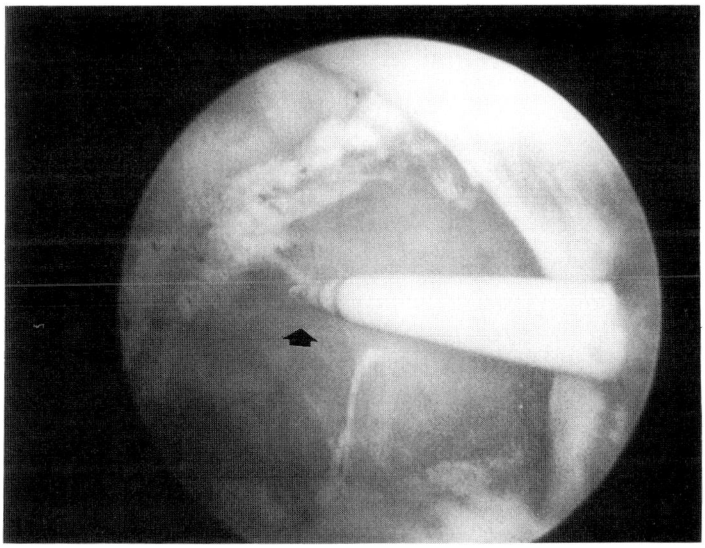

b

FIGURE 10.12. Arthroscopic lateral release performed with electrocautery (a) prior to release and (b) with resection completed.

placed on controlling the hemarthrosis. We prefer to place a light dressing and to use an autochill type of device. The patient is allowed to be full weight bearing and no brace is used. Range of motion is emphasized. As the swelling decreases, emphasis is placed on quadriceps strengthening. Isometric quadriceps exercise is begun to maximize the stress from the quadriceps and minimize the patellofemoral stress. These are performed at full extension. Our patients participate in supervised six-week programs in which home maintenance programs are begun. Patients are allowed to return to sports once their strength is 80% of the opposite leg. Dzioba[57] emphasized the importance of rehabilitation following lateral release, noting that the resolution of tilt did not occur until after an active rehabilitation program was initiated.

Complications can occur with either method of lateral release. Hemarthrosis is the most common complication aside from a poor result. Hemarthrosis may even require aspiration. Often hemarthrosis resolves with time, but rarely, this can lead to arthrofibrosis or loss of motion.[38,58]

An insufficient release may also be noted. Use of the superior medial portal to evaluate patellar tracking at 30° flexion and the "flip test" are guides to an adequate release. The release may need to be extended 1 to 2 cm if lateral tracking remains. Overrelease can lead to a serious complication. Patients may complain of giving way, vague anterior knee pain, and persistent weakness. Physical examination may show 80° to 135° of passive patellar tilt as well as a defect in the vastus lateralis.

Medial patellar subluxation may also develop as a result of lateral release.[59,60] This may be secondary to an excessive lateral release or may occur following lateral release in a patient with subtle preoperative medial subluxation. Cases with increased hypermobility may be at increased risk. Patients with the previous risk factors can be examined preoperatively by observing the patellar tracking as well as the preoperative x-ray. The role of kinematic MRI remains to be established.

Shellock et al.[61] reviewed 40 patients with persistent symptoms following lateral release. Sixty-three percent of these patients had medial subluxation on the operated side, while 43% had medial subluxation on the uninvolved leg. Therefore, the importance of preoperative examination was stressed to rule out medial subluxation prior to undertaking a lateral release. Hughston and Deese[59] examined 54 patients following poor results of arthroscopic lateral release. Thirty of the 54 patients had medial subluxation and computed tomography (CT) scans showed atrophy of the vastus lateralis muscle.

Patella baja is also noted to occur. This may be secondary to adhesions and is termed the *patellar entrapment syndrome.* As scar and adhesions develop, the patellar tendon becomes shortened. This can be worsened by inappropriate rehabilitation. Complaints include pain, weakness, and loss of motion. Reflex sympathetic dystrophy (RSD) may also result following the previous procedure.[62,63] Patients have diffused dysesthetic sensations as well as intolerance to coed. Also noted is a change in knee color with temperature change.

A preventable complication is thermal injury to the skin.[37,64] This can be decreased by maintenance of the equipment as well as using the lowest possible power on the electrode. Avoiding the subcutaneous fat as well as the use of a nonconducting cannula in the anterolateral portal can also decrease this risk. Other complications include deep vein thrombosis (DVT),[40,58,62,63] pulmonary embolus,[62] quadriceps rupture,[65] infection,[66] and adhesions.[37]

One last potential complication is the indiscriminate use of a lateral release. In other words, a lateral release should not be performed on all patellofemoral pain. Lateral release alone is often not enough and may be one aspect of a surgical procedure needed to correct patellar malalignment. Scuderi et al.[67] evaluated the results of lateral release done in conjunction with a proximal realignment. These were done in patients with either patellar subluxation or dislocation, and nine- to ten-years followup was obtained. Eighty-one percent excellent results were obtained, and there was no relationship to the grade of chondromalacia present and the overall success rate. Better results were noted in younger patients, with better results obtained in patients less than 40 years of age. More success was found in males, and this was thought secondary to a broader female pelvis, more femoral anteversion, and genu valgum that may result in an increased lateral pull of the patella.

In a recent article, Brief[68] described a combined open arthroscopic procedure for patellar maltracking, subluxation, and dislocation. This procedure involved a medial tethering of the patellar tendon in those patients with tracking abnormalities as well as patellar hypermobility. A standard arthroscopic lateral release was also performed on these patients. Twenty-nine cases with four- to eight-years followup were obtained. One hundred percent of the patients were noted to be able to return to previous activity levels and 38% improved their preoperative activity levels.

The role of the lateral release in treating pain remains unanswered. The relief of pain can be secondary to the denervation of a previously painful lateral retinaculum or the correction of a mild malalignment. Comparison of the results of arthroscopic release is difficult because various techniques, followup examinations, and selection criteria were used. Most studies show 70% with satisfactory results.[55,57,69–71] In 1989, Aglietti et al.[69] reviewed various techniques and results, and noted a large range from 14% to 99% success rate. The results were noted to be similar in both the open and closed groups. Unfortunately, followup examinations differed and the rate of hemarthrosis was not noted. Gallick et al.[72] reviewed 100 consecutive cases of electrosurgical release and compared them with a similar series of releases performed using arthroscopy without electrocautery. The groups were noted to be comparable regarding sex, age, and activity level. The electrocautery group was performed 100% on an outpatient basis compared with a mean 1.9 days of hospitalization for the arthroscopic-assisted group. The electrocautery group also had a lower hemarthrosis rate of 3% compared with 12% in the other group. All patients achieved greater than 90° flexion by the first week in the electrocautery group and more were able to return to their preoperative activity levels.

Other studies have noted a decrease in the hemarthrosis rate when electrosurgical releases were performed.[73] Sherman et al.[73] had no hemarthrosis in 45 knees treated by this method. Seventy-five percent of the patients showed improvement and an overall 4.4% complication rate was noted.

Small[66] examined 446 patients after lateral release and found the lateral release to have the highest complication rate at 7.2%. The complication rate increased with tourniquet inflation (9.2% versus 3.3%) as well as drain placement (11.8% versus 2.4%). It was felt that placement of suction drain prevents tamponade of ligated vessels from occurring in the knee. The hemarthrosis rate was two times as high in the arthroscopic-assisted group as compared with the intra-articular release group.

Although the surgery techniques have been refined, as can be seen, there still remains some unanswered questions. For example, What is the role in patients with pain and no evidence of instability? Although some authors advocate lateral release,[34,74,75] its role has been questioned.[76]

Mixed results are also present regarding the question, Do results deteriorate with time? While some authors[3,70,77,78] have noted such a trend, the finding has not been universally accepted.[55,57,76] Metcalf[3] noted a decrease in satisfactory results with time in young sedentary females, but no recurrence of patellar dislocation was noted.

Because of the debate on the tests and the results of the procedure, attempts have been made to find the prediction of success. No correlation has been noted with the degree of chondromalacia and postoperative success.[3,34,57,62,63,76–78]

Gecha and Torg[34] found that symptomatic examination, clinical diagnosis of dislocation or subluxation, and x-ray examination are not helpful in predicting success. Some success was noted when tight lateral parapatellar structures (Sage sign) was present as well as the absence of mal-loose signs (increased quadriceps angle, joint laxity, patellar hypermobility, excessive genu valgum, recurvatum, or increased anteversion). Dzioba[57] also looked at predictions of success and found that the quadriceps angle was not significant in predicting success. Factors that were predictors included positive pain with knee flexion against resistive flexion, positive apprehension sign, positive Merchant view, evidence of lateral overhang, and tight lateral stress noted on correcting the lateral retinaculum. The single best predictor was the return of the patella into the femoral groove on the Merchant view. Age is debated as a predictor. Some authors noted a poor outcome with increasing age,[38,58,62,70] while other authors have noted no such trend.[60,63,78] Other poor predictors include more than five dislocations,[69] obesity,[42,62] workmen's compensation,[62,63] contralateral knee pain,[63] and poor quadriceps function.[3,25,58,62]

In closing, it can be seen that much debate exists on the ideal candidate for lateral release to be performed. Since 80% of patellofemoral pain responds without treatment,[30,73] we recommend a trial of three months of physical therapy prior to operative intervention. On clinical examination, we look for normal quadriceps angle as well as a clearly tight lateral retinaculum. On x-ray examination, we look for only mild arthritic changes as well as lateral overhang on the Merchant view. In the future, the role of kinematic MRI may better evaluate maltracking patella.

Arthroscopic Treatment of Acute Patellar Dislocations

The ideal treatment of acute patellar dislocations remains debated. Although often treated in a closed fashion, a new emphasis has been placed on the arthroscopic treatment of the entity. This section will deal with the arthroscopic management of the dislocated patella. The results and findings of arthroscopy; arthroscopy and lateral release; and arthroscopy, lateral release, and medial capsular imbrication will be reviewed.

The natural history of acute patellar dislocations has been shown to have a high recurrence rate, with Cofield and Bryan[79] and Power[80] noting a redislocation rate of approximately 50%. Dainer et al.[81] reviewed 29 arthroscopies performed on acute patellar dislocations with 86% of patients noted to have significant osteochondral fragments. Within this population, 0.15 lateral releases were performed. A 73% good to excellent result was noted with the lateral release group compared with a 93% good to excellent result in the no lateral release group. No recurrences were noted in the no lateral release group compared with four redislocations in the lateral release group. These authors concluded that lateral release is not indicated for acute traumatic dislocation.[81]

Detrisac et al.[82] reported on 77 arthroscopic patellar realignments. This procedure includes an arthroscopic lateral release as well as an arthroscopic imbrication of the medial capsule. Results showed an 80% success rate at one-year followup.[82]

Small et al.[83] reported on arthroscopically assisted proximal realignments, also noting good to excellent results at 18-months followup (92.5%). The indications used for this procedure were recurrent patellar instability and acute initial patellar dislocation. Two recurrent subluxations were noted and the mean time to return to presurgical activities was four months.

At the Insall Scott Kelly Institute, acute patellar dislocations are initially treated closed. If large fragments are noted on the initial films, then arthroscopy is considered. However, we have not found a clinical significance to small osteochondral lesions not seen on initial films treated in a closed fashion. We have no experience with arthroscopically assisted proximal realignments and therefore defer discussion to those authors as noted previously.

References

1. Greenfield MA, Scott WN: Arthroscopic evaluation and treatment of the patellofemoral joint. *Orthop Clin North Am* 1992;23(4):587–599.
2. Casscells SW: The arthroscope in the diagnosis of disorders of the patellofemoral joint. *Clin Orthop* 1979;144:45–50.

3. Metcalf RW: An arthroscopic method for lateral release of the subluxating or dislocating patella. *Clin Orthop* 1982;167:9.
4. Sojbjerg JO, Lauritzen J, Havid I, et al.: Arthroscopic determination of patellofemoral malalignment. *Clin Orthop* 1987;215:243–247.
5. Mayeda P. Ueber das strangartige gebilde in der kniegel-enkhoehle (chordi cavi articularis genu). *Mitt Med Fak Kaisert University Tokyo* 1918;21:507–553.
6. Aoki T: A case of internal derangement of the knee due to so called shelf. *Nippon Seikeigeka Gakka Zasshi* 1965;39:933.
7. Jackson RW, Marshall DJ, Fujisawa Y: The pathological medical shelf. *Orthop Clin North Am* 1982;13:307.
8. Byoung-Hyoun M, Sung-Jae K, Byeong-Mun P, et al.: Arthroscopic anatomy of the infrapatellar plica. American Academy of Orthopaedic Surgeons 61st Annual Meeting Poster Presentation, New Orleans, February 1994.
9. Broom MJ, Fulkerson JP: The plica syndrome: A new perspective. *Orthop Clin North Am* 1986;17(2):279–288.
10. Aprin H, Shapiro J, Gershwind M: Arthrography (plica views). *Clin Orthop* 1984;183:90–95.
11. Pipkin G: Lesions of the suprapatellar plica. *J Bone Joint Surg Am* 1950;32A:363–369.
12. Tasker T, Waugh W: Articular changes associated with internal derangement of the knee. *J Bone Joint Surg Br* 1982;64B:486–488.
13. Patel D: Plica as a cause of anterior knee pain. *Orthop Clin North Am* 1986;17(2):273–277.
14. Denks WMT, DeMooge P, Van Linje B: Ultrasonographic detection of the patellar plica in the knee. *JCU* 1986;14:355–360.
15. Tindel NL, Nisonson B: The plica syndrome. *Orthop Clin North Am* 1992;23(4):613–618.
16. Patel D: Arthroscopy of the plicae—Synovial folds and their significance. *Am J Sports Med* 1978;6:217–225.
17. Nottage WM, Sprague NF, Auerback BJ, et al.: The medial patellar plica syndrome. *Am J Sports Med* 1983;11:211–214.
18. Hardaker WT, Whipple TL, Bassett FH III: Diagnosis and treatment of the plica syndrome of the knee. *J Bone Joint Surg Am* 1980;62A:221–225.
19. Rovere GD, Adair DM: The medial synovial shelf plica syndrome. Treatment by intraplical steroid injection *Am J Sports Med* 1985;13:382–386.
20. Broukhim B, Fox JM, Blazina ME, et al.: The synovial shelf syndrome. *Clin Orthop* 1979;142:135–138.
21. Dandy DJ: Arthroscopy in the treatment of young patients with anterior knee pain. *Orthop Clin North Am* 1986;17(2):221–229.
22. Munzinger U, Ruckstuhl, J, Scherrer H, et al.: Internal derangement of the knee joint due to pathologic synovial folds: The mediopatellar plica syndrome. *Clin Orthop* 1981;155:59–64.
23. Muse GL, Grana WA, Hollingsworth S: Arthroscopic treatment of medial shelf syndrome. *Arthroscopy* 1983;102:67.
24. Johnson DP, Eastwood DM, Witherow PJ: Symptomatic synovial plicae of the knee. *J Bone Joint Surg Am* 1993;75A:1485–1496.
25. Lombardo SJ, Bradley JP: Arthroscopic diagnosis and treatment of patellofemoral disorders, in Scott, WN (ed.): *Arthroscopy of the Knee.* Philadelphia, WB Saunders Co., 1990, pp. 155–171.
26. Schonholtz GJ, Ling B: Arthroscopic chondroplasty of the patella. *Arthroscopy* 1985;1(2):92–96.
27. Wissinger HA: Chondromalacia patellae: A nonoperative program. *Orthopedics* 1982;50:315.
28. Outerbridge RE: The etiology of chondromalacia patellae. *J Bone Joint Surg Br* 1961;43B:752–757.
29. Insall JN: Current concepts review. Patellar pain. *J Bone Joint Surg Am* 1982;64A:147–152.
30. DeHaven KE, Dolan WA, Mayer PJ: Chondromalacia patellae in athletes. Clinical presentation and conservative management. *Am J Sports Med* 1979;7(1):5.
31. Leslie IJ, Bentley G: Arthroscopy in the diagnosis of chondromalacia patellae. *Ann Rheum Dis* 1978;37:540–547.
32. Fisher RL: Conservative treatment of patellofemoral pain. *Orthop Clin North Am* 1986;17(2):269–272.
33. Fulkerson JP, Schutzer SF: After failure of conservative treatment for painful patellofemoral malalignment: Lateral release or realignment? *Orthop Clin North Am* 1986;17(2):283–288.
34. Gecha SR, Torg JS: Clinical prognosticators for the efficacy of retinacular release surgery to treat patellofemoral pain. *Clin Orthop* 1990;253:203–208.
35. Gruber M: The conservative treatment of chondromalacia patellae. *Orthop Clin North Am* 1979;10:105.
36. Bentley G, Dowd G: Current concepts of etiology and treatment of chondromalacia patellae. *Clin Orthop* 1984;189:209–228.

37. Fox J, Ferkel R, Del Pizzo W, et al.: Electrosurgery in orthopaedics. II. Applications to arthroscopy. *Contemp Orthop* 1984;8:37.
38. Grana WA, Hinkley B, Hollingsworth S: Arthroscopic evaluation and treatment of patellar malalignment. *Clin Orthop* 1984; 186: 122–128.
39. Insall JN, Aglietti P, Tria AJ Jr: Patellar pain and incongruence. II: Clinical application. *Clin Orthop* 1983;176:225–232.
40. McGinty JB, McCarthy JC: Endoscopic lateral retinacular release. A preliminary report. *Clin Orthop* 1981;158:120–125.
41. Insall J, Falvo KA, Wise DW: Chondromalacia patellae. *J Bone Joint Surg Am* 1976;58A:1–8.
42. Ogilvie-Harris DJ, Jackson RW: The arthroscopic treatment of chondromalacia patellae. *J Bone Joint Surg Br* 1984;66B:660.
43. Henry JH, Crosland JW: Conservative treatment of patellofemoral subluxation. *Am J Sports Med* 1979;7:12.
44. Sandow MJ, Goodfellow JW: The natural history of anterior knee pain in adolescents. *J Bone Joint Surg Br* 1985;67B:36–38.
45. McCarroll JR, O'Donoghue DH, Grana WA: The surgical treatment of chondromalacia patella. *Clin Orthop* 1983;175:130–134.
46. Hunter W: On the structure and diseases of articulating cartilage. *Philos Trans R Soc Lond Biol* 1743;9:267.
47. Leidy J: On the intimate structure and history of articular cartilage. *Am J Med Sci* 1849;17: 277.
48. Pridie KH: A method of resurfacing osteoarthritic knee joints. *J Bone Joint Surg Br* 1959; 41B:618.
49. Childers JC Jr, Elwood SC: Partial chondrectomy and subchondral bone drilling for chondromalacia. *Clin Orthop* 1979;144:114–120.
50. Roux C: Luxation habituelle de la rotule: Traitemente operatoire. *Rev Chir Orthop* 1888; 8:682–689.
51. Willner P: Recurrent dislocation of the patella. *Clin Orthop* 1970;69:213.
52. Shim SS, Leung G: Blood supply of the knee joint. A microangiographic study in children and adults. *Clin Orthop* 1986;208:119–125.
53. Ficat RP, Hungerford DS: *Disorders of the Patello-Femoral Joint.* Baltimore, Williams & Wilkins Co., 1977.
54. Scuderi GR: Surgical treatment for patellar instability. *Orthop Clin North Am* 1992; 23(4): 619–630.
55. Henry JH, Goletz TH, Williamson B: Lateral retinacular release in patellofemoral subluxation. Indications, results and comparison to open patellofemoral reconstruction. *Am J Sports Med* 1986;14(2):121–129.
56. Fox TM, Ferkel RD: Use of electrosurgery and arthroscopic surgery, in Parisien J (ed.):*Arthroscopic Surgery.* New York, McGraw-Hill Book Co., 1988, pp. 315–330.
57. Dzioba RB: Diagnostic arthroscopy and longitudinal open lateral release: A four year follow-up study to determine predictors of surgical outcome. *Am J Sports Med* 1990; 18(4): 343–348.
58. Simpson L, Barrett T: Factors associated with poor results following arthroscopic subcutaneous lateral release. *Arthroscopy* 1987;3:152.
59. Hughston JC, Deese M: Medial subluxation of the patella as a complication of lateral retinacular release. *Am J Sports Med* 1988; 16(4): 383–388.
60. Kolowich PA, Paulos LE, Rosenberg TO, et al.: Lateral release of the patella: Indications and contraindications. *Am J Sports Med* 1990; 18: 359.
61. Shellock FG, Mink JH, Deutsch A, et al.: Evaluation of patients with persistent symptoms after lateral release by kinematic magnetic resonance imaging of the patellofemoral joint. *Arthroscopy* 1990;6:226.
62. Bray RC, Roth JHT, Jacobsen RP: Arthroscopic lateral release for anterior knee pain: A study comparing patients who are claiming worker's compensation with those who are not. *Arthroscopy* 1987;3:237–247.
63. Busch MT, DeHaven KE: Pitfalls of the lateral retinacular release. *Clin Sports Med* 1989; 8: 279.
64. Lord M, Maltry J, Shall L: Thermal injury resulting from arthroscopic lateral retinacular release by electrocautery: Report of three cases and a review of the literature. *Arthroscopy* 1991;7:33.
65. Bigos, SJ, McBride GG: The isolated lateral retinacular release in the treatment of patellofemoral disorders. *Clin Orthop* 1984; 186: 75–80.
66. Small NC: An analysis of complications in lateral retinacular release procedures. *Arthroscopy* 1989;5:282.
67. Scuderi G, Cuomo F, Scott WN: Lateral release and proximal realignment for patellar subluxation and dislocation. *J Bone Joint Surg Am* 1988;70A:856–861.
68. Brief LP: Lateral patellar instability: Treatment with a combined open-arthroscopic approach. *Arthroscopy* 1993;9(6):617–623.

69. Aglietti P, Pisaneschi A, Buzzi R, et al.: Arthroscopic lateral release for patellar pain or instability. *Arthroscopy* 1989;5:176–183.
70. Betz R, Lonergan R, Patterson R, et al.: The percutaneous lateral retinacular release. *Orthopedics* 1982;5:57.
71. Malek M: Arthroscopic lateral retinacular release: Functional results in series of 67 knees. *Orthop Rev* 1985;14:55.
72. Gallick GS, Bena TA, Fox TM: Electrosurgery in operative arthroscopy. *Clin Sports Med* 1987;6:607.
73. Sherman OH, Fox JM, Sperling H, et al.: Patellar instability: Treatment by arthroscopic electrosurgical lateral release. *Arthroscopy* 1987;3(3):152–160.
74. Krompinger WJ, Fulkerson JP: Lateral retinacular release for intractable lateral retinacular pain. *Clin Orthop* 1983;179:191.
75. Larson RL, Cabaud HE, Slocum DB, et al.: The patellar compression syndrome: Surgical treatment by lateral retinacular release. *Clin Orthop* 1978;134:158–167.
76. Schonholtz GJ, Zahn MG, Magee CM: Lateral retinacular release of the patella. *Arthroscopy* 1987;3:269–272.
77. Christensen F, Soballe K, Snerum L: Treatment of chondromalacia patellae by lateral retinacular release of the patella. *Clin Orthop* 1988;234:145–147.
78. Jackson RW, Kunkel SS, Taylor G: Lateral retinacular release for patellofemoral pain in the older patient. *Arthroscopy* 1991;7:283.
79. Cofield RH, Bryan RS: Acute dislocation of the patella: Results of conservative treatment. *J Trauma* 1977;17(7):526.
80. Power MA: Natural history of recurring dislocation of the patella. *J Bone Joint Surg Br* 1977;59B:107.
81. Dainer RD, Barrack RL, Buckley SL, et al.: Arthroscopy treatment of acute patellar dislocations. *Arthroscopy* 1988;4(4):267.
82. Detrisac DA, Austin MN, Johnson LL: Arthroscopic patellar realignment. Arthroscopy Association of North America Annual Meeting, Washington, DC., March 1988.
83. Small NC, Glogau, AI, Berezin MA: Arthroscopically assisted proximal extensor mechanism realignment of the knee. *Arthroscopy* 1993;9(1):63–67.

11

Surgical Management of Patellar Instability

Giles R. Scuderi

Surgery is not indicated for all cases of patellar malalignment, as the majority of patients with recurrent instability will respond to nonoperative treatment. However, recurrent dislocation requires surgery because of the increased risk of injury to the articular surface. Patellar tilt, abnormal patellofemoral congruence, abnormal quadriceps mechanics, free osteochondral fragments, and chondromalacia have been implicated as contributing factors in the deterioration of the patellofemoral joint.[1] Avoidance of abnormal excursion of the patella, when conservative care fails, should be addressed surgically. Therefore, it is the preservation of normal patellofemoral mechanics that is paramount in the treatment of patellar malalignment and instability.

When considering surgical correction for patellar malalignment or instability, a thorough inspection of the joint should be performed. This can easily be done arthroscopically prior to the arthrotomy, including a superomedial portal that permits an excellent view of the patella.[2] As described in chapter 10, arthroscopic examination can aid in the confirmation of the preoperative diagnosis as well as enable the surgeon to address other disorders within the knee. It is not unusual to find associated injuries that can be easily addressed arthroscopically. Hughston reported 12.8% medial meniscal tears, 13.5% lateral meniscal tears, and 16.5% osteochondral fractures associated with patellar dislocations.[3,4]

Numerous surgical procedures are available for the correction of patellofemoral malalignment and pain (Table 11.1). These procedures release tight contracted soft tissues, including the vastus lateralis and lateral retinaculum; reinforce or transfer medial stabilizing structure; or reorient the insertion of the patellar tendon. The surgical categories include lateral retinacular release, proximal realignment, distal realignment, proximal and distal realignment, tibial tubercle elevation, and patellectomy. Because no single operation corrects all patellofemoral problems, the patient's age, diagnosis, level of activity, and condition of the articular surfaces need to be considered when selecting a surgical procedure.

When planning surgical treatment of patel-

Table 11.1. Patellofemoral diagnosis and suggested surgical treatment.

Diagnosis	Surgical Treatment
Lateral patellar compression syndrome	Lateral release
Patellar subluxation	Lateral release Proximal realignment Proximal and distal realignment
Acute patellar dislocation	Repair medial retinaculum and lateral release Proximal realignment
Recurrent patellar dislocation	Proximal realignment Proximal and distal realignment
Malalignment with severe chondromalacia	Fulkerson anteromedialization Maquet osteotomy Patellectomy

lofemoral disorders, it is important to differentiate the degree of malalignment and the location of patellar articular changes. For those patients with patellofemoral pain and no instability, malposition, or articular changes, treatment should be conservative with no surgical considerations. When the patellofemoral pain is due to articular changes, the surgical treatment should be directed towards the cartilage pathology. For those cases of patellofemoral pain attributed to static malposition of the patella, such as the lateral patellar compression syndrome, treatment is directed to releasing the tight lateral structures. Dynamic patellofemoral instability can be either recurrent subluxation or dislocation with normal or abnormal patellofemoral position. Preoperatively, it is imperative to document patellar malalignment, as a realignment procedure is not indicated for a normally aligned patella.

There are three general principles that should be kept in mind when addressing patellofemoral instability. First, medial instability is rare and is usually iatrogenic, traumatic, or associated with paralysis of the quadriceps. Iatrogenic causes that have been implicated include an extensive lateral retinacular release with complete detachment of the vastus lateralis or a distal realignment procedure in which the tibial tubercle is shifted too far medially (Figure 11.1). Second, it is important to determine preoperatively at which angle of knee flexion the instability occurs. When lateral instability occurs because of abnormal patellofemoral position, it is important to correct all the malalignment factors. The patella should be viewed three dimensionally and not only in the medial–lateral plane. Third, if degenerative articular changes are present, elevation or anteromedialization of the tibial tubercle may relieve pain by redistributing the patellofemoral forces. However, if the superior articular surface of the patella is severely involved, anteriorization is not beneficial. This will be discussed later in chapter 15, Management of Patellofemoral Arthritis.

Acute Dislocations

In most cases, acute dislocations can be treated conservatively. This is usually the case when there is major trauma and no previous history of patellar instability. The following also favor conservative care: a normal patella, little or no swelling, no loose bodies, or severe patellar dysplasia without swelling. For comparison, examination of the contralateral knee is important. If radiographic examination reveals an intra-articular bony fragment, then arthroscopic examination is recommended. Osteochondral fractures of the patella or the lateral femoral condyle represent an important

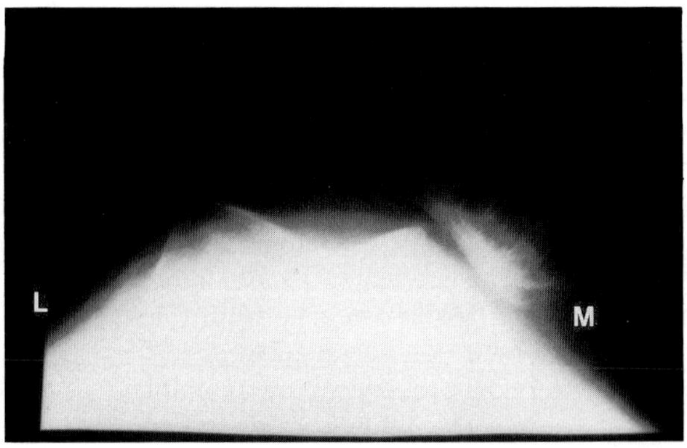

FIGURE 11.1. Iatrogenic medial patellar dislocation following a poorly planned realignment procedure (L = lateral; M = medial).

injury in the course of acute patellar dislocation (Figures 11.2 and 11.3). Vainionpaa et al.[5] reported a 42% incidence of fractures of the medial border of the patella following acute dislocation. In a review of 78 cases of acute patellar dislocation, Krodel and Refior[6] noted that 24 patients (32%) suffered osteochondral fractures. In ten of these cases, the osteochondral fragment was reattached to the patella. These osteochondral injuries also occur with a high frequency on the femoral condyle. In a prospective study of 20 consecutive patients with a clinical diagnosis of acute patellar dislocation, Poggi et al.[7] found 15 patients (75%) with articular cartilage damage to the lateral femoral condyle ranging from condylar abrasions to displaced osteochondral fractures.

Concomitant injuries have also been reported. In addition to bone contusions of the lateral femoral condyle, Poggi et al.[7] noted a significant effusion and a discrete tear of the medial patellofemoral ligament. Vainionpaa et al.[5] observed rupture of the medial retinaculum in 98% of cases. Magnetic resonance imaging (MRI) following an acute dislocation has been helpful in defining associated injuries including contusion of the lateral femoral condyle, tears of the medial retinaculum, and joint effusion[8] (Figure 11.4).

Following a closed reduction of the patella, if an axial radiograph reveals a laterally subluxed or tilted patella, a repair of the medial retinaculum and insertion of the vastus medialis should be performed. Vainionpaa et al.[5] found that following dislocation, a difference in the lateral position of the patella, as seen on an axial radiograph, between the involved and contralateral knee was significant and suggested that surgical repair was indicated. Other variables that influence early surgical intervention include a family history of patellar instability; a history of previous patellar subluxation or dislocation; minimal trauma causing the dislocation; and a young, athletic patient.[9] Steine et al.[10] recently reported that the initial treatment of acute patellar dislocation continues to be conservative, but the presence of an atrophic vastus medialis obliquus (VMO), more than five predisposing anatomic malalignment factors, and a congruence angle greater than 16° correlated with higher rates of recurrence. Despite compliance with a rehabilitation program, 63% of the patients in this study group had recurrent instability, while 18% eventually required surgical correction. It has been suggested that early surgical intervention be considered for those patients with the aforementioned risk factors.

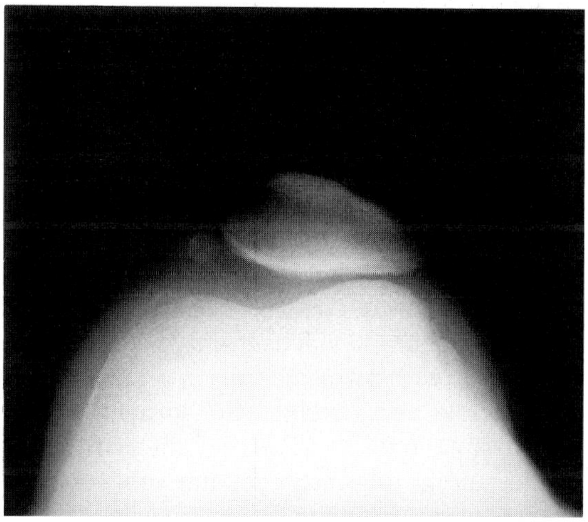

FIGURE 11.2. Osteochondral fracture from the medial border of the patella.

Whether one chooses an arthrotomy or an arthroscopic approach, attention needs to be directed towards repair of the medial retinaculum and imbrication of the VMO, along with a lateral retinacular release. Distal procedures to correct patellar malalignment are not recommended at the time of an acute dislocation because of the increased risk of arthrofibrosis and limited motion.

In 1986, Yamamoto[11] described an arthroscopic technique for the repair of the medial retinaculum and the capsule in acute patellar dislocations. Similarly, Small et al.[12] reported on their technique of arthroscopically assisted proximal patellar realignment performed on 27 knees in 24 patients. The procedure consists of a lateral retinacular release and an arthroscopically controlled plication of the medial retinaculum and the VMO. Subjectively, 92.5% were rated good or excellent, while there were two cases of recurrent subluxation. Following this procedure, the average return to full activities, including sports,

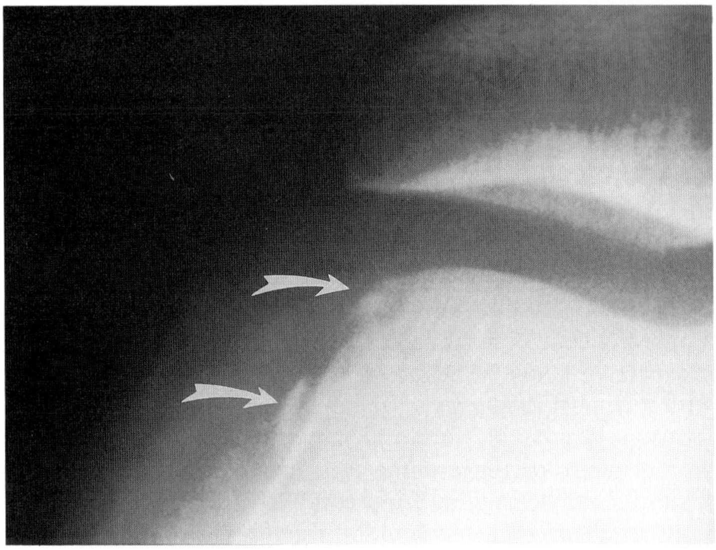

FIGURE 11.3. Osteochondral fracture from the lateral femoral condyle (arrows).

was four months. In another study, Gigli and Mariani[13] found that the arthroscopic technique eliminated postoperative pain and showed the same advantages, as open techniques, in reducing recurrent patellar dislocation.

Technique for Repair of Acute Patellar Dislocation

In the presence of an acute patellar dislocation, the medial retinaculum and the insertion of the VMO are torn and probably avulsed from the medial border of the patella. In performing an open repair, a straight midline incision is the preferred surgical approach. This permits direct exposure to the involved structures. A thorough inspection of the joint is necessary in order to remove any loose fragments that may be present from a chondral injury. Following inspection, the involved medial structures need to be repaired back to the patellar margin and the medial border of the quadriceps tendon with no. 0 nonabsorbable sutures. Soft-tissue anchors, such as the Statak (Zimmer, Warsaw, Ind.) have been helpful in reattaching the medial retinaculum to the medial border of the patella. Prior to closure of the medial defect, a lateral retinacular release should be performed in order to balance the extensor mechanism. Tensioning of the repair and closure of the defect is critical. The repair is placed in enough tension to balance the patella in the femoral sulcus through a full range of motion without a medial or a lateral tilt. Care should also be taken not to overtighten the proximal repair, as this may cause rotation of the patella, or worse, medial subluxation. Following routine wound closure over a drain, which is removed 24 hours later, a soft, bulky dressing is applied. Continuous passive mo-

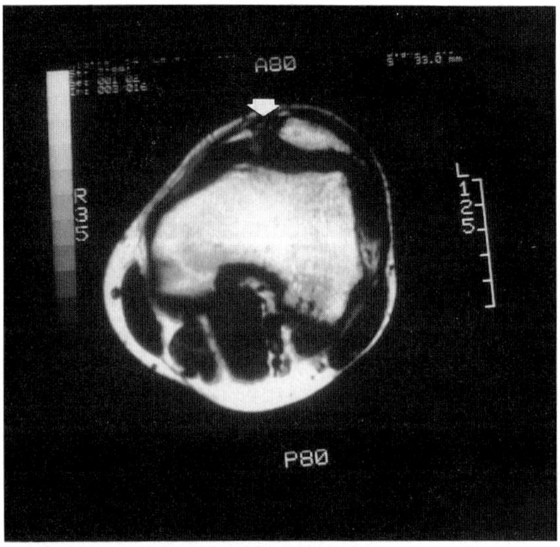

FIGURE 11.4. MRI following an acute dislocation with a torn medial retinaculum.

tion (CPM) and cryotherapy are initiated in the recovery room and the rehabilitation is similar to a proximal patellar realignment, which will be described later in this chapter.

There are certain intraoperative situations that may alter the technique described previously. If a small osteochondral fragment from the medial margin of the patella has avulsed along with the medial retinaculum, it should be excised and the medial retinaculum reattached to the medial border of the patella. This can be achieved by creating a small, bony trough along the medial margin of the patella at the site of the avulsion and placing drill holes along the anterior cortex. Multiple no. 0 nonabsorbable sutures are placed in the medial retinaculum, and are passed into the trough and through the drill holes (Figure 11.5). This permits the medial retinaculum to be drawn into the patella as the sutures are tied. An alternative is to place multiple soft-tissue suture anchors at the base of the bony trough and fix the medial retinaculum in this fashion.

Another intraoperative problem is a large osteochondral fragment. This tends to include the medial and the odd facet of the patella, and should be treated similarly to a medial longitudinal fracture of the patella. Therefore, secure anatomic fixation needs to be performed, similar to intra-articular fractures elsewhere. Once the open reduction is performed, it can be securely held with two bicortical screws (Figure 11.6). Excision of these large osteochondral fragments and imbrication of the medial retinaculum results in overloading of the medial patellofemoral joint. This has been a source of continued pain.

Procedures for Recurrent Instability

Lateral Retinacular Release

In 1974, Merchant and Mercer[14] first described lateral retinacular release. This procedure is indicated for patellofemoral pain with lateral tilt, lateral retinacular pain with lateral patellar position, and lateral patellar compression syndrome. Contraindications include isolated patellofemoral pain without lateral tilt, a hy-

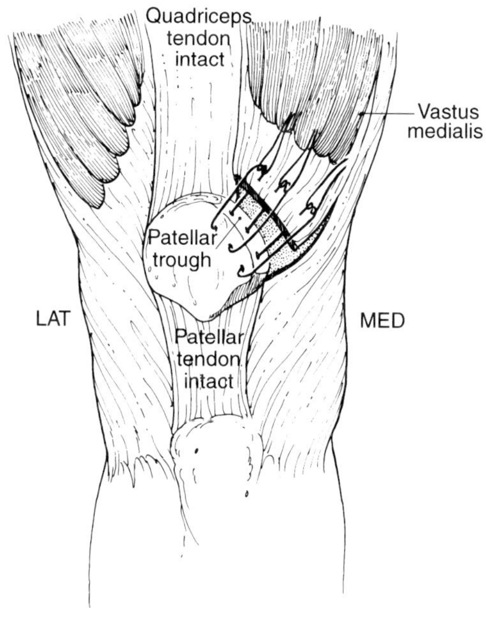

FIGURE 11.5. Medial retinaculum reattached to the patella.

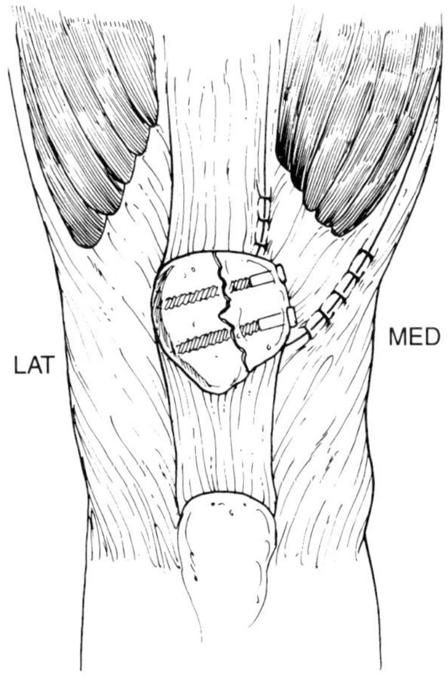

FIGURE 11.6. The large bone fragment is anatomically reattached to the patella and fixed with two bicortical screws.

permobile patella, a normal tracking patella, and significant malalignment with patellar subluxation and dislocation. Acceptable results can be expected in patients who have a tight lateral retinaculum as demonstrated with a Sage sign, limited medial patellar glide, and in patients who have no evidence of patellar malalignment or ligamentous laxity. Clinical prognosticators for the efficacy of lateral retinacular release have been described as the mal-loose signs[15] that include: (1) increased quadriceps angle; (2) generalized hyperlaxity; (3) patellar hypermobility; (4) excessive genu varum, genu valgum, or genu recurvatum; (5) increased femoral anteversion; (6) increased external tibial torsion; and (7) abnormal foot pronation.

Although several arthroscopic techniques for lateral retinacular release have been described,[16] the procedure can be easily performed through a small lateral incision.[17] Since the arthroscopic approach has been described in chapter 10, the following description details the open approach.

Open Lateral Release

After an arthroscopic examination of the knee and under tourniquet control, the leg is positioned in extension. A short, longitudinal skin incision is made along the lateral margin of the patella. The skin above and below the incision is undermined and the lateral capsule, the retinaculum, and the lower fibers of the vastus lateralis are visualized. The lateral retinaculum is then longitudinally divided about 1 to 2 cm from the patellar border including the inferior fibers of the vastus lateralis (Figure 11.7). It is recommended that the synovium be preserved, but at times it may be intimately adherent to the retinaculum and may need to be divided. If the synovium is divided, it is of no clinical significance. Although Ficat et al. recommended excising 5 to 10 mm of the retinaculum to prevent reformation,[18] I have not found this to be necessary. Inevitably, branches of the superior lateral and inferior lateral geniculate vessels are cut and should be cauterized. After the release, the tourniquet is deflated to allow coagulation of these vessels. The wound is closed and a soft compression dressing with a lateral buttress pad is applied. Postoperatively, the patient is allowed full weight bearing as tolerated with crutches and begins a course of physiotherapy within 48 hours.

Proximal Patellar Realignment Procedures

Although lateral release is an appealing procedure, it does not restore normal orientation to a malaligned extensor mechanism. A proximal patellar realignment is indicated for recurrent lateral patellar subluxation or dislocation, especially if the patella fails to centralize after a lateral release or if there is continued lateral subluxation. This procedure releases tight lateral structures and reinforces the pull of the medial supporting structures, especially the VMO. When the proximal pull of the entire quadriceps is altered, both lateral tracking and incongruence move toward normality and a functional reduction of the quadriceps angle is achieved.

The indications for a proximal patellar realignment include: (1) recurrent subluxation that has failed a supervised physiotherapy program; (2) recurrent dislocation; and (3) acute dislocation in a young, athletic patient, especially if there is an avulsion fracture from the medial border of the patella, or the axial radiograph demonstrates lateral subluxation or lateral tilt following a closed reduction.

Historically, in 1975, Madigan et al.[19] described a method of quadricepsplasty with lateral and distal transfer of the vastus medialis (VM) and the VMO with or without a lateral release for recurrent patellar subluxation (Figure 11.8). Because only 58% of patients had excellent or good results, there appeared to be technical problems with reorientation of the pull of the VMO. This led to modifications of the proximal realignment procedures. Insall described the proximal "tube" realignment (Figure 11.9) as a quadricepsplasty,[20] which was later modified to the proximal patellar realignment with advancement of the VM and

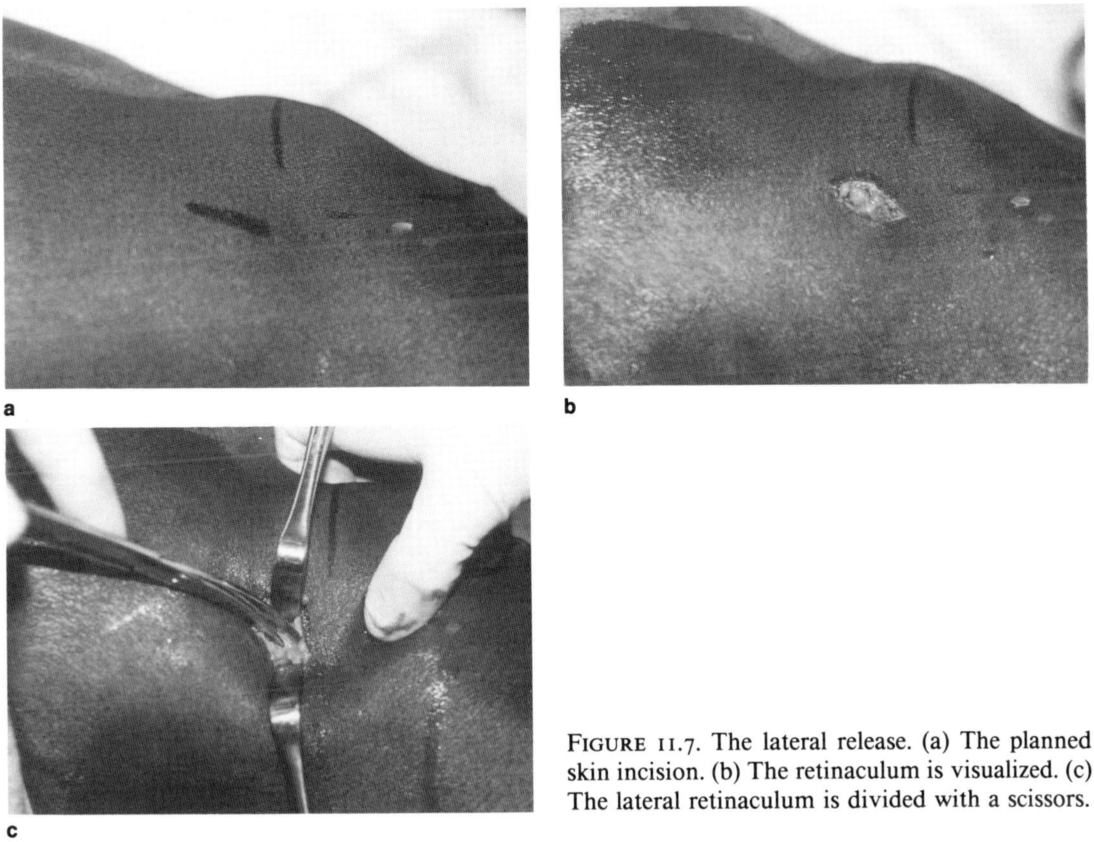

FIGURE 11.7. The lateral release. (a) The planned skin incision. (b) The retinaculum is visualized. (c) The lateral retinaculum is divided with a scissors.

imbrication of the medial capsule[21] (Figure 11.10a and 11.10b)

Proximal Patellar Realignment

Technique

A straight midline skin incision is used starting proximal to the patella and extending distally over the patella to the tibial tubercle. Subcutaneous flaps are developed, exposing the quadriceps tendon and the patellar tendon. A medial parapatellar arthrotomy is performed along the medial border of the quadriceps tendon over the patella and along the medial border of the patellar tendon to the tibial tubercle. This should be almost a straight incision (Figure 11.10c). Fibers of the quadriceps expansion that insert on the medial border of the patella are sharply dissected from the bone so that the patella then can be everted for inspection.

A lateral retinacular release is then performed (Figure 11.10d). The synovium can be preserved; however, if it appears to be a tight restricting band, then it should be incised. The proximal extent of the lateral release should not completely divide the tendon of the vastus lateralis or the quadriceps tendon. Insall has suggested that the lateral retinacular release begin proximally in the fibers of the vastus lateralis and extend distally to the tibial tubercle approximately 1 to 2 cm from the lateral border of the patella.[17] This extensive lateral division may not be necessary in all cases, but in certain situations it should be performed in order to correct patellar tracking. At the time of lateral release, the lateral superior geniculate artery is usually sacrificed and should be cauterized to avoid hemarthrosis.

Medial capsular tightening and advancement of the VM are accomplished by overlapping the medial flap on the patella and the

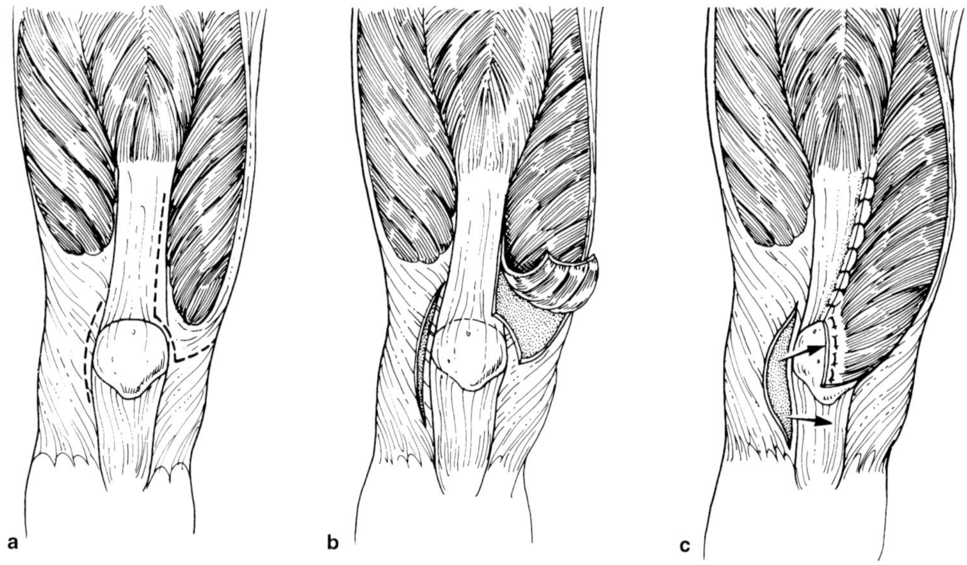

FIGURE 11.8. Quadricepsplasty. Lateral and distal transfer of the vastus medialis with a lateral release. (a) The planned incision along the lateral retinaculum and the VM. (b) The lateral retinacular release is performed, and the VM and the VMO are dissected free from the quadriceps tendon. (c) The VM and VMO are transferred distally and laterally.

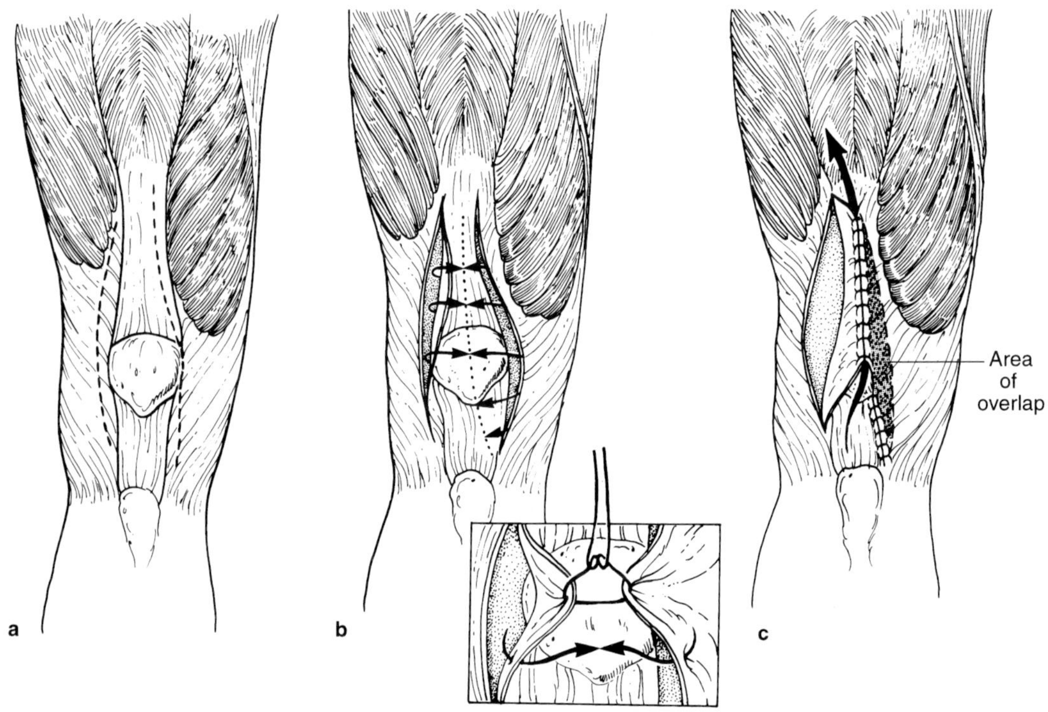

FIGURE 11.9. The Install "tube" realignment. (a) The planned incision for the lateral retinacular release and the medial arthrotomy. (b) The lateral border of the quadriceps tendon is sutured to the medial flap. (c) This creates a tube and proximally realigns the patella.

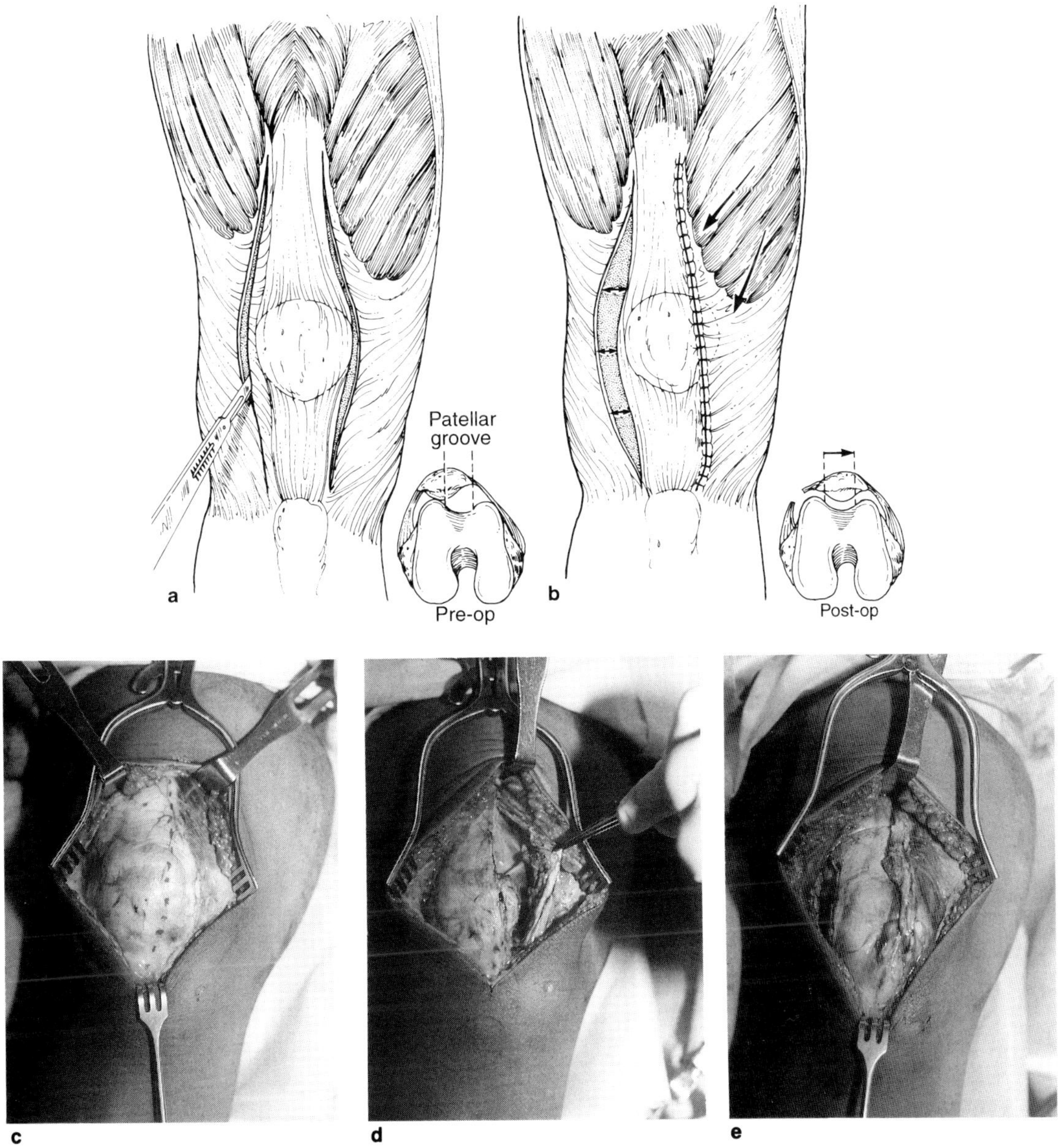

FIGURE 11.10. Proximal realignment. (a) The medial parapatellar arthrotomy and lateral release. (b) The medial flap is advanced laterally. (c) Intraoperative view of the planned arthrotomy. (d) The medial flap. (e) Completion of the proximal realignment with a lateral release.

quadriceps tendon by 1.0 to 1.5 cm (Figure 11.10e). The closure can be performed with absorbable or nonabsorbable no. 0 sutures and moves the insertion of the VM to a more lateral and distal position. Provisional sutures are placed and the pneumatic tourniquet is released so that there is no pressure on the quadriceps expansion during assessment of patellar position. The patella is centralized if it tracks entirely within the intercondylar sulcus with no medial or lateral tilt through a full range of motion. Care should be taken not to overtighten the medial capsule or to rotate the patella at the time of closure. Although Insall reported that the medial capsule could not be overtightened, with a hypermobile patella, overtightening of the medial capsule can result in iatrogenic medial subluxation. The knee is closed in a routine fashion over a Hemovac drain and a soft dressing is applied. A Cryocuff (Aircast, Summit, N.J.) is placed and CPM is initiated in the recovery room. When the patient can achieve 120° of flexion and a straight leg raise, progressive resistive exercises are begun. The patient is allowed to resume recreational activities when the quadriceps strength is 90% of the contralateral quadriceps, as tested by a Cybex (Lomex, Ronkonkoma, N.Y.) dynamometer.

Insall has recommended that the lateral release must extend proximally into the vastus lateralis as far as the medial incision. Unless this is done, a proximal rearrangement of the quadriceps is not possible, and Insall has not observed clinical weakness of the quadriceps with this lateral release. This is dissimilar to the findings of Sherman and colleagues,[22] who reported quadriceps weakness by isokinetic testing in two thirds of patients undergoing lateral release. What is interesting, however, is that this weakness did not correlate with their final subjective results. The fact is that the lateral release should extend as far as necessary into the vastus lateralis in order to centralize the patella.

Results

In a review of 75 cases, Insall et al. reported a 91% incidence of good and excellent results with a followup period of two to ten years.[21] Preoperatively, all patients had dysplasia of the extensor mechanism and complaints of pain or instability for one to five years. The results suggested that clinical improvement correlated with correction of the patellar axial alignment, whereas no correlation existed with the severity of chondromalacia. Additional procedures such as patellar shaving did not influence the final result.

In a review of 60 knees in 52 patients, Scuderi et al. reported that 81% of patients had good or excellent results, regardless of whether the preoperative diagnosis was patellar subluxation or recurrent dislocation, and the successful results appeared to continue for as long as nine years.[23] This study revealed a gender preference, with more excellent results in male patients. In female patients, factors such a broader pelvis, increased femoral anteversion, and genu valgum were speculated to result in residual forces that tend to pull the patella laterally, perpetuating the symptoms. Younger patients also have a better prognosis, which is attributed to less severe chondromalacia. Clinical results correlated more with correction of patellar congruence, assessed with the Merchant view, than with the degree of chondromalacia.

Though redislocation is a common complication of patellar realignment, Scuderi et al. reported a 1.2% rate of redislocation after proximal patellar realignment. This is superior to redislocation rates, noted to be as high as 25% with other procedures.[24,25,26]

Recently, ten patients from our original cohort[23] were reexamined and rated according to a patellar visual analog score (PVAS) (Figure 11.11), as well as the Tegner and Lysholm activity score.[27] This group included one bilateral case for a total of 11 knees. There were eight females and two males with an average followup of 13.8 years (range, 10 to 15 years). The results were 73% excellent or good, 18% fair, and 9% poor. The average postoperative activity score was 5. The number of satisfactory results is only slightly less than our original report.[23] Radiographically, this group demonstrated that the corrected congruence angle was maintained, and that there was no evidence of progressive degenerative changes in the medial patellofemoral joint. No further increase in the incidence of redislocation was revealed in this later review.

Abraham et al. reported similar satisfactory to excellent results in 11 of 12 knees (92%) undergoing proximal realignment for recurrent patellar dislocation.[28] However, when the procedure was performed for chondromalacia, the results seemed to deteriorate with time, with 87% satisfactory to excellent results at two years and 55% satisfactory to excellent results at five to 11 years.

PATELLA SCORE

Name________________ Medical Record No.__________

Date of Surgery__________ Date of Examination__________

Side________ Sex________Age________

Pain with	None									Severe
Run	10	9	8	7	6	5	4	3	2	1
Walk	10	9	8	7	6	5	4	3	2	1
Stairs	10	9	8	7	6	5	4	3	2	1

	None									Constant
Giveway	10	9	8	7	6	5	4	3	2	1
Limp	10	9	8	7	6	5	4	3	2	1
Swelling	10	9	8	7	6	5	4	3	2	1

	No Difficulty									Unable
Run	10	9	8	7	6	5	4	3	2	1
Jump	10	9	8	7	6	5	4	3	2	1
Squat	10	9	8	7	6	5	4	3	2	1
Sit	10	9	8	7	6	5	4	3	2	1

Total Score______

Would you have surgery again?_______
Are you satisfied with the results of the operation?________
Has the knee ever dislocated following surgery?__________

FIGURE 11.11. Patellar visual analog score (PVAS).

Campbell Procedure

Campbell described a technique in the 1930s that addressed recurrent dislocation of the patella by the creation of a proximal medial sling. The procedure was indicated for patients, including adolescents who had attenuated medial structures, no significant patellofemoral arthritic changes, and the rare occurrence of dislocation. This technique was also useful in combination with other realignment procedures, including tibial tubercle transfer.[29] Currently, this procedure is not popular but has historic value.

Technique

An anteromedial skin incision is made from the quadriceps tendon to the tibial tubercle. The exposure is then deepened to the level of the medial capsule and the retinaculum. A proximally based strip of medial capsule, 12.5 cm long and 1.3 cm wide, is then developed. Joint inspection can be performed by incising the synovium in this area, which is then sutured closed. A lateral retinacular release is then performed. This is followed by closure of the medial arthrotomy. The proximally based strip of medial capsule is then passed beneath the quadriceps tendon at the superior pole of the patella from a medial to lateral direction. The flap is then reflected medially over the quadriceps tendon and sutured to the facia in the region of the adductor magnus tendon (Figure 11.12). The wound is then closed in a routine fashion over Hemovac drains. Postoperatively, the knee is immobilized for two weeks followed by a rehabilitation program.

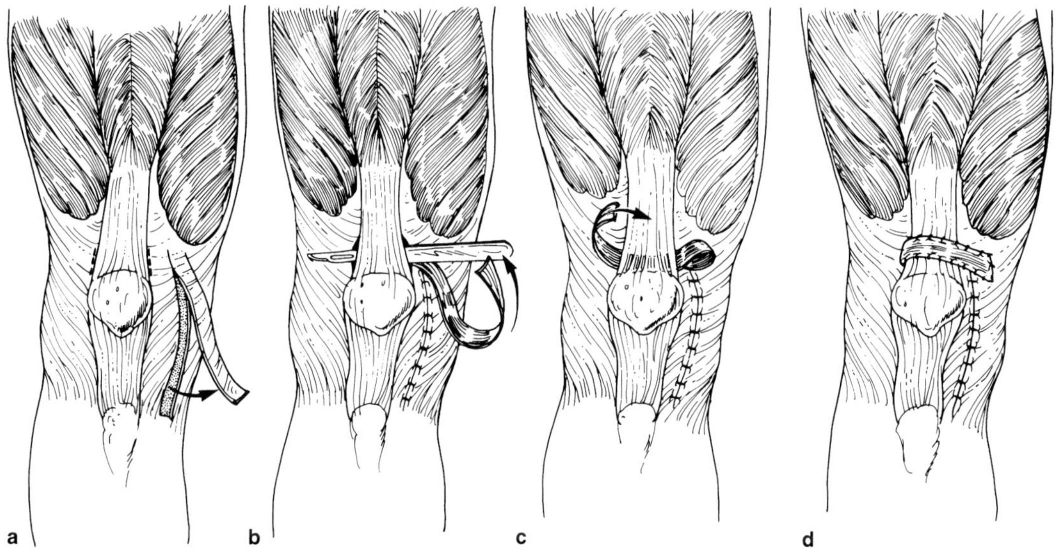

FIGURE 11.12. The Campbell's procedure. Creates a proximal medial sling. (a) A flap of the medial retinaculum is dissected free maintaining a proximal attachment. (b) The medial defect is closed and the medial retinacular flap is passed beneath the quadriceps tendon. (c) The flap is then brought back over the quadriceps tendon. (d) This creates a proximal sling.

Distal Patellar Realignment Procedures

Distal patellar realignment procedures reorient the patellar tendon and tibial tubercle and in the skeletally mature patient, correct recurrent lateral instability. These procedures, which transpose the tibial tubercle, are contraindicated in patients with normal quadriceps angles and in skeletally immature patients with open epiphyseal growth plates. Premature closure of the tibial tubercle with resultant genu varum and genu recurvatum have been reported after distal realignment. Transferring the patellar distally in skeletally immature patients can also cause contracture of the patellar tendon, resulting in patellar infera and chondromalacia patellae.

Hauser Procedure

Numerous techniques have been described for distal realignment of the patella since the early description of Hauser.[30] In this early technique, the insertion of the patellar tendon is freed from the tibial tubercle with a bone block and pulled medially and distally on the tibia. It was recommended that the extensor mechanism be in line with the long axis of the femur and that the tendon not be advanced too distally as to cause increased tension. Ideally, the inferior pole of the patella should lie at the level of the tibial spines with the knee in full extension. The problem with a large bone block as originally described is that there was some difficulty in aligning the patellar tendon. Hughston and Walsh modified this distal bone block by osteotomizing a smaller piece of bone and fixing it to the tibia with a Stone staple.[31] Dougherty et al.[32] introduced another modification that created a keyhole in the proximal medial tibia into which the distal bone block was impacted. Finally, whether the procedure was the original of Hauser or a modified technique, a lateral and a distal advancement of the VM was recommended.

The Hauser technique has become unpopular because of reports of late osteoarthritis caused by excessive distal or medial transfer of the patellar tendon. Since the proximal tibia is triangular in shape, a medial transfer of the patellar tendon is always accompanied by posterior displacement when this technique is used. This position results in a reverse Maquet effect, with increased pressure on the patellofemoral joint and the development of patellofemoral arthritis. For an average of 16 years, Hampson and Hill observed 35 patients who had undergone a Hauser procedure and noted a 70% incidence of degenerative changes.[33] This is similar to the 71% occurrence that Crosby and Insall reported.[25] Contrary to these investigators, DeCesare reported on the late results of the Hauser procedure for recurrent dislocation of the patella.[26] Fifty-two patients were examined at an average followup of 17 years. More than 70% of patients had excellent or good results up to as long as 30 years postoperatively, and there was no predisposition to degenerative arthritis. There did appear to be a gender predisposition, with females, especially those with generalized ligamentous laxity, having a higher incidence of poorer results and redislocation. The overall incidence of redislocation was 7%.

One of the most common technical errors in procedures that realign the patella distally is the failure to correct patellar height.[9] Insufficient correction of patella alta will result in a loose fitting extensor mechanism and potentially recurrent instability. When the tibial tubercle transfer is adjusted for patella alta, it should not be advanced distally more than 2 cm, because this will limit flexion and increase the patellofemoral joint reactive forces.[21] When present preoperatively, patella infera or patella baja can be corrected with proximal displacement of the tibial tubercle. Lengthening of the patellar tendon is not recommended.

Galiazzi Procedure

In 1922, Galiazzi first described his procedure for tenodesis of the semitendinosus to the patella[34] (Figure 11.13). As originally described, the procedure used two separate skin incisions but can easily be performed through a straight midline incision. The semitendinosus tendon is identified and is harvested with as much length as possible—maintaining its distal attachment. Next, a medial parapatellar arthrotomy is performed along with a lateral retinacular release that includes the lower fibers of the vastus lateralis. The medial capsule is then imbricated distally over the patella and sutured in place. An oblique tunnel is then drilled in the patella from its inferomedial to superolateral corners. Care needs to be taken not to violate the anterior cortex or the articular cartilage. The semitendinosus tendon is then passed through the patellar tunnel, brought back over the patella, and sutured onto its distal origin. This technique draws the patella distally and medially. Following routine closure, the knee is immobilized for six weeks in extension. This is then followed by a supervised course of rehabilitation.

Baker et al. recommended this procedure for young patients with open epiphyseal growth plates.[35] In a study of 53 knees in 42 patients with an age range of 5 to 17 years, they reported 81% good or excellent results at an average followup of five years. The recurrent dislocation rate was 4%.

Distal Realignment

Roux–Goldthwait Procedure

Distal transfer of the patellar tendon was first described by Roux in 1888[36] and Goldthwait in 1895.[37] The procedure consists of medial transfer of the lateral half of the patellar tendon. This procedure has fallen out of favor, but at times it has been used in combination with other procedures for the treatment of recurrent patellar subluxation and dislocation.

Technique

The patellar tendon is split longitudinally at the midline and the lateral half is detached from the tibial tubercle. A lateral retinacular release is performed to the vastus lateralis. The detached lateral half of the patellar tendon is then passed beneath the intact medial half and sutured to the medial aspect of the tibia in the region of the pes anserinus tendons. This lateral half should be relocated such that the pull to the extensor mechanism is in line with the femur as the knee flexes (Figure 11.14).

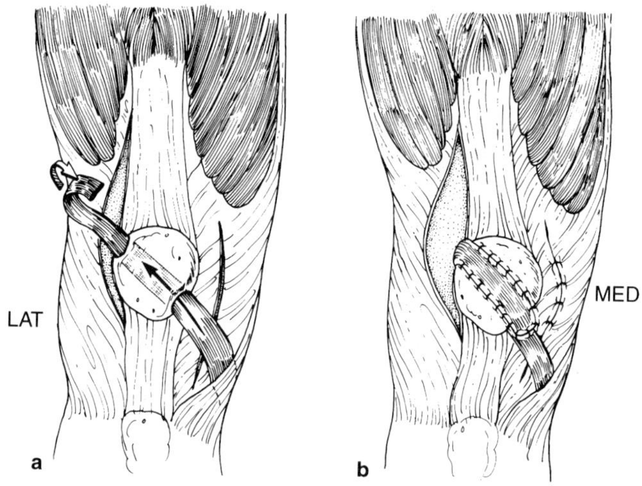

FIGURE 11.13. The Galiazzi procedure. (a) The semitendinosus tendon is passed through an oblique drill hole in the patella and (b) brought back medially to its insertion.

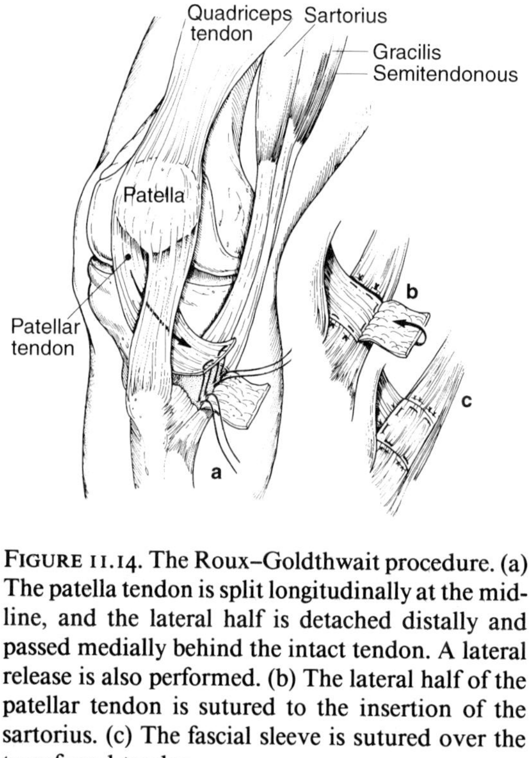

FIGURE 11.14. The Roux–Goldthwait procedure. (a) The patella tendon is split longitudinally at the midline, and the lateral half is detached distally and passed medially behind the intact tendon. A lateral release is also performed. (b) The lateral half of the patellar tendon is sutured to the insertion of the sartorius. (c) The fascial sleeve is sutured over the transferred tendon.

Results

Chrisman et al. reported 93% satisfactory results with this procedure.[24] However, Bowker and Thompson[38] reported a high failure rate, and Hughston and Walsh encountered a rupture of the intact medial half of the tendon following this procedure.[31] It has been recommended that this procedure be avoided in athletic patients with strong, well-developed quadriceps musculature. Fondren et al.[39] reported worse results in knees with severe chondromalacia, with these patients later developing patellofemoral arthritis. Medial transposition of the lateral half of the patellar tendon can cause lateral tilting of the patella, especially if the tendon is pulled too tight.

Hughston Procedure

Hughston and Walsh have described the technique for management of recurrent patellar instability, utilizing a proximal and a distal approach. The indications for this procedure include: (1) failure of nonoperative treatment, (2) dislocation associated with a large osteochondral fracture, (3) patellar instability associated with ligamentous instability, (4) evidence of advancing patellofemoral deterioration, and (5) congenital dislocation of the patella. Similar to other distal procedures, the Hughston technique should be performed in skeletally mature patients with a quadriceps (Q) angle greater than 10°.[31]

Technique

Hughston and Walsh recommended a lateral parapatellar skin incision with the development of medial and lateral skin flaps. However, the procedure can easily be performed through a straight midline incision. Intraoperative measurement of the Q angle determines whether a distal realignment needs to be performed in conjunction with a proximal realignment. If the Q angle is greater than 10°, medial transfer of the patellar tendon was recommended.

With the knee flexed, a lateral retinacular release is performed that extends into the patellar insertion of the vastus lateralis. Next, a medial parapatellar arthrotomy is performed that extends distally to the tibial tubercle. The patellar tendon is then osteotomized from the tibial tubercle with a sliver of bone. Preparation of the new site includes elevating the periosteum medial to the tibial tubercle. The patellar tendon is then transposed medially, usually half the width of the tibial tubercle, and fixed at the new site with a Stone staple or screw. At this point the knee is flexed and extended to ensure that the patellar tracks within the femoral sulcus. Hughston and Walsh commented that the medial transfer of the tibial tubercle rarely exceeds 1 cm. If an adjustment needs to be done, it should be performed at this time. The VM and the medial capsule are now advanced laterally and sutured in place with multiple no. 0 nonabsorbable sutures. This proximal realignment should not overtighten the VM, causing the patella to displace medially. Hughston and Walsh also recommended that the VM not be transferred distal to the midpatella. Once the realignment is complete, the knee is closed in a routine fashion and immobilized in extension (Figure 11.15). The knee is protected in a cast for four to six weeks, followed by a rehabilitation program to restore motion and strength.

Results

Hughston and Walsh reviewed 346 cases over a period of 25 years and reported that 90% of athletes returned to their normal performances.[31] A subjective evaluation, in which a normal knee is considered as an excellent result, demonstrated 22% excellent results, 49% good, 22% fair, and 7% poor. Objectively, 23% were excellent, 43% were good, 26% were fair, and 8% were poor. Although 10% of the patients required further surgery, only 3% needed further surgery for recurrent instability.

Elmslie–Trillat Procedure

Elmslie modified the Roux procedure[36] by transferring the entire tibial tubercle on a distal periosteal hinge. Trillat et al. published the principles of this modification in 1964.[40] Cox has outlined the indications for the Elmslie–Trillat procedure,[41] which include: (1) recurrent patellar subluxation or dislocation, (2) patellofemoral pain with malalignment of the extensor mechanism, and (3) acute dislocation in adults with malalignment of the extensor mechanism.

Technique

The Elmslie–Trillat procedure accomplishes medial repositioning of the patellar tendon, along with a lateral retinacular release and a medial imbrication, while avoiding posterior placement of the tibial tubercle. This procedure uses a lateral parapatellar skin incision that extends to the tibial tubercle. A lateral retinacular release is performed and extends into the tendinous fibers of the vastus lateralis. If possible, the synovium is preserved. Next, the periosteum is elevated from the anteromedial surface of the tibia, in order to prepare the site for later transfer. Using an osteotome, a 4- to 6-cm osteotomy of the tibial tubercle is created maintaining its distal attachment. The tibial tubercle is then rotated medially around its distal attachment and fixed to the anteromedial tibia with a screw. If this distal realignment is not sufficient to centralize the patella, then a medial arthrotomy can be performed, a strip of the medial retinaculum resected, followed by closure under tension (Figure 11.16).

Results

In a review of the Elmslie–Trillat procedure, Cox published a preliminary report in 1976 on 52 knees.[42] At followup to two years, 77% had good or excellent results with a recurrence

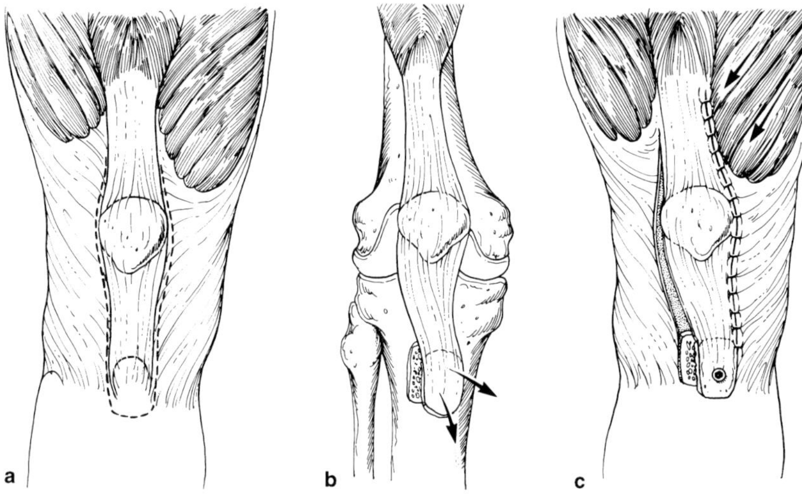

FIGURE 11.15. The Hughston procedure. The procedure incorporates a proximal realignment along with a distal tibial tubercle transfer. (a) The planned incisions for the medial arthrotomy and the lateral release extend to the tibial tubercle. (b) The tibial tubercle is transferred medially (arrows). (c) The transferred tibial tubercle is securely fixed and the VMO is advanced laterally at the time of closure (arrows).

rate of 7%. In a later review of 116 knees with an average followup of three years (one to seven years), Cox reported that 93% had no recurrent subluxation or dislocation.[41] While objective evaluation revealed only 66% good or excellent results, a subjective evaluation by the patients were slightly better at 73% good or excellent. Recurrence was associated with anterior cruciate ligament insufficiency and incomplete correction of a high Q angle. Distal realignment following an acute dislocation was associated with arthrofibrosis, while the degree of chondromalacia at the time of the index procedure directly influenced the end result. In a two-year minimum followup, DeBurge and Chambat reported their results in 114 knees performed for recurrent dislocation.[43] The majority of the patients (81%) were satisfied and the redislocation rate was 1.7%. However, 19% of patients were experiencing pain at followup, which appears to be attributed to the development of degenerative changes. Lateral patellofemoral arthritis was present in 16% at the latest followup. Radiographic examination of the Merchant view demonstrated that 70% were well positioned, 11% were uncorrected with a residual lateral position, and 19% were overcorrected with medial subluxation. More recently, Cerullo et al. compared patients who had the Elmslie–Trillat procedure performed for recurrent patellar dislocation or subluxation.[44] All the patients with dislocating patellae achieved satisfactory results, while the result was slightly less satisfying in the subluxation group.

Fulkerson Procedure

In 1983, Fulkerson first described the oblique osteotomy of the tibial tubercle for anteromedial transfer.[45] The slope of the osteotomy is tailored for the specific needs, depending on the degree of medialization and anteriorization needed. A steeper osteotomy permits greater anteriorization, as much as 17 mm, without adding bone graft.[46] This procedure has several applications and Fulkerson categorizes patients into three treatment groups based on their clinical diagnosis and computed tomography (CT) examination.[46] Patients with lateral subluxation usually benefit from medialization of the tibial tubercle and lateral retinacular release. In patients with minimal patellofemoral articular changes, me-

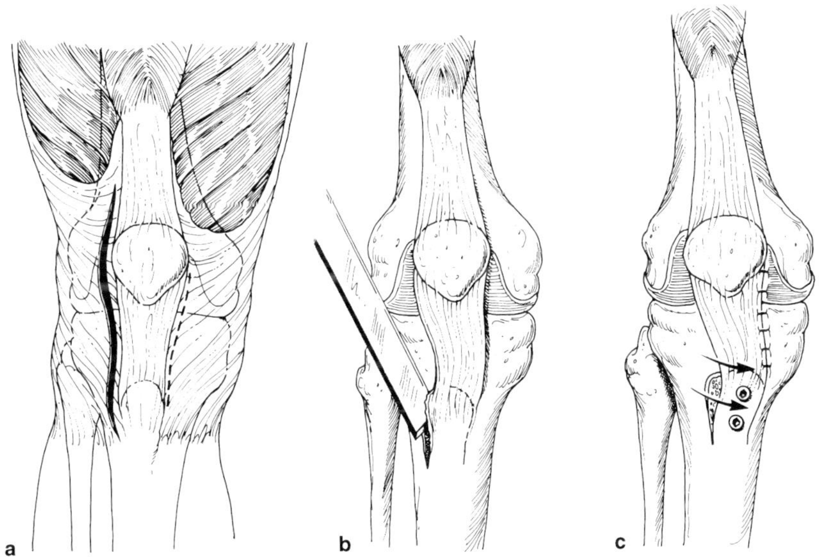

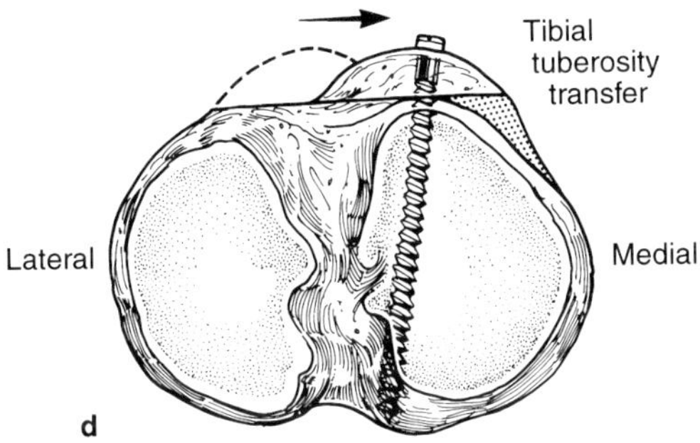

FIGURE 11.16. The Elmslie-Trillat procedure accomplishes medial respositioning of the patellar tendon, along with a lateral release and medial imbrication, while avoiding posterior placement of the tibial tubercle. (a) The planned medial incision and the lateral retinacular release. (b) The tibial tubercle is elevated. (c) The medial displacement of the tibial tubercle. (d) Axial view of the medialized tibial tubercle.

dialization of the tibial tubercle is usually sufficient. However, for more significant degenerative changes, anteromedialization of the tibial tubercle is recommended. The next group of patients are those with lateral subluxation and tilt. Anteromedialization is the recommended procedure, with the degree of anteriorization dictated by the severity of the patellofemoral articular changes, as discussed previously. The last group of patients are those with patellar tilt and degenerative changes. Although lateral release alone is beneficial for those patients with mild degeneration, anteromedialization is required for adequate realignment and pressure relief in patients with severe patellofemoral arthritis.

Technique

The procedure is performed through a straight skin incision from the midlateral patella to a point 5 to 8 cm distal to the tibial tubercle. A lateral retinacular release is performed, including the tendinous fibers of the vastus lateralis. Once the lateral release is performed, the patella is everted and the condition of the articular surface is assessed. The degree of anteromedialization is determined on the extent of the articular changes. The musculature of the anterior compartment is subperiosteally elevated from the tibial crest. The anterior tibial artery and deep peroneal nerve must be carefully protected. The entire patellar tendon is visualized to its insertion on the tibial tubercle. The planned osteotomy is approximately 5 to 8 cm long and is pie shaped, with the distal aspect tapering to 2 to 3 mm. The medial and lateral extent of the osteotomy is outlined with multiple drill holes. The slope of the osteotomy will determine the degree of anteriorization. If no anteriorization is required, the slope of the osteotomy is eliminated. The drill holes are then connected with a sharp osteotomy and care is taken not to injure the patellar tendon. A perfectly flat osteotomy plane is critical for bony opposition and secure fixation. Once completing the osteotomy, the tubercle is hinged distally and pushed up the slope. With the tubercle medialized, the patella tracking is assessed and if it is determined to be appropriate, the position is maintained with two bicortical screws. Anteriorization of 12 to 15 mm is possible without supplemental bone graft. The wound is then closed in a routine fashion over a Hemovac drain (Figure 11.17).

Postoperatively, a soft dressing is used and cryotherapy is begun in the recovery room. Since the osteotomy is securely fixed, active and gentle passive range of motion exercises, along with quadriceps setting exercises, are initiated the day following surgery. The patient is allowed weight bearing as tolerated with a knee immobilizer for comfort and crutches. Usually, by six weeks there is radiographic evidence of bony healing and recovery is generally achieved within four months.[46]

Results

Fulkerson has reported consistent long-term relief of symptoms in patients carefully selected for anteromedialization. Ninety-three percent of patients with patellofemoral pain and degenerative changes demonstrated excellent or good results.[47] Anteromedialization averaged 10.6 mm in this group of 30 patients. The complications with this procedure have been reportedly less when compared with other tubercle osteotomies. Fulkerson has not noted any skin problem, infection, compartment syndrome, or avascular necrosis in 76 consecutive patients. One patient in this group did have displacement of the osteotomized tibial tubercle. However, this case had the fragment fixed with only one screw and since then it has been recommended that the tibial tubercle be secured with two screws. A two-year followup of 26 patients demonstrated 89% good or excellent results, while 75% of patients with severe patellar arthritis had good results. In a group of 11 patients observed for more than five years, 90% had stable results without evidence of deterioration.[48]

Maquet Osteotomy

The Maquet osteotomy[49,50] was originally described in 1963 as an elevation of the tibial tubercle for the management of patellofemoral arthritis and severe chondromalacia patellae (Figure 11.18). Since its introduction, the procedure has been indicated for patellofemoral arthritis, chondromalacia patellae, recurrent patellofemoral instability, and continued anterior knee pain following patellectomy.[51] The clinical results are dependent upon the indications for surgery, length of followup, and clinical rating. Since chapter 15 will describe the operative technique, this current section will evaluate the results of the Maquet osteotomy in patients with recurrent patellar instability.

Theoretically, the Maquet osteotomy anteriorizes the tibial tubercle and does not correct medial or lateral malalignment. Therefore, its indications as a primary procedure for patellar instability are limited. Those cases of patellar instability requiring Maquet osteotomies are usually revision procedures for recurrent patellar instability or patients who have severe chondromalacia. I have found the Maquet osteotomy to be helpful in patients who require revision for a failed Hauser distal realignment or a similar distal procedure that displaces the tibial tubercle posteriorly. Since the proximal aspect of the tibia is triangular in shape, medial transfer of the patellar tendon is potentially accompanied by posterior displacement. This position results in a reverse Maquet effect with patella infera and increased patellofemoral compressive forces. Two patients who each had a prior Hauser procedure, one, ten years prior and the other 20 years prior, underwent Maquet osteotomies because of recurrent anterior knee pain and patellar instability. Preoperative radiographs in both cases demonstrated a medial patellar tilt and narrowing of the medial patellofemoral joint. In both cases, a Maquet osteotomy was performed with elevation of the tibial tubercle 1.2

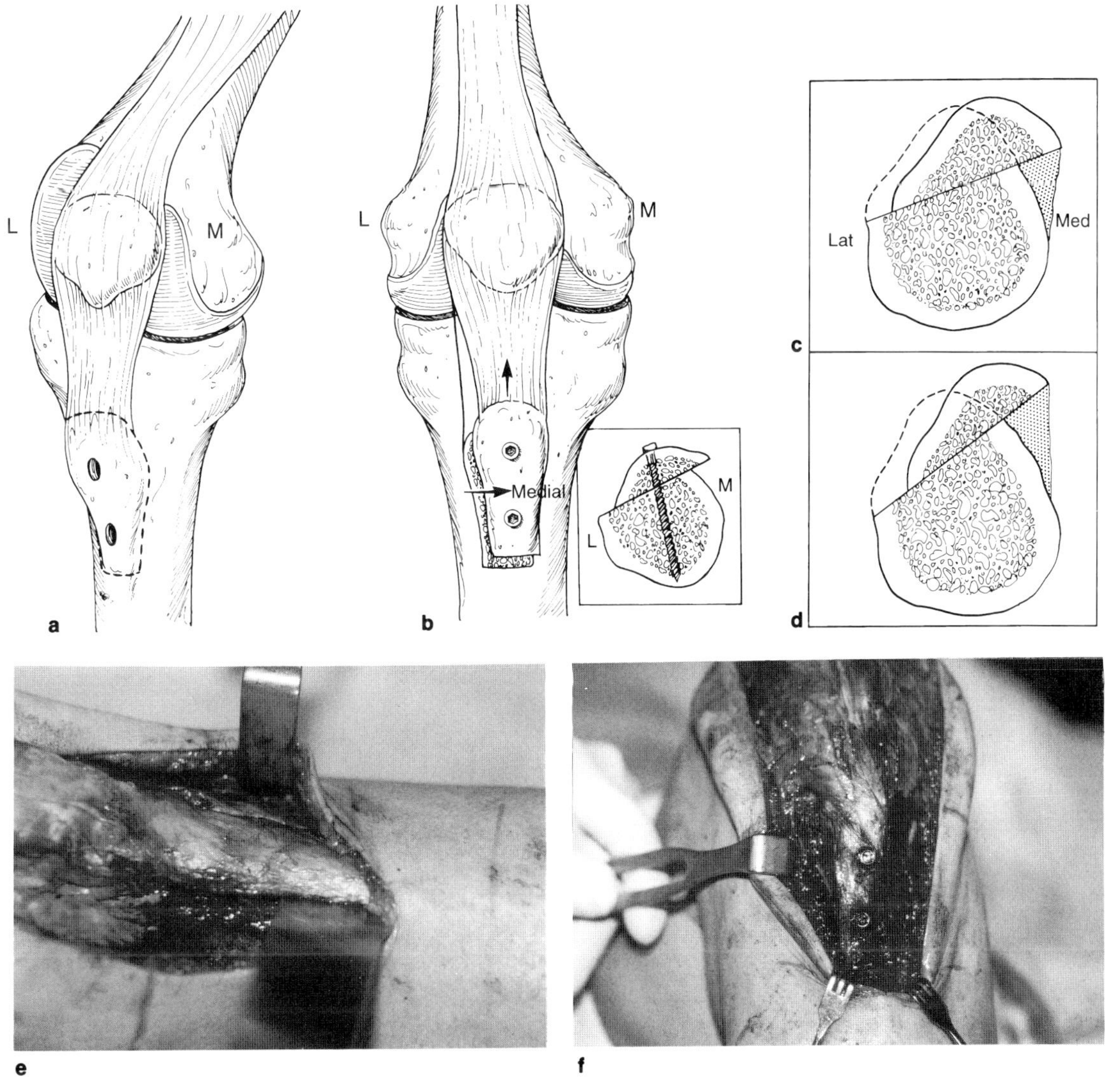

FIGURE 11.17. The Fulkerson procedure. (a, b) Anteromedialization is an oblique osteotomy of the tibial tubercle. (c, d) The slope of the osteotomy determines the degree of anteriorization. (e, f) Intraoperatively, the tubercle is elevated with an osteotome and when in proper position, is secured with two screws.

cm. There were no intraoperative or postoperative complications. At two-years followup, these patients had full range of motion and resolution of the preoperative complaints (Figure 11.19).

Several studies have evaluated the outcome of Maquet osteotomies based on specific diagnoses and have found varying results.[52–55] The poor results in all these studies were directly related to postoperative complications, undiagnosed tibiofemoral osteoarthritis, psychiatric problems, and knee malalignment.

Two studies have reviewed the results of patients with recurrent patellar instability[53,54] (Table 11.2). Radin[53] was able to differentiate the good and the excellent results based on diagnosis at an average followup of 3.5 years. He found that 93% of patients with a prior patellar fracture or traumatic injury had good or excellent results compared with only 81% of patients with recurrent patellar instability. These patients were significantly better than those who had a prior patellectomy with 66% good or excellent results. Similarly, Ferguson[54]

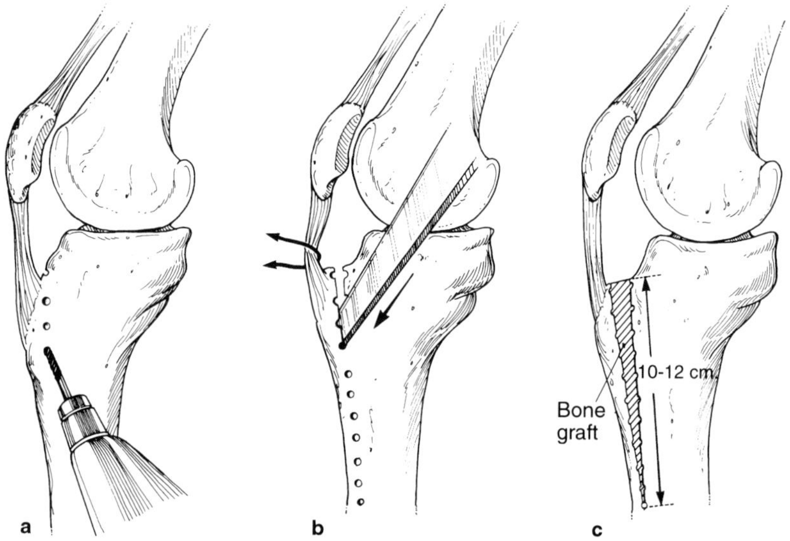

FIGURE 11.18. The Maquet osteotomy elevates the tibial tubercle and is securely held in place with an iliac crest bone graft. (a) The osteotomy site is prepared with multiple drill holes. (b) the completed osteotomy. (c) Elevation of the tibial tubercle is accomplished by insertion of an iliac crest bone graft.

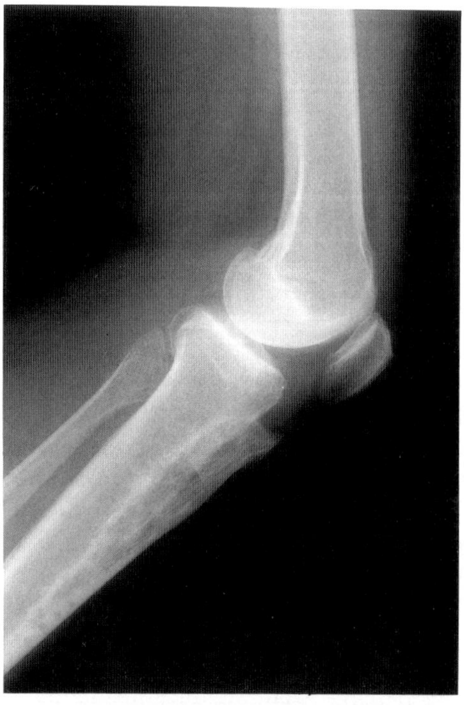

FIGURE 11.19. The healed Maquet osteotomy after a failed Hauser distal realignment.

compared the two- to four-year results and reported that patients with patellar instability had 82% good or excellent results compared with 92% for the patellofemoral osteoarthritis group.

The major criticism of the Maquet osteotomy has been its high complication rate. Depending on the surgeon's technique, the complication rate ranges from 0% to 70%.[50–53,56–58] These range from wound complications, including delayed wound healing, skin necrosis and skin slough requiring muscle flap coverage, wound infections, fractures of the osteotomized tibial tuberosity, and nonunion of the osteotomy site. Modifications in the original technique have reduced the rate of complication.[56,59]

In conclusion, numerous procedures are available for the surgical management of patellar instability as described previously. Because no single procedure corrects all patellofemoral problems, a careful assessment of the etiology of the dysfunction, the condition of the articular surface, and the level of patient activity should influence the treatment.

TABLE 11.2. The results of the Maquet osteotomy for recurrent patellar instability.

Study	No. cases	Average age (years)	Followup (years)	Results	
				Good/excellent	Fair/poor
Radin	16	28	3.5	13 (81%)	3 (19%)
Ferguson	40	21	2–4	33 (82%)	7 (18%)

References

1. MacNab I: Recurrent dislocation of the patella. *J Bone Joint Surg Am* 1952;34A:957.
2. Schreiber SN: Arthroscopic lateral retinacular release using a modified superomedial portal, electrosurgery and postoperative positioning in flexion. *Orthop Rev* 1988;17:375.
3. Hughston JC: Subluxation of the patella. *J Bone Joint Surg Am* 1968;50A:1003–1026.
4. Hughston JC: Reconstruction of the extensor mechanism for subluxing patella. *Am J Sports Med* 1972;1:6–13.
5. Vainionpaa S, Laasonen E, Silvennoinen J, et al.: Acute dislocation of the patella: A prospective review of operative treatment. *J Bone Joint Surg Br* 1990;72B:366–369.
6. Krodel A, Refior HJ: Patellar dislocation as a cause of osteochondral fracture of the femoropatellar joint. Unfallchirurgie 1990;16(1):12–17.
7. Poggi JJ, Garrett WE, Bassett FH, et al.: Presented at the 19th Annual Meeting of the American Orthopaedic Society for Sports Medicine, 1993.
8. Virolainen H, Visuri T, and Kuusela T: Acute dislocation of the patella: MR findings. *Radiology* 1993;189(1):243–246.
9. Scuderi GR: Surgical treatment for patellar instability. *Orthop Clin North Am* 1992;23(4):619–630.
10. Steine HA, Shelbourne KD, Rettig AC, et al.: Conservative treatment of patella dislocations in an athletic population. *Orthop Trans* 1992;16(1):41.
11. Yamamoto RK: Arthroscopic repair of the medial retinaculum and capsule in acute patellar dislocations. *Arthroscopy* 1986;2:125–131.
12. Small NC, Glogau AI, Berezin NA: Arthroscopically assisted proximal extensor mechanism realignment of the knee. *Arthroscopy* 1993;9:63–67.
13. Gigli C, Mariani PP: Arthroscopy in acute dislocation of the patella: A new surgical technique. *G Chir* 1991;12(3):115–117.
14. Merchant AC, Mercer RL: Lateral release of the patella: A preliminary report. *Clin Orthop* 1974;103:40–45.
15. Gecha SR, Torg JS: Clinical prognostications for the efficacy of retinacular release surgery to treat patellofemoral pain. *Clin Orthop* 1990;253:203–208.
16. Metcalf RW: An arthroscopic method for lateral release of the subluxing or dislocating patella. *Clin Orthop* 1982;167:9–18.
17. Insall JN: Disorders of the patella, in Insall JN (ed.): *Surgery of the Knee*. New York, Churchill Livingstone, 1984, pp. 191–260.
18. Ficat P, Phillippe J, Cuzacq JP, et al.: Le syndrome d'hypernession externe de la rotule. *J Radiol* 1972;53:845.
19. Madigan R, Wissinger HA, Donaldson WF: Preliminary experience with a method of quadricepsplasty in recurrent subluxation of the patella. *J Bone Joint Surg Am* 1975;57A:600–607.
20. Insall J, Bullough PG, Burstein AH: Proximal "tube" realignment of the patella for chondromalacia patellae. *Clin Orthop* 1979;244:63–69.
21. Insall JN, Aglietti P, and Tria AJ Jr: Patellar pain and incongruence. II Clinical application. *Clin Orthop* 1983;176:225–232.
22. Sherman OH, Fox J, Sperling H, et al.: Patellar instability: Treatment by arthroscopic electrosurgical lateral release. *Arthroscopy* 1978;3:152.
23. Scuderi G, Cuomo F, Scott WN: Lateral release and proximal realignment for patellar subluxation and dislocation. *J Bone Joint Surg Am* 1988;70A:856–861.
24. Chrisman OD, Snook GA, Wilson TC: A long term prospective study of the Hauser and Roux Goldthwait procedures for recurrent patella dislocation. *Clin Orthop* 1979;244:27–30.
25. Crosby EB, Insall J: Recurrent dislocation of the patella: Relation of treatment to osteoarthritis. *J Bone Joint Surg Am* 1976;58A:9–13.
26. DeCesare WF: Late results of Hauser procedure for recurrent dislocations of the patella. *J Bone Joint Surg Br* 1989;71B:121–125.
27. Tegner Y, Lysholm J: Rating systems in the evaluation of knee ligament injuries. *Clin Orthop* 1985;298:43–49.
28. Abraham E, Washington E, Huang TL: Insall

proximal realignment for disorders of the patella. *Clin Orthop* 1989;248:61–65.
29. Freeman BL: Recurrent dislocations, in Crenshaw AH (ed.): *Campbell's Operative Orthopaedics,* ed. 7. St. Louis, CV Mosby Co., 1987, pp. 2173–2218.
30. Hauser EDW: Total tendon transplant for slipping patella. *Surg Gynecol Obstet* 1938;66:199–214.
31. Hughston JC, Walsh WM: Proximal and distal reconstruction of the extensor mechanism for patellar subluxation. *Clin Orthop* 1979;144:36–42.
32. Dougherty J, Wirth CR, Akbarnia BA: Management of patellar subluxation: A modification of Hauser's technique. *Clin Orthop* 1976; 115:204.
33. Hampson WGJ, Hill P: Late results of transfer of the tibial tubercle for recurrent dislocation of the patella. *J Bone Joint Surg Br* 1975;57B: 209.
34. Galiazzi R: Nuove application del trapianto muscolare e tendineo (XII Congress Societa Italiana di Ortopedia). Archivio Di Ortopedia. 1922, p. 38.
35. Baker RH, Caroll N, Dewar FP, et al.: The semitendinosus tenodesis for recurrent dislocation of the patella. *J Bone Joint Surg Br* 1972;54B: 103.
36. Roux C: Luxation habituelle de la rotule: Traitement operatoire. *Rev Chir Orthop Reparatrice Appar Mot* 1888;8:682.
37. Goldthwait JE: Dislocation of the patella. *Trans Am Orthop Assoc* 1895;8:237.
38. Bowker JH, Thompson EB: Surgical treatment of recurrent dislocation of the patella. *J Bone Joint Surg Am* 1964;46A:1451.
39. Fondren FB, Goldner JL, Bassett FH: Recurrent dislocation of the patella treated by the modified Roux-Goldthwait procedure: A prospective study of 47 knees. *J Bone Joint Surg Am* 1985;67A:993.
40. Trillat A, DeJour H, Couette A: Diagnostic et traitement des sublux-recidivantes de la rotule. *Rev Chir Orthop Reparatrice Appar Mot* 1979; 50:185–191.
41. Cox JS: Evaluation of the Roux-Elmslie-Trillat procedure for knee extensor realignment. *Am J Sports Med* 1982;10(5):303–310.
42. Cox JS: An evaluation of the Elmslie-Trillat procedure for management of patellar dislocations and subluxation. A preliminary report. *Am J Sports Med* 1976;4:72–77.
43. DeBurge A, Chambat P: La transposition de la tuberosite tibiale anterieure. *Rev Chir Orthop Reparatrice Appar Mot* 1980;66(4):218.
44. Cerullo G, Puddu G, Conteduca F, et al.: Evaluation of the results of extensor mechanism reconstruction. *Am J Sports Med* 1988;16(2): 93.
45. Fulkerson JP: Anteromedialization of the tibial tuberosity for patellofemoral malalignment. *Clin Orthop* 1983;177:176–181.
46. Post WR, Fulkerson JP: Distal realignment of the patellofemoral joint: Indications, effects, results and recommendations. *Orthop Clin North Am* 1992;23(4):631–643.
47. Fulkerson JP, Becker GJ, Meaney JA, et al.: Anteromedial tibial tubercle transfer without bone graft. *Am J Sports Med* 1990;18:490–497.
48. Fulkerson JP, Hungerford DS: Surgical treatment of patellofemoral chondrosis and arthrosis, in *Disorders of the Patellofemoral Joint,* ed. 2. Baltimore, Williams & Wilkins Co., 1990, pp. 226–246.
49. Maquet P: Un traitment biomecanique de l'arthrose femoro-patellaire: L'avancement du tendon rotulien. *Rev Rhum Mal Osteoartic* 1963; 30:779.
50. Maquet P: Advancement of the tibial tuberosity. *Clin Orthop* 1976;115:225.
51. Rappoport LH, Browne MG, Wickiewicz TL: The Maquet osteotomy. *Orthop Clin North Am* 1992;23(4):645–656.
52. Rozbruch JD, Campbell RD, Insall J: Tibial tubercle elevation (The Maquet operation): A clinical study of 31 cases. *Orthop Trans* 1979; 3:291.
53. Radin EL: Anterior tibial tubercle elevation in the young adult. *Orthop Clin North Am* 1986; 27:297.
54. Ferguson AB: Elevation of the insertion of the patellar ligament for patellofemoral pain. *J Bone Joint Surg Am* 1982;64A:766.
55. Heatley FW, Allen PR, Patrick JH: Tibial tubercle advancement for anterior knee pain: A temporary or permanent solution. *Clin Orthop* 1986;208:215.
56. Heller H, Hadjipavlou A, Helmy H, et al.: Chondromalacia of the patella treated by the Maquet tibial tubercle osteotomy. *J Bone Joint Surg Br* 1982;65B:262.
57. Hirsh DM, Reddy DK: Experience with Maquet anterior tibial tubercle advancement for patellofemoral arthralgia. *Clin Orthop* 1980; 148:136.
58. Hofmann AA, Wyatt RWB, Jones RE: Combined Coventry-Maquet procedure for two-

compartment degenerative arthritis. *Clin Orthop* 1984;190:186.
59. Radin EL: The Maquet procedure—Anterior displacement of the tibial tubercle: Indications, contraindications, and precautions. *Clin Orthop* 1986;213:241.

12

Osteotomy of the Patellofemoral Joint

Alan Nagel and Giles R. Scuderi

Patellofemoral instability can manifest during flexion, yet most often occurs during early extension when the intrinsic stability of the patellofemoral joint is at a minimum. According to Bohm,[1] the developing fetus has a relatively flat patellar articular surface and corresponding femoral trochlea. It is during the course of development, particularly after ambulation begins, that the femoral condyles become more prominent, the sulcus deepens, and the patella assumes its characteristic bifaceted appearance. According to Malkin,[2] with terminal knee extension, there is external rotation of the tibia upon the femur, known as the *screw home mechanism,* which increases the Q angle. This rotational movement increases the pressure of the lateral femoral condyle. As long as this pressure remains within physiologic limits, growth of the anterior lateral trochlea is stimulated. Though the etiology of patellofemoral dysplasia is unknown, interference with the normal developmental anatomy as detailed previously is a probable contributing factor. In patellofemoral dysplasia, the articular surface of the patella is flat and the anterior lateral condyle, and sometimes the anterior medial condyle, "lie lower" than normal. Consequently, there is no lateral buttress to prevent lateral subluxation or dislocation of the patella. The normal lateral directing forces of the quadriceps mechanism go unrestrained and the patella tracks laterally.

Dysplasias of the patellofemoral joint have been previously described in the literature and implicated in patellar instability. Outerbridge[3] and Brattstrom[4] have reported on dysplasias of the femoral sulcus, while Wiberg[5] has described variation in the patellar shape. It is not rare to encounter a flat sulcus, where patellar stability is dependent upon retinacular attachments and muscle balance.

The intimate relationship between the femoral sulcus and the patella is dependent upon their conformity and constraint. Schultzer et al.[6] have reported that dysplasia of the femoral sulcus mainly occurs proximally with flattening of the anterior aspect of the lateral femoral condyle. In turn, the femoral sulcus normally deepens as it approaches the intercondylar notch, enhancing patellar stability in flexion.

Computed tomography (CT) scan or magnetic resonance imaging (MRI) has been helpful in assessing the morphology of the femoral sulcus. The information gathered from cadaveric measurements and imaging techniques have allowed a set of normal values to be established for the femoral sulcus and the patella. Normally, the femoral sulcus angle decreases from 146° at full extension to 128° at 30° of flexion (Figure 12.1). This reemphasizes the point that the femoral sulcus is broad proximally and deepens as the intercondylar notch is approached. Cadaveric measurements by Keene and Marans[7] have also substantiated the femoral sulcus angle with a range of 130° to 148°; again, these values are dependent upon the degree of knee flexion. It is not unusual to encounter a femoral sulcus angle greater than 148°, which appears as a flat sulcus. However, if there is lack of congruence

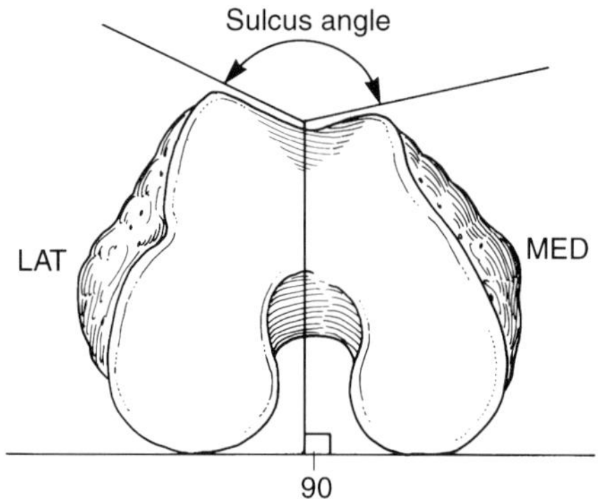

FIGURE 12.1. The femoral sulcus angle.

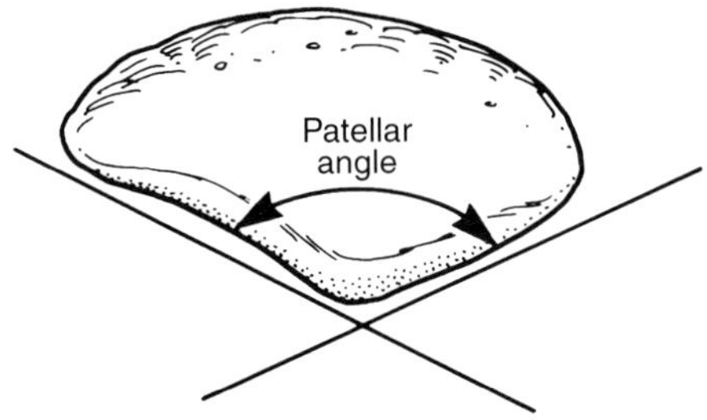

FIGURE 12.2. The patellar angle.

of the patellofemoral articulation and inadequate soft-tissue restraints, then this may lead to recurrent patellar instability.

In a similar fashion, the morphology of the patella influences the stability of the extensor mechanism. In 1941, Wiberg[5] classified the patellar shape on axial radiographic views based on the configuration of the medial and the lateral facets. Later, in 1970, Ficat[8] proposed another radiographic classification based on the angle formed by lines drawn parallel to the medial and the lateral facets. This is termed the *patellar angle* (Figure 12.2) and is dependent upon proximal or distal location at which it is measured. The normal values range from 118° to 127°. Several unusual patellar shapes have also been implicated with instability. The pebble-shaped patella, because of its small size, is unstable. The half-moon patella has a single facet and is often associated with recurrent patellar instability, while the Alpine hunter's cap has an angle of almost 90°, appears as a hemipatella, and is associated with lateral instability (Figure 12.3). Keene and Marans[7] recently measured the patellar angle on CT scans of cadaveric knees and reported that the angle varies from 118° to 127°, depending on the distance from the superior pole of the patella.

Numerous procedures have been described to address patellar instability. The majority of these procedures are directed towards realigning the extensor mechanism, either by releasing tight structures or by reinforcing loose tissues. The challenge is in the presence of patellofemoral dysplasia. These soft-tissue procedures may not be beneficial. Therefore, it may be prudent to direct surgical correction towards the underlying dysplasia.

Historical Perspective

Osteotomy of the patellofemoral joint dates back to 1891, when Pollard[9] "chiseled" out the lateral wall of the trochlea and imbricated the medial capsule in a young girl with chronic dislocation of the patella. In 1904, Graser[10] described a rotational supracondylar osteotomy of the femur for the correction of habitual patellar dislocaters with femoral torsional deformities. Graser felt that this procedure would raise the lateral condylar support, preventing dislocation. From a biomechanical perspective, this would result in an increased Q angle, which may potentiate instability.

In 1914, Luxembourg[11] reported on a "bone barrier" procedure where a fibular strut was placed in a trough created on the anterior lateral trochlea, effectively acting as a buttress to prevent lateral dislocation. In 1915, Albee[12] performed an open-wedge osteotomy of the anterior lateral condyle in patients with patellofemoral dysplasia and recurrent dislocation. In 1950, Brissard[13] performed a variation of Albee's procedure. He created the osteotomy more proximal on the femoral cortex, aiming to give the patella more stability in full extension. He called this the "Albee Superior Osteotomy." In 1978, Morscher[14] reported on the longitudinal open-wedge patellar osteotomy in patients with chondromalacia and ad-

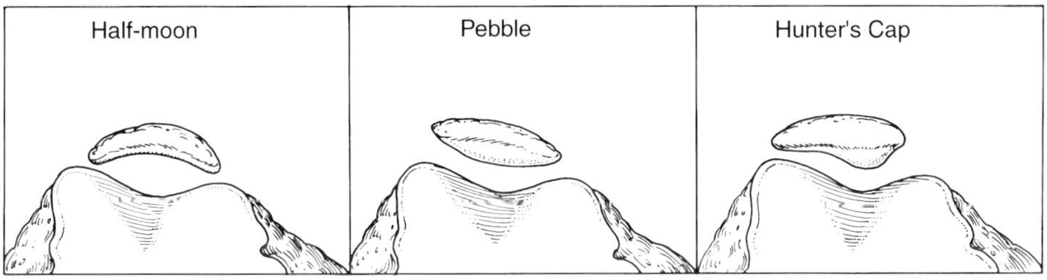

FIGURE 12.3. Variations in patellar shape.

vanced arthritis. In 1988, Peterson et al.[15] reported on a combined procedure where he deepened the femoral trochlea, and performed both proximal and distal realignments, lateral release, medial capsular duplication, and vastus medialis transposition in patients with patellofemoral dysplasia. Most recently, Keene and Marans[7] have described a two-plane sagittal closing wedge osteotomy of the patella and a three-plane radial opening wedge osteotomy of the lateral femoral trochlea. They advocate this procedure for patients with recurrent dislocation secondary to severe patellofemoral dysplasia.

Indications

Keene and Marans[7] have presented the indication for osteotomy of the patella and the femoral sulcus. These include recurrent patella dislocation with radiographic evidence of patellofemoral dysplasia, which is manifested by a sulcus angle greater than 158° and a patellar angle greater than 147°.

Today, osteotomy about the patellofemoral joint is performed for either patellofemoral dysplasia or arthritic conditions. In patellofemoral dysplasia, the osteotomy attempts to restore a more normal anatomy, prevent dislocation, and facilitate improved tracking of the extensor mechanism. In cases of isolated patellofemoral arthritis, the main purpose of osteotomy is to relieve pain. Theoretically, this is accomplished through a reduction of elevated intraosseous pressure, increased patellofemoral contact area, and improved cartilaginous nutrition.

Arnoldi et al.[16,17] have reported extensively on the association of increased juxta-articular medullary pressure and arthritic pain in both the hip and the knee. Björkstrom et al.[18] measured the patella intraosseous pressure in patients with chondromalacia and arthritis, and compared these values to controls. They found that while controls had an average value of 19 mm Hg, patients with chondromalacia averaged 44 mm Hg, and those with arthritis, 37 mm Hg. Nerubay and Katnelson[19] measured the patellar intraosseous pressure in 15 patients prior to and following coronal plane osteotomy. They found that preoperatively, the values averaged 19 mm Hg and post operatively, they fell to 9 mm Hg in both anterior and posterior fragments. They concluded that relief of pain following osteotomy is attributed to a reduction in elevated intraosseous pressure.

Types of Osteotomy

The literature is filled with numerous procedures describing osteotomy about the patellofemoral joint. Those illustrated here have either demonstrated favorable results or reflect sound biomechanical principles.

1. The longitudinal osteotomy was advocated by Morscher.[20] In patients with lateral subluxation, Morscher feels that loss of medial contact pressure with increased lateral contact pressure is the cause of both pain and chondromalacia. Through this osteotomy, Morscher feels that this imbalance will be corrected, increased intraosseous pressure will be reduced, and overall improved cartilaginous nutrition will occur.[20] He reported a four-year followup on 18 osteotomies in 15 patients.

Eleven patients were pain-free, 6 improved, and 1 resulted in persistent pain. Subjectively, eight patients were absolutely enthusiastic and nine were satisfied. One patient had a poor result and underwent a second procedure. Peccina[21] reported 76% excellent results, 20% good, and 4% fair after longitudinal osteotomy. Hejgaard and Arnoldi[22] reported that 37 of 40 patients had highly significant relief of pain five to 19 months following this procedure.

2. The coronal osteotomy and some of its variations have been advocated by several authors.[19,23,24] After a lateral release is carried out, a coronal osteotomy is performed in a lateral to medial direction using an oscillating saw. The displacement is produced by flexing and extending the knee. No internal fixation or cast is used and the patient is mobilized relatively early postoperatively. Nerubay and Katnelson[19] reported 80% good to excellent results, 13% fair, and 7% poor one to five years after coronal plane osteotomy in patients with patellofemoral arthritis. No loss of knee motion was reported, but slight quadriceps atrophy was noted in some patients. Deliss,[23] also reporting on the coronal plane osteotomy for treatment of chondromalacia, found poorer results in females than in males. Further, those males who did well were younger (ages 25 to 29), performed manual labor, had symptoms less than three years, and has no previous knee surgery. Conversely, those who did poorly were older (age greater than 34), had previous knee surgery, and had advanced radiographic evidence of patellofemoral arthritis. In his series there was one nonunion.

3. The technique of Paar[25] combined an open-wedge longitudinal patellar osteotomy with deepening of the femoral trochlea in patients with patellofemoral dysplasia. Currently, this procedure is still experimental, with limited followup. Peterson et al.[15] reported a six-year followup on 21 patients who underwent the combined procedure for instability secondary to dysplasia. In their procedure, Peterson and co-workers added proximal and distal realignments, lateral release, and vastus medialis transposition to femoral trochlea osteotomy. Peterson et al. found that 13 patients had excellent results, 5 good, 2 fair, and 1 poor.

4. In patients with instability because of patellofemoral dysplasia, the technique of Keene and Marans[7] biomechanically addresses the underlying abnormality. Here the patellar osteotomy is a sagittal closing wedge that will decrease the patella angle. Their technique removes a pie-shaped wedge of patellar bone with a width at the anterior cortex of 7 to 9 mm, depending on the degree of angular correction necessary. Keene and Marans found that each millimeter of base width resected decreased the patellar angle 3.5°. The apex of the osteotomy is directed towards the central ridge of the patella and through the subchondral bone. The articular surface should be left intact, acting as a hinge as the osteotomy is closed. With the osteotomy closed, the patella is securely fixed with two screws, maintaining compression of the osteotomy site (Figure 12.4).

The femoral osteotomy, a three-plane radial open wedge, will correspondingly decrease the sulcus angle (Figure 12.5). This femoral osteotomy is based on the nonarticular side of the lateral femoral condyle. The apex of the osteotomy is at the apex of the femoral sulcus, while the inferior portion of the cut penetrates only the subchondral bone with caution not to violate the articular surface. The osteotomy is gently levered open and packed with bone graft; usually the bone from the patella osteotomy is suitable for this purpose. With the bone graft in place, the osteotomy is stable and does not need supplemental fixation.

Postoperatively, the patient is kept partial weight bearing with crutches. Gentle range of motion exercises are allowed until the osteotomy is healed, which usually takes about six weeks. Following complete healing of the osteotomy, strengthening exercises are initiated.

Conclusion

In this chapter, we have discussed two disorders of the patellofemoral joint that remain problematic to the clinician. Our initial approach to these problems is conservative and consists of quadriceps strengthening and re-

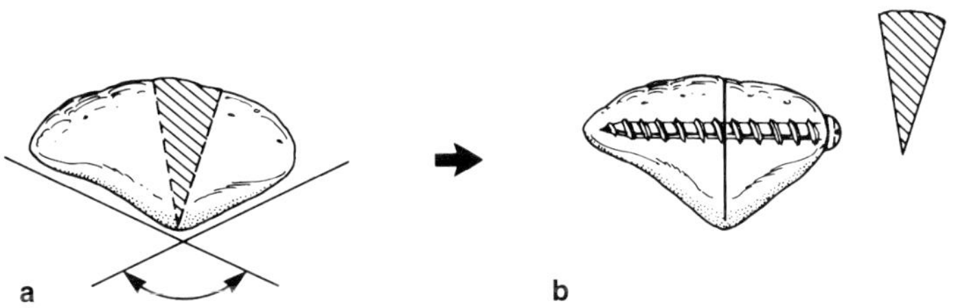

FIGURE 12.4. (a) Closing wedge osteotomy of the patella. (b) The osteomy is securely fixed with a screw.

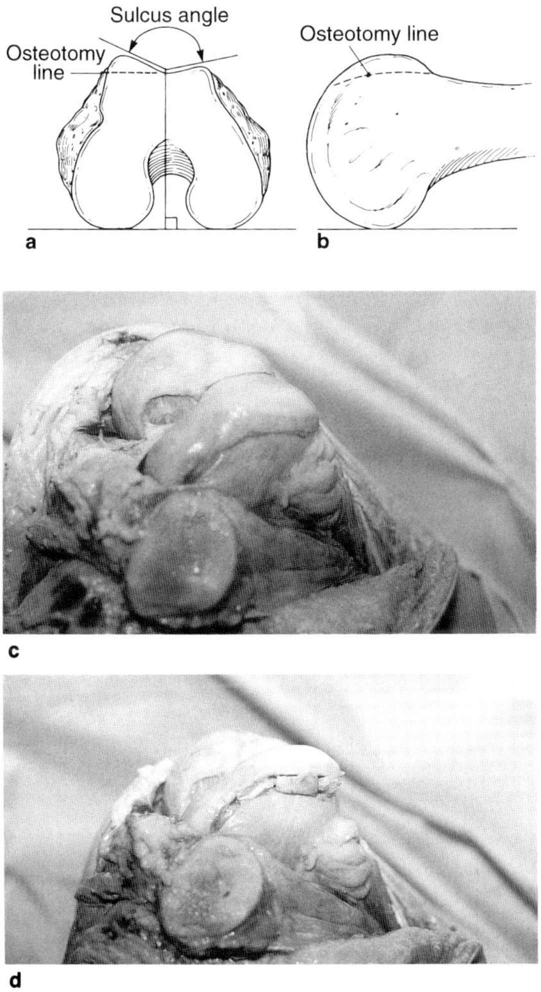

FIGURE 12.5. (a, b) The three-plane femoral osteotomy of Keene and Marans. (c, d) Intraoperative photograph of the planned site of the osteotomy at the lateral femoral condyle. The osteotomy site is levered up and packed with bone graft.

habilitation. If these modalities are unsuccessful, realignment procedures are considered, if appropriate. Osteotomy remains an alternative; however, we feel that more controlled long-term studies with greater numbers are needed before its true value can be measured. Historically, osteotomy has been performed more commonly abroad than here in the United States. Recently, however, there have been reports of more osteotomies of the patellofemoral joint being performed here in North America as clinicians explore new options in treating these difficult disorders.

References

1. Bohm M: Das menschliche bein herman gocht (red) deutsche *Orthopade* 1935.
2. Malkin SA: Dislocation of the patella. *Br Med J* 1932;11:91–94.
3. Outerbridge RE: Further studies on the etiology of chondromalacia patellae. *J Bone Joint Surg Br* 1964;46B:179–190.
4. Brattstrom H: Shape of the intercondylar groove normally and in recurrent dislocation of the patella: A clinical and x-ray anatomical investigation. *Acta Orthop Scand* 1964; 68(suppl.):1.
5. Wiberg G: Roentgenographic and anatomic studies on the femoro-patellar joint. *Acta Orthop Scand* 1941;12:319–410.
6. Schultzer SF, Ramsby GR, Fulkerson JP: Computed tomographic classifications of patellofemoral pain patients. *Orthop Clin North Am* 1986;17:235.
7. Keene GCR, Marans HJ: Osteotomy for patellofemoral dysplasia, in Fox JM, Del Pizzo W (eds.): *The Patellofemoral Joint.* New York, McGraw-Hill Book Co., 1993, pp. 169–176.
8. Ficat P: *Pathologie Femoro-Patellaire.* Paris, Masson et Cie, 1970.
9. Pollard A: An old dislocation of the patella reduced by an intraarticular operation. *Lancet* 1891;1:988.
10. Graser E: Behandlung der Lux. pat. inveterata durch Osteotomie am Femur mit Drehung der

Epiphyse. *Verh Dtsch Ges Chir* 1904;33:II:457–466.
11. Luxembourg H: Zur Behandlung der habit. *Pat Lux Med Klin* 1914;10:I:1013–1014.
12. Albee FM: The bone graft wedge in the treatment of habitual dislocation of the patella. *Med Rec* 1915;88:257–259.
13. Brissard P: Tactique op. dans le traitement des lux cong. et recidiv. de la rotul. *Acta Orthop Belg* 1950;16:452–456.
14. Morscher E: Osteotomy of the patella in chondromalacia preliminary report. *Arch Orthop Trauma Surg* 1978;92:139–147.
15. Peterson L, Karlsson J, Brittberg M: Patellar instability with recurrent dislocation due to patellofemoral dysplasia results after surgical treatment. *Bull Hosp Jt Dis* 1988;48:130–138.
16. Arnoldi CC, Lemperg RK, Linderholm H: Interosseous hypertension and pain in the knee *J Bone Joint Surg* 1975;57B(3):360–363.
17. Arnoldi CC, Lemperg RK, Linderholm H: Immediate effect of osteotomy on the intramedullary pressure of the femoral head and neck in patients with degenerative osteoarthritis. *Acta Orthop Scand* 1971;42:454–455.
18. Björkstrom S, Goldie IF, Wetterquist H: Intramedullary pressure of the patella in chondromalacia. *Arch Orthop Trauma Surg* 1980;97:81–85.
19. Nerubay J, Katnelson A: Osteotomy of the patella. *Clin Orthop* 1986;207:103–107.
20. Morscher E: Indikation und moglichkeiten der patella-keilosteomie. *Orthopade* 1985;14:261–265.
21. Peccina M: Longitudinal osteotomy of the patella and anterior displacement of the patella one stage procedure, in 16th Congress London 1984—poster presentation.
22. Hejgaard N, Arnoldi CC: Osteotomy of the patella in the patella pain syndrome. *Int Orthop* 1984;8:189–194.
23. Deliss L: Coronal patellar osteotomy: Preliminary report of its use in chondromalacia patellae. *Proc R Soc Med* 1977;70:257–259.
24. Vaguero J, and Arriaza R: The patella thinning osteotomy. *Int Orthop* 1992;16:372–376.
25. Paar O: Vertiefung der trochlea femoris und osteotomie der patella als mögliche kausale therapie der rezidivierenden traumatischen patellaluxation. *Unfallchirurgie* 1987; 90: 435–440.

13

Traumatic Maladies of the Extensor Mechanism

James V. Bono, Steven B. Haas, and Giles R. Scuderi

Extensor mechanism injuries can occur in patients of all ages. An understanding of the biomechanics of the patellofemoral joint is essential in diagnosing and treating these conditions. Identification of a mechanical derangement is necessary to correct the underlying cause of the patients complaints. A distinction must be made between bone and soft-tissue injury, and that between acute and chronic injury. There are many causes of extensor mechanism injuries that may be discussed. This chapter will focus on four principal extensor mechanism injuries: (1) patellar and quadriceps tendinitis, (2) quadriceps rupture, (3) patellar tendon rupture, and (4) patellar fractures.

Patellar and Quadriceps Tendinitis

Patellar and quadriceps tendinitis are overuse syndromes defined as repetitive overloading of the patellar tendon and quadriceps tendon. This results in an irritation to the patellar and the quadriceps tendons, as well as the inferior and superior aspect of the patellae, and is related to activity duration and intensity. Typically, patients complain of knee aching; point tenderness may be found along the inferior or superior pole of the patella. Occasionally, patients may experience pain along the tibial tuberosity, peripatellar soft tissues, or along the entire length of the patellar or the quadriceps tendon.

Jumper's knee is a typical functional overload injury because it affects those athletes who submit their knee extensor mechanisms to intense and repeated stress. Defined as an insertional tendinopathy, jumper's knee affects, in order of frequency, the insertion of the patellar tendon into the patella (65% of cases), attachment of the quadriceps tendon to the patella (25%), and the attachment of the patellar tendon to the tibial tuberosity (10%). Tendinitis results from repetitive overloading and therefore presents insidiously, most commonly in athletes participating in running or jumping sports such as basketball, volleyball, high jumping, and aerobic exercise.[1] The type of practice surface and type of footwear, as well as the intensity and the frequency of training are factors that may contribute to the incidence of patellar and quadriceps tendinitis.[1] A high level of performance in these athletes can be maintained, provided they avoid jumping activities. Patellar and quadriceps tendinitis in nonathletes may interfere with activities of daily living, such as stair climbing, kneeling, and getting up from a chair. Ascending and descending stairs frequently are problematic due to the high patellofemoral loads and eccentric loading of the quadriceps that create increased compressive forces across the patellofemoral joint. A thorough history will determine the degree of involvement and aid in organizing a treatment plan.

The bone tendon junction has been implicated as the site of inflammatory injury, presumably from microscopic or macroscopic ruptures of the ligament.[1] This may manifest itself radiographically as elongation or fragmentation of the inferior pole, a periosteal reaction of the anterior patella, or calcification of the patellar tendon.

Biomechanical derangements may also contribute to patellar and quadriceps tendinitis. Poor flexibility of the lower extremity, especially tight quadriceps, creates increased loading of the patellofemoral joint. Any patellofemoral asymmetry is capable of concentrating stresses focally, resulting in local irritation and inflammation. Patella alta, baja, subluxation, and hypermobility all are capable of altering patellofemoral physiology, as are angular and rotational deformities or limb length discrepancies. Malalignment of the patella will predispose the patient to anterior knee pain and the possibility of articular cartilage breakdown.[2]

Blazina et al.[3] have developed a classification system for patellar tendinitis. Phase I is defined as pain after activity only. Phase II describes pain that occurs before and after, but not during the activity. Phase III describes pain occurring during and after activity that results in functional impairment sufficient to interfere with performance. Both phase I and II respond well to conservative treatment; symptoms usually resolve after a period of rest. Activities should be modified to protect the extensor mechanism from eccentric or high loads. Activities that aggravate the patient's symptoms are avoided; other training modalities must be used. All other activities may be continued. A period of warm-up and stretching should occur prior to sports participation. Restoring flexibility and strength are critical if muscle atrophy is to be avoided. All muscle strengthening should be done in the pain-free range, so as not to further injure the inflamed tissues. Isometric exercises are used to minimize compressive forces across the patellofemoral joint. Short arc quadriceps exercises are especially effective in strengthening the vastus medialis obliquus (VMO). It should be emphasized that muscle strengthening and stretching are the mainstay of treatment. Therapeutic modalities such as ultrasound, phonophoresis, or iontophoresis have been used to decrease patellofemoral pain. Ice packs may be applied immediately following activity, and have been advocated by many authors.[4,5] A general conditioning program should be started to improve muscle tone and flexibility. In order for the inflamed tissues to heal, a period of activity modification is necessary. Jumping and eccentric loading of the extensor mechanism is discouraged. A short course of nonsteroidal anti-inflammatory medication may help control swelling and inflammation, and provide pain relief. An external support to provide proprioceptive feedback may be of benefit.

Peripatellar bursitis is a common occupationally related condition that should not be confused with either patellar or quadriceps tendinitis. Soft-tissue irritation in the anterior aspect of the knee has been associated with occupations that require kneeling postures, such as carpet laying and floor laying. "Housemaid's knee" refers to inflammation of the prepatellar bursa, which usually covers the lower half of the patella and the upper half of the patellar tendon. Inflammation of the deep infrapatellar bursa is recognized as pain, tenderness, and swelling localized between the lower part of the patellar tendon and the upper part of the tibia. Treatment of peripatellar bursitis is usually symptomatic, generally responding to conservative measures and avoidance of kneeling postures. Rarely, infection of the deep infrapatellar and prepatellar bursae can develop; these cases require antibiotics and adequate irrigation and drainage.

Soft-Tissue Disruptions

Anatomy

The quadriceps musculature, the quadriceps tendon, the patella, and the patella tendon all contribute to the extensor mechanism of the knee. The structure of the quadriceps musculature is composed of the rectus femoris, the vastus medialis, the vastus lateralis, and the vastus intermedius, which coalesce in a trilaminar fashion to form the quadriceps tendon. The rectus femoris, which is the most superficial component, takes origin from the ilium and narrows to a tendon approximately 3 to 5 cm superior to the patella. The fibers of the quadriceps tendon continue over the anterior surface of the patella and into the patella tendon. The vastus medialis is divided into two groups: (1) the VMO and (2) the vastus medialis longus. These muscle fibers continue toward the superomedial border of the patella and become tendinous a few millimeters before their insertion. In contrast, the muscle fibers of the vastus lateralis terminate more proximally than the vastus medialis, becoming tendinous approximately 3 cm from the superolateral border of the patella. The vastus intermedius lies deep to the other three muscles and its tendinous fibers insert directly into the superior border of the patella, blending medially and laterally with the vastus medialis and the vastus lateralis. The lateral and medial retinaculum receive contributing aponeurotic fibers from both the vastus lateralis and the vastus medialis, respectively.[6]

The patella tendon is primarily derived from the central fibers of the rectus femoris, which extend over the anterior surface of the patella. This condensation of fibers forms a flat tendinous structure that inserts into the tibial tubercle. The patellar tendon narrows approximately 15% as it courses to the tibial tubercle; this represents the anatomic "taper" of the patellar tendon.[7] As the tendon continues past the tubercle, it blends with the iliotibial band on the anterior surface of the tibia. The average length of the patella tendon is 4.3 to 4.6 cm (range 2.0 to 6.5 cm).[7,8]

McMaster experimented with muscle and tendon ruptures in rabbits and showed that normal tendons do not rupture under stress and that linear stress causes disruption at the musculotendinous junction, the muscle belly, or the tendinous insertion into the bone.[9] Therefore, tendinous rupture occurs through the pathologic area of the tendon. It has been shown that the normal quadriceps tendon may be able to tolerate up to 30 kg/mm of longitudinal stress before failing. The estimated force required to disrupt the extensor mechanism of the knee is 17.5 times body weight, and usually occurs during a sudden eccentric contraction of the extensor mechanism with the foot planted and the knee flexed as the person falls. Many pathologic conditions can affect the extensor mechanism including renal disease, diabetes mellitus, hyperparathyroidism, rheumatoid arthritis, systemic lupus erythematous, gout, osteomalacia, infection, obesity, fatty degeneration, tendinous calcifications, tenosynovitis, old fractures, tumor,[9,10] steroid use,[11] and other metabolic diseases. These metabolic diseases cause microscopic damage to the vascular supply to the tendons or alter the architecture of the tendon. Diabetes has been shown to cause arteriosclerotic changes to the tendon vessels, while chronic synovitis causes fibrinoid reactions within the tendon. Muscle fiber atrophy, secondary to renal disease and uremia, will also weaken the tendon. Pathologic changes from advancing age include fatty and cystic degeneration, myxoid degeneration, and calcification, which alter the tendon architecture. Bone resorption and osteopenia can also occur at the osteotendinous junction with advancing age.

Historically, Galen first described extensor mechanism injury.[12] In 1887, McBurney published the first report of surgical treatment.[13] In this report, disruption of the tendon was due to a direct blow to the suprapatellar area. A successful result was achieved using catgut and silver wire. At the time of this first report, the predominant method of treatment was nonoperative. Early in the 20th century, surgical treatment became increasingly advocated. Quenu and Duval published their review of 26 cases treated surgically and recommended this form of treatment of extensor mechanism injuries.[14] In 1927, Gallie and LeMesurier described a technique for repairing the quadriceps tendon using a fascia lata femoris strip and presented a review of six cases.[15] Since the early reports of operative repair, surgical management of quadriceps and patellar tendon disruptions has become generally accepted. Numerous surgeons have described techniques and have presented their results.

There appears to be demographic differences in the occurrence of quadriceps and patellar tendon ruptures. In a review of 117 reported cases of tendon rupture between 1880 and 1978, 88% of quadriceps tendon ruptures were in patients 40 years or older.[16] In contrast, 80% of patients with patella tendon ruptures were less than 40 years old. Quadriceps tendon ruptures are also more common in patients with systemic disease or degenerative changes in the knee. Most spontaneous ruptures of the quadriceps tendon occur within 2 cm of the patella with these pathologic areas. Numerous cases of bilateral extensor mechanism ruptures have been reported and include patients with obesity or systemic illness.[10,17–28] Iatrogenic conditions that may alter the local properties of the extensor mechanism include total knee arthroplasty,[29] lateral retinacular release,[30] and harvesting of the central one third of the patella tendon for ligamentous reconstruction.[7,31,32] Local steroid injection has also been implicated as a cause of tendon rupture. Rupture of the quadriceps tendon has also been reported after patellar dislocation.[33]

Disruption of the extensor mechanism is a significantly disabling injury and should be diagnosed early.[34,35] Patients usually present with the acute onset of knee pain, swelling, and loss of function after a stumble or a fall.[6] On physical examination, a palpable defect in the quadriceps tendon is usually appreciated with a low-lying patella. When asked to perform a straight leg raise, the patient may be unable to do so or demonstrates an extensor lag. A patella tendon rupture presents with similar findings; however, the palpable gap is in the patella tendon with a proximally retracted or high-riding patella (Figure 13.1a). Radiographs provide supporting information, especially on the lateral view with a low position of the patella associated with a quadriceps tendon rupture (Figure 13.1b) and a high patella position associated with a patella tendon rupture (Figure 13.1c).[36,37] If there is any doubt, a lateral radiograph of the contralateral knee is recommended in order to determine the normal patella height. Radiographic findings in patients with quadriceps ruptures frequently include degenerative spurring of the patella seen on the tangential view of the patella (tooth sign).[37,38] If there is any doubt to the diagnoses, some authors have suggested that an arthrogram be performed that may reveal extravasation of the dye into the defect.[39] More recently, ultrasound and magnetic resonance imaging (MRI)[40] have aided in making the diagnosis in the partially torn or difficult cases (Figure 13.1d and 13.1e). However, clinically, the examination is specific and these studies are rarely indicated.

Quadriceps Tendon Rupture

Quadriceps tendon ruptures usually occur at the osteotendinous junction or through an area of degenerative tendon. The rupture originates in the tendon of the rectus femoris, often extending into the vastus intermedius tendon or transversely into the medial and lateral retinaculum.[9] Surgical repair should be performed as soon as possible following injury in order to obtain the best results. Cases in which surgery was delayed beyond six weeks have been shown to have inferior results.

Numerous techniques have been described in the literature for the repair of acute and chronic ruptures of the quadriceps tendon.[9,14,16,36,41–44] Over the years, the repair techniques have progressed from simple suture with catgut or silk[13] to wire-reinforced repairs, autografts,[15] xenografts, allografts, and synthetic materials. Conwell and Alldrege,[9] in 1937, described the use of kangaroo tendon for repair, while Gallie and LeMesurier[15] described the use of free fascial grafts. McLaughlin reported on an operative technique in which a traction suture is used to approximate the tendon rupture.[45–47] Using a transverse incision, the tendon ends were debrided. A bolt was passed transversely through the patella and stainless steal suture was then placed across the musculotendinous junction and anchored to the bolt. Limited motion at the knee joint was allowed and the internal fixation was removed at eight weeks postoperatively. McLaughlin has even recommended a two-stage procedure with traction for better approximation of the tendon.[45–47] When there is an acute rupture, direct repair may be obtained.

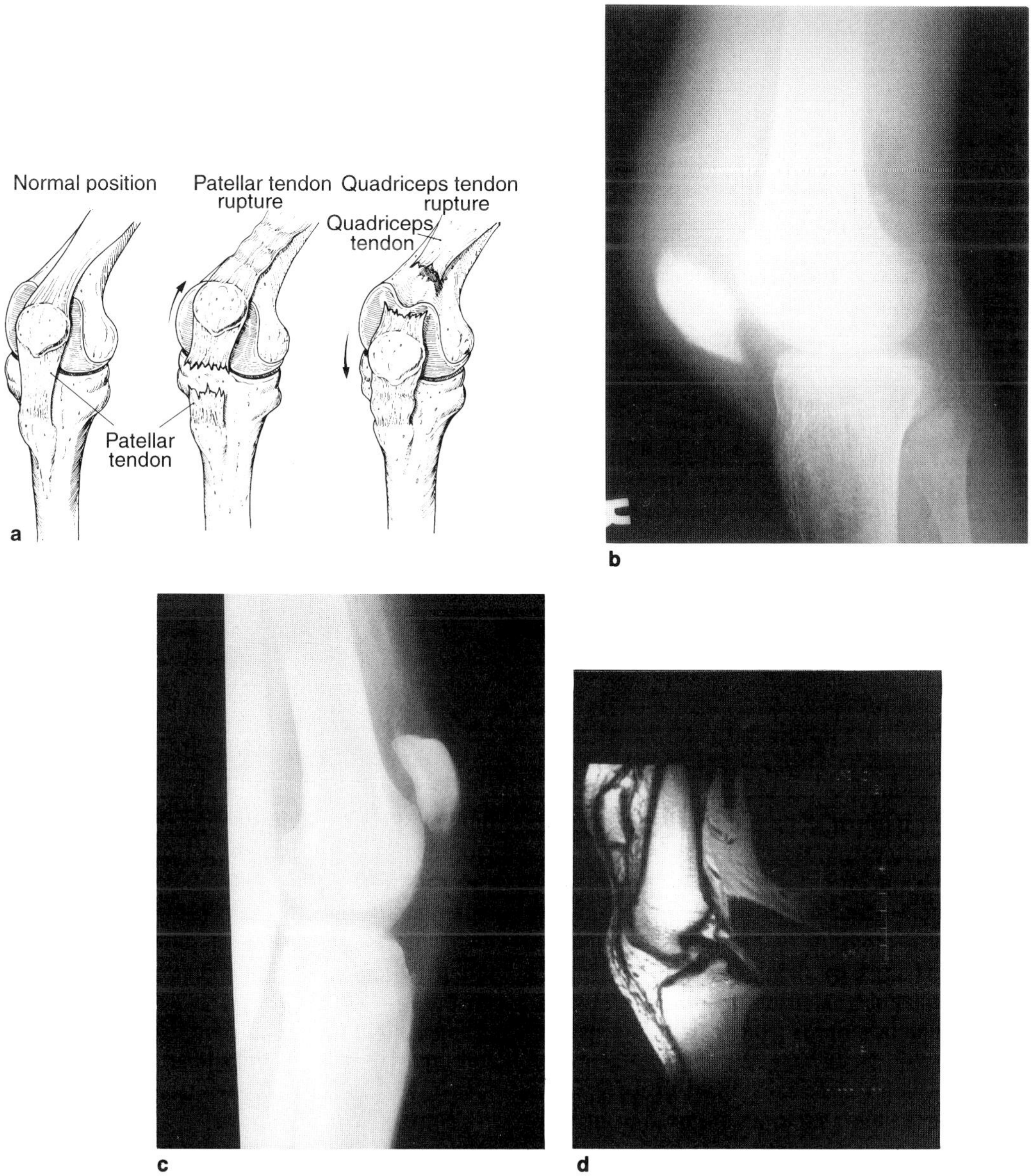

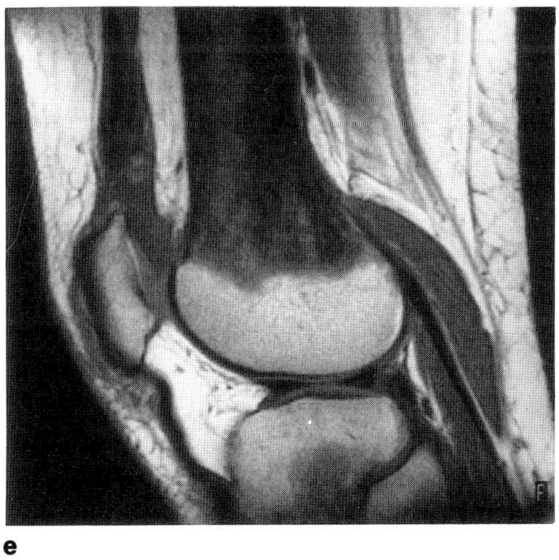

FIGURE 13.1. (a) Diagram of normal position of patellar tendon, the patellar tendon rupture, and the quadriceps tendon rupture. (b) Low position of the patella associated with a quadriceps tendon rupture. (c) High patella position associated with a patella tendon rupture. (d) MRI of a torn patellar tendon. (e) MRI of a torn quadriceps tendon.

Technique

A straight midline incision will expose the quadriceps tendon rupture, which is irrigated of hematoma. The tendon edges are debrided back to healthy tissue; care should be taken to avoid excising an excessive amount of the tendon. If there is sufficient tendon proximally and distally, an end-to-end repair is performed with multiple interrupted no. 2 nonabsorbable sutures, while the retinaculum is repaired with multiple interrupted no. 0 absorbable sutures. Once the repair is complete, careful assessment of patella rotation and tracking should be performed. The knee is then extended and the repair may be protected with a cerclage wire or nonabsorbable suture. The wound is closed in layers and the leg is placed in a cylinder cast for six weeks. When the cast is removed, a control-dial hinged knee orthosis (Figure 13.2) is used so that flexion can be gradually increased. The brace is discontinued when greater than 90° of flexion has been achieved and the quadriceps strength is sufficient to support the limb.

When the rupture occurs at the osteotendinous junction, the proximal end of the rectus femoris and the vastus intermedius tendon is cut fresh to normal tendon, while the superior pole of the patella is debrided of residual tendon. A transverse trough is then made in the superior pole of the patella with a high-speed burr (Figure 13.3a and 13.3b). To avoid patella tilt, the trough should not be placed near the anterior surface. Three or four longitudinal drill holes are then made at the base of the trough approximately 1 to 1.5 cm apart and exiting at the inferior pole of the patella (Figure 13.3c). A no. 5 nonabsorbable suture is secured with an interlocking stitch along the lateral portion of the tendon. The two free ends are then passed through the longitudinal drill holes at the base of the trough with a suture passer. A second no. 5 nonabsorbable suture is placed in a similar fashion along the medial tendon and passed through the patella drill holes (Figure 13.3d). The proximal end of the tendon is then pulled into the trough and the sutures are held provisionally with a hemostat. The knee is then flexed so that patella tracking and rotation can be assessed. The repair is then completed by tying the no. 5 nonabsorbable suture distally and repairing the medial and lateral retinaculum with multiple interrupted no. 0 absorbable sutures (Figure 13.3e). After closure of the subcutaneous layer and skin, a cylinder cast is applied with the knee in full extension. Postoperatively, the cylinder cast is maintained for six weeks and the patient is allowed weight bearing as tolerated with a walker or crutches. Once the cast is removed, a control-dial hinged knee orthosis is used until 90° of flexion is achieved and the quadriceps strength returns.

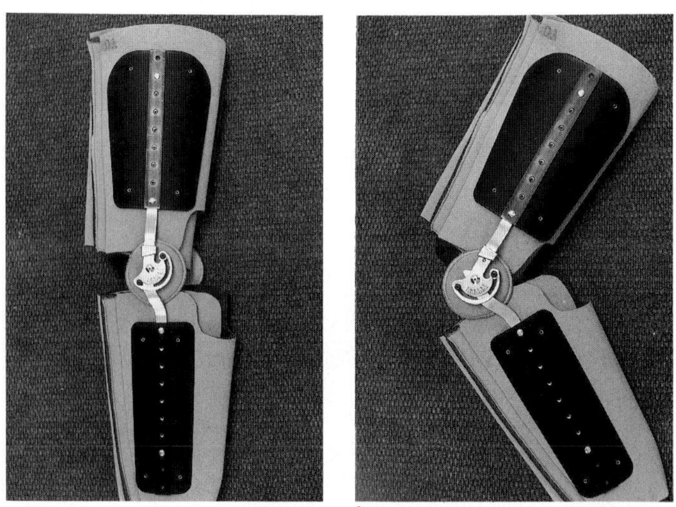

a b

FIGURE 13.2. A control-dial hinged knee orthosis with a drop lock to keep the knee in extension (a) during early ambulation and to allow flexion when exercising (b). (Photo courtesy of NBB Orthotics, Rockville Centre, N.Y.)

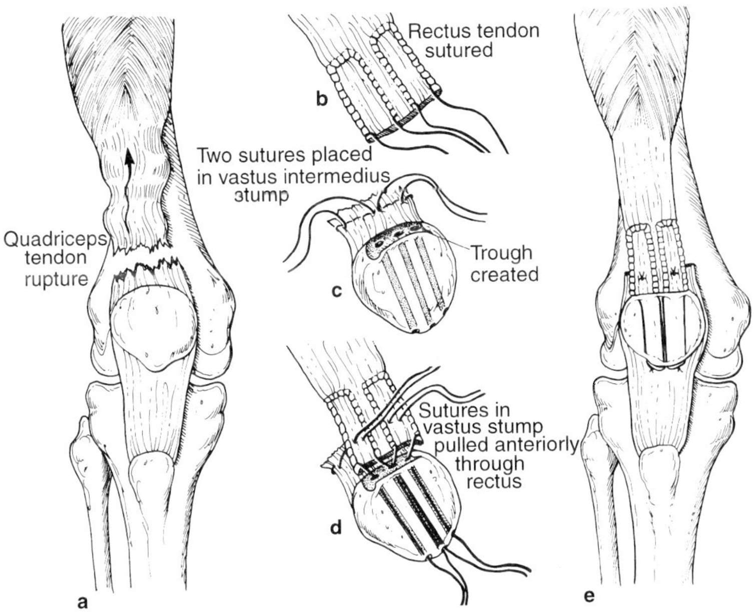

FIGURE 13.3. Acute repair of the quadriceps tendon. (a) The retracted quadriceps tendon; (b) an interlocking stitch is secured along the medial and lateral border of the tendon; (c) a trough is made along the superior pole of the patella and three longitudinal drill holes are made at the base of the trough exiting at the inferior pole of the patella; (d) the sutures are then pulled through the drill holes; and (e) the sutures are tied distally and the retinaculum is repaired.

The Scuderi technique[48,49] for repairing acute repairs of the quadriceps tendon has been popular (Figure 13.4). Using a midline longitudinal incision, the tendon rupture is exposed and the tendon edges are debrided until solid tendinous material is achieved. The knee is extended and the tendon edges are pulled with clamps, overlapped, and repaired with interrupted absorbable sutures. A triangular flap, measuring 2.4 to 3.2 mm thick, 7.5 cm long on each side, and 5 cm at the base, is fabricated from the anterior surface of the proximal tendon. The base of the flap is left attached about 5 cm proximal to the rupture. The flap is folded distally over the rupture and sutured in place. A Bunnell pullout wire is placed along the medial and lateral side of the quadriceps tendon, patella, and patella tendon. The distal end of the wire is tied over a 1-in (2.5 cm) pearl button. Before Scuderi would pull down the wire over the buttons, he would place five to six layers of gauze or sterilized sponge rubber in order to avoid skin necrosis. The wound is closed in layers and the leg is placed in a cylinder cast with the knee in the extended position. Postoperatively, the cylinder cast is maintained for six weeks and at three weeks the pullout wires are removed. When the cast is removed, a control-

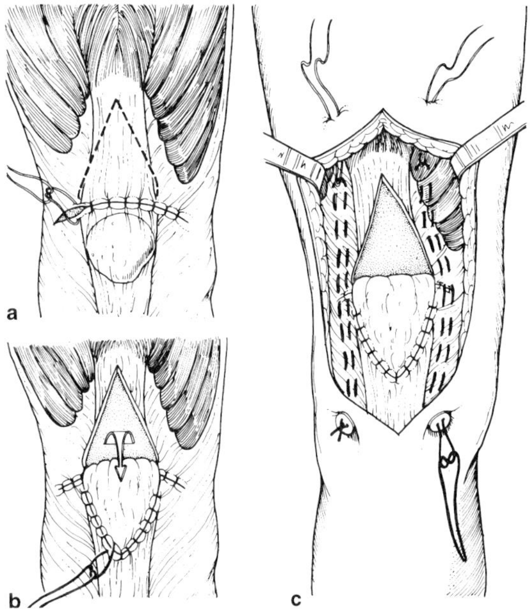

FIGURE 13.4. The Scuderi technique for repairing acute tears of the quadriceps tendon. (a) The torn tendon edges are debrided and repaired. (b) A triangular flap is developed from the anterior surface of the proximal tendon, folded distally over the rupture and sutured in place. (c) Prior to closure, pullout sutures are placed along the medial and lateral retinaculum. From G.R. Scuderi [35], adapted by permission of Mosby—Year Book, Inc., © 1991.

dial hinged knee orthosis is used so that flexion can be gradually increased. It is also recommend that the patient undergo physiotherapy, especially a quadriceps strengthening program.

Neglected or chronic ruptures of the quadriceps tendon present a difficult reconstruction and the results for these chronic tears are less satisfactory than the treatment of acute tears. A longitudinal midline incision is the preferred approach and the exposure may reveal a large gap between the tendon edges. When the tendon can be apposed, the ends are debrided and repaired with the Scuderi technique, as described previously. However, when there is a contraction of the tendon and a large gap, the Codivilla tendon lengthening and repair are recommended (Figure 13.5). An inverted V is cut through the full thickness of the proximal quadriceps tendon with the lower margin of the V ending approximately 1.3 cm proximal to the rupture. The tendon ends are apposed and repaired with multiple no. 0 nonabsorbable sutures. The medial and lateral retinaculum is also repaired at this time with multiple interrupted no. 0 absorbable sutures. The flap is then brought distally and sutured directly to the patella through drill holes as described. The open upper portion of the V is closed with interrupted no. 0 absorbable sutures. If there is any doubt about the integrity of the repair, it should be reinforced with a Scuderi flap or with strips of fascia lata femoris.[49] The reconstruction should be protected with a pullout cerclage wire. The postoperative treatment is similar to that with the Scuderi procedure.

Results

Using their technique, Scuderi and Schrey reported good or excellent results in seven of nine patients.[49] Ramsey and Muller did not feel that reinforcement of the suture line or Bunnell pullout sutures were necessary if the quadriceps repair was performed within the first week.[34] Ramsey and Muller reported the results of 17 patients. Ten patients were treated during the first week after injury and the remaining seven were treated between two weeks and one year postinjury. Acute repairs were performed through a transverse incision. After debridement, the tendon ends were approximated with interrupted mattress sutures and immobilized for six weeks. Delayed repairs were performed with some type of reinforcement of the suture line, such as Bunnell pullout wires. Nine of ten patients treated

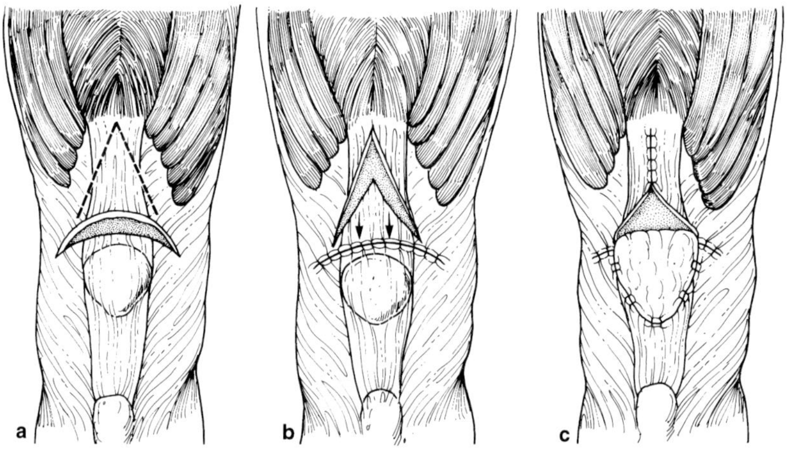

FIGURE 13.5. The Codivilla quadriceps tendon lengthening and repair for chronic ruptures. (a) The torn tendon edges are debrided and repaired. (b) An inverted V is cut through ther proximal tendon. (c) The flap is brought distally and sutured in place. The open upper portion of the V defect is closed. Reprinted with permission from ref. [49]. Copyright © 1950, American Medical Association.

acutely regained full motion, while loss of motion was common after delayed repair. Of the seven delayed repairs in this series, four patients lost between 10° and 20° of full active extension.

Miskew et al. described the use of Mersilene strip sutures to repair quadriceps and patellar tendon disruptions.[50] The authors used a transverse incision made 0.5 inch (1.3 cm) proximal to the patella for the quadriceps tendon and a longitudinal incision for the patellar tendon. If avulsion of the quadriceps tendon has occurred, the tendon ends are first debrided. Drill holes are then placed in the patella approximately 1 cm from the its edge. The Mersilene sutures are passed first through the drill holes and then through the tendon 1 cm proximal to the rupture. In most cases, four or five sutures were necessary for repair of the quadriceps tendon and three to four sutures for the patellar tendon. Postoperative management included cast immobilization for six weeks followed by nonrestricted quadriceps strengthening. Ten patients with 12 ruptures were included in this series. Full range of motion was obtained in nine repairs. Prior infection or fracture were present in the three cases where range of motion was lost.

In 1981, Siwek and Rao published the largest series of extensor mechanism ruptures, which included 67 patients with 72 ruptures.[16] The study included 34 patients with 36 quadriceps ruptures. Immediate repair of the quadriceps tendon was performed in 30 patients. Several different techniques were used to repair the tendon. In most cases, the tendon was repaired by directly suturing the defect with no. 2 silk or chromic sutures. Reinforcement of the tendon was performed in some patients, although the exact number was not specified in the article. The techniques used to reinforce the repair included the following: a circumferential wire passed through the quadriceps tendon and anchored to a bolt placed through the patella, a Bunnell pullout wire in conjunction with a bolt through the proximal tibia, a circumferential wire placed proximal to the rupture and attached to a Steinmann pin inserted through the proximal tibia, and a Scuderi-type flap. Delayed repairs (beyond two weeks) were performed in six patients in whom the diagnosis was initially missed. One patient required a Codivilla lengthening in order to approximate the tendon ends. In the other five patients, the tendon ends were debrided and then approximated with mattress sutures of heavy braided silk or no. 2 chromic. Results were rated as excellent, good, or unsatisfactory, based on the patients' quadriceps muscle strength and range of motion of the knee. All 30 patients who had immediate repair of the quadriceps tendon had good or excellent results with full extension and 120° or more of flexion. Despite good functional results, approximately 75% of these patients had persistent quadriceps muscle atrophy. Of the six patients who had delayed repairs, three were graded as having good results and three had unsatisfactory results. Only one patient in this group had greater than 90° of flexion and five had persistent quadriceps atrophy. The results of this study confirmed the importance of early diagnosis and treatment of extensor mechanism disruption. The authors also concluded that acute quadriceps tendon repairs could be performed successfully with the end-to-end sutures followed by immobilization for six to eight weeks. They felt that fixation that required surgical removal was not necessary.

Ruptures of the Patella Tendon

Rupture of the patella tendon is less common than that of the quadriceps and usually occurs at the insertion into the patella. In general, patients are also younger and less likely to have degenerative changes of the knee or systemic illness. The patella may displace 5 cm proximally because of associated retinacular and capsular disruption caused by the strong pull of the quadriceps mechanism. Disruptions that occur through the substance of the patella tendon can happen spontaneously, however, they more often occur with trauma or laceration. Some authors have noted an increase risk for patellar tendon rupture after steroid injections.[31] Early diagnoses and treatment provide the best results.

Historically, McLaughlin[45–47] recommended

that repair of the patellar tendon be reinforced with the use of stainless steel wire anchored to a bolt placed in the tibial tubercle. He used a longitudinal medial parapatellar incision. The tendon ends are identified, debrided, and mobilized. A stainless steel wire is then placed through the quadriceps tendon just proximal to the patella. A bolt is placed transversely across the tibial tubercle. Using the wire to pull the patella and proximal portion of the tendon distally, the torn ends are reapproximated. The wire is then anchored to the bolt and the tendon is repaired with fine silk sutures. McLaughlin removed the wire at eight weeks, however, other authors have recommended ten to 12 weeks. Siwek and Rao[16] also recommended that all immediate repair of the patella tendon be reinforced by external devices. Several reports have described reinforcing the repair with various augmentation grafts including allografts[51,52] (fascia lata femoris, semitendinosus, and gracilis) and synthetic grafts (Mersilene,[50] Dacron,[53,54] and carbon fiber[55]).

Kelikian et al. was the first to describe the use of the semitendinosus tendon for reconstruction of the patella tendon.[52] A preliminary surgical procedure was used to mobilize the patella and a traction pin was placed. When the patella had descended to a level 1 inch (2.5 cm) proximal to the articular surface, the reconstruction was performed. Through a proximal incision the semitendinosus tendon was then divided at its musculotendinous junction. A longitudinal paramedial incision was made and drill holes were then made in the tibial tubercle and the distal third of the patella. The free end of the tendon was passed from medial to lateral through the tibial tunnel and then from lateral to medial through the patellar tunnel. The tendon end was then brought down and sutured onto itself. The patient was placed in a cylinder cast that incorporates the tibial traction pin. The cast and the pin were removed at six weeks, and therapy was begun.

Technique

Once the patella tendon ruptures are diagnosed, surgical intervention is indicated. A straight midline incision is made and, with careful dissection, the peritenon is opened longitudinally. Rupture of the patella tendon usually occurs at the osteotendinous junction. When this is the case, a horizontal trough is then made along the inferior pole of the patella (Figure 13.6). Four longitudinal drill holes are placed at the base of the trough, exiting at the superior pole of the patella (Figure 13.7). Several no. 2 nonabsorbable sutures, using a Kessler stitch, are placed in the patella tendon and the free ends are passed through the longitudinal drill holes. The stitches are pulled taut and the free end of the patella tendon should be seated within the trough. The sutures are provisionally held with a hemostat in order to assess patella tracking and rotation. It is important to make sure that patella infera has not been produced by the repair. At 45° of flexion, the inferior pole of the patella should be above the roof of the intercondylar notch. The medial and lateral retinaculum are repaired with no. 0 absorbable suture. The wound is then closed in layers and a cylinder cast with the knee in extension is applied and maintained for six weeks. The patient may ambulate full weight bearing as tolerated with crutches. When the cast is removed, the control-dial hinged knee orthosis is used, allowing progressive flexion of the knee. When the patient has achieved greater than 90° of flexion and sufficient quadriceps strength to support the limb, it is discontinued.

Acute ruptures that occur within the substance of the patella tendon can be repaired with running interlocking sutures of no. 2 nonabsorbable suture material (Figure 13.8). The distally based tendon is reinforced through longitudinal drill holes in the patella, while the proximally based tendon is repaired through a horizontal drill hole in the tibial tubercle. Each flap is repaired side-to-side with interrupted no. 0 absorbable sutures. The medial and lateral retinaculum is also repaired with no. 0 absorbable sutures at this time. The postoperative course is similar to that described previously.

In treating midsubstance tears of the patellar tendon, augmentation with the semitendinosus or gracilis tendon is recommended

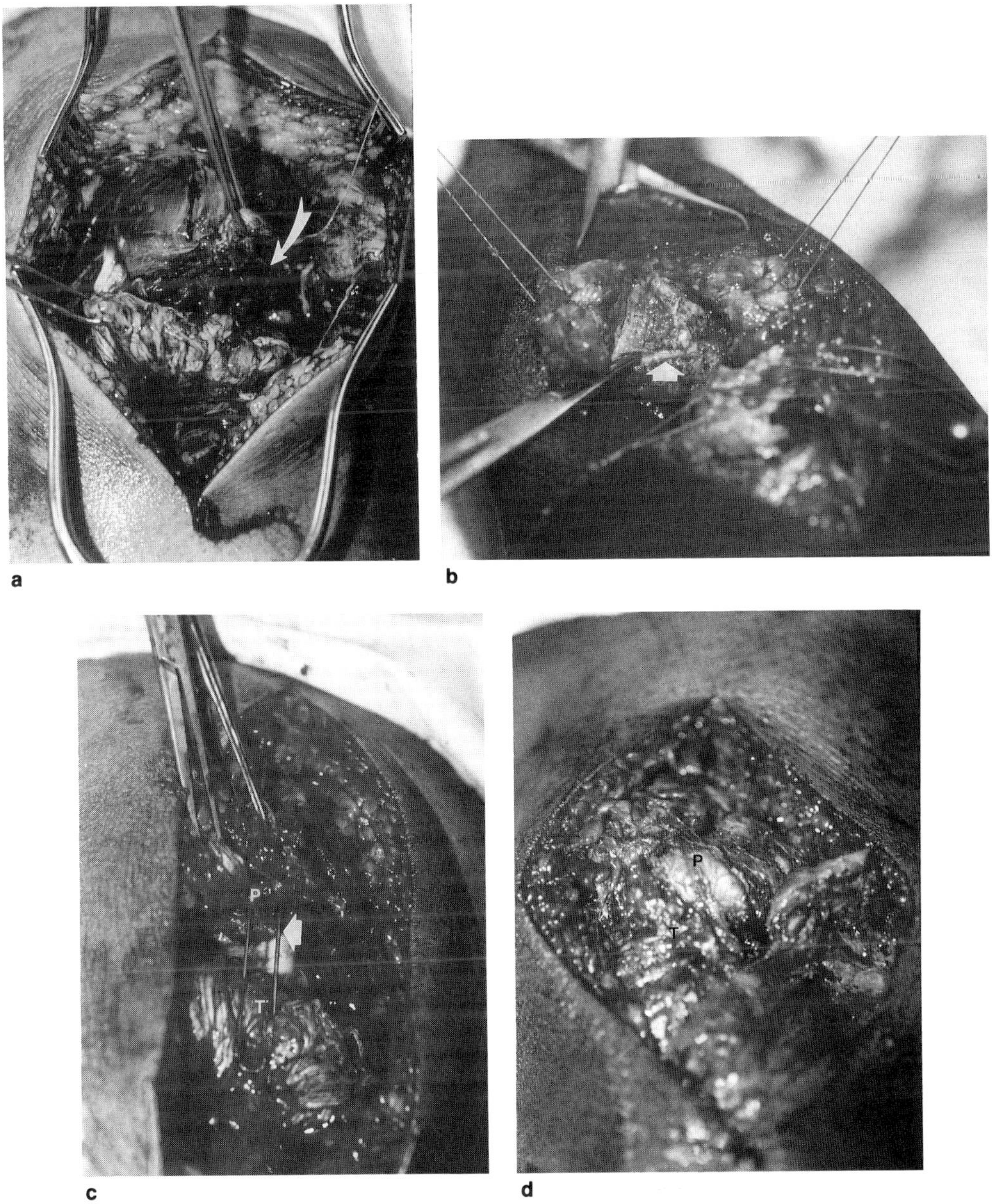

FIGURE 13.6. (a) Intraoperative photograph of an acute patella tendon rupture (arrow). (b) The bony trough (arrow) is created along the inferior border of the patella. (c) Sutures are passed through multiple drill holes in the base of the bony trough (P = patella; T = patella tendon; arrow = suture needle). (d) The sutures are pulled taut and the free end of the patella tendon is seated within the trough (P = patella; T = patella tendon).

(Figure 13.9). Through the original midline incision, the insertion sites of the semitendinosus and the gracilis tendons are identified. Preserving the distal insertion, a tendon stripper is used to divide the tendon proximally. If a tendon stripper is unavailable, a second incision is made along the distal medial thigh and the semitendinosus and the gracilis tendons are divided at their musculotendinous junction (Figure 13.10). The tendons are

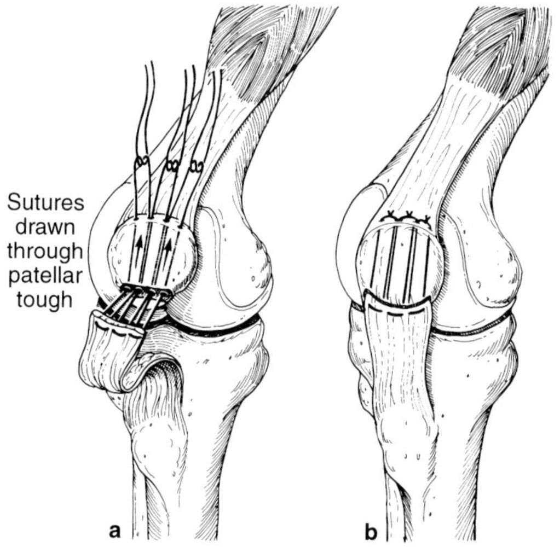

FIGURE 13.7. Technique for acute repair of the patella tendon into a bony trough. (a) A trough is made along the inferior border of the patella and four longitudinal drill holes are made at the base of the trough exiting at the superior pole of the patella. (b) Several interlocking sutures are placed in the patellar tendon, passed to the drill holes, and tied securely at the superior border of the patella.

trimmed of any muscle and sutured together. If only the semitendinosus is used for augmentation, it should be passed through an oblique drill hole at the tibial tubercle from the medial to lateral direction. The graft is then pulled superiorly and passes lateral to medial through a transverse drill hole in the inferior aspect of the patella to then be sutured to the origin of the semitendinosus with no. 0 nonabsorbable suture. This creates a circle around the patella tendon. The corners of the graft are sutured with nonabsorbable suture to prevent slippage. If the semitendinosus tendon is thin and further augmentation is needed, the gracilis tendon can also be used. The gracilis tendon origin is maintained distally and the tendon is passed medial to lateral through a second horizontal drill hole in the patella, circling the patella tendon and returning lateral to medial through the oblique tibial drill hole. The postoperative course is similar to that described previously with six weeks of immobilization in a cylinder cast. In cases in which the patient is found to have a large semitendinosus tendon, it may be used alone for augmentation (Figure 13.11). We prefer the use of this biologic augmentation over a wire because it avoids the risk of wire breakage and does not require a second procedure for removal.

Chronic ruptures of the patella tendon pose a particular problem, especially if there is retraction of the quadriceps tendon with proximal migration of the patella. Previously, a two-stage reconstruction with preoperative traction through a transverse Steinmann pin placed in the patella was described.

Mobilization of the patella and the quadriceps tendon can be obtained by clearing the medial and lateral gutters into the suprapatellar pouch and subperiosteally elevating the vastus intermedius from the anterior femur.[26] A lateral retinacular release is also performed. If necessary, a medial retinacular release can be performed, but this may increase the risk of avascular necrosis of the patella.[56,57] Several techniques have been described for reconstruction of chronic tears of the patella tendon including direct repair with augmentation, allograft, and synthetic grafts. Regardless of the technique performed, it is important that care be taken to maintain normal patella tracking, rotation, and height. Preoperative planning should include a lateral radiograph of the contralateral knee to determine patella height. Intraoperatively, the inferior pole of the patella should be above the roof of the intercondylar notch at 45° of flexion. The knee should be able to achieve 90° of flexion and when in full extension, the patella tendon should be lax approximately 1 to 1.5 cm.

Reconstruction of chronic patella tendon ruptures is performed through a longitudinal midline incision. The peritenon is incised longitudinally, exposing the patella tendon. If there is sufficient tendon, the ends are cut fresh and sutured as described previously for the acute repair. However, augmentation with the semitendinosus and the gracilis is necessary. A bone tenaculum can be used to pull the patella distally, and the semitendinosus and the gracilis are sutured under tension.

When there is a deficiency of remaining tendon or the remaining tendon is attenuated and

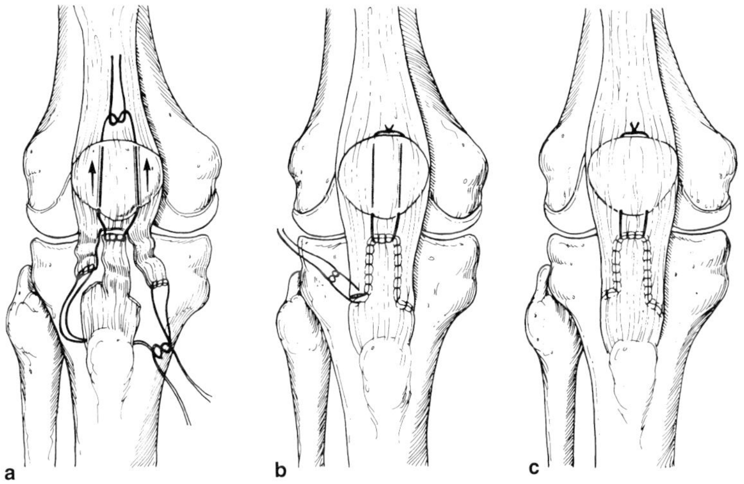

FIGURE 13.8. Technique for acute repair of intrasubstance tears of the patella tendon. (a) Two longitudinal drill holes are placed in the patella while a transverse drill hole is made at the level of the tibial tubercle. (b) The distally based tendon is reinforced through the longitudinal patellar drill holes, while the proximally based tendon is repaired through the transverse drill hole in the tibial tubercle. (c) Each flap is then repaired side to side.

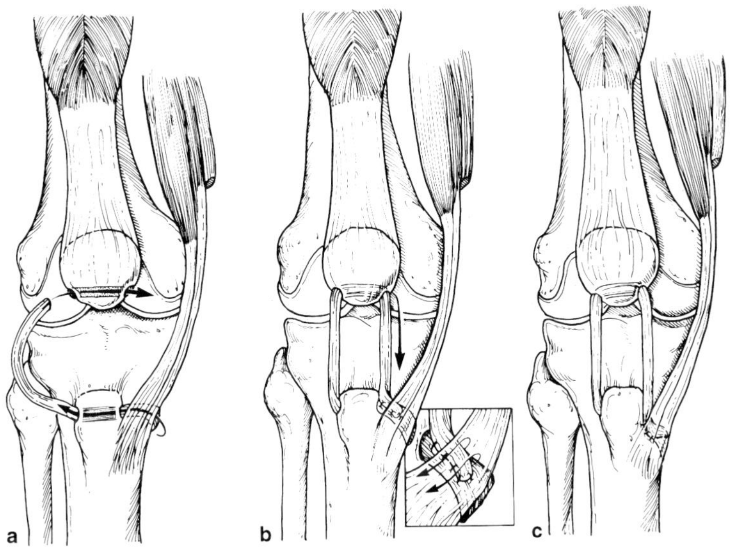

FIGURE 13.9. Augmentation of the patella tendon repair with the semitendinosus tendon. (a) the semitendinosus tendon is harvested maintaining its distal attachment. The proximal end is passed through a drill hole at the tibial tubercle from a medial to lateral direction. (b) The graft is pulled superiorly and passes lateral to medial through a drill hole in the inferior aspect of the patella. (c) The remaining tendon is pulled inferiorly and sutured to its site of origin. From G.R. Scuderi [35], adapted by permission of Mosby—Year Book, Inc., © 1991.

scarred, a Z shortening of the patella tendon in a Z lengthening of the quadriceps tendon can be performed (Figure 13.12). This technique requires intraoperative radiographs to determine appropriate patella height and position because essentially you are sliding the patella distally toward the tibia with a high likelihood of creating a patella infera. Once the proper position of the patella has been determined, the Z plasty is reinforced with multiple interrupted no. 0 nonabsorbable sutures. This reconstruction requires augmentation with the semitendinosus and the gracilis tendons, which are harvested as two free tendons and sutured end to end. The hamstring tendons pass through a transverse drill hole in the midportion of the patella and then through a transverse hole in the tibial tubercle in a figure-eight fashion. The semitendinosus and the gracilis grafts are secured to the patella tendon with absorbable sutures. The postoperative course is similar to that described previously.

Recently, allografts[58] have been used for reconstruction of the neglected patella tendon ruptures (Figure 13.13). The Achilles tendon with a cortical cancellous calcaneal bone block

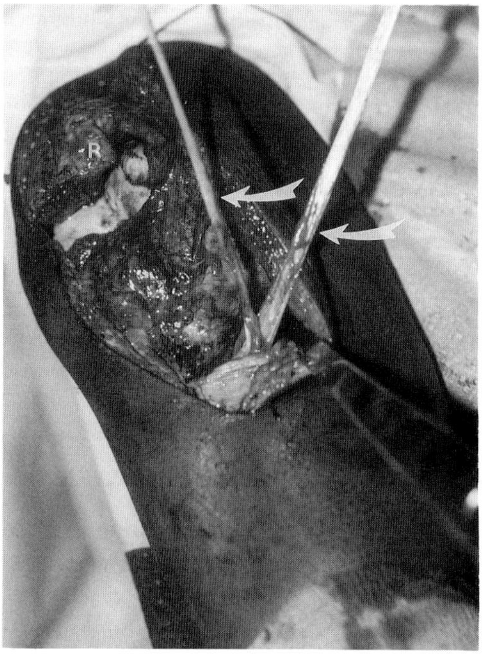

FIGURE 13.10. Harvesting the semitendinosus and the gracilis tendons (arrows) (P = patella).

is a convenient allograft. The tibial tubercle is prepared with an oscillating saw or a burr, creating a trough measuring 2.5 to 3 cm long, 1.5 to 2 cm wide, and 1.5 cm deep. The bone block is contoured and press-fit into the trough. It is then secured with two 4.0 cancellous screws. The Achilles tendon graft is divided into thirds. The central third, which should measure 8 to 9 mm in width, is then pulled through a slit in the residual patella tendon. The graft is then passed through a longitudinal drill hole in the patella, measuring 8 to 9 mm wide. This drill hole enters the inferior pole of the patella and exits at the superior border proximally 3 mm posterior to the central portion of the quadriceps tendon. The tendon is then pulled through a vertical slit in the quadriceps tendon. The tendon is sutured at the inferior pole of the patella and at the quadriceps tendon with multiple interrupted no. 0 nonabsorbable sutures. The patella height should be determined at this time. The knee should flex to 90° and at 45° of flexion, the inferior pole of the patella should be superior to the roof of the intercondylar notch. Once the patella position has been determined correct, the medial and lateral flaps are sutured to the medial and lateral retinaculum with multiple no. 0 nonabsorbable sutures. If the peritenon is present, it should be closed over the graft with 2–0 absorbable sutures. The wound is closed in layers and a cylinder cast is applied. The cast is worn for five weeks and a control-dial hinged knee orthosis is worn until 90° of flexion has been achieved and the quadriceps strength is strong enough to support the limb during ambulation.

Results

In Siwek and Rao's review of 67 patients with extensor mechanism ruptures, 31 were patellar tendon ruptures.[16] Twenty-five patients had immediate repair and six had delayed reconstruction of the patellar tendon. All immediate repairs were reinforced by external devices, which include Bunnell pullout wires, pullout wire with a Steinmann pin through the tibia, or with Steinmann pin through both the tibia and the patella connected with wire. Postoperative management of these patients included casting the knee in extension for six to 11 weeks. Twenty of the 26 patients with immediate repairs regained full motion and were considered to have excellent results. Four patients had some loss of flexion and were graded as good. Rerupture occurred in one patient at eight weeks after surgery. Preoperative traction was used in three of five patients with delayed repair in Siwek and Rao's series.[16] A Steinmann pin was placed transversely through the proximal portion of the patella and 5 lb (2.25 kg) of traction was then applied. Knee ranges of motion exercises were also initiated. The authors felt that preoperative traction was advisable in the following circumstances: neglected rupture of the patellar tendon, great clinical and radiographic displacement, inability to manually move the patella distally, and loss of free passive side-to-side motion. All repairs were augmented; a fascial graft plus pins and wire were used in three patients, a Bunnell wire plus a pin was used in one patient, and a flap of rectus femoris plus a Bunnell wire was used in one

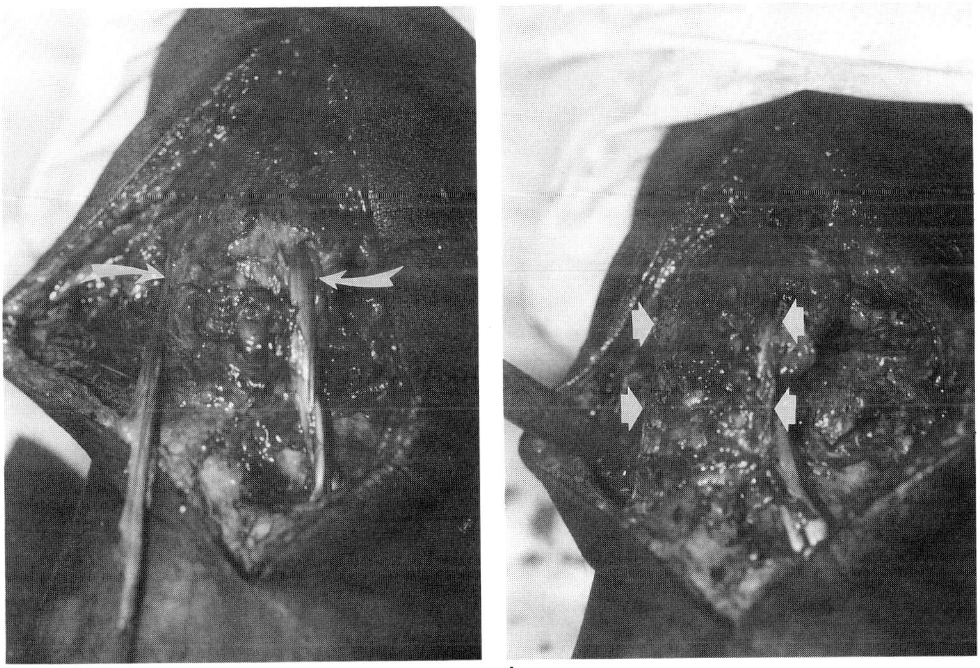

a b

FIGURE 13.11. (a) The semitendinosus and the gracilis tendons can also remain attached distally and pass through a transverse drill hole in the patella medial to lateral (arrows). (b) The tendons are then sutured in place with nonabsorbable suture material, forming a circle around the patella tendon (arrows).

patient. Good or excellent results were obtained in four of five patients, while one patient with bilateral ruptures that were repaired after 13 weeks had an unsatisfactory result with limited knee flexion.

Miskew et al. described the use of Mersilene strips for the repair of extensor mechanism injuries.[50] For patellar tendon avulsions, the debrided ends of the tendon are repaired with three to four Mersilene sutures through drill holes in the patella or two Mersilene sutures through the tibial tubercle. A cylinder cast was then applied for six weeks. This technique was used for both immediate and delayed repairs. Four of six patients had full extension and greater than 130° of flexion. One patient had full extension and 100° of flexion, while one patient who had a six-week-old septic rupture developed a 15° extension lag and only 80° of flexion. Phillip has recommended the use of Mersilene suture repair of fresh avulsions of the patellar tendon.[58] A transverse or longitudinal incision may be used. A small horizontal trough is made in the inferior pole of the patella. Three horizontal mattress sutures of no. 2 Mersilene are placed through the end of the tendon. Three longitudinal drill holes are placed through the patella, and the sutures are then passed through the holes and tied. Care must be taken to avoid shortening the tendon and causing patella baja. Phillip did not think that augmentation was necessary if the secure fixation was achieved, however, intrasubstance tears or those with extensively frayed ends generally require augmentation.

Kelly et al. reported on ten patients with patellar tendon repair.[36] All had a history of symptoms and/or findings consistent with jumper's knee prior to rupture. The ruptures were repaired with nonabsorbable sutures passed through drill holes in the patella. Two patients had augmentation of the repair, one with a wire loop and another with umbilical tape. Good or excellent clinical results were obtained in eight of ten patients. Cybex testing showed good or excellent strength in only four of nine patients.

Frazier and Clark have described the use 5-mm Dacron vascular graft to repair acute ruptures of the patellar tendon.[53,54] The authors report four cases with good results at four months. Two of these patients were felt to have excellent long-term results.

Ecker et al. reported on four patients who underwent late reconstruction of the patellar tendon using the semitendinosus and the gracilis tendons.[51] The patella had retracted proximally in all four cases; however, preoperative traction was not required. After exposure and mobilization of the patella, the quadriceps, and the tibial tubercle were achieved, a Steinmann pin was placed transversely through the proximal portion of the patella and traction was exerted distally. The Insall–Salvati ratio was used to determine the correct height of the patella. The semitendinosus and the gracilis tendons were harvested, leaving their distal insertion intact. Two large drill holes were then transversely placed through the distal patella and an oblique was then made through the tibial tubercle. The semitendinosus tendon was inserted from medial to lateral through the tibial hole and then from lateral to medial through the patella hole. The gracilis was next passed from medial to lateral through the other patellar hole. A heavy-gauge wire placed through the tibial tubercle and the patella was then used to hold the position of the patella. With the patella held in position, the two tendons were sutured to each other. A cylinder cast was placed for six weeks following the procedure. The patient was then readmitted, and under general anesthesia the knee was manipulated and the wire was removed. The authors caution that active knee motion should not be initiated prior to removal of the wire. Results using this technique were satisfactory and all four patients were able to return to work. All patients had full active extension and were able to flex beyond 100°. One patient regained 135° of motion and was able to return to sports activity.

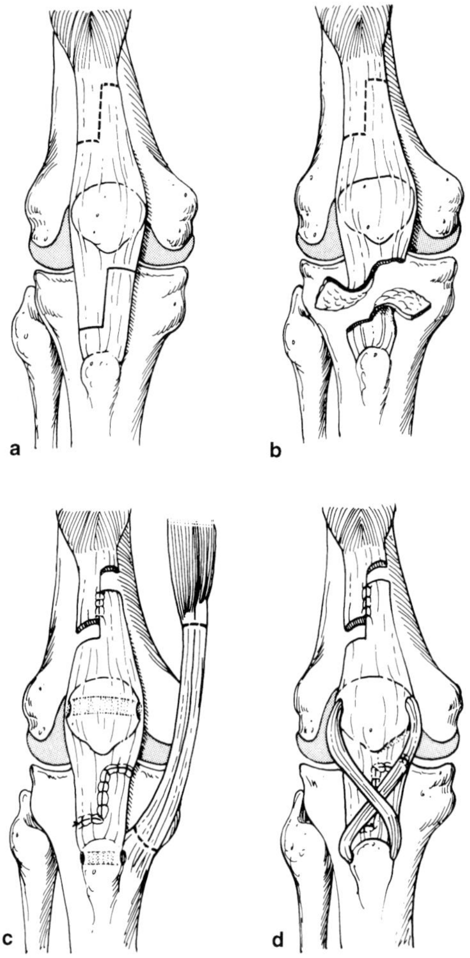

FIGURE 13.12. Repair of a chronic patella tendon rupture with a Z shortening of the patella tendon and a Z lengthening of the quadriceps tendon. Augmentation with the semitendinosus and the gracilis tendons sutured end to end. (a) The planned z incisions along the quadriceps and patella tendons. (b) the Z incision of the patella tendon. (c) the Z shortening of the patella tendon and a Z lengthening of the quadriceps tendon. (d) Augmentation of the repair with the semitendinosus and the gracilis tendons sutured end to end and passed in a figure-eight fashion through the tibial tubercle and transverse patella drill holes.

Patellar Fractures

The patella acts to increase the moment arm of the quadriceps mechanism. Tensile stresses occur on the patella with the knee in extension; in flexion, the tensile stresses about the patella are counterbalanced by the joint reactive force of the distal femur, creating a three-point bending model. This accounts for

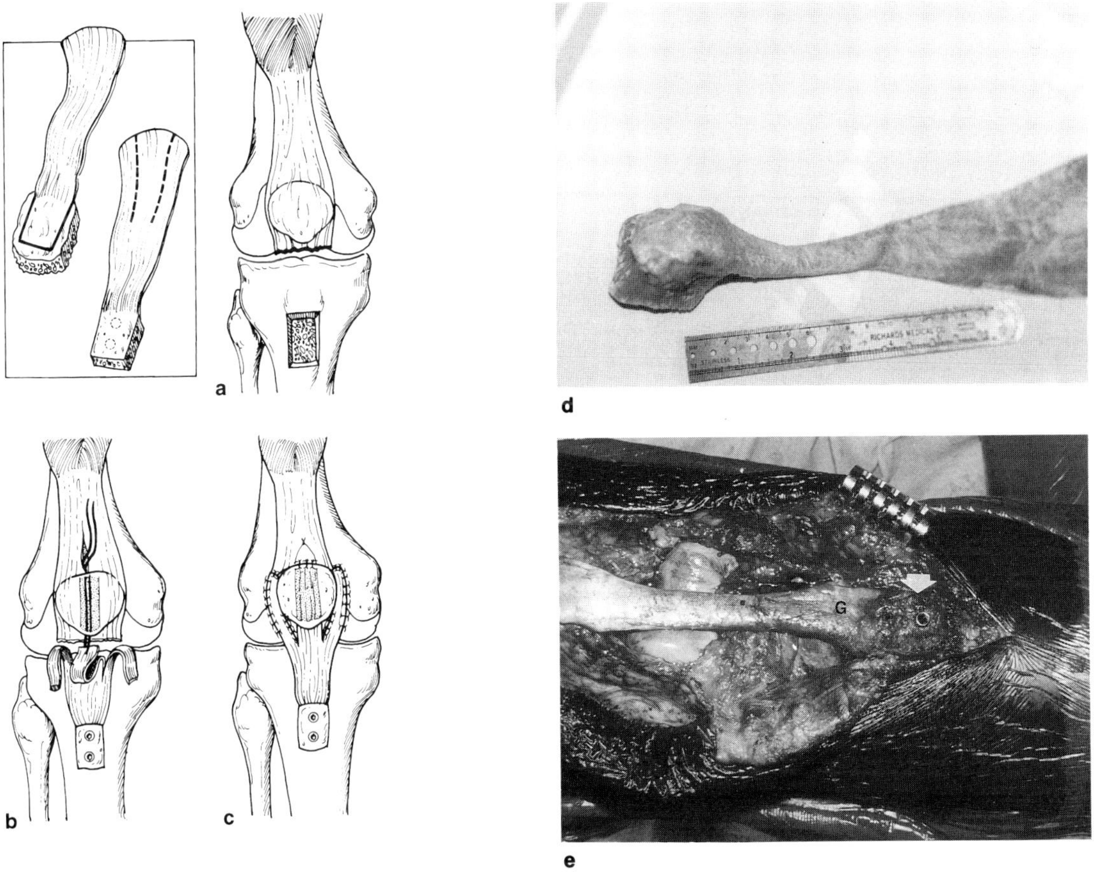

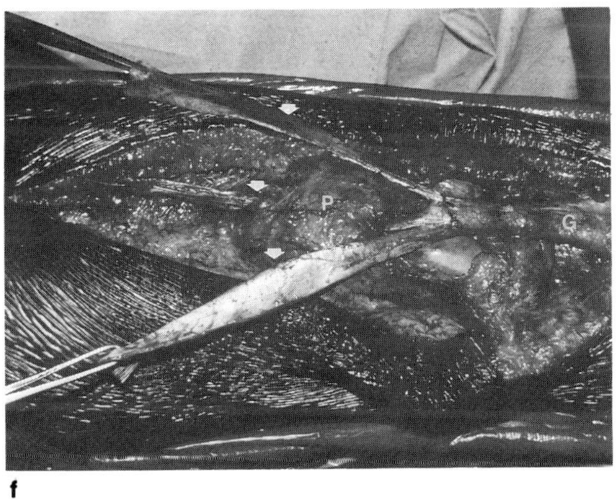

FIGURE 13.13. (a, b, c) Allograft reconstruction for neglected patella tendon ruptures. (d) An Achilles tendon allograft is sizable and suitable for reconstruction of chronic tears. (e) The allograft is fixed in a bony trough at the tibial tubercle (arrow) (G = graft). (f) the Achilles allograft (G) is split in thirds (arrows) with the central third passing through a vertical drill hole in the patella (P) and the outside thirds secured along the medial and lateral retinaculum.

the primary mode of failure of indirect injuries to the extensor mechanism; when the extensor mechanism is eccentrically overloaded, failure will occur at either the quadriceps tendon, the patella, the patellar ligament, or the tibial tubercle.

Diagnosis of patellar fractures can be easily missed. A complete history should be obtained, with particular attention paid to knee position and activity when the injury occurred. A direct blow to the knee, or a sudden episode of giving way following eccentric loading of the knee while the quadriceps was contracted, followed by immediate pain, swelling,

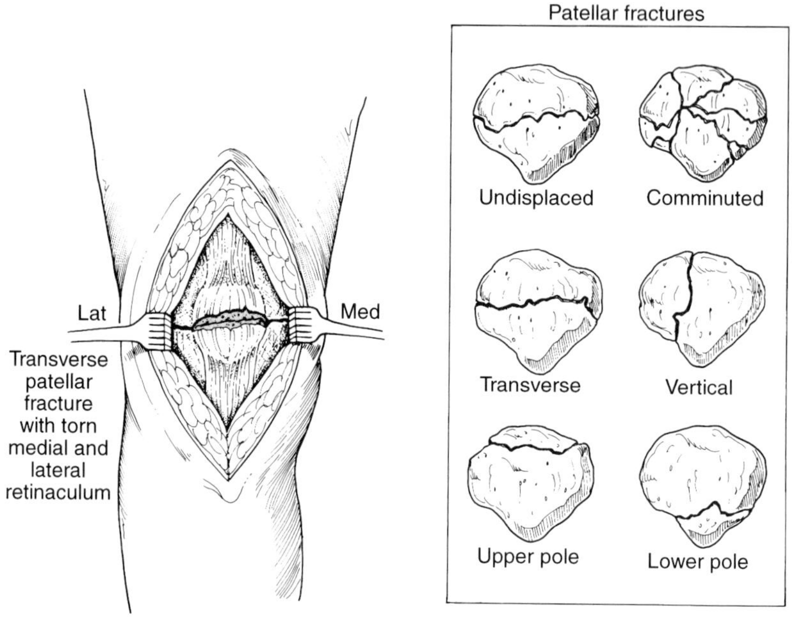

FIGURE 13.14. Classification of patellar fractures.

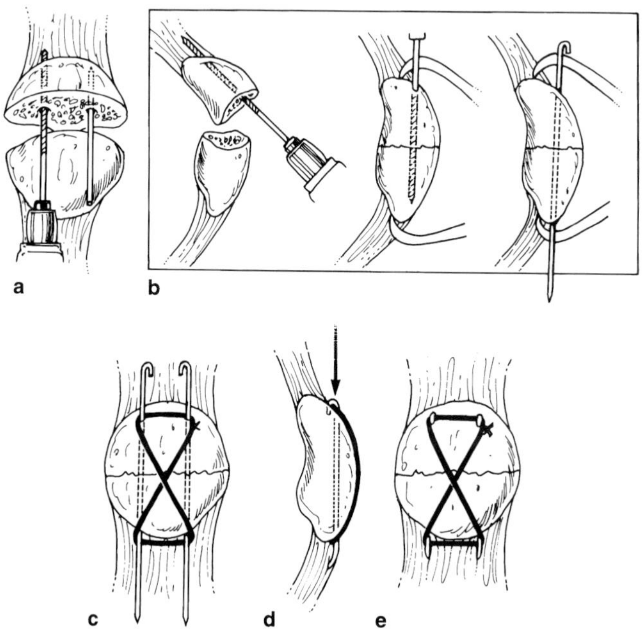

FIGURE 13.15. The tension band technique for open reduction and internal fixation of patella fractures as popularized by the AO/ASIF group.[63] (a) Two longitudinal drill holes are made in the proximal fragment from a distal to proximal direction. (b) The fracture is reduced and held with bone clamps. The drill bit is then passed through the proximal drill hole and into the distal fragment. Two Kirschner wires are then inserted into the drill holes. (c) A figure-eight tension band wire is passed around the K wires and tightened. (d) The reduction is maintained as the Kirschner wires are countersunk proximally. (e) The figure-eight configuration maintains the reduction.

and extensor weakness, should alert the practitioner to the possibility of an extensor mechanism injury. The knee must be examined for any palpable soft tissue or bony defects. Loss of active knee extension with a palpable defect in the patella is pathognomonic of a patellar fracture. Anteroposterior, lateral, and tangential views of the knee are confirmatory. Views of the contralateral knee are helpful in differentiating a bipartite patella from a genuine fracture.

Because the patella is a prominent subcutaneous structure, it is susceptible to direct injury as well. Any fall on the knee results in a direct blow to the patella with little soft-tissue protection. High-speed motor vehicle trauma often results in patellar fractures that result from a direct blow against the automobile dashboard. These injuries often result in greater articular cartilage damage than indirect injuries resulting from eccentric overload.

Patellar fractures often are a result of a combined injury composed of direct and indirect loading. Therefore, when devising a classification scheme, one has to account for some overlap. Patellar fractures may be classified according to morphology (Figure 13.14), which often indicates the mechanism of injury. Major classification phenotypes include transverse, vertical, comminuted, undisplaced, upper pole, and lower pole. Further classification must include a description of articular congruity of displacement. A history of patellar dislocation or subluxation is associated with a high incidence of osteochondral fractures.[59]

Treatment of patellar fractures is based on displacement of the fracture fragments, articular congruity, and the status of the extensor mechanism. As a general rule, nondisplaced or minimally displaced fractures with less than 2 mm or less of articular incongruity are best treated by a period of immobilization. A well-padded cylinder cast applied for four to six weeks, followed by gentle range-of-motion exercises, generally produces satisfactory results.

Operative treatment is reserved for displaced fractures with articular incongruities. The patella should be preserved if at all possible to retain its biomechanical advantage. Comminution may be severe enough to preclude fixation; partial patellectomy may be considered for this situation. Following excision of all comminuted fragments, the remaining patellar segment is reattached to the adjacent quadriceps or patellar ligament with the use of multiple drill holes with heavy nonabsorbable suture. Attention should be given to correct rotation and alignment of the existing patellar remnant; the repair should result in little incongruity between the remaining articular surface and the soft tissue. A heavy-gauge wire may be used to reinforce the repair. Rarely, comminution may be so severe that partial patellectomy alone is inadequate. In this setting, no viable choice exists other that complete patellectomy. The results following total patellectomy, however, are uniformly disappointing, often resulting in decreased strength, persistent discomfort, and an extensor lag.[60–62]

The decision to operate should be made expeditiously. The subcutaneous location of the patella makes it prone to concomitant soft-tissue injury. Open fractures should be taken to the operating room for irrigation and debridement as soon as possible after the injury. A midline incision is the most versatile and utilitarian when addressing fractures of the patella. Complete exposure of the patella and the extensor mechanism is mandatory to determine the full extent of injury to the extensor mechanism.

Many forms of internal fixation for patellar fractures have been described in the literature. Fixation may be achieved with wires or screws, either alone or in combination. Regardless of the method of fixation, an anatomic reduction of the articular surface must be achieved. Reduction of the fracture, along the anterior extra-articular surface, does not guarantee a congruous articular reduction; a miniarthrotomy allows direct visualization of the fracture site to ensure articular congruity and can prevent violation of the articular surface by fixation devices. The Swiss Association for the Study of Internal Fixation (AO/ASIF) has popularized the modified tension-band technique as a method of fixation (Figure 13.15).[63] In this technique, two parallel Kirschner wires are passed longitudinally through

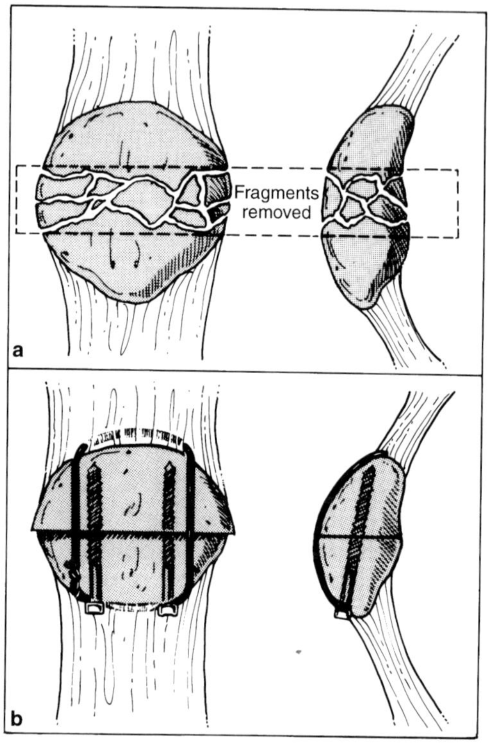

FIGURE 13.16. A partial patellectomy and repair for a comminuted patella fracture recommended by the AO/ASIF group.[63] (a) The comminuated fragments are removed and the proximal and distal fragments are cut level. (b) The proximal and distal fragments are secured with two compression screws and augmented with a circlage wire.

the midportion of the patella following anatomic reduction. An 18-gauge wire is then looped around the wires and symmetrically tightened. By neutralizing the distraction force that acts on the anterior surface of the patella with flexion, a compressive force is created along the articular surface of the fracture which acts to improve stability. Comminuted fractures can be fixed by a similar technique along with a partial patellectomy (Figure 13.16). Avulsion fractures can be easily repaired with internal fixation (Figure 13.17).

Recently, a technique combining cannulated screws in conjunction with tension-band wiring has been reported.[64] In this technique, two parallel cannulated lag screws (4.0 to 4.5 mm) are placed across the fracture. An 18-gauge tension-band wire is placed through one of the cannulated screws, then over the anterior surface of the patella, through the center of the other cannulated screw, and then back over the anterior surface of the patella, where it is twisted to the other end of the wire.[64] Theoretically, this construct should provide resistance to fracture displacement from anterior distraction when the knee is in extension as well as resistance to displacement as the knee moves into flexion.[64]

Conclusion

In summary, extensor mechanism injuries represent a challenging problem for the orthopedic surgeon. Accurate diagnosis is essential, since the best results are obtained with early diagnosis and treatment. Numerous

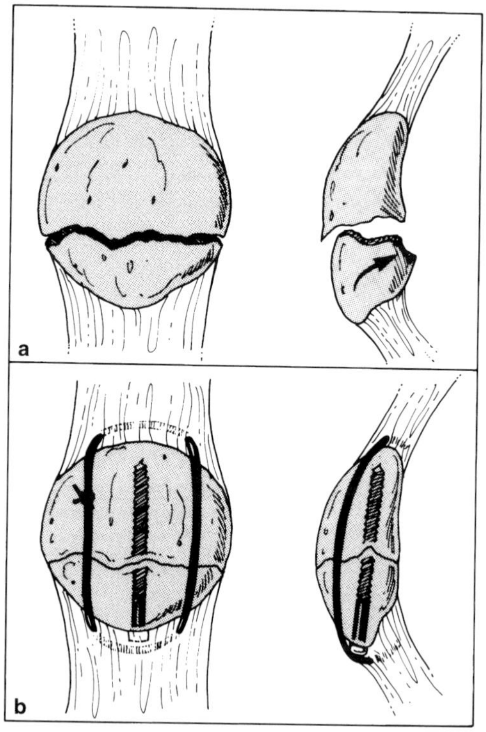

FIGURE 13.17. Internal fixation for an avulsion fracture of the distal pole of the patella. (a) The displaced avulsion of the distal pole of the patella. (b) Following anatomic reduction the fragment is secured with a compression screw and augmented with a circlage wire.

techniques have been described for both early and late repairs. The choice of which repair to use is dependent upon the location of the extensor mechanism disruption, the time interval between injury and repair, and the degree of secondary contractures. Despite these difficulties, satisfactory results can be achieved.

References

1. Feritti A: Epidemiology of jumper's knee. *Sports Med* 1986;3:289–295.
2. Woodall W, Welsh J: A biomechanical basis for rehabilitation program involving the patellofemoral joint. *J Orthop Sports Phys Ther* 1990;11:535–542.
3. Blazina ME, Kerlan RK, Jobe FW, et al.: Jumper's knee. *Orthop Clin North Am* 1973;4:665–673.
4. Antich TJ, Brewster CE: Modification of quadriceps femoris muscle exercises during knee rehabilitation. *Phys Ther* 1986;66:1246–1251.
5. Antich TJ, Randall, CC, Westbrook, RA, et al.: Treatment of knee extensor mechanism disorders: Comparison of four treatment modalities. *J Orthop Sports Phys Ther* 1986;8:225–259.
6. Scuderi GR: Quadriceps and patellar tendon disruptions, in Scott WN (ed.): *The Knee.* St. Louis, Mosby, 1994, pp. 469–478.
7. Bono JV, Teixeira K, Roger DJ, et al.: Central third patellar ligament graft: The anatomic "taper." *Am J Knee Surg* 1994;7(1):36–38.
8. Reider B, Marshall JL, Koslin B, et al.: The anterior aspect of the knee joint. An anatomic study. *J Bone Joint Surg* 63:351–356.
9. Hohl M, Larson RL, Jones DC: Disruption of the extensor mechanism, in Rockwood, Green (eds.): *Fractures in Adults.* Philadelphia, JB Lippincott Co., 1984.
10. Preston FT: Avulsions of both quadriceps tendons in hyperparathyroidism. *JAMA* 1972; 221(4):406–407.
11. Miles JW, Grana WA, Egle D, et al.: The effect of anabolic steroids on the biomechanical and histological properties of patella tendon. *J Bone Joint Surg* 1992;74:411–422.
12. Galen: De usu partium corpus huminis librae. 1533.
13. McBurney C: Suture of the divided ends of a ruptured quadriceps extensor tendon with perfect recovery. *Ann Surg* 1887;6:170.
14. Quenu E, Duval P: Traitement operatoire des ruptures sousrotuliennes du quadriceps. *Rev Chir Orthop Reparatrice Appar Mot* 1905; 31:169–194.
15. Gallie WE, LeMesurier AB: The late repair of fractures of the patella and of rupture of the ligamentum patellae and quadriceps tendon. *J Bone Joint Surg* 1927;9(1):47–54.
16. Siwek CW, Rao JP: Ruptures of the extensor mechanism of the knee joint. *J Bone Joint Surg Am* 1981;63A(6):932–937.
17. Anderson WE, Habermann ET: Spontaneous bilateral quadriceps tendon rupture in a patient on hemodialysis. *Orthop Rev* 1988;17:411.
18. Bhole R, Johnson JC: Bilateral simultaneous spontaneous rupture of quadriceps tendons in a diabetic patient. *South Med J* 1985;78:486.
19. Goodrich A, Difiore RJ, Tippens JK: Bilateral simultaneous rupture of the infrapatellar tendon: A case report and literature review. *Orthopedics* 1983;6(1):1472–1474.
20. Kamali M: Bilateral traumatic rupture of the infrapatellar tendon. *Clin Orthop* 1979; 142:131–134.
21. Keogh P, Shanker SJ, Burke T, et al.: Bilateral simultaneous rupture of the quadriceps tendons. *Clin Orthop* 1988;234:139.
22. Lavalee C, Aparicio LA, Moreno J, et al.: Bilateral avulsion of quadriceps tendons in primary hyperparathyroidism. *J Rheum* 1985; 12:596.
23. MacEachern AG, Plewes JL: Bilateral simultaneous spontaneous rupture of the quadriceps tendons: Five case reports and a review of the literature. *J Bone Joint Surg Br* 1984; 66B(1):81–83.
24. Margles SW, Lewis MM: Bilateral spontaneous concurrent rupture of the patellar tendon without apparent associated systemic disease: A case report. *Clin Orthop* 1978;136:186.
25. Razzano CD, Wilde AH, Phalen GH: Bilateral rupture of the infrapatellar tendon in rheumatoid arthritis. *Clin Orthop* 1973;91:158–161.
26. Stern RE, Harwin SF: Spontaneous and simultaneous rupture of both quadriceps tendons. *Clin Orthop* 1980;147:188–189.
27. Walker LG, Glick H: Bilateral spontaneous quadriceps tendon ruptures. A case report and review of literature. *Orthop Rev* 1989;18:867.
28. Webb LX, Toby EB: Bilateral rupture of the patella tendon in an otherwise healthy male patient following minor trauma. *J Trauma* 1986; 26:1045.

29. Lynch AF, Rorabeck CH, Bourne RB: Extensor mechanism complications following total knee arthroplasty. *J Arthroplasty* 1987;2:135.
30. Blaiser RB, Ciullo JV: Rupture of the quadriceps tendon after arthroscopic lateral release. *Arthroscopy* 1986;2:262–263.
31. Bonamo J, Krinick R, Sparn A: Rupture of the patellar ligament after use of its central third for anterior cruciate reconstruction. *J Bone Joint Surg Am* 1984;66A:1294.
32. Longan P, Fontanetta AP: Rupture of the patella tendon after use of its central third. *Orthop Rev* 1987;16:317.
33. Naver L, Aalberg JR: Rupture of the quadriceps tendon following dislocation of the patella. A case report. *J Bone Joint Surg Am* 1985; 67A:324.
34. Ramsey RH, Muller: Quadriceps tendon rupture: A diagnostic trap. *Clin Orthop* 1970; 70:161–164.
35. Scuderi GR: Extensor mechanism injuries: Treatment, in Scott WN (ed.): *Ligament and Extensor Mechanism Injuries of the Knee.* St. Louis, Mosby–Year Book, 1991, pp. 183–193.
36. Kelly DW, Carter VS, Jobe FW, et al.: Patella and quadriceps tendon ruptures—Jumper's knee. *Am J Sports Med* 1984;12(5):375–380.
37. Nance EP, Kaye JJ: Injuries of the quadriceps mechanism. *Radiology* 1982;142:301–307.
38. Kelly DW, Godfrey KD, Johanson PH, et al.: Quadriceps rupture in association with the roentgenographic "tooth" sign: A case report. *Orthopedics* 1980;3(12):1206–1208.
39. Aprin H, Broukhim B: Early diagnosis of acute rupture of the quadriceps tendon by arthrography. *Clin Orthop* 1985;195:185.
40. Daffner RH, Riemer BL, Lupetin AR, et al.: Magnetic resonance imaging in acute tendon ruptures. *Skeletal Radiol* 1986;15:619.
41. Dabezies EJ, Schutte J: Orthopedic grand rounds: Quadriceps rupture: Case report. Orthopedics 1981;4(3):357–359.
42. Larsen L, Lund PM: Ruptures of the extensor mechanism of the knee joint. *Clin Orthop* 1986; 213:150.
43. Levy M, Goldstein J, Rosner M: A method of repair for quadriceps tendon or patellar ligament (tendon) ruptures without cast immobilization. *Clin Orthop* 1987;218:297.
44. Oni OO, Ahmad SH: The vastus lateralis derived flap for repair of neglected rupture of the quadriceps femoris tendon. *Surg Gynecol Obstet* 1985;161:385.
45. McLaughlin HL: Repair of ruptures through the larger tendons by removable staple suture. *Arch Surg* 1946;52:547–556.
46. McLaughlin HL: Repair of major tendon rupture by buried removable suture. *Am J Surg* 1947;74(5):758–764.
47. McLaughlin HL, Francis KC: Operative repair of injuries to the quadriceps extensor mechanism. *Am J Surg* 1956;91:651–653.
48. Scuderi C: Ruptures of the quadriceps tendon: Study of 20 tendon ruptures. *Am J Surg* 1958; 95(4):626–635.
49. Scuderi C, and Schrey EL: Ruptures of the quadriceps tendon: Study of 14 tendon ruptures. *Arch Surg* 1950;61:42–54.
50. Miskew WBW, Pearson RL, Pankowvich AM: Mersilene strip suture in repair of disruptions of the quadriceps and patellar tendons. *J Trauma* 1980;20(10):867–872.
51. Ecker ML, Lotke PA, Glazer RM: Late reconstruction of the patellar tendon. *J Bone Joint Surg Am* 1979;61A(6):884–886.
52. Kelikian H, Riashi E, Gleason J: Restoration of quadriceps function in neglected tear of the patellar tendon. *Surg Gynecol Obstet* 1957; 104(2):200–204.
53. Frazier CH: Tendon repairs with dacron vascular graft suture: A follow up report. *Orthopedics* 1981;4(5):539–540.
54. Frazier CH, Clark EM: Major tendon repairs with dacron vascular graft suture. *Orthopedics* 1981;3(4):539–540.
55. Evans PD, Pritchard GA, Jenkins DH: Carbon fibre used in the late reconstruction of rupture of the extensor mechanism of the knee. *Injury* 1987;18:57.
56. Scuderi GR, Scharf SC, Meltzer LP, et al.: The relationship of lateral releases to patella viability in total knee arthroplasty. *J Arthroplasty* 1987;2:209–214.
57. Scuderi G, Scharf SC, Meltzer LP, et al.: Evaluation of patella viability after disruption of the arterial circulation. *Am J Sports Med* 1987; 15:490–493.
58. Phillip BB: Knee injuries, in *Campbell's Operative Orthopedics,* ed. 8. St. Louis, CV Mosby Co., 1992, pp. 1895–1938.
59. Hughston JC: Subluxation of the patella. *J Bone Joint Surg Am* 1968;50A:1003–1026.
60. Einola S, Aho AJ, Kallio P: Patellectomy after fracture. Long-term follow-up results with special reference to functional disability. *Acta Orthop Scand* 1976;47:441–447.
61. Jakobsen J, Christensen KS, Rasmussen OS: Patellectomy. A 20-year follow-up. *Acta Orthop Scand* 1985;56:430–432.

62. Peeples RE, Margo MK: Function after patellectomy. *Clin Orthop* 1978;132:180–186.
63. Muller ME, Allgower M, Schneider R, et al.: in Schatzker J (translated by): *Manual of Internal Fixation: Techniques Recommended by the AO Group*, ed. 2. New York, Springer-Verlag, 1979, pp. 348–352.
64. Carpenter JE, Kasman R, Matthews LS: Fractures of the patella. *J Bone Joint Surg Am* 1993; 75A:1550–1562.

14

Complications of Patellofemoral Surgery

David C. Hillsgrove and Lonnie E. Paulos

With a better understanding of the anatomy and biomechanics of the patellofemoral joint and the more specific indications for surgical intervention, complications of patellofemoral surgery should become less frequent. However, seemingly innocuous procedures can result in severe functional disability if complications arise. Nothing can substitute for carefully planned and performed procedures in avoiding such complications. This chapter will address the complications of patellofemoral surgery, their avoidance, and guidelines for treating complications that may occur.

As a sesamoid bone within the quadriceps tendon, the patella floats in the femoral groove with increasing degrees of flexion. Normally, the patella is well seated in the groove by 30° of flexion. Both static and dynamic restraints influence patellar tracking and thus extensor mechanism function. The static restraints include the bony congruence and geometry, as well as the knee ligaments. A dysplastic femoral sulcus will predispose to patellar subluxation and dislocation. Excessive femoral anteversion or tibial external rotation will result in an increase in the lateral vector pull on the patella during flexion, leading to lateral tracking. Rotational stability afforded the knee by the anterior cruciate ligament and medial collateral ligament prevent excessive valgus and external rotation that can contribute to abnormal patellofemoral articulation. The patellofemoral ligaments are significant restraints to medial and lateral patellar glide. Overrestraint or underrestraint can influence patellar tracking and alter normal articular pressures. The dynamic stabilizers are the quadriceps muscle, most importantly the vastus medialis obliquus (VMO). Deficiency of the VMO because of developmental abnormality or acquired atrophy lead to further lateral subluxation of the patella.[1]

The common complaints of patellofemoral problems include pain, grinding, giving way, subluxation, and dislocation. These are the end result of several etiologies including developmental and acquired abnormalities. A systematic history and physical examination will most often delineate the primary cause. At times, more than one abnormality can be identified. Developmental problems include lateral patellar compression syndrome (LPCS), malalignment, and patellofemoral dysplasia. LPCS is the result of a tight lateral retinaculum that inhibits the normal distribution of joint reactive forces in the patellofemoral joint, leading to an overload of the lateral patellar facet and the lateral femoral condyle. Passive patellar tilt is 0° or less, patellar glide is less than two quadrants, and the lateral retinaculum is often tender to palpation. A patient presenting with these findings without significant malalignment is a candidate for a lateral release if conservative measures fail. Malalignment may be diagnosed proximally, distally, or both. It is characterized by examining the proximal soft-tissue restraints and the tubercle sulcus angle at 90°. By determining the site or sites of abnormality, a proximal realignment, including lateral release and medial reefing, may be necessary with a distal procedure such as a tibial tubercle osteotomy, if indicated. Patellofemoral dysplasia encompasses abnormalities of the patella or the femoral sulcus, excessive femoral anteversion, and excessive tibial external rotation. No predictable surgical option exists; however, derotational osteotomies are occasionally performed. Injury to the extensor mechanism, arthritides, and failed complicated surgical intervention represent acquired disorders of the patellofemoral joint. Open reduction and internal fixation offers the best results following patella fractures amenable to holding fixation. Partial or total patellectomy remains an option in highly comminuted fractures. Ruptures of the patellar tendon or quadriceps tendon are best treated with early repair. Isolated posttraumatic arthritis or osteoarthritis of the patellofemoral joint may be treated with anteriorization of the tibial tubercle or, less desirably, by partial or total patellectomy. Such procedures are contraindicated in multicompartment osteoarthritis or inflammatory arthritis. In these cases, total knee replacement may be required if symptoms warrant. Patellofemoral replacement is still considered to be experimental.

The patellofemoral joint often assumes a passive role in reconstructive procedures such as anterior cruciate ligament or posterior cruciate ligament surgery. However, the central third patellar tendon used as autogenous graft is popular. Transpatellar tendon exposures for tibial plateau and distal femoral procedures have limited applications. As demonstrated, several conditions may require direct or indirect alteration of the patellofemoral joint (Table 14.1). Complications may occur and must be dealt with as meticulously as the original surgery if a satisfactory outcome is to be obtained.

Complications of Lateral Release

Release of the lateral retinaculum and capsule was first described in the English literature in 1974 by Merchant and Mercer for patients with recurrent subluxation or dislocation of the patella.[2] Arthroscopic lateral release was further championed by Metcalf in 1982.[3] Small retrospectively reviewed 10,262 knee arthroscopies for complication including 446 lateral releases.[4] Complications developed in 7.2% of patients of which 65% were hemarthroses. Other complications include deep vein thrombosis (DVT) and infection. Direct correlation of lateral release to incidence of hemarthrosis was found with the use of a tourniquet, subcutaneous technique, and the use of a drain for 24 hours. Hemarthrosis inhibits forceful contraction of the quadriceps leading to atrophy, which is most pronounced in the vastus medialis.[5,6] Small recommended release of the tourniquet prior to closure in order to examine the superior lateral genicular artery for bleeding and also the use of a drain for 2 to 3 hours postoperatively.

Should a tense hemarthrosis develop, consideration should be given to sterile aspiration. This is performed with an 18- or 16-gauge needle placed superolaterally in the suprapatellar pouch. A 1% lidocaine with epinephrine may be instilled followed by a compressive dressing and application of ice to prevent recurrence. Surgical exploration is rarely indicated. Treatment of DVT and infection are based on local and systemic factors.

The goal of lateral release is to lessen the restraining factor of the distal aspect of the vastus lateralis origin from the intermuscular septum and the epicondyle. Extensive release of the vastus lateralis, as advocated by some, has led to pronounced quadriceps weakness, medial subluxation of the patella, quadriceps tendon rupture, and patellar hypermobility.[7–12] Hughston and Deese retrospectively reviewed 54 patients who underwent lateral release 6 to 8 cm above the superior pole of the patella and failed to improve or had worsening symptoms following release.[9] Clinically detectable medial subluxation was found in 50% of patients. Atrophy and retraction of the vastus lateralis were also found. In another study of patients with failed lateral release, Shellock et al. used kinematic magnetic resonance imaging (MRI) to demonstrate medial subluxa-

TABLE 14.1. Summary of complications of patellofemoral surgery.

Diagnosis	Procedure	Complications
Malalignment	Lateral release	Hemarthrosis Tendon rupture Quadriceps weakness Medial patellar subluxation
	Proximal realignment	Recurrent instability Medial patellar subluxation Patellar malrotation Arthrofibrosis
	Proximal/distal realignment	Nonunion Physeal closure Neurovascular injury Recurrent instability Arthrofibrosis Osteoarthritis
Lateral patellar compression syndrome (LPCS)	Lateral release	See previous description
Patellofemoral dysplasia	None	
Patellar arthrosis, chondromalacia	Maquet procedure	See proximal/distal realignment
	Patellectomy partial/total	Extensor weakness Tendon rupture Tendon calcification Extensor mechanism instability Compromise arthroplasty
Patella fracture	Open reduction, internal fixation	Nonunion Malunion Osteoarthritis Avascular necrosis
	Patellectomy	See previous description
Tendon rupture	Tendon repair/reconstruction	Rerupture Quadriceps atrophy Loss of motion Patella baja/patella alta
Graft source	Harvest of central third of tendon	Quadriceps weakness Infrapatellar contraction syndrome

tion in 63% of the knees with continued symptoms following lateral release.[12]

Worsening of patellar hypermobility with recurrent subluxation or dislocation may result from lateral release in patients with marginal or incompetent medial restraints.[9-12] Adequate assessment of preoperative patellar glide is imperative to avoid this complication. Kolowich et al. compared two groups of patients who had undergone lateral release and were entirely satisfied or were complete failures to define more objective criteria for this procedure.[10] Negative passive patellar tilt was the most predictable criterion for success. In addition, medial and lateral patellar glides of less than two quadrants and a normal tubercle sulcus angle at 90° correlated with the more favorable outcome. Radiographic criteria of congruence angle was not a reliable predictor of outcome.

While initial results of isolated lateral release were up to 85% good or excellent, these numbers have not withstood the test of time.[3,13-16] Specific complications such as hemarthrosis, infection, and DVT may be preventable as stated previously. However, patient selection and the avoidance of an overzealous release prevent failure to relieve symptoms or onset of medial subluxation.

When performing lateral release, both the retinaculum and the synovium should be incised up to the level of the vastus lateralis.[10] Tracking of the patella may then be observed through the superolateral portal. If the patella continues to track laterally, the insertion of the vastus lateralis should not be released more proximally. Complete release of the vastus lateralis insertion is contraindicated and medial reefing should be considered if the patella does not center adequately. Should medial tracking be noted, reattachment or repair of the superior aspect of the release is considered using a suture anchor in the midcoronal plane of the patella to prevent lateral tilt because of anteriorization of the retinaculum.

Complications of Proximal Realignment

Along with the previously described lateral release, proximal realignment also involves medial plication of the vastus medialis insertion. Patients must be examined for increased tubercle sulcus angle, as failure to perform a distal osteotomy in these patients will lead to recurrent instability. Other complications include medial subluxation, arthrofibrosis, and patellar malrotation and tilt.[16,17]

Medial reefing most often follows lateral release in patients with a normal tubercle sulcus angle when the patella continues to track laterally after adequate release of the capsule and the synovium. Medial subluxation results from overadvancement of the vastus medialis as Hughston and Walsh reported.[16] Patients with hypermobile patella, that is, greater than three quadrants of patellar glide, are at greatest risk for this complication.

Malrotation and excessive tilt of the patella can lead to increased contact pressures because of reduced surface area contact in the patellofemoral joint. In a study of the contact pressure changes following capsular reconstruction procedure, Huberti and Hayes demonstrated increased contact stresses on the lateral side after medial capsular plication.[18] Malrotation may result from misplacement of the VMO advancement sutures by as little as 1 to 2 mm.[16] Potentially, malrotation and tilt can lead to accelerated patellofemoral arthrosis.

To prevent such misadventures, Hughston and Walsh have recommended placing provisional sutures when performing medial plication.[16] The knee is then repeatedly flexed and extended to evaluate tracking and presence of tilt. Use of a suture anchor to advance the VMO into a midcoronal bony trough and avoiding advancement below the equator of the patella will prevent inadvertent introduction of medial tilt or rotation of the patella. One must also keep in mind that evaluation of tracking in an anesthetized patient eliminates the dynamic effect the quadriceps has on patellofemoral articulation. Thus, optimal alignment of the static restraints is extremely important.

Complications of Combined Proximal and Distal Realignment

Patients with a history of recurrent subluxation or dislocation of the patella and a tubercle sulcus angle of greater than 5° may benefit from a combined proximal and distal realignment procedure.[10,19] In addition to the previously described complications associated with proximal realignment, distal osteotomy offers further risks. Nonunion, physeal arrest, loss of motion, patellar tendon injury, neurovascular injury, accelerated arthrosis, and recurrent instability are complications associated with distal realignment.[20–33]

Infrapatellar contraction syndrome (IPCS) is characterized by significant restriction in knee flexion and extension, as well as compromised patellar mobility.[20] This will be discussed as a separate section. There is a significant relationship of development of ankylosis to the timing of surgery. Distal realignment performed soon after acute dislocation with an associated hemarthrosis is at increased risk for development of ankylosis as Cox reported.[21] Current recommendations of delay in surgery until the hemarthrosis resolves and range of motion has been regained may help decrease the incidence of fibrous ankylosis.

Nonunion of the distal bony block with displacement has been reported with high incidence in some studies.[22–24] With early mobilization rehabilitation protocols to prevent loss of motion, internal fixation is strongly recommended. Should displacement or nonunion occur, revision with the use of rigid internal fixation and autogenous bone grafting may salvage the outcome.

Arrest of the tibial tubercle physis may result from bony distal realignment procedures in skeletally immature patients and is mentioned only to condemn this operation in this patient population. Physeal closure can result in angular deformity, recurvatum, and distal migration of the patellar tendon with patella baja.[16,21–27] Osteotomy with or without completion of epiphysiodesis would be required to correct the resultant deformity if indicated.[23,27]

Neurovascular injury with resultant palsy or compartment syndrome have been reported. Garland and Hughston reviewed four cases of peroneal nerve palsy after performing a Hauser procedure.[28] The palsies were the result of hematoma compression of the peroneal nerve in patients who did not have the tourniquet released prior to closure. They recommend release of the tourniquet prior to closure to establish adequate hemostasis. Evacuation of hematoma should be accomplished with limited exploration of the peroneal nerve in this setting. Vascular complications resulting in compartment syndrome following a Hauser procedure were reported by Wall[29] and Wiggins.[30] In Wall's review, 11 patients suffered residual disabilities ranging from mild weakness to above-knee amputations in two patients.[29] Through cadaveric dissection, Wall postulated that a leash of recurrent anterior tibial vessels may be ligated at the time of surgery. The vessels retract posteriorly out of site and continue to bleed. Ischemic necrosis of the anterior compartment may ensue followed by development of elevated compartment pressures in the other lower-leg compartments. Failure to recognize the cardinal signs of compartment syndrome can lead to delay in diagnosis and treatment, with a greater loss of function. If compartment syndrome is suspected on the basis of physical examination, dressings should be released and compartment pressures measured. Four-compartment fasciotomy leaving the skin open followed by delayed closure or split-thickness skin grafting is indicated in symptomatic patients with pressures greater than 30 mm Hg.

Correction of the tubercle sulcus angle to 0° avoids medial patellar subluxation and recurrent lateral subluxation associated with overcorrection and undercorrection, respectively.[10,22,25] Tibial tubercle osteotomy can be better controlled by beginning the osteotomy on the lateral cortex and extending distally 6 to 8 cm below the proximal edge, leaving the distal and medial periosteal hinges intact. Medial displacement is accomplished with thumb pressure. The knee is then flexed and extended to find the optimal position of the tubercle following centralization of the patella in the femoral groove. If revision is necessary due to recurrent instability, Templeman and McBeath describe a technique of correction under local anesthesia to preserve the dynamic function of quadriceps in selection of a more appropriate tubercle sulcus angle.[31]

Finally, suboptimal alteration of the patellofemoral contact forces can lead to accelerated arthrosis. Again, this complication is most closely associated with the Hauser procedure. Patella baja because of distalization of the tubercle results in immediate disability following surgery, retropatellar pain, and loss of motion.[16,25,32,33,34] Diagnosis is based on radiographic comparison with the contralateral knee. Excessive posteriorization of the tubercle along the medial cortex of the tibia results in increased joint reactive forces by shortening the moment arm of the patellofemoral joint and long-term moderate to severe patellofemoral arthrosis is seen in up to 70% of patients.[23,33] Early recognition of patella baja and posterior placement of the tubercle warrant immediate revision to a more optimal position.

Complications of Salvage Procedures

When nonoperative measures are unsuccessful for intractable pain because of isolated patellofemoral arthrosis, salvage procedures such as the Maquet procedure, patellofemoral arthroplasty, and total patellectomy are considered.

Maquet Procedure

Maquet described the anteriorization of the tibial tubercle to reduce the loads on the patellofemoral joint and thus slow the progress of patellofemoral arthrosis.[35] The original recommendation of 2 cm of elevation led to wound-healing problems in 9.7% of patients.[36,37] Several other reviews have reported complications in up to 56% of patients, with most related to skin necrosis or wound dehiscence.[36,38–42] More recent work evaluated the need for anteriorization beyond 1.5 cm.[39,43] Heatley et al. found a diminishing mechanical benefit beyond 1.25 to 1.5 cm, concluding that the risks of wound-healing problems outweigh the benefit of the extra elevation of the tibial tubercle.[34] Other recommendations to limit wound-healing problems include relaxing incisions, use of tissue expanders in patients with previous anterior knee scars and inadequate soft tissue, and the use of drains to avoid hematoma formation leading to compromise of local circulation.[40] Radin and Labosky routinely use oblique incisions to limit flap creation and to avoid extensive soft-tissue dissection, preserving the local blood supply.[42] While the presence of previous scars is a relative contraindication to a Maquet procedure, skin extensibility, evaluated by an adequate pinch test described by Mendes et al., may serve as an indication that the tissues are relatively safe and the procedure may be performed.[40] Skin necrosis with subsequent slough should be treated aggressively and coverage should be obtained as soon as possible to avoid increased risk of developing osteomyelitis. Plastic surgery consultation is recommended as needed. Graft displacement and nonunion of the osteotomy site have been reported in up to 5% of patients undergoing the Maquet procedure.[38–40] Internal fixation of the graft and osteotomy reduce the incidence of this complication. However, several authors have recommended against the use of hardware because it may increase the risk of wound-healing problems.[38,41] Internal fixation has the advantage of allowing early motion, which reduces the risk of arthrofibrosis. Less micromotion at the osteotomy site will allow for more predictable healing and graft incorporation. Radin and Labosky stressed the importance of fitting the graft flush with the proximal edge of the osteotomy shingle.[42] This reduces the chances of osteotomy fracture and subsequent displacement of the graft and the tubercle. The knee should be placed through a full range of motion intraoperatively to ensure adequate stability of the graft. Routine use of a low-profile screw is recommended to prevent graft or tubercle displacement and to avoid local wound complications. If graft displacement, tubercle fracture, or symptomatic nonunion occur, early revision with the use of autogenous bone graft and rigid internal fixation are recommended. A Kennedy ligament augmentation device may be used as a stent to protect the healing osteotomy site if adequate internal fixation of the bony fragments is not obtained.

Complications of iliac bone graft harvest also exist with the Maquet procedure. While most are relatively minor complaints of prolonged pain usually resolving after one to two years, others are severe. Mendes et al. had two patients with incisional hernias at the graft harvest site.[40] One patient required repair with a Dacron mesh graft. Proper planning and surgical technique including tight closure of the deep fascia can circumvent most serious complications.

Patellofemoral Arthroplasty

Isolated patellofemoral resurfacing remains investigational. Early designs were associated with unpredictable outcome and various complications leading to early failure and revision. Loosening, patellar subluxation, maltracking, and loss of motion were reported in a series of 85 patellofemoral arthroplasties by Blazina et al.[44] A total of 101 secondary procedures were performed to correct complications. Furthermore, 42% of patients with long-term followup continued to have mild to moderate pain.

Insall et al. had a 45% failure rate in a series of 28 patients undergoing patellar resurfacing.[45] Recurrent effusion, instability, and great quadriceps atrophy also occurred in many patients. Revision to total knee replacement or patellectomy are possible salvage procedures for failed patellofemoral resurfacing.

Patellectomy

Once a common procedure for treatment of patellofemoral arthrosis, total patellectomy is rarely indicated, except in severely comminuted patellar fractures.[46–48] Complications following patellectomy include extensor mechanism weakness, extensor lag, subluxation of the quadriceps tendon, degenerative changes of the femoral groove, and rupture of the quadriceps tendon.[14,36,37,48–55] Extensive work has been done to study the effects of patellectomy on the efficiency and the strength of the extensor mechanism. The mechanical advantage of a longer lever arm is lost after patellectomy, requiring a large force to be generated by the quadriceps muscle in order to extend the knee.[37] Clinical manifestations include difficulty ascending and descending stairs, progressive knee recurvatum because of instability in stance, and quadriceps atrophy as a result of pain from excessive friction at the abnormal tendon–femoral groove articulation. The average loss of strength following patellectomy is approximately 50%.[49] Kaufer showed a 30% decrease in quadriceps efficiency in the terminal 60° of knee extension.[50] As a result, extensor lag averaging 18° requires approximately a 15% increase in quadriceps contraction force to compensate for the loss of the patella. Maquet has reported quadriceps rupture following patellectomy resulting from such increased force.[36] Anteriorization of the tibial tubercle has been suggested to compensate for the loss of the normal lever arm and thus increase the efficiency of the extensor mechanism following patellectomy. No long-term clinical data exist for this set of circumstances at this time.

Subluxation of the quadriceps tendon may occur postpatellectomy.[14,51] Failure to balance the medial and lateral constraints can lead to subluxation with further compromise of the extensor strength and excessive wear of the femoral condyles. Release of tight retinacular tissues or plication of incompetent restraints may be required. However, if the tubercle sulcus angle is increased, distal realignment is considered.

Quadriceps tendon calcification may occur following patellectomy. While some studies suggest that calcification correlates with poorer results, others have refuted this association. Compere et al. describe a method of protecting the trochlear groove if calcification occurs.[48] They suggest tubing the quadriceps tendon to prevent damaging the cartilage of the trochlear groove if calcification develops.

Accelerated medial and lateral compartment arthrosis following patellectomy is the result of an altered angle of pull. Tibiofemoral compressive forces have been shown to increase in the postpatellectomy knee.[37,52,53] Total knee replacement results are worse in postpatellectomy knees. Component loosening, instability, continued pain, and weakness in extension contribute to less predictable outcomes in these patients.[54] Beuchel described a technique of implanting a small bone graft in the anatomic location of the patella to reestablish the mechanical advantage of the quadriceps.[55] In six of seven patients, normal gait and extension were restored.

Partial patellectomy offers an attractive alternative to total patellectomy. Indications include painful, impinging facet with loss of cartilage on the patella and in fractures with severely comminuted inferior or superior poles having a significant remaining uninvolved fragment. In the arthritic knee, only the impinging portion of the patella is resected. This may be performed open or arthroscopically. Complications are failure to remove enough patella or removing too much patella so as to compromise future total knee replacement. With patellar fractures requiring resection of a comminuted pole, failure of the tendon to bone repair is managed with early reoperation. Suture anchors and autogenous graft with semitendinosus or gracilis tendons may be used to supplement primary repair.

Complications of Patellar Fracture Treatment

Patellar fractures occur as a result of a direct blow to the anterior knee or a sudden, forceful contraction of the quadriceps exceeding the strength of the patella in osteoporotic patients. Operative intervention is required if the extensor mechanism is incompetent, or a step off or separation of fragments exceeds 2 mm.[56] Methods of surgical treatment include open reduction and internal fixation, partial patellectomy with repair of the tendon to the remaining patella, or total patellectomy.

Open reduction and internal fixation is most often accomplished with a tension band as described by the Swiss Association for the Study of Internal Fixation (AO/ASIF).[57] Complications include nonunion, malunion with posttraumatic arthrosis, avascular necrosis, hardware problems, and loss of motion. The incidence of nonunion is low at 2.4%.[56] Often patients are minimally symptomatic. Nummi reported 14 of 17 nonunions as having satisfactory results without operative intervention, thus repeat osteosynthesis is advised only if patients are significantly symptomatic and fragments are amenable to fixation.[58] Displacement of fragments was reported at 11% in Nummi's review after initial osteosynthesis. Again, intervention should be individualized to those patients who are symptomatic. Hardware complications are common and usually are related to tendon irritation with motion or prominence in the subcutaneous tissues.[59] These problems are managed by removal of the hardware when the fracture has healed. Scapinelli reported avascular necrosis in 25% of patellar fractures treated by open reduction internal fixation.[60] Treatment is observation, as most will spontaneously revascularize by two years.

Complications of Tendon Rupture Repair

Ruptures of the quadriceps tendon and the patellar tendon occur as the result of direct injury or indirectly from forceful quadriceps contraction. Significant hematoma and quadriceps inhibition make diagnosis difficult in some cases, leading to delay in treatment. Most satisfactory results are obtained with early recognition and surgical repair of the rupture. Complications associated with repair include rerupture, loss of motion, heterotopic ossification, patella alta, patella baja, and quadriceps atrophy.[61,62]

Siwek and Rao reviewed 34 patients with 36 quadriceps tendon ruptures and 33 patients with 36 ruptures of the patellar tendon treated surgically.[61] Motion loss was pronounced in the group undergoing delayed repair of the quadriceps tendon rupture. Only one of six patients regained more than 90° of flexion. Quadriceps atrophy was more common in patients with quadriceps rupture than in those with patellar tendon rupture. Regaining motion in this setting is difficult. Intra-articular adhesions may be lysed arthroscopically with the re-creation of the suprapatellar pouch. Extra-articular scarring is addressed with a quadricepsplasty. The use of continuous passive motion is encouraged in the immediate postoperative period.[61]

Rerupture of the repaired tendon is relatively infrequent. It most often occurs because of early active motion in a recently repaired tendon. Again, early recognition and reoperation are recommended. Augmentation of repairs has been described with wire through the extensor mechanism and tibial shaft below the tubercle. Complications of such augmentation include wire breakage and patella baja in cases of overtightening. A second operation may be needed to remove retained, bothersome hardware. Levy et al. used a 4-mm Dacron vascular graft to reinforce repairs with no noted complications and were able to institute early mobilization.[62] Our practice has been to use the Kennedy ligament augmentation device to protect the repair of the quadriceps or the patellar tendon. Passive motion is begun early to avoid loss of motion. Patella baja with resultant increased patellar forces is avoided by anatomic repair, and early diagnosis and treatment. A lateral radiograph may be taken to compare with the contralateral side in cases of delayed diagnosis and treatment.

Complications of Ligament Surgery

As surgical technique and results of anterior cruciate ligament and posterior cruciate ligament reconstruction improve, the indications for these procedures has been expanded to include a larger population of patients. The central third bone–patellar tendon–bone composite is the most widely used graft for intra-articular reconstruction. However, donor site morbidity is a major concern that is often overlooked. Complications of patellar tendon harvest include patellar tendinitis, quadriceps tendon rupture, patellar tendon rupture, patellar fracture, patellar instability, decreased quadriceps strength, patella baja, and IPCS.[63–70]

Management of quadriceps and patellar tendon rupture have been discussed. Some mention of contributing factors and avoidance of these complications is warranted. Bonamo et al. reported on two patients with patellar tendon rupture following anterior cruciate ligament (ACL) reconstruction with the central third patellar tendon and the quadriceps aponeurosis; no bone block was used.[63] Both patients suffered falls at 3.5 and 8.0 months postoperatively, resulting in patellar tendon avulsion from the inferior pole of the patella. The defect created by tendon harvest was noted to be completely healed at reoperation. The authors postulated that there was reduced tensile strength as a result of compromised vascularity to the remaining tendon and they recommended leaving the defect open. Burks et al. studied the dog model after removal of the central third patellar tendon.[64] They demonstrated a 30% decrease in stiffness and a 66% decrease in modulus of elasticity of the remaining tendon six months after graft harvest. The histologic analysis revealed poorly organized collagen in the area of the healing tendon, which helps explain the decreased tensile strength. No significant difference was found in those tendons that were closed and those left open. DeLee and Craviotto reported on a patient sustaining a quadriceps tendon avulsion six weeks after ACL reconstruction with central third bone–patellar tendon–bone autograft.[65] They cautioned against taking too long of a bone plug from the patella because this may weaken the insertion of the quadriceps tendon. Patellar fracture may occur as a result of graft harvest intraoperatively or in a delayed fashion up to six months postoperatively. Graf and Uhr reviewed the complications of intra-articular ACL reconstruction and reported the occurrence of patellar fractures intraoperatively.[66] No long-term sequelae were noted if the fracture was recognized and adequately stabilized allowing early motion. McCarroll reported a case of transverse patellar fracture occurring six months after ACL reconstruction with the central third bone–patellar tendon–bone autograft.[67] The author postulated that the fracture was due to fatigue of relatively osteoporotic bone resulting from graft harvest. Patellar fractures in this setting are best managed by internal fixation with a tension band configuration using 16- or 18-gauge wire or no. 5 Ti-Cron suture to avoid the need for hardware removal. Early motion is begun if the goal of stable fixation has been obtained. Fractures may be avoided by making the depth of the patellar bone block shallow and the shape of the block a square or trapezoid. A triangular-shaped graft creates a significant stress riser in the patella. In addition, bone graft from the tibial donor site, notchplasty, and tunnel drillings may be used to fill the patellar defect.

Patellar instability can result or be exacerbated by harvest of the medial or lateral third of the patellar tendon.[68] Patients with preexisting patellofemoral malalignment of hypermobile patella are at risk for this complication. At least 1 cm of medial tendon should be retained. Patellar tilt and glides should be assessed following ACL reconstruction. If the tilt is negative and the glide of the patella is reduced, a lateral release is performed.

Patellofemoral crepitation and residual anterior knee pain are common sequelae following ACL reconstruction with the central third patellar tendon autograft. Sachs et al. reported activity-limiting pain in 19% of patients and flexion contracture of greater than 5° in 24% of patients.[69] Quadriceps weakness was present in 65% of patients at one-year followup. Rosenberg et al. reported on a group of patients 12 to 24 months after ACL reconstruction in an accelerated postoperative protocol.[70] Complaints of anterior knee pain, crepitus, and weakness were common, with only one third of patients returning to preinjury sports despite ligamentous stability. The use of alternative graft sources such as semitendinosus or gracilis tendons may alleviate much of these problems.

Infrapatellar Contraction Syndrome

Infrapatellar Contraction Syndrome (IPCS) is a subcategory of arthrofibrosis, which is characterized by significantly restricted patellar mobility, loss of flexion of greater than 25°, and loss of extension of greater than 10°.[20] The use of the patellar tendon as an autogenous graft in ligament reconstruction has been the most commonly associated surgical procedure preceding IPCS.[20,71,72] Lateral release and patellar realignment have also been associated with IPCS. Paulos et al. described patellar entrapment by hyperplasia of the fat pad and retinacular tissues as a result of both injury and immobilization.[20] Patients complain of stiffness, pain, and swelling after prolonged standing or walking. Physical examination reveals patellofemoral crepitation, loss of motion, moderate to severe quadriceps atrophy, and "shelf sign" describing the abrupt drop-off from the patellar tendon to the tibial tubercle because of induration of swollen anterior tissues. Furthermore, patients were unable to sustain a strong contraction of the quadriceps and a tendency toward patella infera was noted.

IPCS may be due to primary infrapatellar contraction or secondary infrapatellar contraction resulting from prolonged immobility, nonisometric ligament reconstruction, or extensive injury to the retropatellar fat pad. Three stages of IPCS are described, with treatment based on the stage at diagnosis. Stage I, or the prodromal stage, develops two to eight weeks after surgery or injury and is characterized by diffuse edema, abnormally prolonged pain, quadriceps weakness, and decreased patellar glide and tilt. Aggressive, supervised rehabilitation emphasizing patellar mobilization, active motion to regain full extension, and use of anti-inflammatory medications are effective at this stage of IPCS.

Stage II, or the active stage, develops in approximately 5% of patients and generally requires surgical intervention. Patients fail to respond to conservative measures. Manual manipulation, forced passive motion, and traction should be avoided because the knee may become more inflamed. Timing of the surgery is delayed until inflammation decreases and a sustained forceful quadriceps contraction is obtained, which may require months of waiting. In a recent followup of 75 patients with IPCS treated surgically, Paulos et al. describe the evaluation and treatment of IPCS.[73] Evaluation of patellar mobility is most important. With true IPCS, superior patellar glide is significantly reduced. After allowing time for the inflammation to reduce, intra-articular and extra-articular releases are performed with debridement of all adhesions. Most importantly, the retropatellar fat pad is resected and the patellar tendon is freed from the anterior, proximal tibia to its insertion. If a patella infera of 8 mm or greater is noted on preoperative radiographs, a tibial tubercle osteotomy with proximal advancement is performed. Manipulation of the knee must be avoided following this procedure because of the risk of fracture through the osteotomy site.

Postoperatively, continuous passive motion, neuromuscular stimulation of the quadriceps, cold therapy, and night extension splints are employed to maintain motion gains with emphasis on full extension. Corticosteroid dose packs may be used as well. If knee flexion is lost as a consequence of maintaining extension, arthroscopic lysis of adhesions and manipulation may be performed six to nine months later to gain flexion. Following this protocol, Paulos et al. reported average extension gains of 14.2° and flexion gains of 32.5°.[73] Modest gains in patellar mobility were also attained. Sixty-one patients had intra-articular ACL reconstruction, predominately with autogenous bone–patellar tendon–bone as the inciting procedure in the development of IPCS. Nonisometric graft placement and impingement of the graft were noted in most cases. Graft resection was performed along with debridement of adhesions. KT-1000 measurements revealed an average side-to-side difference of 3.08 mm in those patients with resected grafts. Despite large gains in motion and objective stability in the treated knees, 88% of patients remained below their preinjury activity level at an average of 53 months following their initial (inciting) surgical procedure.

Stage III IPCS, or the residual stage, presents eight months to one year after the onset of stage I. Physical examination will be less dramatic than stage II, with reduced inflammation and induration of the tissues. Significant patella infera and patellofemoral arthrosis may be the only remaining symptoms. Treatment is directed toward pain control and only salvage procedures such as tubercle advancement, patellectomy, Maquet procedure, and total knee replacement are considered if warranted.

Obviously, avoidance of IPCS is most desirable. Paulos et al. have found that 5% of patients demonstrate abnormal fibrosclerotic healing and may develop IPCS following surgery or injury. There is no test or screening method presently available to detect those patients that are susceptible to developing IPCS. Knowledge of significant associated factors may help reduce the risk of developing IPCS. Avoid surgery on the acutely injured knee if possible until near-normal motion returns and there is minimal inflammation. Perform fewer extra-articular procedures on older and/or acutely injured patients. Risks of using central third bone–patellar tendon–bone composite for ligament reconstruction must be realized and anticipated. Near-isometric graft placement is essential with adequate notchplasty to avoid impingement. Early range of motion, patellar mobilization techniques, and functional rehabilitation as soon as possible are important postoperative considerations. Early recognition of IPCS in the prodromal stage is possible with careful examination of the post-surgical knee. Steps to resolve the problem, often decreasing painful, forceful physical therapy modalities, can be instituted.[20,73]

Reflex Sympathetic Dystrophy

Reflex sympathetic dystrophy (RSD) may occur as the result of any knee surgery or injury, but there appears to be a higher incidence following patellofemoral surgery. Katz and Hungerford reported patellofemoral surgery or injury as the precipitating event in 64% of patients in their series.[74] Cooper et al. reported on 14 patients with RSD of the knee, 11 of which had previous patellar procedures.[75] Clinical manifestations of RSD include unduly prolonged pain, vasomotor disturbances, delayed functional recovery, and trophic changes. Diagnosis is based upon clinical suspicion and is confirmed by relief of symptoms with sympathetic block. Bone scan, thermography, and diffuse osteopenia on x-ray may also aid in the diagnosis. Early diagnosis and treatment correlate with improved outcome.

Treatment includes physical therapy, with emphasis on active range of motion, functional weight bearing, and patellar mobility. Cooper et al. used an indwelling epidural catheter to induce a sympathetic block combined with continuous passive motion, manipulation, stimulation of muscles, and alternating hot and cold soaks. The investigators reported complete resolution in 11 of 14 patients.[75]

References

1. Evans IK, Paulos LE: Complications of patellofemoral joint surgery. *Orthop Clin North Am* 1992;3:697–709.
2. Merchant AC, Mercer RL: Lateral release of the patella: A preliminary report. *Clin Orthop* 1974;103:40–45.
3. Metcalf RW: An arthroscopic method for lateral release of the subluxating or dislocating patella. *Clin Orthop* 1982;167:9–18.
4. Small NC: An analysis of complications in lateral retinacular release procedures. *Arthroscopy* 1989;5:282–286.
5. Dzioba RB: Diagnostic arthroscopy and longitudinal lateral release: A four year follow-up study to determine predictors of surgical outcome. *Am J Sports Med* 1990;18:343–348.
6. Kennedy JC, Alexander IJ, Hayes KC: Nerve supply of the human knee and its functional importance. *Am J Sports Med* 1982; 10:329–335.
7. Betz RR, MaGill JT, Lonergan RP: The percutaneous lateral retinacular release. *Am J Sports Med* 1987;15:477–482.
8. Blasier RB, Ciullo JV: Rupture of the quadriceps tendon after lateral release: A case report. *Arthroscopy* 1986;2:262–263.
9. Hughston JC, Deese M: Medial subluxation of the patella as a complication of lateral retinacular release. *Am J Sports Med* 1988;16:383–388.
10. Kolowich PA, Paulos LE, Rosenberg TD, et al.: Lateral release of the patella: Indications and contraindications. *Am J Sports Med* 1990; 18:359–365.
11. Langeland N: Recurrent dislocation of the patella following lateral retinacular release: A case report. *Arch Orthop Trauma Surg* 1983; 102:65–66.
12. Shellock FG, Mink JH, Dutsch A, et al.: Evaluation of patients with persistent symptoms after lateral retinacular release by kinematic MRI of the patellofemoral joint. *Arthroscopy* 1990; 6:226–234.
13. Ceder LC, Larson RL: Z-plasty lateral retinacular release for the treatment of patellar compression syndrome. *Clin Orthop* 1979; 144:110–113.
14. Kettlekamp DB: Current concepts review: Management of patellar malalignment. *J Bone Joint Surg Am* 1987;63A:1344–1348.
15. McGinty JB, McCarthy JC: Endoscopic lateral retinacular release: A preliminary report. *Clin Orthop* 1981;158:120–125.
16. Hughston JC, Walsh WM: Proximal and distal reconstruction of the extensor mechanism for patellar subluxation. *Clin Orthop* 1979;144:36–42.
17. Larson RL: Subluxation-dislocation of the patella, in Kennedy JC (ed.): *The Injured Adolescent Knee.* Baltimore: Williams & Wilkins Co., 1979;pp. 161–204.
18. Huberti HH, Hayes WC: Contact pressure in chondromalacia patellae and the effects of capsular reconstructive procedures. *J Orthop Res* 1988;6:499–508.
19. Brown DE, Alexander AH, Lichtman DM: The Elmslie-Trillat procedure: Evaluation in patellar dislocation and subluxation. *Am J Sports Med* 1984;12:104–109.
20. Paulos LE, Rosenberg TD, Draubach J, et al.: Infrapatellar contraction syndrome: An unrecognized cause of knee stiffness with patella entrapment and patella infera. *Am J Sports Med* 1987;15:331–341.
21. Cox JS: Evaluation of the Rous-Elmslie-Trillat procedure for knee extensor realignment. *Am J Sports Med* 1982;10:303–310.
22. Barbari S, Raugstad TS, Lichtensberg N: The Hauser operation for patellar dislocation: 3–32 year results in 63 knees. *Acta Orthop Scand* 1990;61:32–35.
23. Crosby EB, Insall J: Recurrent dislocation of the patella. *J Bone Joint Surg Am* 1976;58A:9–13.
24. Fulkerson JP, Becker GJ, Meaney JA, et al.: Anteromedial tibial tubercle transfer without bone graft. *Am J Sports Med* 1990;18:490–497.
25. Hughston JC, Walsh W, Puddu G: in Sledge CB (ed.): *Patellar Subluxation and Dislocation.* Philadelphia, WB Saunders Co., 1984, pp. 87–128.
26. Macnab I: Recurrent dislocation of the patella. *J Bone Joint Surg Am* 1952;34A:957–967.
27. Noyes FR, Wojtys EM, Marshall MT: The early diagnosis and treatment of developmental patella infera syndrome. *Clin Orthop* 1991;265:241–252.
28. Garland DE, Hughston JC: Peroneal nerve paralysis: Complications of extensor mechanism reconstruction of the knee. *Clin Orthop* 1979; 140:169–171.
29. Wall JJ: Compartment syndrome as a complication of the Hauser procedure. *J Bone Joint Surg Am* 1979;61A:185–191.
30. Wiggins HW: The anterior tibial compartment syndrome: A complication of the Hauser procedure. *Clin Orthop* 1975;113:90–92.
31. Templeman D, McBeath A: Iatrogenic patella

malalignment following the Roux-Goldthwait procedure, corrected by dynamic intraoperative realignment. *J Bone Joint Surg Am* 1986; 68A:1096–1098.
32. Blazina ME, Fox JM, Carlson GJ, et al.: Patella baja: A technical consideration in evaluating results of tibial tubercle transplantation. *J Bone Joint Surg Am* 1975;57A:1027–1032.
33. Linclau L, Dokter G: Iatrogenic patella baja. *J Bone Joint Surg Am* 1976;58A:9–13.
34. Hampson WG, Hill P: Late results of transfer of the tibial tubercle for recurrent dislocation of the patella. *J Bone Joint Surg Br* 1975; 57B:209–213.
35. Maquet PGJ: Consideration biomechanique sur, l'arthrose du genou. *Rev Rheum* 1963; 30:779.
36. Maquet PGJ: Pathomechanics of osteoarthritis of the knee, in *Biomechanics of the Knee, with Application to the Pathogenesis and Surgical Treatment of Osteoarthritis,* ed. 2. Berlin, Springer-Verlag, 1984, pp. 107–109.
37. Maquet PGJ: Mechanics and osteoarthritis of the patellofemoral joint. *Clin Orthop* 1979; 155:70–73.
38. Bessette GC, Hunter RE: The Maquet procedure: A retrospective review. *Clin Orthop* 1988; 232:159–167.
39. Ferguson AB, Brown TD, Fu FH, et al.: Relief of patellofemoral contact stress by anterior displacement of the tibial tubercle. *J Bone Joint Surg Am* 1979;61A:159–166.
40. Mendes DG, Soudray M, Iusim M: Clinical assessment of Maquet tibial tuberosity advancement. *Clin Orthop* 1987;222:228–238.
41. Radin EL: Anterior tibial tubercle elevation in the young adult. *Orthop Clin North Am* 1976; 17:297–302.
42. Radin EL, Labosky DA: Avoiding complications associated with the Maquet procedure. *Comp Orthop* 1989;2:48–53.
43. Heatley FW, Allen PR, Patrick JH: Tibial tubercle advancement for anterior knee pain: A temporary or permanent solution. *Clin Orthop* 1986;208:215–224.
44. Blazina ME, Fox JM, Del Pizzo W, et al.: Patellofemoral replacement. *Clin Orthop* 1979; 144:98–103.
45. Insall J, Tria AJ, Aglietti P: Resurfacing of the patella. *J Bone Joint Surg Am* 1980;62A:933–936.
46. Baker CL, Hughston JC: Miyakawa patellectomy. *J Bone Joint Surg Am* 1988;70A:1489–1494.
47. Bentley G, Dowd, G: Current concepts of etiology and treatment of chondromalacia patellae. *Clin Orthop* 1984;189:209–228.
48. Compere CL, Hill JA, Lewinek GE, et al.: A new method of patellectomy for patellofemoral arthritis. *J Bone Joint Surg Am* 1979;61A:714–719.
49. Sutton FS, Thompson CH, Lipke J, et al.: Effect of patellectomy on knee function. *J Bone Joint Surg Am* 1976;58A:537–540.
50. Kaufer H: Mechanical function of the patella. *J Bone Joint Surg Am* 1971;53A:1551–1560.
51. Kelly MA, Insall JN: Patellectomy. *Orthop Clin North Am* 1986;17:289–295.
52. Steurer PA, Gradisar IA, Hoyt WA, et al.: Patellectomy: A clinical study and biomechanical evaluation. *Clin Orthop* 1979;144:84–90.
53. Watkins MP, Harris BA, Wender S, et al.: Effect of patellectomy on the function of the quadriceps and hamstrings. *J Bone Joint Surg Am* 1983;65A:390–395.
54. Larson KR, Cracchiolo A, Dorey FJ, et al.: Total knee arthroplasty in patients after patellectomy. *Clin Orthop* 1991;264:243–254.
55. Beuchel FF: Patellar tendon bone grafting for patellectomized patients having total knee arthroplasty. *Clin Orthop* 1991;271:72–78.
56. Johnson EE: Fractures of the patella, in Rockwood CA, Green DP, Bucholz RW (eds.): *Fractures in Adults.* Philadelphia: JB Lippincott Co., 1991, pp. 1762–1777.
57. Muller ME, Allgower M, Willinegger H: *Manual of Internal Fixation: Technique Recommended by the AO Group.* New York, Springer-Verlag, 1979.
58. Nummi J: Fracture of the patella: A clinical study of 707 patellar fractures. *Ann Chir Gynaecol* 1971;60(suppl.):179–189.
59. Hung LK, Chan KM, Chow YN, et al.: Fractured patella: Operative treatment using the tension band principle. *Injury* 1985; 16:343–347.
60. Scapinelli R: Blood supply of the patella: Its relation to ischemic necrosis after fracture. *J Bone Joint Surg Br* 1967;49B:563–570.
61. Siwek CW, Rao JP: Ruptures of the extensor mechanism of the knee joint. *J Bone Joint Surg Am* 1981;63A:932–937.
62. Levy M, Goldstein J, Rosner M: A method of repair for quadriceps tendon or patella ligament ruptures without cast immobilization. *Clin Orthop* 1987;281:297–301.
63. Bonamo JJ, Krinick RM, Sporn AA: Rupture of the patellar ligament after use of its central third for anterior cruciate reconstruction: A re-

port of two cases. *J Bone Joint Surg Am* 1984; 66A:1294–1297.
64. Burks RT, Haut RE, Lancaster RL: Biomechanical and histological observations of the dog patellar tendon after removal of its central one-third. *Am J Sports Med* 1990;18:146–153.
65. DeLee JC, Craviotto DF: Rupture of the quadriceps tendon after a central third patellar tendon ACL reconstruction. *Am J Sports Med* 1991;19:415–416.
66. Graf B, Uhr F: Complications of intra-articular ACL reconstruction. *Clin Sports Med* 1988; 7:835–848.
67. McCarroll JR: Fracture of the patella during a golf swing following reconstruction of the ACL: A case report. *Am J Sports Med* 1983;11:26–27.
68. Hughston JC: Complications of ACL surgery. *Orthop Clin North Am* 1985;16:237–240.
69. Sachs RA, Daniel DM, Stone MI, et al.: Patellofemoral problems after ACL reconstruction. *Am J Sports Med* 1989;17:760–765.
70. Rosenberg TD, Franklin JL, Bladwin GN, et al.: Extensor mechanism function after patellar tendon graft harvest for ACL reconstruction. *Am J Sports Med* 1992;20:519–526.
71. Richmond JC, Assal MA: Arthroscopic management of arthrofibrosis of the knee, including infrapatellar contraction syndrome. *Arthroscopy* 1991;7:144–147.
72. Sprague NF, O'Connor RL, Fox JM: Arthroscopic treatment of postoperative knee arthrofibrosis. *Clin Orthop* 1982;166:165–172.
73. Paulos LE, Wnorowski DC, Greenwald A: Infrapatellar contracture syndrome: Diagnosis, treatment, long-term follow-up. Submitted for publication 1993.
74. Katz MM, Hungerford DS: Reflex sympathetic dystrophy affecting the knee. *J Bone Joint Surg Br* 1987;69B:797–803.
75. Cooper DE, DeLee JC, Ramamurthy S: Reflex sympathetic dystrophy of the knee. *J Bone Joint Surg Am* 1989;71A:365–369.

15

Management of Patellofemoral Arthritis

David D. Bullek and Michael A. Kelly

Patellofemoral arthritis is most often associated with tibiofemoral arthritis.[1] Surgical treatment of these patients with tricompartmental replacement has proven to be successful.[2–8] Isolated patellofemoral arthritis is much less common. A large retrospective review of patients with idiopathic osteoarthritis showed only 3.8% to have isolated patellofemoral arthritis.[9] These patients were predominantly elderly women with bilateral disease in a majority of cases. Surgical treatment of these patients is more difficult and less reliable than the long-term clinical success reported with total knee arthroplasty in cases of tricompartmental disease. The problem is even more difficult in the young patient for which tricompartmental replacement is to be avoided when possible. Multiple procedures have been described to treat isolated patellofemoral arthrosis, ranging from arthroscopic debridement to patellar arthroplasty. The purpose of this chapter is to review pertinent operative treatment of this entity and present a logical treatment regimen based upon detailed patient examination and sound mechanical principles.

Patellofemoral arthritis is typically idiopathic or secondary to malalignment and is found to involve primarily the lateral facet. An example of this is shown in Figure 15.1. Usually the lateral joint space of the patellofemoral articulation is narrowed, with osteophyte formation evident on the lateral patella and the trochlea. Subchondral sclerosis and cyst formation are evident in severe cases. Patellofemoral arthritis secondary to trauma or iatrogenic causes may present with medial or global arthritis, such as that reported with distal realignment.[10] Medial tilt and luxation may also be theoretically seen in "overtightening" of the medial retinaculum.

It is commonly assumed that osteoarthritis of the patellofemoral joint is a continuation of chondromalacic changes found in young patients. In a long-term retrospective study, Karlson showed that most persons treated nonoperatively for chondromalacia did not ultimately develop patellofemoral arthritis.[11] It does seem logical that arthritis would follow from lesser cartilage damage. Histologically, cartilage at the periphery of osteoarthritic ulcers is indistinguishable from chondromalacia.[12] Ficat et al. believe that a tight lateral retinaculum leads to overload of the lateral facet and subsequent arthrosis.[13] Aglietti et al. believe that lateral facet erosion simply reflects the normal valgus vector of the patellofemoral articulation.[1] It remains difficult to explain why few people with patellofemoral arthritis have not had a long history of instability or patellar pain.[1]

Treatment choices of patellofemoral arthritis are difficult. Surgical options are based upon the extent of cartilage damage, patellofemoral mechanics, patient's age, activity level, and any associated structural abnormality. Decision making must be individualized based upon the patient's needs and the surgeon's preferences. Historically, several procedures have been described to directly ad-

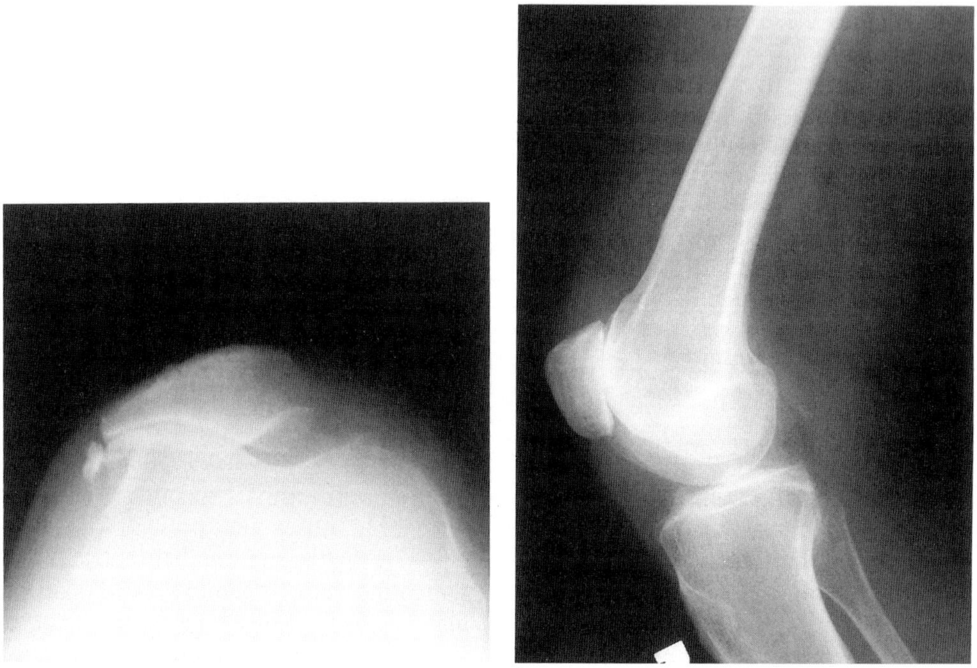

a b

FIGURE 15.1. (a) Axial and (b) lateral radiographs of narrowing of the lateral joint space and malalignment of the patellofemoral articulation, typical of patellofemoral arthritis.

dress patellar arthritis. Arthritis can be addressed primarily by arthroscopic debridement, subchondral drilling, spongialization, or abrasion arthroplasty. More recently, the focus has shifted towards surgical alteration of patellar malalignment and biomechanics. Operative procedures that alter biomechanics and alignment are lateral release, tibial tubercle elevation, or anteromedialization. Patellar hemiarthroplasty, patellofemoral arthroplasty, and patellectomy have been advocated in more advanced cases of patellar arthritis. With the advent of successful tricompartmental knee replacements, the elderly patient with severe patellofemoral arthritis may be best suited for total knee replacement. The younger patient with severe isolated patellofemoral arthritis presents the most difficult problem. Options for this patient population are limited. A better understanding of the biomechanics and complex pathophysiology of this problem may aid in improved management of this difficult problem. The goal of this chapter is to review the operative procedures described to address patellofemoral arthritis. A historic review of these procedures, along with their indications, operative techniques, and reported results, are presented.

Patient Examination

Evaluation of chronic anterior knee pain is sometimes difficult. The symptoms of patellofemoral arthritis are dominated by pain. However, distinguishing the patient with chronic pain from those with arthritis is important. The patient with multiple operations and pain without significant arthritis is a different entity and should not be approached in the same manner as those patients with true arthritis. Arthritis typically presents with anterior knee pain, but in more advanced degenerative arthritis involving the femoral groove, patients may complain of posterior pain as well. Daily activities, especially those that stress the patellofemoral articulation, exacerbate the pain. Physical examination of the patient with patellar pain has been previously described in chapter 5 and will not be discussed here in detail. Care should be taken in patient examination to exclude other causes of pain such as patellar tendinitis, prepatellar bursitis, pathologic plica, and quadriceps tendinitis. Some patients with patellofemoral arthritis may have had multiple previous surgical procedures. The surgical scars should be examined for possible neuromata. Psychologic examination as well as workup for reflex sympathetic dystrophy should be considered in these complex cases. Consultation with a pain specialist may be considered preoperatively.

In addition to comprehensive history and physical examination, radiographic examination is necessary to aid in establishing the proper diagnosis. Attention should be paid to both the tibiofemoral joint and the patellofemoral compartment. We routinely obtain standing anteroposterior, lateral, and modified Merchant radiographs of all patients presenting to our institution. A 45° posterior–anterior view may be helpful to further evaluate tibiofemoral disease, especially in the valgus knee. Specific cases may warrant the use of magnetic resonance imaging (MRI) and bone scans. Although computed tomography (CT) scanning of the patellofemoral joint has been useful in evaluating malalignment, it is seldom indicated in the examination of patients with patellofemoral arthritis.

The status of the tibiofemoral joint is important in the selection of treatment recommendations. Older patients with arthritis involving other compartments are usually considered for tricompartmental replacement. This may also be the preferred treatment of patients older than 60 years of age with isolated patellofemoral arthritis.

Surgical Treatment

Our surgical management is based upon patient's age, activity level, severity and location of arthritis, and structural abnormality. After detailed examination is completed, all patients are initially started on a rehabilitation regimen emphasizing activity modification, pain control, and isometric muscle strengthening. Exercises are advanced to short arc isotonic and closed chain exercises as pain permits. Our rehabilitation regimen has been previously described in detail.[14] A detailed therapeutic approach is presented earlier in chapter 8. All patients are encouraged to continue physical therapy for six months prior to considering operative treatment.

Several surgical procedures have been described in the treatment of patellofemoral arthritis. One category of procedures involve direct treatment of the articular cartilage changes on the patella. Historically, these procedures have included spongialization and drilling of the exposed subchondral bone. More recently, arthroscopic techniques have renewed interest in patellar debridement with chondral shaving and abrasion arthroplasty. The second category of procedures are directed to improve the abnormal mechanics at the patellofemoral articulation. Lateral retinacular release and patellar realignment procedures, both proximal and distal, have been used in the setting of malalignment. Anteriorization[15] and anteromedialization[16] procedures have been developed to reduce stresses across the patellofemoral joint and to relieve pain.[17–19] A third category of procedures would include patellar resurfacing, patellofemoral arthroplasty, and patellectomy. These procedures are typically considered salvage in nature and are associated with controversial results.

Arthroscopy

Arthroscopic treatment is often the initial step in the evaluation and treatment of patellofemoral arthritis. As a diagnostic tool, arthroscopy allows an accurate assessment of articular cartilage changes in both the patellofemoral and the tibiofemoral compartments. The extent of articular cartilage change may prove critical in surgical decision making in anteriorization or anteromedialization procedures designed to alter patellar contact patterns. Additionally, arthroscopic procedures are often employed in conjunction with procedures designed to alter patellar mechanics.

Perhaps the most common arthroscopic procedure performed is a debridement procedure with patellar shaving. The rationale for this treatment is twofold: (1) to remove any mechanical element to the patient's pain and (2) to decrease the cartilage breakdown products associated with synovitis of the knee.[20–23]

Our technique of debridement is to conduct a standard diagnostic arthroscopic examination through our anterior lateral and medial portals. An accessory lateral supra patellar portal is made to examine the patellofemoral articulation and to evaluate patellar tracking. Arthroscopic assessment of the patellofemoral compartment is described in detail earlier in this text. We refer the reader to chapter 10 for a more detailed explanation. A conservative approach is used with respect to chondral shaving. No attempt is made to stimulate cartilage repair with a more aggressive technique. The loose flaps and fibrillations are debrided using a synovial resector. Care is taken not to violate the subchondral bone. The joint is then copiously irrigated and a compressive dressing is applied. The patient is then started on an aggressive rehabilitation program. Our success with this type of procedure is unpredictable and the patient's understanding of the surgical goals is critical. Despite this, many patients will opt for this approach prior to considering tibial tubercle elevation or other more extensive procedures.

Review of the orthopedic literature reveals few articles on this subject. Ogilvie-Harris and Jackson reported a five-years result in a posttraumatic group of 42 knees treated by debridement and lavage.[24] Only 20% of patients with exposed subchondral bone had satisfactory results. Schonholtz and Ling reported a 78% patient satisfaction rate with debridement but only 45% of patients had good or excellent results at 40 months. Only three of 41 patients had exposed subchondral bone in this series.[25]

Arthroscopic debridement in the patient with Outerbridge grade III changes of the patellar articular surface is a temporizing measure in the posttraumatic patient. Debridement in the face of malalignment is also unpredictable. Less than one third of cases of unstable patellae treated with debridement have good results.[24] The indication for arthroscopic debridement and chondral shaving are not clear. Malalignment and advanced degenerative disease are poor prognostic indicators. The procedure should involve a conservative approach to management of the articular cartilage changes and should use a postoperative strengthening program. Clinical results are variable. Limited goals of arthroscopic debridement should be discussed with patients preoperatively.

Pridie originally proposed drilling of the subchondral bone to underlying cancellous bone to encourage fibrous ingrowth in areas of cartilage degeneration.[26] Variations of this technique include spongialization, as Ficat et al.[27] described, and abrasion arthroplasty, as Johnson[28] described. Ficat et al. described a technique done as an open procedure with removal of all subchondral bone, not just drilling as Pridie described. Johnson used an arthroscopic technique with a burr to remove subchondral bone. All these techniques result in cartilage defects being filled by fibrous tissue or fibrocartilage that is mechanically inferior to normal hyaline cartilage.[29]

Results of these techniques are variable and unpredictable. Ficat et al. reported on their technique in the treatment of 85 patients of various ages and extents of the disease. With 15-month average followup, 79% reported good or excellent results.[27] Bentley reported only 35% satisfactory results at seven-year average followup.[30] Beltran reported on resection arthroplasty of the patella in which the patella was cut level to the quadriceps tendon. He operated on patients from Saudi Arabia who have high function demands upon their patellofemoral joints. He reported that 60% of patients were pain-free at 60 months.[31] Important biomechanical studies dispute the usefulness of these techniques, especially in early cartilage lesions. Hayes et al. reported that early cartilage lesions still transfer load, whereas Outerbridge grades III and IV changes have no load transmission.[32] Therefore, it is desirable not to convert partial thickness cartilage lesions to full thickness lesions during one of these procedures. It is also advisable to preserve the margins of cartilage unless there are loose flaps to assist in load transfer. Our current use of these techniques is only in cases of isolated small lesions where we drill the subchondral bone and preserve the intact cartilage rim. In larger lesions, we use these techniques only in conjunction with unloading procedures.

Lateral Release

Arthroscopy has also been used to perform lateral retinacular release in the treatment of patellofemoral arthritis. Multiple authors have recommended this approach based on the theory that it will "unload" the lateral facet of the patella.[33-36] Both arthroscopic and open techniques for lateral release have been described and are both well described in previous chapters 10 and 11. In patellofemoral arthritis, lateral release has usually been combined with arthroscopic debridement. Reported results of lateral release in patients with patellofemoral arthritis are variable. Jackson et al. reported the results of patients with unremitting patellofemoral pain in the presence of malalignment. Severity of articular cartilage changes was not documented. The average age of the patients was 42 years. He reported 75% good and excellent results at four years, which deteriorated to 56% at six years. Eventually, 31% of patients required further operative treatment.[33] Aglietti et al. reported only one patient in six with patellofemoral arthritis improved with isolated lateral release at four-year followup.[37] Scuderi et al. reported poor results in patients more than 30 years of age.[38]

The results of the isolated lateral release in patellofemoral arthrosis are poor. Patients with tilt and early degenerative disease are reasonable candidates for lateral retinacular release and debridement with good chances of success. Patient education concerning unpredictable outcome and need for extensive post-operative rehabilitation is crucial. Patient symptoms and functional needs are important in the surgical decision-making process. We view this approach as one with limited goals. The patient's realistic expectation of the surgical outcome is important.

Tibial Tubercle Elevation or Transfer

Tibial tubercle elevation was originally advocated as an alternative to patellectomy in patients with patellofemoral pain unresponsive to rehabilitation by Maquet in 1963.[39] Bandi described a similar procedure.[40] Fulkerson described a combination of tubercle elevation and medialization to address arthrosis and malalignment.[16,41] The biomechanical rationale for anterior displacement was originally described by Maquet in 1979.[42] Figure 15.2 shows the diagrammatic changes in forces

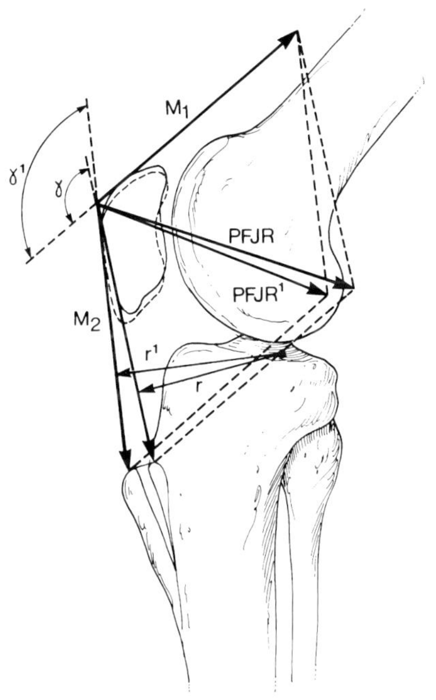

FIGURE 15.2. Biomechanical analysis of tibial tubercle advancement. M_1, quadriceps force; M_2, patellar tendon force; r, patellar tendon moment arm; r^1, patellar tendon moment arm after tubercle elevation. Elevation of the tibial tubercle causes an anterior displacement of the patellar tendon vector (M_2). This decreases the resultant vector, the patellofemoral joint reaction force (PFJRF) to PFJRF^1, at every angle of flexion.

about the patellofemoral joint as Maquet described. Elevation of the tibial tubercle increases the lever arm of the patellar tendon. This reduces the resultant forces across the patellofemoral articulation. Maquet calculated a 50% reduction in patellofemoral forces with a 2-cm advancement of the tibial tubercle. He also advised medialization of the tubercle and lateral release in the malaligned arthritic patella.

Multiple authors have since investigated the biomechanics of the anteriorization of the patellofemoral joint. Ferguson et al. reported that most of the reduction of forces across the patellofemoral joint occur in the first 1.25 cm of elevation. They also noted a shift of forces to the superior pole of the patella and elevation of the distal pole with increasing elevations.[17] Nakamura et al. confirmed that load is shifted proximally. They reported 1 cm of elevation to be biomechanically optimal. They also demonstrated significant decreases in contact areas that act to increase the force per unit area with increasing elevations of the tibial tubercle.[43] Fernandez et al. confirmed the work of Nakamura et al. and warned of shifting loads proximally in the patient with significant superior and lateral patellar arthritis. They also concluded 1 cm of tibial tubercle elevation to be optimal.[44] Hayes et al. investigated patellofemoral forces in cadaver knees in normal, 1.25 cm, and 2.5 cm of elevation. They concluded that forces are shifted proximal and lateral, and that no consistent reduction in contact pressure can be obtained.[32] This is due to the fact that as loads decrease, a concomitant decrease in contact area occurs. Therefore, total contact pressures are not significantly changed. Fulkerson et al. evaluated the effects of anteromedialization of the tibial tubercle in cadaver knees. They concluded that load on the lateral facet decreases in the first 0° to 30° of motion. At flexion greater than 30°, there was no significant reduction of forces compared with preoperative values. The load was shifted proximally at all degrees of flexion.[45]

The improvement in the understanding of the biomechanics of the patellofemoral articulation can only serve to assist surgeons in selecting better treatment options for their patients. Proximal and lateral shifting of joint forces is a valuable point from most of the cited studies. With these principles in mind, a patient with proximal arthrosis may not be suitable for treatment by tibial tubercle elevation. Arthroplasty or patellectomy may be the only choices available to a surgeon in this circumstance.

Clinical reports on the results of anterior tibial tubercle transfer are numerous. Maquet reported on 37 knees with isolated tibial tubercle elevation and an average followup of 4.7 years. At last followup, 36 knees were found to have satisfactory results. One knee had skin necrosis over the tibial tubercle requiring the graft to be removed.[46] Hirsch and Reddy reported on nine knees in eight patients followed at 13 to 72 months. They reported 7 excellent, 1 good, and 1 fair result. They noted one skin complication in the area of elevation.[47] Rozbruch et al. reported a 60% satisfactory rating on 30 knees with average followup of one to five years. They also noted significant complications of skin necrosis in four patients, a stress fracture of the tibial tubercle, and a tibial shaft fracture.[48] Heatley et al. reported on 29 cases of a modified Maquet procedure with an average followup of six years. They reported 65% excellent or good results at three years that decreased to 54% at six-years followup. They also reported a 13% complication rate.[49] Ferguson reported on 184 patients who had undergone his modification of the Maquet procedure. He advocated a transverse incision with 1.25 cm of elevation of the tubercle. His patients were divided into the following five groups: (1) chondromalacia, (2) patellofemoral arthrosis, (3) patellar dislocation, (4) previous trauma, and (5) prior patellectomy. Overall, 85% of patients had satisfactory results at two-years followup. The patients with isolated patellofemoral arthrosis had 92% relief of pain and improvement of function. Ferguson also noted that the alignment of the patella did not change with this procedure and that it took up to six months for the patients to reach maximal benefit from the procedure.[50] Mendes et al. reported on 25 patients with average followup of 5.5 years.

Only 14 had isolated tibial tubercle elevation. Eleven of 14 patients had good or excellent results. The complication rate was 55%. Eight patients developed skin problems, two of which required rotational flap for coverage. One graft displaced requiring reoperation. Two grafts went on the nonunion.[51] Radin reported on his modified Maquet at 3.5 years of followup. All patients had at least 2 cm of elevation. He reported a 94% success rate, a 19% minor complication rate, and a 5% serious complication rate.[52] Bassette and Hunter reviewed the results of 21 knees with a minimum followup of one year. Best results were found in male patients with a Q angle less than 20° and followup of less than three years. They also reported a 40% complication rate.[53] Engelbretsen et al. reported on 33 patients with an average followup of five years. Ten patients were improved, 17 patients were unchanged, and six patients had worsening of symptoms following tibial tubercle elevation. More favorable results were reported in patients with advanced lateral facet arthrosis. No patient with less than 15 mm of tibial tubercle elevation had improvement postoperatively.[54] Friedman et al. reported on 51 patients who had a modified Maquet as Ferguson described.[50] Seventy-three percent of patients reported significant improvement in pain at 38-months average followup. Success was higher in patients who had lateral retinacular releases, medialization of the tubercle, and greater preoperative arthrosis.[55]

The studies cited have a satisfactory outcome that varies from 54% to 95%. The major problems reported have been significant rates of skin and graft complications. Patients also complain of difficulty kneeling after tubercle elevation. Limiting the amount of elevation as Ferguson advocated significantly decreased wound complications.[50] A significant shortcoming of the Maquet procedure is that elevation alone does not alter patellofemoral tracking.

Fulkerson described an anteromedial tibial tubercle transfer to address both arthrosis and malalignment of the patella. Fulkerson described an oblique osteotomy that accomplishes elevation and medial transfer without bone graft.[16] This procedure is often used in conjunction with a lateral retinacular release. Fulkerson reported his results in 30 patients at two-years followup. Subjective results were good and excellent in 93% of patients. All 12 patients examined at five years maintained the good result. Of patients with severe patellofemoral arthritis, 75% had good results but there were no excellent results. There were no reported complications of skin necrosis, compartment syndrome, or infection.[45] Miller and LaRochelle reported on anteromedial tubercle transfer by an alternative technique in 38 knees at 2.5-years average followup. There were 33 good and excellent results, and five failures. The failures were patients with no improvement over preoperative status. No wound complications were noted.[56] Morshuis et al. reported on 25 knees treated by the Fulkerson technique of anteromedial tibial tubercle transfer. At 12-month followup, 84% showed satisfactory results, while at 30 months, only 70% satisfactory results remain. The best results were obtained in knees with patellofemoral pain and no signs of arthritis. No skin or tubercle complications were reported.[57]

The results of the Fulkerson technique are similar to those reported in the review of the Maquet and modified Maquet procedures but with much lower complication rates. There are several other advantages: no bone graft is usually required, malalignment is addressed directly by medialization of the tubercle, and postoperative skin complications are reduced. The major risk inherent in the Fulkerson technique is to anterior tibial artery and deep peroneal nerve.

Operative Technique

Both the Maquet tibial tubercle advancement and the Fulkerson anteromedial tubercle transfer are technically demanding procedures. In-depth knowledge of the technical aspects of both procedures is necessary for the surgeon caring for patients with patellofemoral arthritis.

Maquet Tibial Tubercle Advancement

Maquet's original surgical technique was reported in 1963.[39] The tibial tubercle was osteotomized and the osteotomy was extended approximately 12 cm distally. He advocated anterior displacement of 2 to 3 cm using a wedged block of iliac crest bone graft. No internal fixation was used.

The authors' preferred technique varies from Maquet's original description. Careful preoperative assessment of any existing surgical scars is critical. Tenuous blood supply locally may increase the risks of skin and wound-healing problems following anteriorization of the tibial tubercle. Plastic surgery consultation may be useful in these cases. Radin and Leach have described "fish-mouthing" technique[58] to gain skin laxity, while others have reported using skin expanders.

We prefer a long, anterolateral skin incision when possible extending from the superior pole of the patella to near the distal extent of the proposed osteotomy. The lateral retinaculum is divided and the lateral genicular vessels are coagulated. The lateral release is continued distally to the tibia. Arthroscopic examination is typically performed as the initial step of the procedure. If necessary, the patellar articular surface can be further inspected at this time. Great care is taken to develop the medial skin flap. The anterior compartment of the calf is released. The exposure should allow good visualization of the patellar tendon insertion and the tibial crest. The osteotomy is performed at a depth approximately 8 mm posterior to the tibial crest using either an osteotome or an oscillating saw. Two osteotomes are then inserted at the medial and lateral aspects of the osteotomy. They are oriented longitudinally. They are then driven incrementally distal in alternating fashion. The distal extent of the osteotomy is approximately 10 cm, as shown in Figure 15.3. Great care is taken to preserve the distal cortex. Maquet recommended a graft measuring from 2 to 3 cm.[46] We seek an elevation of 15 mm and iliac crest graft is harvested to this proportion. The osteotomy is carefully levered forward and the block of bone inserted flush with the tip of the tibial tubercle. More distal graft placement had been associated with fracture at the more proximal aspect of the tubercle. The remaining area posterior to the osteotomy is filled in with morsalized bone graft.

The bone graft is typically stable without internal fixation. Fracture of the distal cortex of the osteotomy may necessitate the use of screw fixation. One or two cancellous screws countersunk into the proximal tibia may be used. Careful attention should be paid to wound closure, which may be difficult. The skin is closed and the patient is splinted in extension until the skin heals, at which time weight bearing and motion are permitted. Aggressive rehabilitation based on closed chain exercises are started at six weeks postoperatively. A radiographic example of a healed Maquet tibial tubercle elevation is shown in Figure 15.4.

Fulkerson Anteromedial Tibial Tubercle Transfer

An anterolateral skin incision is made, extending from the superior pole of the patellar to the distal extent of the planned tubercle osteotomy approximately 5 cm. The lateral retinaculum is released and the patellar articular surface is inspected. Appropriate debridement or drilling is then done. The anterior compartment musculature is then reflected in a subperiosteal fashion off the lateral tibia to the posterior cortex. Care must be taken to protect the anterior tibial artery and the peroneal nerve. Exposure of the lateral and posterior cortex is necessary for a length of approximately 5 to 7 cm. The medial tibia should also be exposed at this time in a subperiosteal fashion. Both borders of the patellar tendon should be well visualized. Guide pins are then placed from anteromedially to posterolaterally. The osteotomy is tapered distally to a thickness of 2 to 3 mm, as shown in Figure 15.5. To ensure that the osteotomy plane is perfectly flat, Fulkerson and Hungerford have recommended the use of a Hoffman drill guide to place the guide pins.[41] The osteotomy can then be completed using an oscillating saw.

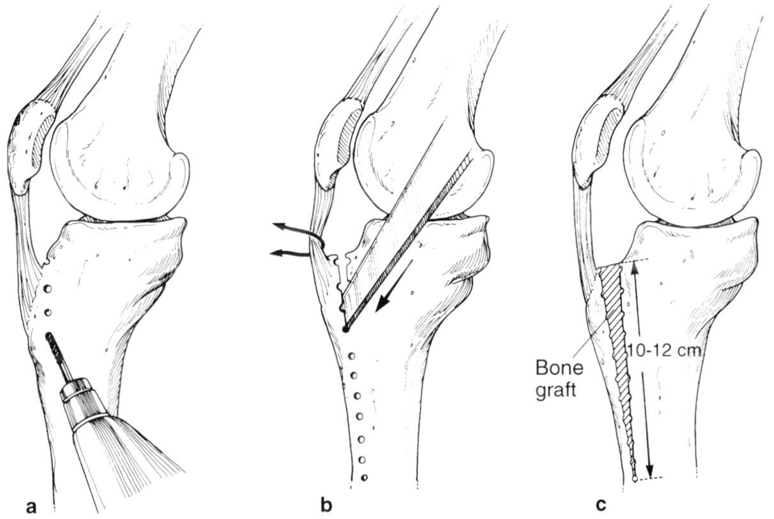

FIGURE 15.3. The Maquet technique of tibial tubercle elevation. (a) Multiple drill holes are useful in marking the line of the osteotomy. A split 10 to 12 cm is necessary. (b) Care is taken to preserve the distal bone bridge while elevating the tubercle. (c) The bone graft is placed with the distal gap filled with morselized bone graft.

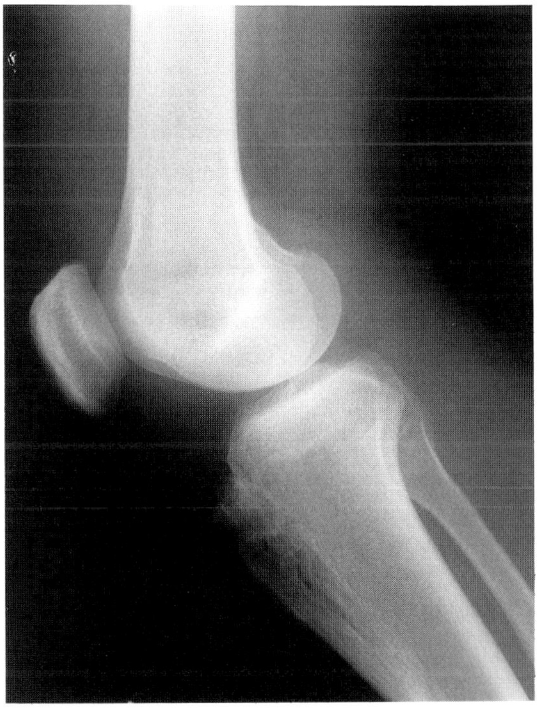

FIGURE 15.4. Lateral radiograph of a tibial tubercle elevation.

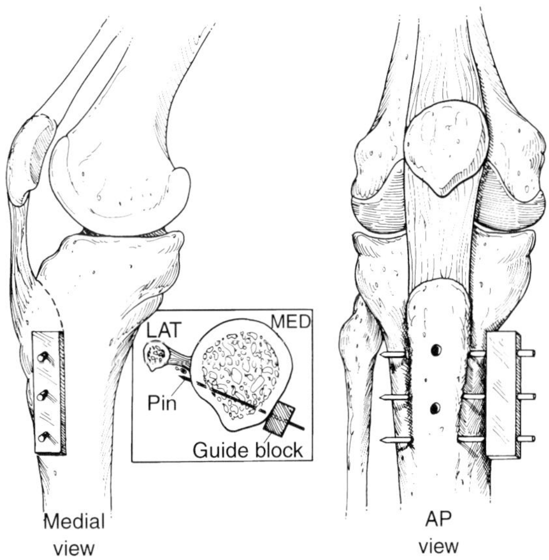

FIGURE 15.5. The guide pins are placed in a parallel fashion to ensure a flat cut of the osteotomy.

The patellar tendon must be protected at all times. A lateral cut is also made proximally to prevent extension of the osteotomy into the joint, as shown in Figure 15.6. An osteotome is then used to complete the osteotomy behind the patellar tendon. The obliquity of the osteotomy plane can be varied to change the amount of both anterior and medial displacement (Figure 15.7).

Once the osteotomy is complete, the tubercle is rotated medially and anterior. The proper position is determined by the amount of anterior displacement necessary and the patellar tracking after medialization. The tubercle is then secured by two bicortical screws, as shown in Figure 15.8. Fulkerson et al. report that 12 to 15 mm of displacement can be routinely achieved without bone graft with this technique.[45] The fixation with two screws is usually secure, enabling early range of motion. We routinely place these patients in continuous passive motion postoperatively and in a drop lock postoperative brace. Patients are instructed in non-weight-bearing crutch ambulation and are encouraged to bend the knee by releasing the drop lock. Continuous passive motion is continued until 90° of passive motion is obtained. Progressive weight bearing is allowed at one month and crutches are discarded by six to eight weeks.

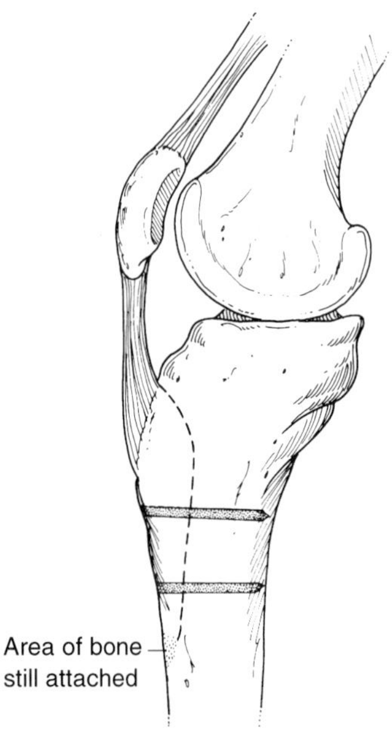

FIGURE 15.6. Lateral view of the osteotomy plane. Note the proximal limb extending from the most posterior portion of the osteotomy anteriorly to just behind the patellar tendon.

Patellar and Patellofemoral Arthroplasty

Patellar hemiarthroplasty and patellofemoral arthroplasty are considerations in the younger patient with severe arthritis of the entire articular surface of the patella and/or the trochlea. They serve as alternatives to patellectomy. Patients with involvement of the proximal pole of the patella and severe arthritis of the trochlea are not good candidates for tibial tubercle elevation. In the elderly patient with or without arthritic changes in the tibiofemoral compartments, tricompartmental replacement is our preferred treatment. Surgical decision making is much more difficult in the younger patient with advanced patellofemoral degenerative changes. Several options have been described including patellar hemiarthroplasty and patellofemoral replacement.

McKeever reported on the results of the first patellar hemiarthroplasty in 1955. The McKeever prosthesis is a cobalt–chromium anatomic patella secured to the patella by a transfixing screw. He reported on the results of 40 patients with the longest followup being five years. There were four failures due to infection and none due to mechanical failure. His results were otherwise described as satisfactory. The patient population was largely severe degenerative panarthritis, rheumatoid arthritis, and posttraumatic arthritis.[59] Most of these patients would not be candidates for isolated patellar hemiarthroplasty today. Depalma et al. reported results on 17 patients with a similar dome-shaped prosthesis. They reported satisfactory results with short followup.[60] Levitt reported on the long-term results with the Depalma patellar hemiarthroplasty. He reported greater than 50% unsatisfactory results. He noted successful results with

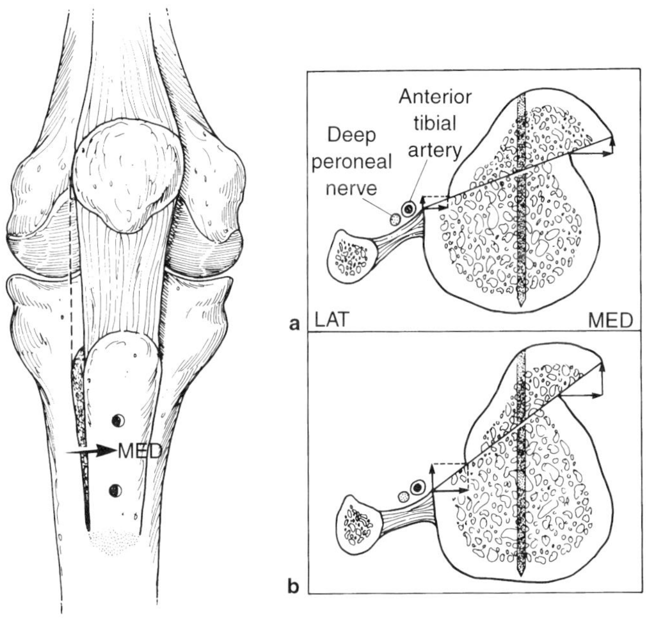

FIGURE 15.7. The obliquity of the osteotomy plane can be varied to alter the relative amount of medial and anterior displacement of the tibial tubercle. (a) Medial displacement that can be obtained by a flatter osteotomy. As the obliquity of the osteotomy increases, more anterior displacement can be obtained (b).

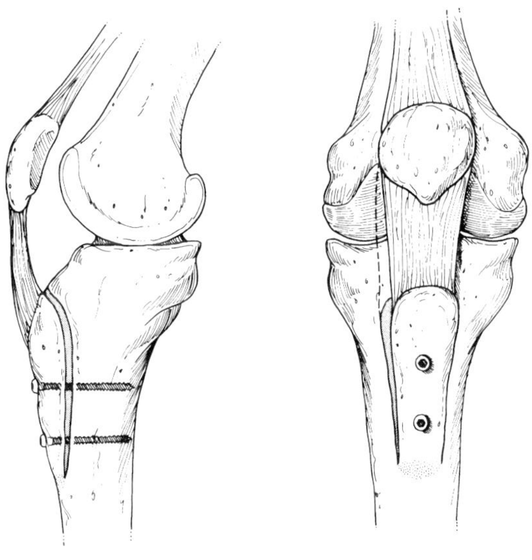

FIGURE 15.8. The bone pedicle is hinged anterior and medial, and is fixed with two cancellous screws.

early, localized arthritis of the patella.[61] More recently, Harrington reported results of the McKeever prosthesis at an average followup of eight years. Twenty-eight patients were reviewed, all had preoperative grades III and IV changes of the patellar articular surface. The patients had an average of 1.8 operations prior to hemiarthroplasty. The patients were reviewed at five and eight years. At five years, 70% had good or excellent results by the Hospital for Special Surgery Knee Rating Scale. Of these, 17 all had normal or grade I changes of the femoral trochlear cartilage at the time of operation. There were three poor results. Two of the poor results had tricompartmental arthritis, which were ultimately revised to total knee arthroplasty. One poor result was a compensation case that improved to a fair rating at eight years after his case was settled. There were no complications and no evidence of prosthetic loosening. At eight years, 80% of patients had good or excellent results. Harrington concluded that patellar hemiarthroplasty is appropriate in patients with grade III or IV articular cartilage changes of the patella and near-normal femoral articular surfaces.[62]

In 1973, a new cobalt–chromium patellar prosthesis was designed at the Hospital for Special Surgery. It was dome shaped and available in two sizes[63] (Figure 15.9). Bone cement was used for fixation in contrast to both the McKeever and Depalma patellar prostheses. Insall et al. reported on the result of this prosthesis on 29 knees at three- to six-year followup. They found only 55% to have

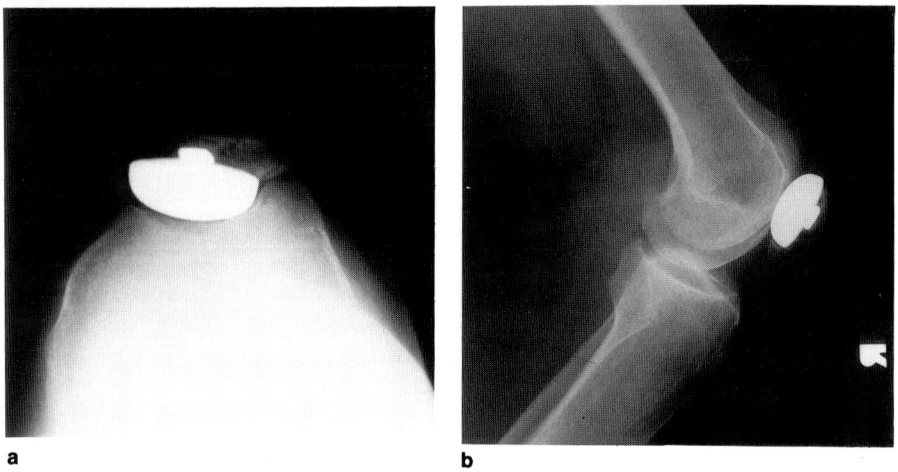

FIGURE 15.9. (a) Axial and (b) lateral radiograph of patellar prosthesis developed at The Hospital for Special Surgery.

good or excellent results. Those patients with no tibiofemoral arthritis had 67% satisfactory results.[64] Worrell reported on his cobalt–chromium anatomic patellar prosthesis in 1979. He also cemented the prosthesis in place. Early results showed eight excellent and five good results in 14 knees.[65] In 1986, he reported his results with this prosthesis on patients less than 40 years of age. All patients had patellar arthritis and were candidates for patellectomy. There was no documentation of the condition of the femoral trochlear articular cartilage. With followup ranging from six weeks to eight years, there were 3 good or excellent results, 8 fair, and 4 poor results. Fair results were defined as full or limited range of motion with occasional episodes of pain that is not disabling.[66] By this definition most patients in this study would have satisfactory outcomes.

Overall, the results of patellar hemiarthroplasty have been unpredictable. Recent studies suggest that with proper patient selection, improved clinical results can be obtained. Additionally, improved prosthetic design and surgical technique may also contribute to improved results. Patellar hemiarthroplasty may be considered in the younger patient with severe global patellar arthritis with minimally involved femoral trochlear articular cartilage. Failed patellar replacements may be salvaged with patellectomy. However, advanced degenerative changes on the corresponding femoral groove may lead to less than excellent results. Further investigation is necessary to determine the long-term outcomes in properly selected patients.

In those patients with severe arthritis of the patella and the trochlea, isolated patellofemoral arthroplasty has been reported. The original reports on patellofemoral arthroplasty were by Blazina et al. in 1979. They believe that patellofemoral arthroplasty is indicated when there is severe arthritis of the femoral groove and patellectomy is not advised. The prosthesis used in this study has a cemented polyethylene patellar button and a metallic trochlear implant. Subjective and objective examination of 57 replacements revealed that 78% were improved at 21-month followup. Thirty of 85 total patients had a subsequent operative procedure. They concluded the results to be unpredictable and to be considered only in cases of severe isolated arthritis involving both the patella and the trochlea.[67] Arciero and Toomey reported on the results of 25 patellofemoral arthroplasties with an average followup of 64 months. Excellent or good results were found in 72% of patients.[68] The authors noted better results in females. Tibiofemoral arthritis, malalignment, and component malposition contributed to unsuccessful results. Cartier et al. reported on the results of patellofemoral arthroplasty in 72 knees with an average followup of four years. All had grade IV chondromalacia and complete disappearance of the patellofemoral joint line. Thirty-six knees had concomitant unicompartmental replacements. All patients with malalignment had proximal realignments with tibial tubercle transfer if the Q angle was increased. They reported 85% satisfactory results. There were 14 complications; one half of which were secondary to the implant. They consider patella baja and age of less than 50 years to be contraindications for the procedure.[69] The concurrent operative procedures in this series make it difficult to evaluate the reported results with respect to patellofemoral arthroplasty.

Operative Technique

The surgical technique for a patellar hemiarthroplasty is similar to that used in standard total knee arthroplasty. Proper alignment of the extensor mechanism is critical in the surgical technique. Although the optimal prosthetic design is debatable, attention to the thickness of the patella at resurfacing appears to be important. Our own approach is to avoid increasing the composite thickness greater the original patella, attempting to restore near-normal patellar mechanics.

The operative technique of patellofemoral arthroplasty has been well described by Cartier et al.[69] They advise the use of a nonanatomic trochlea with a corresponding V-shaped patellar button. A standard anterior midline incision is used and initially the trochlea is inspected. Notch osteophytes are removed to prevent impingement on the tibial spines. The trochlear component is implanted, with care taken not to tilt the component to fit a dysplastic trochlea. The surgeon must be willing to accept cement under one side of the implant if necessary. The tip of the trochlear component should not overhang into the notch. This will cause impingement with the tibial spines. The patellar component is then implanted, with care taken to restore the normal thickness. The V-shaped patella component must be aligned correctly to articulate well with the trochlear component. Extensor mechanism realignment is usually necessary to have the patella track normally. This is a critical part of the procedure. The knee should then be put through a range of motion. If catching is apparent past 110°, this is usually indicative of patella baja. In this circumstance, Cartier et al. recommend a proximal transfer of the tibial tubercle.

Patellectomy

Patellectomy has been used in the surgical management of patellofemoral arthritis. It is typically considered as a salvage procedure for advanced degenerative disease of the patella. There is little doubt regarding the important role of the patella in normal biomechanics of the knee. Conflicting reports regarding the efficacy of patellectomy in treating patellar arthritis exist in the literature.[70–73] Some have favorable reports. Haggart reported on 20 patients with degenerative arthritis of the knee who underwent patellectomy. Nineteen patients noted improved range of motion and diminished knee pain.[73] Boucher noted favorable results with patellectomy in a series of 76 patients who were 50 years or older.[71] Others have noted less favorable reports. Ackroyd and Polyzoides found that approximately one half of their patients had improvement in pain following patellectomy. Additionally, they observed more favorable results in patients with minimal tibiofemoral disease.[70] Kelly and Insall noted 72% good to excellent results in reviewing 100 patellectomies for arthritis or patellar fracture. Failure was almost always due to unrelieved pain and was associated with concurrent tibiofemoral disease.[74] Although there is no consensus of opinion regarding the efficacy of patellectomy for patellofemoral arthritis, the results do appear better if degenerative changes of the knee are restricted to the patellofemoral compartment.

Operative Technique

Several surgical techniques have been described to perform excision of the patella. Perhaps the most common involves enucleation of the patella through a transverse incision in the quadriceps expansion. In his study on the mechanical function of the patella, Kaufer reported less reduction of extensor power with this technique compared with longitudinal closures. An additional 30% of quadriceps force was required to extend the knee with a longitudinal repair compared with 15% with a transverse repair.[75] Boyd and Hawkins reported on a longitudinal technique of patellectomy. This technique employs a side-to-side or imbricated closure, permitting early knee motion with minimal tension on the repair.[76] Fulkerson and Hungerford reported no extensor lag in their patients when an imbricated longitudinal closure was used as Boyd and Hawkins described. This surgical technique divides the fibers of the quadriceps and the patella longitudinally. The patella is divided in halves with an osteotomy after a malleable retractor has been introduced into the joint to protect the trochlear surface. The patellar halves are now enucleated with sharp dissection, carefully preserving the fibers of the quadriceps expansion. The wound is closed by imbricating one side over the other in a double row of interrupted sutures. Flexion to 90° without stressing the repair should be present. A lateral retinacular release may be required to centralize the repaired tendon. Proper tracking is critical. Early range of motion and quadriceps strengthening are instituted postoperatively.[41]

Compere et al. described a technique of patellectomy creating a "tube" within which any bone regeneration would be contained.[77] This technique permits enucleation of the patella through medial and lateral parapatellar incisions. The medial border of the quadriceps is then brought underneath and is sutured to the lateral border, creating a tube. The vastus medialis is then advanced distally and laterally, and is sutured to the tube. Care is taken to ensure proper tracking of the tube centrally in the femoral groove. The technique is illustrated in Figure 15.10. Again early range of motion and quadriceps strengthening are employed postoperatively. Compere et al. reported 90% good or excellent clinical results with this technique. We have favored this technique, also noting an improved cosmetic appearance to the patellectomized knee.

Other techniques of patellectomy have been described including those that reinforce the patellar defect. Baker and Hughston reported excellent long-term results with the Miyakawa technique.[78] In this technique, the vastus medialis and the vastus lateralis are advanced with a strip of quadriceps tendon used to fill the patellar defect. Regardless of the surgical technique, Kaufer has demonstrated a decreased lever arm of the quadriceps extensor power. He suggested that anteriorization of the tibial tubercle may be useful in lengthening the extensor moment arm, mitigating some of the ill effects of patellectomy.[75] Radin and Leach reported good results in six of nine knees following anteriorization of the tibial tubercle for failed patellectomy.[79]

Patellectomy is rightfully considered as a last resort in the surgical treatment of patellofemoral arthritis. The patella serves an integral role in the biomechanics of the knee. Loss of the patella alters these mechanics in several ways. The most significant change is the reduction of quadriceps force lever arm. An additional 15 to 30 quadriceps force is required following patellectomy to maintain the same torque during knee extension. Additional alterations include decreased stance-phase flexion and decreased flexion with stair climbing, compromised function of the quadriceps and hamstring muscle groups, an increased incidence of knee instability, and the obvious cosmetic alteration in the knee. Following patellectomy, less satisfactory results with total knee arthroplasty have been reported. We believe that the patella should be preserved when possible and alternatives should be sought in the setting of patellar arthrosis. Similar to Fulkerson, we believe that a good patellectomy may be indicated to improve function and relieve pain in selected patients such as younger patients with severe, symptomatic patellofemoral arthrosis.

Summary

The treatment of isolated patellofemoral arthritis in the young patient is a great clinical

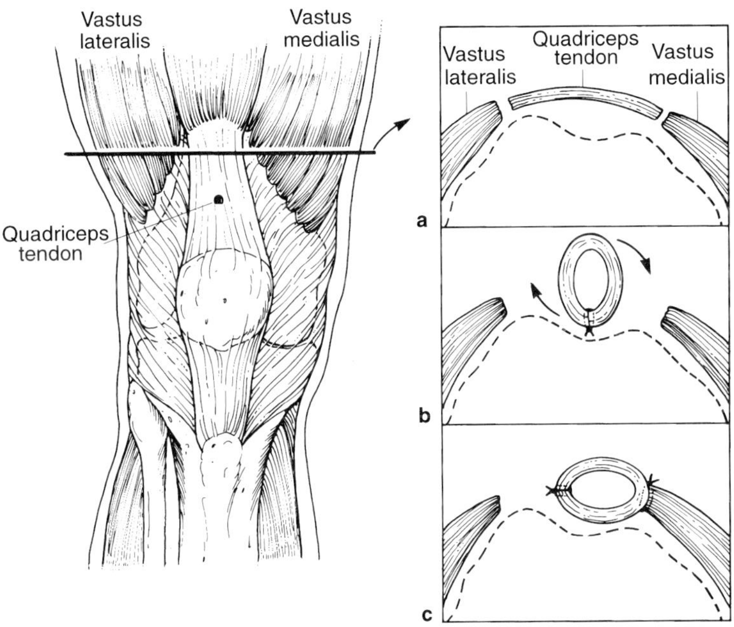

FIGURE 15.10. Technique of the Compere patellectomy. (a) The Patella is enucleated through medial and lateral parapatellar incisions. (b) The medial border is brought underneath and sutured to the lateral border to form a tube. (c) The vastus medialis is advanced and sutured to the tube.

challenge. The older patient with patellofemoral arthritis can be offered total knee arthroplasty with reliable success. Of course, it would be preferable in all patients to address the isolated arthritis directly. Unfortunately, the results of patellofemoral replacement are unpredictable. The true dilemma is present in the younger patient with significant patellar or patellofemoral arthritis. Present treatment courses are improving, but clinical studies with specific selection criteria are sparse. Further evaluation of present treatment courses is necessary to better define treatment indications and outcomes for this patient population. Advancements in understanding of patellofemoral pathophysiology and biomechanics will aid in more logical treatment recommendations. Our hope is that future research can increase successful treatment options available to these patients.

References

1. Aglietti P, Buzzi R, Insall JN: Disorders of the patellofemoral joint, in Insall JI (ed.) *Surgery of the Knee,* ed. 2. New York, Churchill Livingstone, 1993, pp. 241–386.
2. Aglietti P, Buzzi R, Gaudeni A: Patellofemoral functional results and complications with the posterior stabilized total condylar knee prosthesis. *J Arthroplasty* 1988;3(1):17–23.
3. Aglietti P, Buzzi R: Posterior stabilized total condylar knee replacement: Three to 8 years follow up of 85 knees. *J Bone Joint Surg Br* 1988; 70B:211–216.
4. Groh GI, Parker J, Elliott J, et al.: Results of total knee arthroplasty using the posterior stabilized condylar prosthesis: A report of 137 consecutive cases. *Clin Orthop* 1991;269:58–62.
5. Insall JN, Lachiewicz PF, Burstein AH: The posterior stabilized condylar prosthesis: A modification of the total condylar design. *J Bone Joint Surg Am* 1982;64A:1317–1323.
6. Scuderi GR, Insall JN, Windsor RE, et al.: Survivorship of cemented knee replacement. *J Bone Joint Surg Br* 1989;71B:798–803.
7. Stern SH, Insall JN: Posterior stabilized prosthesis: Results after follow-up of 9 to 12 years. *J Bone Joint Surg Am* 1992;74A:980–985.
8. Scott RD, Volatile TB: Twelve years experience with posterior cruciate-retaining total knee arthroplasty. *Clin Orthop* 1986;206:100–107.
9. Barrett JP, Rashkoff E, Sirna EC, et al.: Correlation of roentgenographic patterns and clinical manifestations of symptomatic idiopathic osteoarthritis of the knee. *Clin Orthop* 1990;253: 179–183.

10. Crosby EB, Insall JI: Recurrent dislocation of the patella. Relation of treatment to osteoarthritis. *J Bone Joint Surg Am* 1976;58(A):9–13.
11. Karlson S: Chondromalacia patellae. *Acta Chir Scand* 1940;83:347–381.
12. Wiles P, Andrews PS, Devas MB: Chondromalacia of the patella. *J Bone Joint Surg Br* 1956;38B:95–113.
13. Ficat D, Ficat C, Bailleux A: Syndrome d'hyperpression externe de la rotule (shpe): son interet pour la connaissance de l'arthrose. *Rev Chir Orthop Reparatrice Appar Mot* 1975;61: 39–59.
14. Bullek DD, Kelly MA: Nonoperative treatment of patellofemoral pain, in Scott WN (ed.): *The Knee,* St. Louis, Mosby–Year Book, 1994, pp. 415–440.
15. Maquet P: Advancement of the tibial tubercle. *Clin Orthop* 1976;115:225–230.
16. Fulkerson JP: Anteromedialization of the tibial tubercle for patellofemoral malalignment. *Clin Orthop* 1983;177:176–181.
17. Ferguson AB, Brown TD, Fu FH, et al.: Relief of patellofemoral contact stress by anterior displacement of the tibial tubercle. *J Bone Joint Surg Am* 1979;61A:159–166.
18. Nakamura N, Ellis M, Seedhom BB: Advancement of the tibial tuberosity: A biomechanical study. *J Bone Joint Surg Br* 1985;67B:255–260.
19. Lewallen DG, Reigger CL, Myers ER, et al.: Effects of the retinacular release and tibial tubercle elevation in patellofemoral degenerative joint disease. *J Orthop Res* 1990;8(6):856–862.
20. Chrisman OD, Ladenbauer Bellis IM, et al.: The relationship of mechanical trauma and the early reactions of osteoarthritic cartilage. *Clin Orthop* 1981;161:275–284.
21. Chrisman OD: The role of articular cartilage in patellofemoral pain. *Orthop Clin North Am* 1986;17(2):231–234.
22. Chrisman OD: Biomechanical aspects of degenerative joint disease. *Clin Orthop* 1969;64: 77–86.
23. Shoji H, Granada JL: Acid hydrolases in the articular cartilage of the patella. *Clin Orthop* 1974;99:293–297
24. Ogilvie-Harris DJ, Jackson RW: The arthroscopic treatment of chondromalacia patellae. *J Bone Joint Surg Br* 1984;66B:660–665.
25. Schonholtz GJ, Ling B: Arthroscopic chondroplasty of the patella. *Arthroscopy* 1985;1(2):92–96.
26. Pridie KH: A method of resurfacing osteoarthritic knee joints. *J Bone Joint Surg Br* 1959; 41B:618–619.
27. Ficat RP, Ficat C, Gedeon P, et al.: Spongialization: A new treatment for diseased patella. *Clin Orthop* 1979;144:74–83.
28. Johnson LL: *Arthroscopic Surgery, Principles and Practice,* ed. 3. St. Louis, CV Mosby Co., 1986.
29. Mitchell M, Shepard N: The resurfacing of adult rabbit articular cartilage by multiple perforations through the subchondral bone. *J Bone Joint Surg Am* 1976;58A:230–233.
30. Bentley G: The surgical treatment of chondromalacia patella. *J Bone Joint Surg Br* 1978;60B: 74–81.
31. Beltran JE: Resection arthroplasty of the patella. *J Bone Joint Surg Br* 1987;69B:604–608.
32. Hayes WC, Huberti HH, Lewallen DG, et al.: Patellofemoral contact pressures and the effects of surgical reconstructive procedures, in Ewing JW (ed.): *Articular Cartilage and Knee Joint Function: Basic Science and Arthroscopy,* New York, Raven Press, 1990.
33. Jackson RW, Kunkel SS, Taylor GJ: Lateral retinacular release for patellofemoral pain in the older patient. *Arthroscopy* 1991;7(3):283–286.
34. Fox JM, Ferkel RD: Use of electrosurgery in arthroscopic surgery, in Pariesien J (ed.): *Arthroscopic Surgery,* New York, McGraw-Hill Book Co., 1988, pp. 313–330.
35. Sherman OH, Fox JM, Sperling H: Patellar instability: Treatment by arthroscopic electrosurgical lateral release. *Arthroscopy* 1987;3(3): 152–160.
36. Schonholtz GJ, Zahn MG, Magee CM, et al.: Lateral release of the patella. *Arthroscopy* 1987; 3:269–272.
37. Aglietti P, Pisaneschi A, Buzzi R, et al.: Arthroscopic lateral release for patellar pain or instability. *Arthroscopy* 1989;5(3):176–183.
38. Scuderi G, Cuomo F, Scott WN: Lateral release and proximal realignment for patella subluxation and dislocation. A long term follow-up. *J Bone Joint Surg Am* 1988;70A:856–861.
39. Maquet P: Un traitement biomecanique de l'arthrose femero-patellaire. *Rev Rhum Mal Osteoartic* 1963;30:779–783.
40. Bandi W: Chondromalacia patellae and femoropatellar arthrosis. *Helv Chir Acta* 1972; 1(Suppl.):3.
41. Fulkerson JP, Hungerford DS: *Disorders of the Patellofemoral Joint,* Baltimore, Williams & Wilkins Co., 1990.
42. Maquet P: Mechanics and osteoarthritis of the patellofemoral joint. *Clin Orthop* 1979;144:70–73.

43. Nakamura N, Ellis M, Seedhom BB: Advancement of the tibial tubercle. A biomechanical study. *J Bone Joint Surg Br* 1985;67B:255–260.
44. Fernandez L, Usabaga J, Yubero J, et al.: An experimental study of the redistribution of patellofemoral pressure by the anterior displacement of the anterior tuberosity of the tibia. *Clin Orthop* 1989;238:183–194.
45. Fulkerson JP, Becker GJ, Meaney JA, et al.: Anteromedial tibial tubercle transfer without bone graft. *Am J Sports Med* 1990;18:490–497.
46. Maquet P: Advancement of the tibial tuberosity. *Clin Orthop* 1976;115:225–230.
47. Hirsch PM, Reddy DK: Experience with Maquet anterior tibial tubercle advancement for patellofemoral arthraglia. *Clin Orthop* 1980; 148:136–139.
48. Rozbruch JD, Campbell RD, Insall JN: Tibial tubercle elevation (the Maquet operation): A clinical study of 31 patients. *Orthop Trans* 1979;3:291.
49. Heatley FW, Allen PR, Patrick JH: Tibial tubercle advancement for anterior knee pain. *Clin Orthop* 1986;208:215–224.
50. Ferguson AB: Elevation of the insertion of the patellar ligament for patellofemoral pain. *J Bone Joint Surg Am* 1982;64A:766–771.
51. Mendes DG, Soudry M, Iusim M: Clinical assessment of Maquet tibial tuberosity advancement. *Clin Orthop* 1987;222:228–238.
52. Radin EL: Anterior tibial tubercle elevation in the young adult. *Orthop Clin North Am* 1986; 17(2):297–301.
53. Bassette G, Hunter RE: The Maquet procedure: A retrospective review. *Clin Orthop* 1988;232: 159–166.
54. Engelbretsen L, Svenningsen S, Benum P: Advancement of the tibial tuberosity for patellar pain. A five-year follow-up. *Acta Orthop Scand* 1989;60(1):20–22.
55. Friedman MJ, Pachelli AF, Fox JM, et al.: Modified Maquet tibial tubercle elevation: A retrospective review. *Am J Knee Surg* 1990;3: 114–118.
56. Miller BJ, LaRochelle PJ: The treatment of patellofemoral pain by combined rotation and elevation of the tibial tubercle. *J Bone Joint Surg Am* 1986;68A:419–423.
57. Morshuis WJ, Pavlov PW, DeRooy KP: Anteromedialization of the tibial tubercle in the treatment of patellofemoral pain and malalignment. *Clin Orthop* 1990;255:242–250.
58. Radin E, Leach R: Anterior displacement of the tibial tubercle for patellofemoral arthrosis. *Orthop Trans* 1979;3:291.
59. McKeever DC: Patellar prosthesis. *J Bone Joint Surg Am* 1955;37A:1074–1084.
60. Depalma AF, Sawyer B, Hoffman JD: Reconsiderations of lesions affecting the patellofemoral joint. *Clin Orthop* 1962;18:63–85.
61. Levitt RL: A long term evaluation of patellar prosthesis. *Clin Orthop* 1973;97:153–157.
62. Harrington KD: Long term results for the McKeever patellar resurfacing prosthesis used as a salvage procedure for severe chondromalacia patellae. *Clin Orthop* 1992;279:201–213.
63. Aglietti P, Insall JN, Walker PS, et al.: A new patellar prosthesis. Design and application. *Clin Orthop* 1975;107:175–187.
64. Insall JN, Tria AJ, Aglietti P: Resurfacing of the patella. *J Bone Joint Surg Am* 1980;62A: 933–936.
65. Worrell RV: Prosthetic resurfacing of the patella. *Clin Orthop* 1979;144:91–97.
66. Worrell RV: Resurfacing of the patella in young patients. *Orthop Clin North Am* 1986; 17(2): 303–309.
67. Blazina ME, Fox JM, Del Pizzo W, et al.: Patellofemoral replacement. *Clin Orthop* 1979; 144:98–102.
68. Arciero RA, Toomey HE: Patellofemoral arthroplasty. A three to nine year follow-up study. *Clin Orthop* 1975;107:175–187.
69. Cartier P, Sanouiler JL, Grelsamer R: Patellofemoral arthroplasty. Two to 12 Year follow-up study. *J Arthroplasty* 1990;5(1):49–55.
70. Ackroyd CE, Polyzoides AJ: Patellectomy for osteoarthritis. *J Bone Joint Surg Br* 1978;60B: 353–357.
71. Boucher HH: Results of excision of the patella. *J Bone Joint Surg Br* 1952;34B:516–521.
72. Geckler EO, Queranta AV: Patellectomy for degenerative arthritis of the knee—Late results. *J Bone Joint Surg Am* 1962;44A:1109–1112.
73. Haggart GE: The surgical treatment of degenerative arthritis of the knee joint. *J Bone Joint Surg Am* 1940;22:717–725.
74. Kelly MA, Insall JI: Patellectomy. *Orthop Clin North Am* 1986;17:289–295.
75. Kaufer H: Mechanical function of the patella. *J Bone Joint Surg Am* 1971;53A:1551–1560.
76. Boyd HB, Hawkins BL: Patellectomy: A simplified technique. *Surg Gynecol Obstet* 1948;86: 357–367.
77. Compere CL, Hill JA, Lewinnek GE, et al.: A new method of patellectomy for patellofemoral arthritis. *J Bone Joint Surg Am* 1979;61A:714–719.
78. Baker CL, Hughston JC: Miyakawa patellec-

tomy. *J Bone Joint Surg Am* 1988;70A:1489–1494.
79. Radin E, Leach R: Anterior displacement of the tibial tubercle for patellofemoral arthrosis. *Orthop Trans* 1979;3:291.

16

Patellar Considerations in Total Knee Replacement

Andrew I. Spitzer and Kelly G. Vince

Successful resurfacing of the patellofemoral articulation in total knee replacement is a crucial aspect of successful arthroplasty. Although it was the last of the knee compartments to be addressed by arthroplasty, its role in the overall function of knee replacement cannot be overemphasized. Proper attention to detail in the management of the patellofemoral joint in total knee arthroplasty can avoid a myriad of potential complications.

History

The early designs of knee replacements did not specifically address the patellofemoral articulation.[1] Options for management of the arthritic patella in a resurfaced knee included only patellectomy, patelloplasty, or benign neglect. However, residual anterior knee pain attributed to the patella persisted in a high percentage of patients in whom those early designs of knee arthroplasty were implanted. In many instances, patellectomy did not alleviate the problem.[2] Furthermore, maltracking, subluxation, and dislocation of thc unresurfaced patellae were documented in a large number of these early knee arthroplasties.[2,3]

In response to the failures of these early designs, anterior flanges were added to the femoral components for articulation with a resurfaced patella, and patellar resurfacing became available. The total condylar prosthesis and its cruciate sparing cousin, the duopatellar prosthesis were designed to accommodate a dome-shaped patellar button.[1,4] Patellofemoral pain became a much more predictably manageable issue in the arthritic knee, but resurfacing introduced many new issues and potential complications to the field of knee arthroplasty.

Currently, patellar resurfacing is an option with all total knee systems. A femoral flange covers the anterior femur and provides an articulating trochlea for the patella. Patellar and femoral component design have evolved with the overriding principle being maximizing proper tracking while minimizing contact stresses in an effort to avoid component wear and breakage, and bony fracture. Proper preparation of the patella, careful axial and rotary alignment of the femoral and the tibial components, and special attention to soft tissue balance in order to optimize patellar tracking have become basic principles in total knee replacement. Despite all of these advances, avoidance of complications related to the patella and the extensor mechanism remain a contemporary challenge.

Design of Patellofemoral Resurfacing Components

Patellar Button

The original design for the patellar button consisted of a symmetric polyethylene dome with a central fixation lug for use with cement on the prepared undersurface of the patella.[1] The dome shape did not require any rotational alignment. However, this shape has been shown to sustain high contact stresses and to experience significant point loading.[5–8] This raised concern regarding wear, deformation, and early failure of this design.

One solution to this problem was to create a more anatomic design that would articulate with a more constraining femoral trochlea. The advantages to this design are lower contact stresses, reduced wear and deformation, and theoretically greater longevity.[6–8] While perfect tracking is a constant goal, it is rarely achieved in the clinical setting, and the majority of patellae tilt from the ideal orientation after implantation, regardless of design.[9] Therefore, the added constraint of an anatomic patella, particularly in the presence of poor soft-tissue balance, may significantly increase the shear at the bone-prosthesis interface, and in fact, can asymmetrically load the facets of the patellar component.[5] This compounds the risk of wear with the risk of osseous patellar fracture. One attempt at addressing this concern is the "congruent-contact, metal-backed, rotating bearing patellar prosthesis," designed by Buechel and associates. This consists of a congruent patellofemoral design, but the polyethylene is free to slide on a smooth metal backing that is affixed to the patella. No failures have been reported in 515 arthroplasties at six-months to 11-years followup.[10]

Other variations of the aforementioned designs include asymmetric, oval components, sombrero type, and biconvex patellar buttons.[11] The oval designs, either anatomic or dome shaped, allow more complete coverage of the bony patella and theoretically distribute stress more uniformly to the patellar bone. The articulating surface is translated medially in order to avoid tightening the lateral structures, but the articulation itself is no different than the equivalent symmetric, nonoval design. The sombrero type may distribute forces more evenly over the surface of the button by modulating the contact points of the patellofemoral articulation over the range of motion of the knee. Biconvex patellae require either reaming or insetting of the button into the patellar cancellous bed. This has particular application in deficient patellae, especially in revision situations. No specific complications related to this design have yet been identified.[12,13]

The method for fixation of the patellar button to the bony patella has also undergone some modifications. The initial large-sized, central single lug has largely been abandoned in favor of smaller and peripheral fixation lugs. The central large lug was associated with osseous patellar fracture.[11,14] Smaller single central lugs have been associated with loosening.[11,14,15] The peripheral lugs, particularly when oriented in a transverse fashion, provide excellent stability with reduced risk of fracture.[16] A three-year followup of three pegged patellae shows a complication rate of only 0.86% in 577 total knees.[17] In addition, many of the currently available buttons have a contoured undersurface with undercut regions to provide for better cement interlock to the component.

Interest in porous ingrowth fixation techniques spawned the development of metal-backed patellar components.[18,19] This technology had the additional theoretic advantage of distributing the contact stresses evenly over the polyethylene and the bone, and was shown to reduce anterior surface strain when compared with all polyethylene patellar components.[7,19,20] Unfortunately, many reports of dissociation of the polyethylene from the metal backing, catastrophic wear of the peripheral thin polyethylene against the metal and subsequent metal on metal abrasion of the femoral component, and broken patellar components have resulted in significantly reduced enthusiasm for these prostheses.[21–31] Attempts are currently underway to improve this design. These include newer methods for securing the polyethylene to the metal backing, and recessing the metal backing into the patellar bone, allowing for thicker polyethylene surfaces without increasing the overall thickness of the patellar button–patella complex.[19] Nevertheless, caution must be exercised when applying this newer technology.

In summary, while some advances have been made in patellar button design, the predictions of catastrophic failure of the initial dome designs have not proved clinically correct.[32-34] As well, the predicted solutions to the theoretic design flaws of those early designs have created nothing less than clinical disasters. A measured enthusiasm for newer technologies must be recommended.

Femoral Trochlea

The design of the femoral component has also evolved. While some designs have been absolutely flat, without any constraint,[35] most have had a trochlear groove designed to articulate with a corresponding patellar button. The struggle between maximizing congruency and constraint in order to optimize tracking, and minimizing contact stress in order to avoid wear, breakage, and fracture has resulted in several variations in flange design. Increasing the height of the lateral ridge of the flange and thickening the anterolateral aspect of the femoral component improves tracking by constraining the patella.[35,36] However, it also tightens the lateral structures, and potentially increases the total and point contact stresses on the lateral surface of the patella. The added constraint also increases shear at the bone prosthesis interface with the potential for osseous patellar fracture.[36] Deepening the trochlear groove without lateral buildup also increases constraint but does not increase contact stress and shear as significantly.[35,37] Finally, regarding materials, titanium femoral components, even when ion bombarded for surface hardening and smoothness, may produce more polyethylene wear debris than comparable chromium–cobalt surfaces.[38,39]

In summary, design of the patellofemoral articulation must resolve the conflict between constraint to optimize tracking and reduction of contact stress to minimize wear. Probably the more important issue is the overall balance of patellofemoral tracking, which has less to do with the design of the articulation itself and more to do with tibial, femoral, and patellar component positioning, and soft-tissue balance. As noted, even when intraoperative attention to all of these details is meticulous, the dynamic interactions of the soft tissues, which cannot be assessed intraoperatively, may tilt, or otherwise alter a patella that has perfect passive tracking.[9]

Resurfacing Controversy

Although not resurfacing the patella in early knee arthroplasty designs resulted in an incidence of residual pain as high as 58%,[40] there is still not uniform agreement that patellar resurfacing is universally necessary.

Because resurfacing the patella created a whole series of new complications, including loosening, fracture, wear, maltracking, and extensor mechanism disruptions, comparison of the risks of resurfacing versus the risks of residual patellofemoral pain became important. Early data indicated that the incidence of secondary resurfacing because of residual patellofemoral pain after bicompartmental arthroplasty exceeded the incidence of complications after primary tricompartmental arthroplasty.[41] This was further supported by data that directly compared a resurfaced group with an unresurfaced group using the same total condylar prosthesis. Fully one third of those not receiving patellar resurfacing were unable to ascend stairs. The resurfaced group had improved stair climbing and less pain.[42] Interestingly, these authors were unable to correlate the gross assessment of chondromalacia at surgery with postoperative anterior knee pain.

More recent and longer-term data support the claim that all knees undergoing knee replacement, whether for osteoarthritis or rheumatoid arthritis, should have the patellae resurfaced.[43,44] Complications are believed to result from technical errors; therefore, attention to technical detail should avoid the majority of complications.[45] There has been no documented decrease in postarthroplasty range of motion with resurfacing.[15] Those that favor resurfacing feel that the overall quality of the knee replacement is improved.[32,33,46] Even when selective resurfacing is undertaken, and only the healthiest patellae are left unresurfaced, the unresurfaced group has a statistically higher revision and complication rate. Intractable patellofemoral pain necessitated patellar resurfacing in this unresurfaced group at an average of five years following the index procedure.[44] It follows that even a selection process carried out by the experienced arthritis surgeons performing this study may not be adequate to exclude those at risk for residual anterior knee pain. Other authors have also documented recurrence of anterior knee pain three to five years following bicompartmental arthroplasty with modern designs.[15]

Despite these compelling arguments, some still advocate selective resurfacing.[14] Several studies have directly compared bilateral knee replacements in the same patients in whom one knee has had the patella left unresurfaced while the other knee has had patellar resurfacing. Even when both knees had severe patellofemoral disease, only nine of 25 patients unequivocally preferred the resurfaced knee at three-years followup.[47] Another series of 17 bilateral knees with two-year followup indicated no difference between the knees at all.[48] Even at 7.5-years followup, as many as 92% of unresurfaced knees with osteoarthritis had no more than mild anterior knee pain.[49] Proponents of not resurfacing will also point out that resurfacing patellae increases anterior surface strain,[50] and that the incidence of patellar fracture after knee arthroplasty is greater (0.33% versus 0.05%) in resurfaced patellae.[51]

There is, however, almost undisputed agreement that all patellae in knees with inflammatory arthritides should be resurfaced at the index operation. Articular cartilage is believed to be an antigenic stimulus for synovial inflammation.[52] Any remaining cartilage in a knee may allow recurrence of inflammatory synovitis. A propensity for recurrence of synovitis has been demonstrated in rheumatoid knees without patellar resurfacing.[14,53–55] Nevertheless, one study comparing bilateral rheumatoid knees, both with relatively spared patellae, in which one patella was resurfaced and the other was not, could not document a difference in outcome at 2.7-years followup.[56]

The controversy is obviously not resolved. How long even normal cartilage will wear comfortably against metal is not currently known. Presumably, some of the theoretic concerns applicable to patellar components are also applicable to unresurfaced patellae. Ensuring proper tracking will undoubtedly prove to be an important factor for both resurfaced and unresurfaced patellae.[57] Femoral design, congruence of the articulation, and contact stresses will inevitably affect longevity of patellar cartilage and buttons.[35] Certain guidelines for resurfacing can, however, reliably be stated. Most would agree that patellae afflicted with inflammatory arthritis should be resurfaced. Any significant arthritis in the patellofemoral articulation of any kind should mandate resurfacing. Even for those most committed to selective resurfacing, certain criteria must be met in order not to resurface. There must be symmetrical cartilage on preoperative skyline radiographs; absence of eburnated bone at surgery; an anatomic shape of the patella that is congruent with the trochlear groove of the femoral trochlear flange; normal tracking that may be achieved by lateral release; and absence of inflammatory synovium, pyrophosphate deposition, or gout.[14] At most, 15% to 20% of patients will satisfy these criteria.

Complications of Patellofemoral Resurfacing

Complications of patellofemoral resurfacing account for as many as 50% of all revision knee surgeries.[11,58–60] Significantly, patellar maltracking is implicated as an etiologic factor of many of these complications. Although some complications cannot be attributed directly to technical error, the majority of complications can be avoided or at least minimized with careful attention to technical details, and to intraoperative patellar preparation and tracking.

Maltracking

Etiology

There are numerous explanations for maltracking of the patella. It is important to understand that maltracking is not simply a complication of patellar resurfacing. On the contrary, it is equally a problem for the unresurfaced patella.[57] General issues to be considered are axial and rotary alignment of the limb, and those factors that either statically or dynamically affect the tightness of the lateral retinacular structures.

Overall limb alignment of more than 10° of valgus and femoral component valgus of more than 7° increase the risk of maltracking.[61,62] This increased Q angle results in a laterally directed vector sum of the quadriceps and patellar tendons, tending to subluxate or dislocate the patella. Similarly, internal rotation of the tibial component functionally externally rotates the tibia with an increase in the Q angle. As in valgus alignment, this increases the laterally directed vector, tending to subluxate the patella.[62–64] Internal rotation of the femoral component stretches the lateral retinaculum and increases the tendency of the patella to track laterally[36,63,65] (Figure 16.1). Medial displacement of the femoral component as little as 5 mm significantly tightens the lateral retinaculum, increasing contact stresses and lateral tracking.[36,66] A similar effect is observed with lateralization of the patellar button.[37] As the button articulates with the trochlear groove, the lateral structures are stretched over the lateral trochlear flange and contact stresses are increased. In contrast, lateralization of the femoral component and medialization of the patellar button reduce the tension in the lateral structures and improve tracking.[36,37,63,66]

Component design is an important variable in patellar tracking. A flat, totally unconstrained trochlear surface provides no centralizing forces to the patella, and even physiologic valgus may cause the patella to track laterally.[35,67] In contrast, a high, lateral trochlear ridge and a deep groove will hold a more constrained patella centrally.[36,37] It is wrong, however, to rely on the constraint alone to centralize the patella. If the soft tissue is not balanced, the increased contact stresses and the increased shear at the bone prosthesis interface may lead to increased polyethylene wear, and prosthetic and osseous patellar fractures. Patellar shape can affect tracking, particularly if an anatomic or asymmetric component is improperly oriented.[68,69] More important, though, is the overall thickness of the patellar prosthesis–bone complex. Thickening the patellofemoral complex either by a thick component, insufficient bony resection, or a thick or anteriorly placed femoral component can tighten the lateral structures and lead to maltracking. In addition, asymmetric

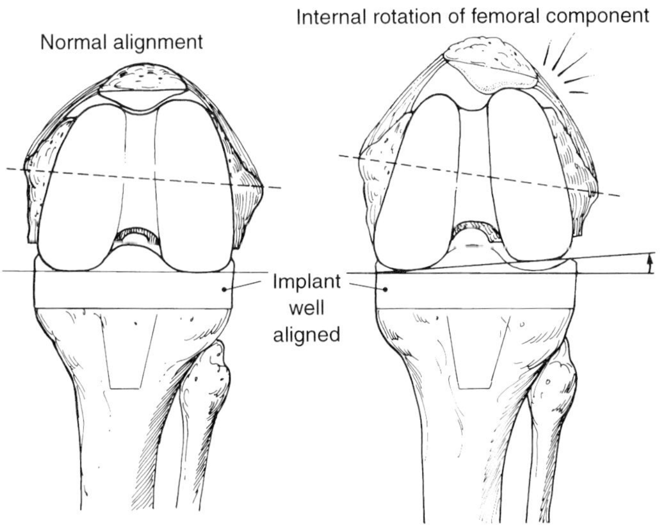

FIGURE 16.1. Internal rotation of the femoral component significantly increases the tendency for lateral tracking by tenting the lateral soft tissues over a prominent lateral trochlear ridge. Constraint maintains the patella centrally but at a cost of increased point loading of the lateral patellar facet against the lateral femoral trochlear ridge. (a) Normal alignment of the femoral component. (b) Internal rotation of the femoral component.

patellar resection with the lateral facet left thick and the medial facet preferentially resected can tighten the lateral structures and lead to subluxation.[11,14,61]

Finally, the soft-tissue structures themselves can contribute to lateral tracking of the patella. A tight lateral retinaculum in a valgus knee may pull the patella laterally as the knee is returned to more anatomic alignment.[11,14] Late maltracking can occur because of dehiscence of the medial retinacular repair or traumatic rupture of the medial retinaculum.[11,14,15,61]

Unfortunately, despite careful assessment of all of these static factors, the dynamic balance of the muscles powering the knee and acting on the patella may favor lateral tracking of the patella. This dynamic instability is impossible to detect or to assess in the operating room.[9]

Evaluation

It is a luxury to optimize patellar tracking in the operating room at the time of the primary arthroplasty. Unfortunately, patellar tracking problems often do not present until after the wound is well healed. As in any disorder, a proper history is essential. Subjective sensation of subluxation or frank dislocation, poor motion, and pain over the medial or lateral retinacula may all be heralds of patellar maltracking. New onset of symptoms after either trauma or a sense of tearing or popping in the knee may signal retinacular dehiscence.

The physical examination should be directed at detecting the exact cause of the maltracking. Limb alignment and Q angle should be measured. Rotation of the components is difficult to assess. Mobility of the patella and tightness of the lateral retinaculum should be assessed. Certainly, tracking with both active and passive range of motion should be observed. Maltracking only with active bending probably indicates a dynamic rather than a static imbalance. Radiographs can be helpful in confirming the diagnosis. The Merchant[70] or the sunrise view can document the statically subluxed patella. Patellar tilt and asymmetric patellar resection is easily identified. Rotational malalignment can sometimes be appreciated on standard radiographs.

Treatment

The purpose of optimizing tracking is to reduce the contact stress at the patellofemoral articulation, to maximize the longevity of the arthroplasty by avoiding associated complications, and to avoid the clinical discomfort associated with patellar maltracking. It must be understood that abnormal forces tending to force the patella from its trochlear articulation must be minimized. Countering the forces with more constraint simply increases the stresses in the whole system. Ultimately, if constraint and not reduction of deforming forces is the methodology used to achieve proper patellar tracking, some link in the system should be expected to fail. This mechanism probably contributes significantly to increased contact stresses, patellar polyethylene wear, breakage, dissociation from metal backing, and shear at the bone-prosthesis interface causing osseous patellar fracture. Therefore, treatment should be specifically directed at the cause rather than compensating one abnormality with another.[63]

The best treatment for this complication, and of course for all others, is prevention. Careful implantation at the initial arthroplasty will enhance the likelihood of achieving adequate patellar tracking. The femoral component should be externally rotated on the femur and should never be internally rotated.[36,65,66] Care should be taken not to reference off a deficient posterolateral condyle, as in a valgus knee, because this can easily lead to internal rotation of the femoral component.[63] The femoral component should also be lateralized maximally without overhang.[36,65,66] The tibial component should be aligned with the crest of the tibia, avoiding internal rotation of the component[62] (Figure 16.2). Excessive external rotation should also be avoided, however, in order to avoid overloading the lateral tibial–femoral articulation by tightening the lateral structures.[61] The combined angle of the femoral and the tibial cuts should not exceed 10° of valgus,[62] and the femoral component itself should not be in more than 7° of valgus.[61] The thickness of the patella should be measured prior to resection, and enough bone should be

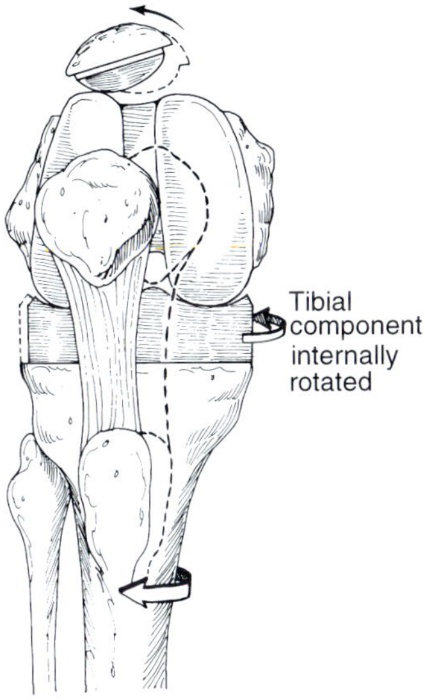

FIGURE 16.2. Aligning the tibial component over the crest of the tibia is preferred. Internally rotating the tibial component functionally externally rotates the tibia, increasing the Q angle, and leading to lateral tracking and increased lateral contact stresses of the patella.

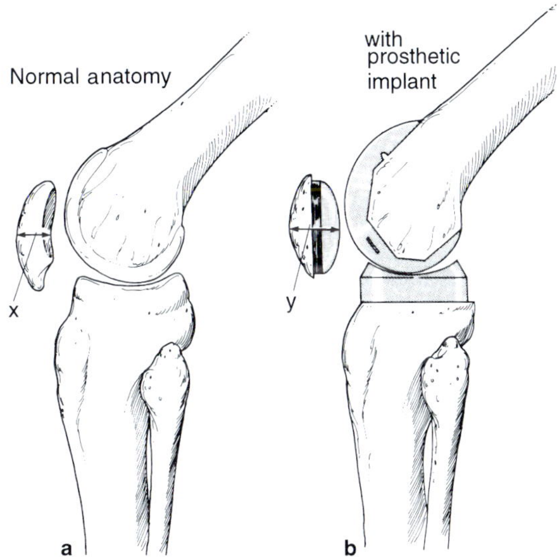

FIGURE 16.3. The thickness of the native patella should be assessed prior to resurfacing in order to estimate the amount of necessary bony resection to accommodate the patellar button without thickening the overall construct (x, patella thickness; y, patella-component composite. (a) Preoperative patella anatomy. (b) Anatomy with component in place.

resected in order to provide adequate space for the patellar button, without thickening the complex[45] (Figure 16.3). A symmetric cut of the patella should be performed, and certainly the lateral facet should not be left thicker than the medial facet,[61] as this may tighten the lateral structures and increase the tendency toward subluxation (Figure 16.4). Although the patellar cut is important, it may be possible to obtain excellent central tracking with minimal constraint even with a poorly cut patella as long as the other components have been properly aligned and the soft tissue has been correctly balanced (Figure 16.5). Medial placement of the button on the patella will reduce stress on the lateral structures[37,63] (Figure 16.6). Finally, assessing patellar tracking with either the real or trial components in place is essential prior to soft-tissue balancing. The patella should track centrally without tendency toward lateral subluxation or lateral tilt in full flexion. The "rule of no thumbs" should pertain; that is, central patellar tracking should occur without requiring the surgeon's thumb or any other external force to stabilize the patella within its articulation.[71,72] A variant of this rule is the one-stitch technique in which no more than one stitch is necessary to maintain proper, central patellar tracking.[73] Careful soft-tissue balancing, including patellofemoral ligament release, lateral retinacular release, possible proximal realignment with medial retinacular, or vastus medialis advancement, should be performed as necessary to optimize

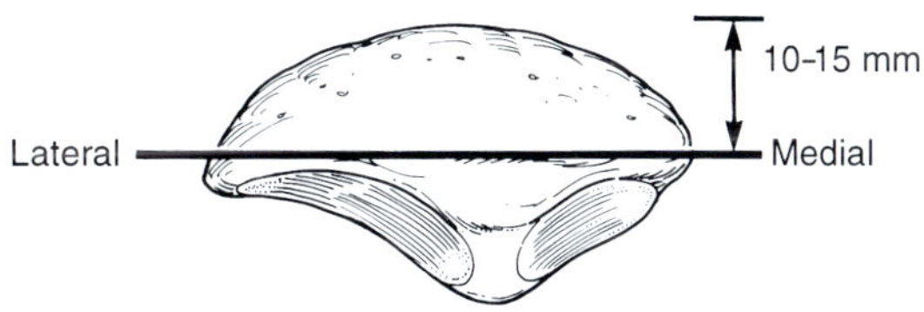

FIGURE 16.4. Resection of the patella from medial osteochondral junction to lateral osteochondral junction will usually produce a flat cut parallel to the anterior patellar surface. This avoids over, under, or asymmetric resection of the patella, which can lead to tracking or fracture complications.

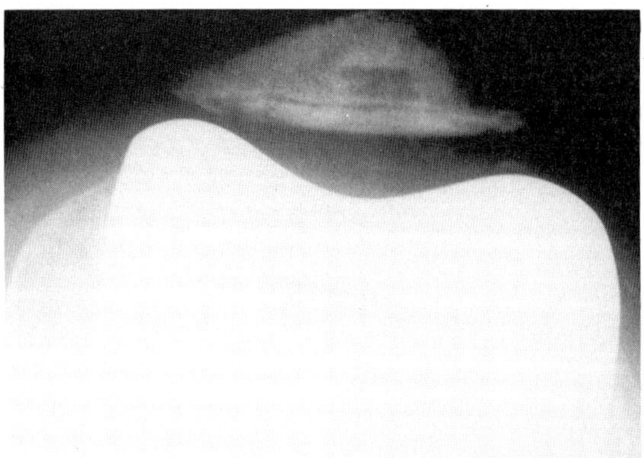

FIGURE 16.5. Although patellar cut is important to optimize tracking, a poorly prepared patella can still track centrally with proper alignment of the tibial and the femoral components, and careful soft-tissue balancing.

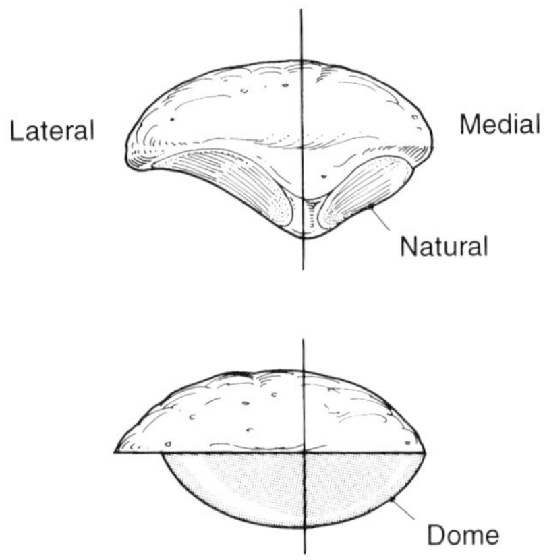

FIGURE 16.6. Medializing the patellar button on the cut surface of the patella improves patellar tracking and reduces forces on the lateral patella by allowing the osseous patella to track somewhat laterally while allowing the button to articulate centrally in the trochlear groove.

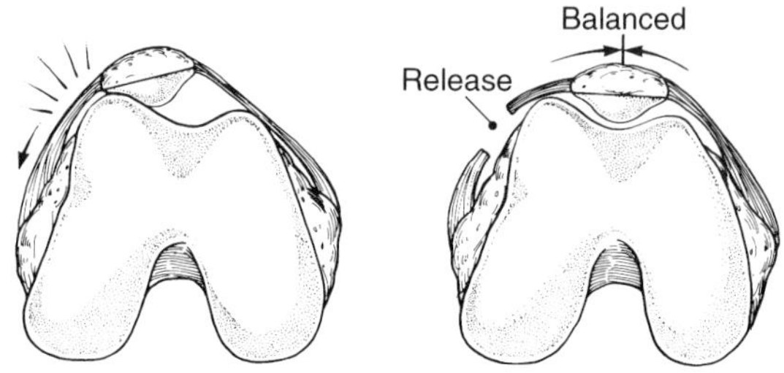

FIGURE 16.7. Lateral retinacular release is an important maneuver to both optimize patellar tracking and to reduce loads on the lateral patellar facet caused by maltracking.

patellar tracking[11,14,58,62,71–73] (Figure 16.7). Distal bony realignment should rarely be necessary at primary arthroplasty if the remainder of the details have been properly addressed, and is generally discouraged due to its causal association with extensor mechanism disruption.[58,74]

When diagnosed late, the usual hierarchy of treatment should be observed. Conservative treatment consisting of vastus medialis obliquus (VMO) strengthening and bracing is rarely successful[4] but certainly should be attempted. Because the instability is rarely dynamic, addressing the static problem will usually require surgical intervention. Arthroscopy has been used successfully to perform lateral releases and to treat patellar maltracking.[75] A lateral release alone may be inadequate to correct the problem if the cause is one of component malalignment. Formal arthrotomy may be necessary. A thorough inspection of the components and a search for the etiology of maltracking should be undertaken. If there is clear component malposition, the offending components, and in some cases the whole knee, must be revised.[61,76] In the absence of significant component malposition, proximal realignment consisting of advancement of the vastus medialis and the medial retinaculum combined with lateral release has been successful at restoring central tracking[62,76] (Figure 16.8). Distal realignment procedures in which the tibial tubercle is elevated and repositioned, or in which the patellar tendon or a portion of it is rerouted have been frought with complications including patellar tendon rupture, one of the most difficult to treat and catastrophic complications of total knee replacement.[11,58,74,77] Despite these risks, there are those who favor distal realignment, because it allows direct alteration of the Q angle.[63,78,79] Newer methods for elevation of the tubercle using a long and relatively thick tubercle osteotomy, maintaining the distal bony attachment as a hinge, and preserving the lateral soft-tissue attachments may im-

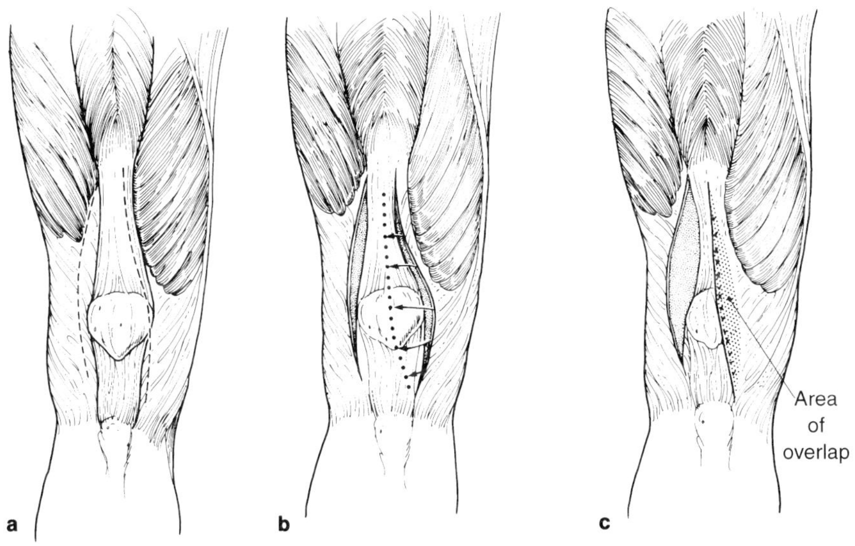

FIGURE 16.8. Proximal realignment for patellar maltracking consists of (a) a lateral relase, (b) a medial retinacular incision, and (c) a reefing of the medial retinaculum over the lateral flap.

prove healing, allow secure fixation, and reduce complications.[80,81]

Patellar Fracture

Etiology

Patellar fracture has been attributed to a large number of etiologic factors. These factors can be subclassified into a few general categories (Table 16.1).

The patella experiences forces as much as seven times the body weight with certain activities.[82,83] Intuitively, anything that either increases these forces or compromises the bone's ability to withstand them should be expected to increase the risk of patellar fracture. Similarly, increasing the stresses in the lateral structures while constraining the patellar component would be expected to increase the shear at the bone-cement or bone-prosthesis interface and ultimately result in failure of the lateral soft tissue or the fragment of patellar bone to which they attach.

Increased weight and activity level have been associated with an increased risk of fracture.[84–86] In addition, excessive flexion has been implicated[85,87]; however, others have found that extent of flexion has no bearing on fracture.[88] Osteopenia of any etiology will increase the risk of patellar fracture.[53]

Component design has an impact on patellar fracture. Large central fixation lugs, particularly when long or if they cause anterior patellar perforation during preparation, can increase the risk of fracture.[11,53,89,90] Increased thickness of the patellofemoral articulation as a result of errors of preparation, an anteriorly translated femoral component, a thick button, or a large lateral femoral flange, increases the stresses in the lateral structures and has been associated with patellar fracture.[51,91]

Those factors within the surgeon's control become the most important, because their impact can be significantly reduced by careful technique. Patellar preparation should avoid excessive bone removal. Patellar resurfacing of any kind increases patellar surface strain.[7,50] A very thin fragment of remaining patella after resection of too much bone or peripheral bone may not be able to withstand the increased surface strains and may fracture.[53,83,86,92,93] At least 1.5-cm of host patella should remain after resection.[93] Similarly, too little resection can thicken the patellar construct, increase the forces on the lateral retinaculum, and, particularly if a constrained patella is used, those forces can increase the shear between the component and the bone

TABLE 16.1. Etiology of patellar fractures.

Category	Description
Patient characteristics	1. Weight 2. Activity level 3. Flexion 4. Osteopenia (steroids)
Component design	1. Large central lug 2. Constrained patella (shear at bone-prosthesis interface) 3. Increased thickness 4. Lug length
Surgical consequences	1. Avascular necrosis (AVN) • Lateral superior genicular artery cut during lateral release • Thermal necrosis due to PMMA 2. Maltracking/malalignment • Lateral shear of patella • Malalignment of any of the components • Anterior tibial displacement and increased distance from the tibial tubercle to origin of extensors causing increased tension in the extensor mechanism 3. Patellar preparation • Excessive bone resection • Insufficient bone resection • Removal of peripheral bone • Removal of lateral facet subchondral bone • Perforation of the anterior cortex of the patella 4. Loosening of the patellar component
Trauma	1. Direct 2. Indirect

Adapted from Vince and McPherson.[4]

and lead to bony fracture.[5,11,14,61,64,86,91,94,95] Some of this shear can be reduced by medializing the patellar button in order to relax the lateral structures.[37,63] Asymmetric resection in which the lateral subchondral bone is removed weakens the bone and may lead to fracture.[33] Excessive cement use should be avoided as thermal necrosis of the bone, and cytotoxic and lipolytic effects of the PMMA can result.[90,96,97] Optimum fixation should be a priority, though, because patellar loosening, while rare, can lead to osseous fracture.[86]

Maltracking because of malalignment or malposition of any of the prosthetic components can increase the forces the patella must withstand and lead to patellar fracture.[88,98,99] When maltracking exists, careful attention must be paid to soft-tissue balancing. Even in a constrained system, contact stresses and lateral tracking must be reduced in order to reduce shear at the bone-prosthesis interface, which can result in bone literally pulling away from the prosthesis as a fracture.[61] Lateral retinacular release is an important step that optimizes tracking and can reduce contact stresses[100] (Figure 16.7). (Avascular necrosis) has been documented following laceration of the superior lateral genicular artery during lateral release,[90,101–104] especially in association with medial arthrotomy.[101,103,105] This is felt by many to be an additional risk factor for patellar fracture. While there are those who dispute this claim,[95,106] it is straightforward and advisable[107] to preserve this vessel during lateral release. The vessel can be found 1 to 2 cm distal to the inferior border of the vastus lateralis muscle[11] (Figure 16.9). If the vessel continues to represent a significant tether to the patella after adequate release, it then can be sacrificed because central tracking of the patella should take precedence.[4,62] Finally, trauma of any sort can cause a fracture of the patella, whether violent or relatively controlled as in manipulation under anesthesia.[11]

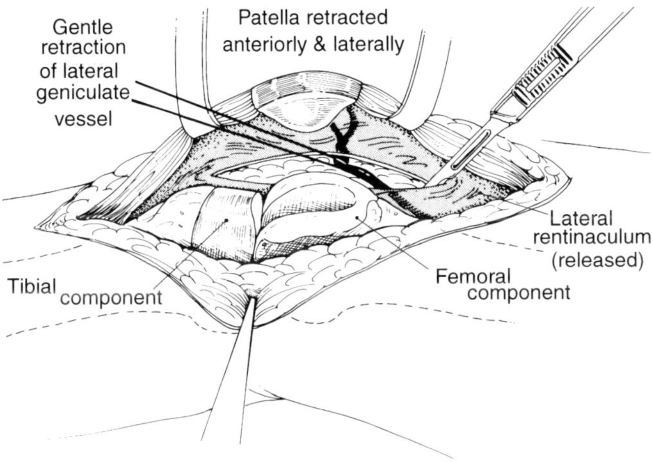

FIGURE 16.9. Lateral retinacular release should be performed from inside the joint. The lateral superior geniculate artery can be found and protected at 1 to 2 cm distal to the inferior border of the vastus lateralis muscle.

Evaluation

A history of chronic subluxation or dislocation, or trauma should alert the surgeon to the possibility of a fracture in a patient complaining of pain in a total knee replacement. New onset of pain or crepitus, particularly about the patella or the lateral retinaculum, also raises the suspicion. Physical examination should be remarkable for crepitus and pain. The competence of the extensor mechanism and patellar tracking should be assessed without causing displacement of a fracture. Clues to etiology should be sought both during the physical and the radiographic examinations. X-rays should demonstrate a fracture, particularly on the sunrise view. Important prognostic factors include displacement, comminution, and component loosening.

Treatment

Management certainly must be guided by the character of the fracture. In the absence of loosening and wide displacement, nonoperative treatment in the form of cast or brace immobilization should be undertaken. In contrast, if the extensor mechanism is disrupted, fragments are displaced by more than 2 cm, or if the component is loose, surgical management will undoubtedly be necessary.[11,14,15,51,108–110]

Although operative fixation of the fracture may seem irresistible, poor results have generally been reported from open reduction and internal fixation.[51,108,110] The bone's ability to heal may be compromised by AVN and generalized osteopenia; the bone's ability to accept fixation devices may be poor; and rigid stability may be unachievable at surgery. For these reasons, even when the fracture has resulted in component loosening, a period of nonoperative treatment may be indicated to enable the fracture to consolidate. Although this may result in a malunion by conventional standards, when surgery is then undertaken, options for resurfacing the bony mass may be greater than in the acute setting. When fixation is attempted, cerclage wiring may be preferable to and more realistically achievable than tension-band wiring or screw fixation.[4] At surgery, if fixation is impossible, and resurfacing is simply not feasible, patelloplasty or partial patellectomy is functionally and biomechanically much preferred over complete patellectomy.[4,111] The biomechanical advantages of the patella are well described and they should be preserved when possible.[112,113] Furthermore, patellectomy can result in tendon rupture[4] and in instability of the total knee arthroplasty.[114]

Implant Failure and Broken Components

Etiology

Although patellar component breakage has been reported for a polyethylene component,[115] it has been encountered, along with other modes of component failure, overwhelmingly with metal-backed components of multiple designs.[18,21–26,28–30] The metal backing was initially introduced as a method for more evenly distributing stresses and to provide a mechanism for fixation of the component without cement.[7,18–20] In order to accommodate the thickness of the metal backing, however, the polyethylene was made thinner. Resecting more patella represented a dangerous solution to the thickness issue, because this would leave a thin wafer of bone to bear the large forces transmitted across the patellofemoral joint. Similarly, thickening the overall construct was undesirable, because this would tighten the extensor mechanism, increase stresses, diminish motion, and produce maltracking. Therefore, the thinner polyethylene remained and became a source for many problems that followed.

In particular, while the whole polyethylene was thinner, the thickness at the periphery, where forces are concentrated particularly with any lateral tracking, was only 1 to 2 mm.[21,22,98] This simply was not enough material to withstand the cyclic loading within the joint. The result was many reports of fracture and wear through of the polyethylene (Figure 16.10). In addition, dissociation of the polyethylene button from the metal backing also occurred, attributed to poor linking of the metal and the plastic.[21,22,25,26,29,30] As a result of both of these complications, metal from the patellar component was exposed to the femoral component, resulting in audible grating, metal synovitis, and pain.[22] This converted the patellar problem into a global joint problem with wear of metal against metal, creating a vicious cycle of rapid failure.

These components have also failed by breakage of the metal itself. Fixation lugs have fractured off the metal base plates.[16,22,23,25,28] This has been associated with preferential ingrowth of the lugs without fixation of the base plate.[28] Although metal-backed patellae have been plagued by this litany of failures, some still maintain that improvement in design, insetting the patellar back into the bony patella, and attention to technical detail to optimize tracking increase the success rate.[19] In general, however, use of metal-backed patellae should be discouraged and avoided.[27]

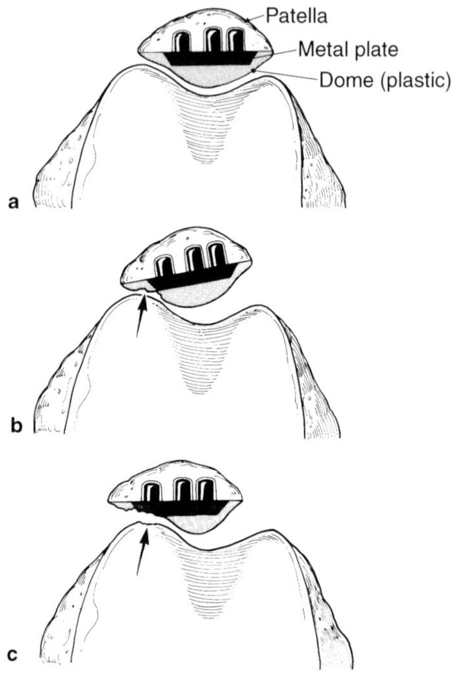

FIGURE 16.10. Lateral tracking of a metal-backed patella can significantly load the thin peripheral polyethylene, leading to catastrophic wear of the polyethylene, scoring of the femoral component against the exposed metal base plate, and precipitous deterioration of the knee anthroplasty.

Evaluation

The new onset of pain and swelling in a patient with a metal-backed patella should be a herald of patellar failure. Audible grating of metal against metal confirms the diagnosis. The physical examination may elicit pain about the patella or the retinaculum. Synovitis and effusion will often be observed. If complete wear through or fracture of the polyethylene has occurred, palpable grating will be present. Radiographic assessment may show a metal synovitis,[116] with outline of the synovial pouch by a radiodense shadow. In addition, metal-to-metal contact may sometimes be seen. Breakage of the metal may be observed. Even in the absence of conclusive findings, evidence of lateral tracking should raise the suspicion of asymmetric wear and attrition of the thin polyethylene. Aspiration will yield a darkly stained synovial fluid containing polyethylene and metal debris, and arthrography may reveal loose bodies of polyethylene.[4] If the diagnosis is still not evident, arthroscopy can delineate the lesion under direct vision.[117,118]

Treatment

The solution to failure or impending failure of a metal-backed component is revision surgery. Often the tissues will be stained black from the metal debris and a synovectomy of this abnormal tissue should be performed.[4,15] Management options depend largely on the appearance of the joint and the other components at surgery. If complete wear through has not occurred, or if the femoral component is not significantly scored, revision of the patella alone is feasible.[119,120] This will entail either conversion to a cemented all-polyethylene component, using either a flat base or a biconvex patella to fill bony defects, or patelloplasty with shaping of the remaining bone to articulate directly against the intact femoral component. If the femoral component is significantly damaged, or if any of the components are loose or require revision, full knee revision will be necessary.[4,15] A new technology may permit intraoperative polishing of a scuffed femoral component and may avoid the morbidity of revising a well-fixed, but damaged, femoral component.[121] The utility of this technology remains to be proven.

Loosening

Etiology

Component loosening has been associated with small, central fixation lugs. Poor technical fixation with inadequate cement technique, or poor bone preparation or quality can compromise initial and long-term fixation.[11,14,15] Failure of ingrowth certainly is possible as with any other porous ingrowth technology.[18] Even without contributing prosthetic or osseous factors, high activity level, particularly when coupled with excessive flexion, can loosen a well-fixed patellar component. High contact or shear stresses as a result of maltracking can also contribute to component loosening.[11,14,15]

Evaluation

Loosening tends to be symptomatic.[11,14] History will reveal patellar pain, and perhaps swelling and synovitis from debris. Physical examination should isolate the pain to the patella unless other components are loose or symptomatic as well. Radiographs may reveal alteration of the position of the component, or a radiolucent line between the bone and the cement or between the cement and the prosthesis.

Treatment

The symptomatic loose patellar button requires revision surgery to either implant a new component, or to perform a patelloplasty or a patellectomy. Choice of procedure as well as of revision component depends on the quality and the quantity of bone present at revision surgery.[12,13] Attention to patellar tracking and fixation should be fastidious, and the need for revision of the other components should be assessed. (See section ????? on The Patella in Revision Total Knee Arthroplasty.)

Extensor Mechanism Rupture

Etiology

Rupture of the extensor mechanism following total knee arthroplasty is a devastating complication. It most frequently occurs distally with either the soft tissue peeling away from the tibial tubercle or the tubercle itself avulsing.[14,74] This has been correlated with distal realignment procedures.[58,74] Increased stresses in the extensor mechanism either from maltracking, an overly thick patellofemoral joint, or from excessive scarring can also cause rupture of the extensor mechanism, particularly if flexion is forced. Attrition of the patellar and quadriceps tendons can occur over sharp or abraded components, particularly if the soft tissue is already compromised as in diabetes mellitus, collagen vascular diseases, or chronic corticosteroid use.[74]

Evaluation

History will elicit either an acute or a subacute onset of extensor lag, usually associated with discomfort if not frank pain. Complete inability to extend the knee may be present. A palpable defect either in the suprapatellar or the infrapatellar region will be present. Relative patella infera or alta may also be present. Radiography should confirm the patella alta or infera and may show soft-tissue defects.

Treatment

The first step in management must be avoidance. In any knee surgery, the skin incision should generously avoid the tibial tubercle in order not to create damage to the patellar tendon or its blood supply.[4] Exposure of a knee with poor flexion or difficult patellar eversion necessitates a patellar turndown, a rectus snip, or a tibial tubercle osteotomy in order to avoid avulsion of the patellar tendon[80,81,122–125] (Figure 16.11). Although tubercle osteotomy has generally been discouraged, newer techniques of extended tibial tubercle osteotomies with maintenance of the lateral and the distal soft-tissue attachments may improve fixation and healing, and reduce the risk of subsequent avulsion.[80,81]

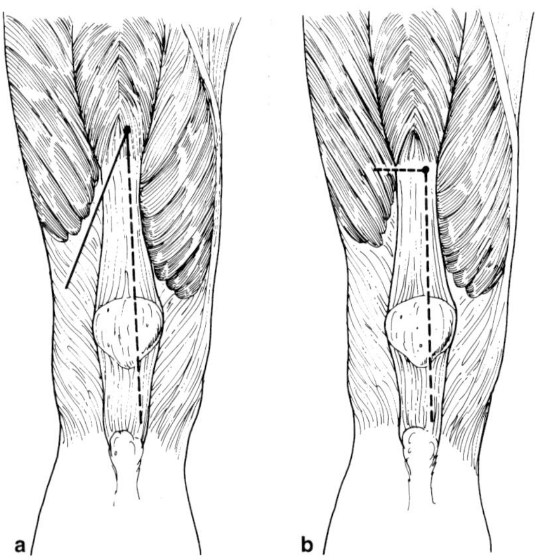

FIGURE 16.11. Exposure of the stiff knee by (a) a modified quadriceps turndown or (b) a rectus snip.

The literature reports are generally discouraging regarding the results of repair of the ruptured extensor mechanism. As in any repair, the goal must be to obtain secure fixation to bone of either the tendon itself or the bony avulsion fragment. Sutures, staples, and tendinous reconstructions all have failed in a large percentage of attempts reported.[3,4,74,126] Newer technology consisting of suture anchors may provide a valuable addition to the treatment methods. Reinforcements or augmentations of the repair with semitendinosus and gracilis tendons, or tensor fascia lata may be used to protect against recurrent rupture.[4,74,127] The Swiss Association for the Study of Internal Fixation (AO/ASIF) techniques useful for protection of patellar fracture fixation or traumatic patellar tendon rupture repair during healing may also be beneficial.[128]

A fundamentally different approach to the problem is allograft replacement of the extensor mechanism. In the technique that Emerson et al. described, the entire extensor mechanism is replaced by an allograft consisting of the quadriceps tendon, the patella with cemented polyethylene button, the patella tendon, and the tibial tubercle. This has been successfully accomplished in 11 of 13 patients with improvement in active extension.[129]

Soft-Tissue Impingement

Etiology

Some soft-tissue scarring and fibrous tissue occurs in the majority of knees following total knee arthroplasty, and can form a "patellar meniscus."[130] This may act as a shock absorber and distribute stresses evenly over the patella, much as does the tibiofemoral menisci. However, abnormal scar and fibrous tissues can create symptomatic tracking abnormalities—clicks and clunks—that can compromise the result of an otherwise successful total knee replacement. The stimulus for this abnormal scarring is not well understood, but it could be a response to maltracking and increased contact stresses between prosthetic components.[61]

Various different configurations of fibrous

tissue have been implicated. Thorpe et al. classified fibrous bands as type I, superior and transverse; type II, lateral; and type III, inferior.[131] They felt that these tethered the patella and prevented smooth, unrestricted motion. The patellar clunk syndrome occurs because of a fibrous mass of tissue just superior to the patella on the undersurface of the quadriceps tendon, similar to Thorpe's type I band, which catches on the distal intercondylar edge of posterior stabilized femoral components during active extension from the acutely flexed position.[132,133] The tibial eminence has also been implicated as the impingement site for the hypertrophic scar tissue.[134] Aberrant scarring in the infrapatellar fat pad, similar to Thorpe's type III band, as well as posterior scarring have also been implicated in postoperative anterior knee pain in total knee arthroplasty.[94,135] Progressive patella baja has been documented along with this infrapatellar scarring.[135,136] Alteration of the joint line at the time of surgery with resultant patella baja creates a construct conducive to this scarring.[87,99]

Evaluation

History reveals anterior knee pain, often worse at the extremes of flexion or extension, in many of the soft-tissue scarring syndromes.[135] A report of painful and audible catching and clunking when actively extending the knee from a flexed position, particularly in the presence of a posterior stabilized prosthesis, is virtually diagnostic of the patellar clunk syndrome.[4,132,133] It should be difficult to reproduce clunking passively, but the patient may demonstrate this with active extension. Examination may reveal point tenderness, or elicitable tenderness at specific locations of popping or clicking. A "rubbery" bulge in the infrapatellar area may be palpable.[15] Patella baja may be noted. Radiographs may show progressive or static patella baja. Aspiration should routinely be performed to rule out the possibility of infection.[15]

Treatment

Beight et al. outlined a stepwise treatment protocol.[132] Although most of these syndromes do not respond to conservative therapy, a trial of physical therapy, steroid injection, and antiinflammatory medications is warranted. Arthroscopy has been successfully employed in the management of all of these syndromes.[131,137] If relief of symptoms is not obtained, or recurs after arthroscopy, open surgery may be necessary and may include resecting the fibrous tissue and hypertrophic fat pad, freeing up the scarred patella and patellar tendon, and possibly revision of components if tracking is felt to contribute to the problem.[14,15,132] Usually, symptoms resolve with arthroscopy alone and rarely recur.

Technique of Patellar Resurfacing

Exposure

Exposure in the routine total knee arthroplasty is rarely difficult and can be adequately performed through a transpatellar, medial parapatellar, or subvastus exposure.[123,138,139] In the tight knee, however, with limited flexion, additional maneuvers may be necessary. Although a complete quadriceps turndown is rarely necessary,[122] it is often useful to utilize a V–Y quadricepsplasty, a modification of the turndown.[124] Alternatively, simple transection of the quadriceps tendon with a rectus snip may provide comparable exposure with no additional morbidity[123,125] (Figure 16.11). Tibial tubercle elevation is less desirable because of the risk of subsequent extensor mechanism rupture.[58,74] Recently described techniques in which the lateral soft-tissue attachments are maintained with a long, extended tubercle osteotomy, and rigid fixation of the bone is obtained at closure may reduce some of the risk to rupture and improve healing.[80,81] Controlled exposure by any method is certainly preferable to uncontrolled exposure. When a tight extensor mechanism creates difficulty in everting the patella, and extensor mechanism rupture is a risk, one of these techniques should be used. Once the patella is everted, the synovium, which often obscures the medial facet of the patella, should be either resected or reflected back so that the undersurface of the patella and the osteochondral junction is completely visible circumferentially.

Resection

The goal of resurfacing the patella should be to reestablish the thickness of the original patella (Figure 16.3). The thickness of the patella should be measured with a caliper prior to resection.[45] Thickening should be meticulously avoided because of the adverse effects it may have on tracking, contact stresses, and the risk for fracture.[11,14,25,61,140] Similarly, excessive bone should not be resected. A thin wafer of remaining bone may be inadequate to withstand the stresses placed across the patellofemoral joint.[53,83,86,92,93] Furthermore, adequate fixation may be impossible to achieve in a very thin remaining patella, with the risk of anterior perforation of the fixation lug holes, and creation of stress risers being prohibitively high.[11,53,89,90] At least 1.5 cm of patella bone should remain after resection, because less than this significantly increases anterior surface strain on the patella.[93]

There are many jigs that are designed to cut the patella. They are replete with cutting slots, cutting platforms, reamers with stops, and guides to prevent excessive resection. Most are difficult and cumbersome to use, if not altogether impossible. Furthermore, grip on the patella is often achieved maximally over a narrow range of actual bone. Repositioning the jig when recutting the patella is necessary can therefore be a significant challenge. Freehand resection is preferred by many. Nevertheless, interest persists in developing a reliable cutting guide to reproducibly prepare the patella.[141]

The patella can be cut in flexion with the benefit of more rigid immobilization of the bone. It may also be cut in extension with the benefit of easier positioning and jig placement. In either position, care should be taken to create a symmetric, flat cut, leaving as much of the firm subchondral bone as possible.[142] This allows for solid fixation of the patellar component and avoids tracking problems from either tightening or loosening the extensor mechanism. Generally, cutting from the medial to lateral osteochondral junctions will resect the appropriate amount of bone and provide a symmetric cut (Figure 16.4). This can be assessed on the preoperative sunrise or the Merchant view.[70] Once the cut is made, its symmetry should be verified both with the surgeon's fingers and with the caliper.[45] Adjustments should be made as necessary.

Choosing the appropriate size button usually follows initial resection and is based on the size of the remaining patellar surface, less osteophytes. Maximal coverage should be sought that also allows for some medialization of the patellar button to optimize patellar tracking[123] (Figure 16.6). Overhang is probably undesirable. The cut surface of the patella should then be prepared, usually with the aid of a drill guide, to accept the fixation lugs of the patellar button. Trials can be placed to assess tracking prior to actual component implantation and to assess the thickness of the bone–patellar component composite. Pulsatile irrigation of the surface and drying in preparation for cementing should be performed. The actual component is then implanted.

Of course, attention to the details of patellar preparation is just one step in avoiding postoperative complications attributable to the patella. Careful alignment and rotation of the femoral and the tibial components are essential to proper patellar function after total knee arthroplasty. It certainly may be possible to achieve proper tracking of a poorly prepared patella if the other components are implanted properly and the soft tissues are properly balanced (Figure 16.5).

Soft-Tissue Balancing

Soft-tissue balance is crucial to proper patellar tracking. Even when the components are all implanted with great care, there may still be a relative imbalance causing patellar maltracking. The rule of no thumbs[71,72] or the one-stitch technique[73] should apply. That is, minimal external force, if any, should be necessary to maintain central tracking of the patella. A stepwise approach to soft-tissue releases should be followed, beginning with patellofemoral ligament release. If necessary, a lateral retinacular release should be performed. In order to reduce the possibility of patellar AVN, the release should be performed from within the joint and at 1.5 to 2.0 cm posterior and lateral to the patella between the vastus lateralis and the iliotibial band.[62,102] The lateral superior genicular artery, located near the inferior border of the vastus lateralis,[11] should be preserved if it does not represent a significant lateral tether to the patella[4,62,107] (Figure 16.9). Medial reefing can be added to further stabilize the patella medially.

The Patella in Revision Total Knee Arthroplasty

When the revision arthroplasty is being performed specifically for patellar failure, addressing the patellar component is inevitable. However, a well-fixed patella need not always be resurfaced when revision for other purposes is undertaken. If the revision prosthesis will accommodate the old patellar button design with adequate tracking and acceptable contact stresses as judged at the time of surgery, it is preferable to retain the old patella rather than to create a potentially unsalvageable situation by removing a well-fixed component.

Ideally, the patella at revision will retain enough bone stock to support a revision of the patellar button. Certainly, if the patella will accommodate resurfacing in the standard fashion, then a standard resurfacing should be performed. However, bone stock will often be deficient. For central deficiency, a biconvex patella may fill the defect while still maintaining patellar height.[12,13] Bone grafting of contained defects may also be acceptable, but there are no reports of this technique to the best of our knowledge. For the extremely deficient patella, patelloplasty without resurfacing is preferable to patellectomy.[4,111] At least some thickness to the extensor mechanism and therefore some mechanical advantage is retained. The surface should be smoothed and shaped in order to avoid gross incongruency and high contact stresses. Good long-term results with this technique have been reported.[143] For the unsalvageable patella or an extremely comminuted fracture, patellectomy may be the only real alternative. In these situations, consideration should be given to extensor mechanism allografting techniques and to intratendinous allografts[129,144] to restore the mechanical advantage normally provided by the patella.[112,113] This also may be desirable from the standpoint of the stability of the tibial femoral articulation, because total knee replacement in the patellectomized patient has often been complicated by instability.[114]

Patellar revision and resurfacing is certainly desirable from the standpoint of knee function. However, several recent series have documented a high complication rate in isolated patellar revisions, with only 75% good to excellent results.[119,120]

Total Knee Replacement after Patellectomy

Total knee arthroplasty following patellectomy has been complicated by instability, residual anterior knee pain, and poor results.[89,114,145] Sledge and Ewald have described the importance of the four-bar linkage to stability of the knee following total knee arthroplasty, with the patella acting to position the quadriceps and the patellar tendons parallel to the anterior and the posterior cruciate ligaments, respectively.[146] With the absence of the patella, this relationship is disrupted. The anterior cruciate ligament is usually sacrificed in current total knee arthroplasty designs, leaving only the posterior cruciate ligament to provide stability after knee arthroplasty. If the posterior cruciate ligament is attenuated, tensioned improperly, or sacrificed, stability of the knee arthroplasty lacking a patella can be severely compromised.[147] This has led some to suggest the use of a hinged prosthesis in this clinical situation.[114]

While most agree that overall results tend to be poorer in patients undergoing total knee arthroplasty following patellectomy, several series have reported adequate results. Railton et al. reported pain-free status in six out of seven patients implanted with unconstrained knee replacements sacrificing both cruciate ligaments. They stressed the importance of careful soft-tissue tensioning in flexion in order to avoid instability.[148] Larson et al. reported seven of 14 good to excellent primary knee replacements in patellectomized patients, and seven of 12 good to excellent results in revision situations. While Larson et al. recognized poorer results than in a control group, they felt that the satisfactory results justified total knee arthroplasty in this population, particularly in lower-demand, more debilitated patients with inflammatory arthritides. They warned that patients with posttraumatic osteoarthritis and concurrent patellectomy were at high risk for failure, and that, in general, "patients without patellae may be at a higher risk for failure of the prosthesis." Larson et al. suggested use of a prosthesis with some intrinsic stability for these patients.[147] Cameron and Jung agreed with the recommendation for a stabilized prosthesis, particularly if the cruciates were absent.[149] Szalapski et al. reported 18 of 22 patients with good to excellent results who were implanted with cruciate, sparing unconstrained devices at average five-years followup. They noted that only 30% of their patients were able to stair climb normally compared with 60% of a control group of osteoarthritics. No instability was noted in this series.[150] Reporting only five of 11 good to excellent results, Lennox et al. have warned that:

> The patient with a painful knee with a previous patellectomy and a number of other previous knee procedures, none of which provided pain relief, with minimal or moderate tibiofemoral arthritic changes and with severely compromised quadriceps function, is unlikely to achieve an acceptable result from total knee arthroplasty.

Positive prognostic factors in their series included less than three previous knee procedures, an arthritic tibiofemoral joint, and quadriceps performance greater than 40 ft-lb at 30°/s testing speed.[145] They also used a minimally constrained device and underscored proper soft-tissue tensioning to avoid instability.

In summary, the consensus seems to be that while complications are frequent, total knee arthroplasty in the well-selected patient with a patellectomy can be successful. Special attention to soft-tissue tensioning, particularly in flexion, can avoid postoperative instability and enable use of a minimally constrained device. A posterior stabilized prosthesis, however, may represent a safer and more predictably stable choice in these patients.

Conclusions

The role of the patella in total knee replacement has been a topic of great controversy and debate. While some still selectively resurface the patella, the overwhelming majority of authors recommend universal resurfacing in order to avoid postoperative anterior knee pain. The design of patellar components has undergone many changes, some of which, like metal backing, have created more problems than they have solved. Nevertheless, components are available today that better resolve the conflict between constraint for the purposes of tracking and minimizing contact stresses. Maltracking has emerged as one of the most crucial elements contributing to patellar complications. Management of these complications successfully can be a major challenge for the reconstructive knee surgeon. Although patellar complications have accounted for the majority of revisions of total knee replacements in many series, a better understanding of the mechanics of the patellofemoral articulation in total knee replacement, and of the effects that component alignment, rotation, and position have on patellar tracking and function should reduce the complications related to the patella in total knee replacement in the future.

References

1. Insall JN: Historical development, classification, and characteristics of knee prostheses, in Insall JN, Windsor RE, Scott WN, et al. (eds.): *Surgery of the Knee.* New York, Churchill Livingstone, 1993, pp. 677–718.

2. Insall JN, Ranawat CS, Aglietti P, et al.: A comparison of four models of total knee replacement prostheses. *J Bone Joint Surg Am* 1976; 58A:754–765.
3. Jones EC, Insall JN, Inglis AE, et al.: GUEPAR knee arthroplasty results and late complications. *Clin Orthop* 1979;140:145–152.
4. Vince KG, McPherson EJ: The patella in total knee arthroplasty. *Orthop Clin North Am* 1992; 23:675–686.
5. Buechel FF, Pappas MJ, Makris G: Evaluation of contact stress in metal-backed patellar replacements. A predictor of survivorship. *Clin Orthop* 1991;273:190–197.
6. Collier JP, McNamara JL, Surprenant VA, et al.: All-polyethylene patellar components are not the answer. *Clin Orthop* 1991;273:198–203.
7. Goldstein SA, Coale E, Weiss A, et al.: Patellar surface strain. *J Orthop Res* 1986;4:372–377.
8. Hsu HP, Walker PS: Wear and deformation of patellar components in total knee arthroplasty. *Clin Orthop* 1989;246:260–265.
9. Bindelglass DF, Cohen JL, Dorr LD: Patellar tilt and subluxation in total knee arthroplasty. Relationship to pain, fixation, and design. *Clin Orthop* 1993;286:103–109.
10. Buechel FF, Rosa RA, Pappas MJ: A metal-backed, rotating-bearing patellar prosthesis to lower contact stress. An 11-year clinical study. *Clin Orthop* 1989;248:34–49.
11. Brick GW, Scott RD: The patellofemoral component of total knee arthroplasty. *Clin Orthop* 1988;231:163–178.
12. Rand JA, Gustilo RB: Technique of patellar resurfacing in total knee arthroplasty. *Tech Orthop* 1988;3:57–66.
13. Gomes LS, Bechtold JE, Gustilo RB: Patellar prosthesis positioning in total knee arthroplasty. A roentgenographic study. *Clin Orthop* 1988;236:72–81.
14. Barnes CL, Scott RD: Patellofemoral complications of total knee replacement, in Heckman, JD (ed.): *Instructional Course Lectures*. Chicago, American Academy of Orthopaedic Surgeons, 1993, pp. 303-308.
15. Rand JA: Extensor mechanism, in Morrey BF (ed.): Joint replacement arthroplasty. New York, Churchill Livingstone, 1991, pp. 1039–1049.
16. Cheal EJ, Hayes WC, Harry JD, et al.: *Influence of Component Orientation on Peg Failure of Patellar Surface Replacements*. New Orleans, Orthopaedic Research Society, 1986.
17. Ridhalgh M, Scott RD, Brick GW, et al.: *Three-Pegged All-Plastic Patella Components in Total Knee Arthroplasty*. San Francisco, American Academy of Orthopaedic Surgeons, 1993.
18. Firestone TP, Teeny SM, Krackow KA, et al.: The clinical and roentgenographic results of cementless porous-coated patellar fixation. *Clin Orthop* 1991;273:184–189.
19. Laskin RS, Bucknell A: The use of metal-backed patellar prostheses in total knee arthroplasty. *Clin Orthop* 1990;260:52–55.
20. Hayes WC, Levine BM: *Finite Element Analysis of Patellar Resurfacing Procedures*. Atlanta, Orthopaedic Research Society, 1980.
21. Bayley JC, Scott RD: Further observations on metal-backed patellar component failure. *Clin Orthop* 1988;236:82–87.
22. Bayley JC, Scott RD, Ewald FC, et al.: Failure of the metal-backed patellar component after total knee replacement. *J Bone Joint Surg AM* 1988;70A:668–674.
23. Felmet G, de Nicola U, Springorum HW: Failure of metal-backed uncemented patellar components. Report on three cases. *Acta Orthop Scand* 1989;60:715–717.
24. Halbrecht J, Giordano CP, Jaffe WL: Metal-backed patellar component failure and metallic synovitis in total knee arthroplasty: A case report. *Bull Hosp Jt Dis* 1989;49:48–54.
25. Lewallen DG, Rand JA: *Failure of Metal Backed Patellae in Total Knee Arthroplasty*. New Orleans, American Academy of Orthopaedic Surgeons, 1990.
26. Lombardi AJ, Engh GA, Volz RG, et al.: Fracture/dissociation of the polyethylene in metal-backed patellar components in total knee arthroplasty. *J Bone Joint Surg Am* 1988; 70A: 675–679.
27. Peters JD, Engh GA, Corpe RS: The metal-backed patella. An invitation for failure? *J Arthroplasty* 1991;6:221–228.
28. Rosenberg AG, Andriacchi TP, Barden R, et al.: Patellar component failure in cementless total knee arthroplasty. *Clin Orthop* 1988;236: 106–114.
29. Stulberg SD, Stulberg BN, Hamati Y, et al.: Failure mechanisms of metal-backed patellar components. *Clin Orthop* 1988;236:88–105.
30. Sutherland CJ: Patellar component dissociation in total knee arthroplasty. A report of two cases. *Clin Orthop* 1988;228:178–181.
31. Wright TM, Bartel DL: The problem of surface damage in polyethylene total knee components. *Clin Orthop* 1986;205:67–74.
32. Ranawat CS, Rose HA, Bryan WJ: Replacement of the patello-femoral joint with the total

condylar knee arthroplasty. *Int Orthop* 1984;8: 61–65.
33. Ranawat CS: The patellofemoral joint in total condylar knee arthroplasty. Pros and cons based on five- to ten-year follow-up observations. *Clin Orthop* 1986;205:93–99.
34. Ranawat CS, Flynn WF, Saddler S, et al.: Long-term results of the total condylar knee arthroplasty: A 15-year survivorship study. *Clin Orthop* 1993;286:94–102.
35. Freeman MA, Samuelson KM, Elias SG, et al.: The patellofemoral joint in total knee prostheses. Design considerations. *J Arthroplasty* 1989;4:(Suppl.):69–74.
36. Rhoads DD, Noble PC, Reuben JD, et al.: The effect of femoral component position on the kinematics of total knee arthroplasty. *Clin Orthop* 1993;286:122–129.
37. Yoshii I, Whiteside LA, Anouchi YS: The effect of patellar button placement and femoral component design on patellar tracking in total knee arthroplasty. *Clin Orthop* 1992;275:211–219.
38. Milliano MT, Whiteside LA: Articular surface material effect on metal-backed patellar components. A microscopic evaluation. *Clin Orthop* 1991;273:204–214.
39. Milliano MT, Whiteside LA, Kaiser AD, et al.: Evaluation of the effect of the femoral articular surface material on the wear of a metal-backed patellar component. *Clin Orthop* 1993; 287: 178–186.
40. Picetti G, McGann WA, Welch RB: The patellofemoral joint after total knee arthroplasty without patellar resurfacing. *J Bone Joint Surg Am* 1990;72A:1379–1382.
41. Scott WN, Rozbruch JD, Otis JC, et al.: Clinical and biomechanical evaluation of patella replacement in total knee arthroplasty. *Orthop Trans* 1978;2:203.
42. Soudry M, Mestriner LA, Binazzi R, et al.: Total knee arthroplasty without patellar resurfacing. *Clin Orthop* 1986;205:166–170.
43. Boyd A Jr., Ewald F, Thomas W, et al.: Long term complications of the resurfaced and unsurfaced patella in total knee arthroplasty. *Orthop Trans* 1991;15:725.
44. Boyd A Jr., Ewald FC, Thomas WH, et al.: Long-term complications after total knee arthroplasty with or without resurfacing of the patella. *J Bone Joint Surg Am* 1993;75A:674–681.
45. Rand JA: Patellar resurfacing in total knee arthroplasty. *Clin Orthop* 1990;260:110–117.
46. Cameron HU: Comparison between patellar resurfacing with an inset plastic button and patelloplasty. *Can J Surg* 1991;34:49–52.
47. Enis JE, Gardner R, Robledo MA, et al.: Comparison of patellar resurfacing versus nonresurfacing in bilateral total knee arthroplasty. *Clin Orthop* 1990;260:38–42.
48. Greenky B, Hostein E, Scott R, et al.: Bilateral knee replacement, with and without patella resurfacing. *Orthop Trans* 1991;15:726.
49. Levitzky KA, Harris WJ, McManus J, et al.: Total knee arthroplasty without patellar resurfacing. Clinical outcomes and long-term follow-up evaluation. *Clin Orthop* 1993;286:116–121.
50. McLain RF, Bargar WF: The effect of total knee design on patellar strain. *J Arthroplasty* 1986; 1:91–98.
51. Grace JN, Sim FH: Fracture of the patella after total knee arthroplasty. *Clin Orthop* 1988;230: 168–175.
52. Steinberg J, Sledge CB, Noble J, et al.: A tissue-culture model of cartilage breakdown in rheumatoid arthritis: Quantitative aspects of proteoglycan release. *Biochem J* 1979; 180: 403–412.
53. Scott RD: Duopatellar total knee replacement: The Brigham experience. *Orthop Clin North Am* 1982;13:89–102.
54. Scott RD, Reilly DT: Pros and cons of patellar resurfacing in total knee replacement. *Orthop Trans* 1980;4:328.
55. Thomas WH, Ewald FC, Poss R, et al.: Duopatella total knee arthroplasty. *Orthop Trans* 1980;4:329–330.
56. Shoji H, Yoshino S, Kajino A: Patellar replacement in bilateral total knee arthroplasty. A study of patients who had rheumatoid arthritis and no gross deformity of the patella. *J Bone Joint Surg Am* 1989;71A:853–856.
57. Smith SR, Stuart P, Pinder IM: Nonresurfaced patella in total knee arthroplasty. *J Arthroplasty* 1989;4(Suppl.)81–86.
58. Grace JN, Rand JA: Patellar instability after total knee arthroplasty. *Clin Orthop* 1988;237: 184–189.
59. Malkani AL, Rand JA: *Long-Term Results of Kinematic Condylar Total Knee Arthroplasty.* San Francisco, American Academy of Orthopaedic Surgeons 1993.
60. Mason MD, Ewald FC, Poss R, et al.: *Ten to 14 Year Review of a Posterior Cruciate, Nonconstrained Condylar Total Knee Arthroplasty.* San Francisco, American Academy of Orthopaedic Surgeons, 1993.
61. Hozack WJ: Patellar complications related to

tracking, in Vince KG (ed.): *Knee Surgery*. Baltimore, Williams & Wilkins Co., 1994, in press.
62. Merkow RL, Soudry M, Insall JN: Patellar dislocation following total knee replacement. *J Bone Joint Surg Am* 1985;67A:1321–1327.
63. Briard JL, Hungerford DS: Patellofemoral instability in total knee arthroplasty. *J Arthroplasty* 1989;4(Suppl.):87–97.
64. Nagamine R, Whiteside LA: The effect of tibial tray malrotation on patellar tracking in total knee arthroplasty. *Trans Orthop Res Soc* 1992; 38:271.
65. Anouchi YS, Whiteside LA, Kaiser AD, et al.: The effects of axial rotational alignment of the femoral component on knee stability and patellar tracking in total knee arthroplasty demonstrated on autopsy specimens. *Clin Orthop* 1993;287:170–177.
66. Rhoads DD, Noble PC, Reuben JD, et al.: The effect of femoral component position on patellar tracking after total knee arthroplasty. *Clin Orthop* 1990;260:43–51.
67. Goldberg VM, Henderson BT: The Freeman-Swanson ICLH total knee arthroplasty: Complications and problems. *J Bone Joint Surg Am* 1980;62A:1338–1344.
68. Flandry F, Harding AF, Kester MA, et al.: A chronically dislocating prosthetic patella. A case report. *Orthopedics* 1988;11:457–460.
69. MacCollum MS, Karpman RR: Complications of the PCA anatomic patella. *Orthopedics* 1989; 12:1423–1428.
70. Merchant AC, Mercer RL, Jacobsen RH, et al.: Roentgenographic analysis of patellofemoral congruence. *J Bone Joint Surg Am* 1974;56A: 1391–1396.
71. Scott RD: Prosthetic replacement of the patellofemoral joint. *Orthop Clin North Am* 1979; 10:129–137.
72. Ewald FC: Leg-lift technique for simultaneous femoral, tibial, and patellar prosthetic cementing: "Rule of no thumb" for patellar tracking, and steel rod rule for ligament tension. *Tech Orthop* 1991;6:44–46.
73. Rae PJ, Noble J, Hodgkinson JP: Patellar resurfacing in total condylar knee arthroplasty. Technique and results. *J Arthroplasty* 1990;5: 259–265.
74. Rand JA, Morrey BF, Bryan RS: Patellar tendon rupture following total knee arthroplasty. *Tech Orthop* 1988;3:45–48.
75. Bocell JR, Thorpe CD, Tullos HS: Arthroscopic treatment of symptomatic total knee arthroplasty. *Clin Orthop* 1991;271:125–134.
76. Scott RD: Treatment of patellar instability associated with total knee replacement. *Tech Orthop* 1988;3:9–14.
77. Doolittle K, Turner RH: Patellofemoral problems following total knee arthroplasty. *Orthop Rev* 1988;17:696–702.
78. Kirk P, Rorabeck CH, Bourne RB, et al.: Management of recurrent dislocation of the patella following total knee arthroplasty. *J Arthroplasty* 1992;7:229–233.
79. Mochizuki RM, Schurman DJ: Patellar complications following total knee arthroplasty. *J Bone Joint Surg Am* 1979;61A:879–883.
80. Masini MA, Stulgerg SD: A new surgical technique for tibial tubercle transfer in total knee arthroplasty. *J Arthroplasty* 1992;7:81–86.
81. Whiteside LA, Ohl MD: Tibial tubercle osteotomy for exposure of the difficult total knee arthroplasty. *Clin Orthop* 1990;260:6–9.
82. Huberti HH, Hayes WC: Patellofemoral contact pressures: The influence of Q-angle and tendofemoral contact. *J Bone Joint Surg Am* 1984;66:715–724.
83. Reilly DT, Martens M: Experimental analysis of the quadriceps muscle force and patello-femoral joint reaction force for various activities. *Acta Orthop Scand* 1972;43:126–137.
84. Dupont JA, Baker SA: Complications of patellofemoral resurfacing in total knee arthroplasty. *Orthop Trans* 1982;6:369.
85. Insall JN, Dethmers DA: Revision of total knee arthroplasty. *Clin Orthop* 1982;170:123–130.
86. Thompson FM, Hood RW, Insall JN: Patellar fractures in total knee arthroplasty. *Orthop Trans* 1981;5:490.
87. Aglietti P, Buzzi R, Gaudenzi A: Patellofemoral funcional results and complications with the posterior stabilized total condylar prosthesis. *J Arthroplasty* 1988;3:17–25.
88. Simison AJM, Noble J, Harding K: Complications of the Attenborough knee replacement. *J Bone Joint Surg Br* 1986;68B:100–105.
89. Cameron H, Fedorkow DM: The patella in total knee arthroplasty. *Clin Orthop* 1982;165: 197–199.
90. Clayton ML, Thirupathi R: Patellar complications after total condylar arthroplasty. *Clin Orthop* 1982;170:152–155.
91. Scott WN, Schosheim P: Posterior stabilized knee arthroplasty. *Orthop Clin North Am* 1982;13:131–139.
92. Levai JP, McLeod HC, Freeman MA: Why not resurface the patella? *J Bone Joint Surg Br* 1983;65B:448–451.

93. Reuben JD, McDonald CL, Woodard PL, et al.: Effect of patella thickness on patella strain following total knee arthroplasty. *J Arthroplasty* 1991;6:251–258.
94. Bryan RS: Patellar infera and fat-pad hypertrophy after total knee arthroplasty. *Tech Orthop* 1988;3:29–33.
95. Ritter MA, Campbell ED: Postoperative patellar complications with or without lateral release during total knee arthroplasty. *Clin Orthop* 1987;219:163–168.
96. Berman AT, Reid JS, Yanicko DR, et al.: Thermally induced bone necrosis in rabbits: Relation to implant failure in humans. *Clin Orthop* 1984;186:284–292.
97. Willert HG, Ludwig J, Semlitsch M: Reaction of bone to methacrylate after hip arthroplasty: A long-term gross, light microscopic, and scanning electron microscopic study. *J Bone Joint Surg Am* 1974;56A:1368–1382.
98. Figgie HE, Goldberg VM, Figgie MP, et al.: The effect of alignment of the implant on fractures of the patella after condylar total knee arthroplasty. *J Bone Joint Surg Am* 1989;71A: 1031–1039.
99. Figgie HE, Goldberg VM, Heiple KG, et al.: The influence of tibial-patellofemoral location on function of the knee in patients with the posterior stabilized condylar knee prosthesis. *J Bone Joint Surg Am* 1986;68A:1035–1040.
100. Wackerhagen A, Bodem F, Hopf C, et al.: The influence of lateral release on patello-femoral joint loading in knee arthroplasty. An experimental in vitro study. *Int Orthop* 1992;16:19–24.
101. Brick GW, Scott RD: Blood supply to the patella. Significance in total knee arthroplasty. *J Arthroplasty* 1989;4(suppl.):75–79.
102. Kayler DE, Lyttle D: Surgical interruption of patellar blood supply by total knee arthroplasty. *Clin Orthop* 1988;229:221–227.
103. McMahon MS, Scuderi GR, Glashow JL, et al.: Scintigraphic determination of patellar viability after excision of infrapatellar fat pad and/or lateral retinacular release in total knee arthroplasty. *Clin Orthop* 1990;260:10–16.
104. Wetzner SM, Bezreh JS, Scott RD, et al.: Bone scanning in the assessment of patellar viability following knee replacement. *Clin Orthop* 1985;199:215–219.
105. Scuderi G, Scharf SC, Meltzer LP, et al.: The relationship of lateral releases to patella viability in total knee arthroplasty. *J Arthroplasty* 1987;2:209–214.
106. Ritter MA, Keating EM, Faris PM: Clinical, roentgenographic, and scintigraphic results after interruption of the superior lateral genicular artery during total knee arthroplasty. *Clin Orthop* 1989;248:145–151.
107. Tria AJ, Harwood DA, Alicea JA, et al.: Patellar fractures in posterior stabilized knee arthroplasties. *Clin Orthop* 1994;299:131–138.
108. Goldberg VM, Figgie HE, Inglis AE, et al.: Patellar fracture type and prognosis in condylar total knee arthroplasy. *Clin Orthop* 1988;236:115–122.
109. Goldberg VM, Figgie HE, Figgie MP: Technical considerations in total knee surgery. Management of patella problems. *Orthop Clin North Am* 1989;20:189–199.
110. Hozack WJ, Goll SR, Lotke PA, et al.: The treatment of patellar fractures after total knee arthroplasty. *Clin Orthop* 1988;236:123–127.
111. Albanese SA, Livermore JT, Werner FW, et al.: Knee extensor mechanics after subtotal excision of the patella. *Clin Orthop* 1992;285: 217–222.
112. Kaufer H: Mechanical function of the patella. *J Bone Joint Surg Am* 1971;53A:1551–1560.
113. Kaufer H: Patellar biomechanics. *Clin Orthop* 1979;144:51–54.
114. Bayne O, Cameron HU: Total knee arthroplasty following patellectomy. *Clin Orthop* 1984;186:112–114.
115. Conway WF, Gilula LA, Serot DI: Breakage of the patellar component of a kinematic total knee arthroplasty: A case report. *Orthopedics* 1986;9:532–534.
116. Weissman BN, Scott RD, Brick GW, et al.: Radiographic detection of metal-induced synovitis as a complication of arthroplasty of the knee. *J Bone Joint Surg Am* 1991;73A:1002–1007.
117. Wasilewski SA, Frankl U: Fracture of polyethylene of patellar component in total knee arthroplasty, diagnosed by arthroscopy. *J Arthroplasty* 1989;4(suppl.):19–22.
118. Johnson DR, McGinty JB, Mason JL, et al.: The role of arthroscopy in the problem total knee replacement. *Arthroscopy* 1990;6:30–32.
119. Berry DJ, Rand JA: Isolated patellar component revision of total knee arthroplasty. *Clin Orthop* 1993;286:110–115.
120. Lynch JA, Baker PL, Lepse PS, et al.: *Solitary Patellar Component Revision Following Total Knee Arthroplasty.* San Francisco, American Academy of Orthopaedic Surgeons, 1993.
121. Taylor JK, Yerby SA, Fisk T, et al.: *Intraoperative Femoral Component Polishing: Addressing Wear through of Metal-Backed Pa-*

tellae. San Francisco, American Academy of Orthopaedic Surgeons, 1993.
122. Coonse K, Adams JD: A new operative approach to the knee joint. *Surg Gynecol Obstet* 1943;77:344.
123. Insall JN: Surgical techniques and instrumentation in total knee arthroplasty, in Insall JN, Windsor RE, Scott WN, et al. (eds.): *Surgery of the Knee.* New York, Churchill Livingstone, 1993, pp. 739–804.
124. Scott RD, Siliski JM: The use of a modified V-Y quadricepsplasty during total knee replacement to gain exposure and improve flexion in the ankylosed knee. *Orthopedics* 1985; 8:45–48.
125. Vince KG: Arthritis surgery of the knee. *Curr Opin Orthop* 1991;2:22–30.
126. Gustilo RD, Thompson R: Quadriceps and patellar tendon ruptures following total knee arthroplasty, in Rand JA, Dorr L (ed.): *Total Arthroplasty of the Knee.* Rockville, Md., Aspen Publishers, 1986, pp. 41–47.
127. Haas SB, Callaway H: Disruptions of the extensor mechanism. *Orthop Clin North Am* 1992;23:687–695.
128. Szyszkowitz R: Patella and tibia, in Muller ME, Allgower M, Schneider R, et al. (eds.): *Manual of Internal Fixation.* Berlin, Springer-Verlag, 1990, pp. 553–594.
129. Emerson RJ, Head WC, Malinin TI: Reconstruction of patellar tendon rupture after total knee arthroplasty with an extensor mechanism allograft. *Clin Orthop* 1990; 260: 154–161.
130. Cameron HU, Cameron GM: The patellar meniscus in total knee replacement. *Orthop Rev* 1987;16:170–172.
131. Thorpe CD, Bocell JR, Tullos HS: Intra-articular fibrous bands. Patellar complications after total knee replacement. *J Bone Joint Surg Am* 1990;72A:811–814.
132. Beight JL, Yao B, Hozack WJ, et al.: The patellar clunk syndrome after posterior stabilized total knee arthroplasty. *Clin Orthop* 1994;299:139–142.
133. Hozack WJ, Rothman RH, Booth RJ, et al.: The patellar clunk syndrome. A complication of posterior stabilized total knee arthroplasty. *Clin Orthop* 1989;241:203–208.
134. Hirsh DM, Sallis JG: Pain after total knee arthroplasty caused by soft tissue impingement. *J Bone Joint Surg Br* 1989;71B:591–592.
135. Pettine KA, Bryan RS: A previously unreported cause of pain after total knee arthroplasty. *J Arthroplasty* 1986;1:29–33.
136. Koshino T, Ejima M, Okamoto R, et al.: Gradual low riding of the patella during postoperative course after total knee arthroplasty in osteoarthritis and rheumatoid arthritis. *J Arthroplasty* 1990;5:323–327.
137. Vernace JV, Rothman RH, Booth RJ, et al.: Arthroscopic management of the patellar clunk syndrome following posterior stabilized total knee arthroplasty. *J Arthroplasty* 1989; 4:179–182.
138. Hofmann AA, Plaster RL, Murdock LE: Subvastus (southern) approach for primary total knee arthroplasty. *Clin Orthop* 1991;269:70–77.
139. Hoppenfeld S, DeBoer P: The knee, in *Surgical Exposures in Orthopaedics: The Anatomic Approach.* Philadelphia, JB Lippincott Co., 1984, pp. 389–442.
140. Reithmeier E, Plitz W: A theoretical and numerical approach to optimal positioning of the patellar surface replacement in a total knee endoprosthesis. *J Biomech* 1990;23:883–892.
141. Bartlett DH, Franzen J: Accurate preparation of the patella during total knee arthroplasty. *J Arthroplasty* 1993;8:75–82.
142. Josefchak RG, Finlay JB, Bourne RB, et al.: Cancellous bone support for patellar resurfacing. *Clin Orthop* 1987;220:192–199.
143. Drakeford MK, Hungerford DS, Krackow KA, et al.: Resection arthroplasty for failed patellar components. San Francisco, American Academy of Orthopaedic Surgeons, 1993.
144. Buechel FF: Patellar tendon bone grafting for patellectomized patients having total knee arthroplasty. *Clin Orthop* 1991;271:72–78.
145. Lennox DW, Hungerford DS, Krackow KA: Total knee arthroplasty following patellectomy. *Clin Orthop* 1987;223:220–224.
146. Sledge C, Ewald F: Total knee arthroplasty experience at the Robert Breck Brigham hospital. *Clin Orthop* 1979;145:78–84.
147. Larson KR, Cracchiolo A, Dorey FJ, et al.: Total knee arthroplasty in patients after patellectomy. *Clin Orthop* 1991;264:243–254.
148. Railton GT, Levack B, Freeman MA: Unconstrained knee arthroplasty after patellectomy. *J Arthroplasty* 1990;5:255–257.
149. Cameron HU, Jung YB: Prosthetic replacement of the arthritic knee after patellectomy. *Can J Surg* 1990;33:119–121.
150. Szalapski EW Jr., King TV, Siliski J, et al.: Total knee replacement in the patellectomized knee. *Orthop Trans* 1991;15:725.

17

Reflex Sympathetic Dystrophy of the Knee

Jeffrey Y. Ngeow

Until recently, medical literature about reflex sympathetic dystrophy (RSD) tended to treat the upper or the lower extremities as a whole. The knee joint was seldom mentioned in isolation. Many clinicians doubt that an "RSD knee" is truly an entity that exists. This impression is reinforced by the fact that, to date, there are only a handful of clinical reports that specifically address RSD found in the knee joint.

This chapter is intended to provide a brief overview of the published data concerning RSD of the knee joint, calling attention to the fact that this condition is not a rarity. In addition, it is hoped to add some insights obtained through the treatment of several of such cases. Such experience came from patients seen in the pain management program of a single orthopedic institution. Admittedly, patient population is preselected and therefore personal opinions expressed herein are made from a rather narrow-angled perspective. It is also assumed in the discussions that follow, that the patella is included as part of the knee even though in some of the cases a patellectomy may have been done, for example, after total knee replacement.

Overview

Actual incidence of RSD limited to the knee is at best conjectural. From the few published series available, nearly all are retrospective reviews. This is hardly surprising since there is a great divergence of opinions regarding the incidence of RSD in the body as a whole. A case in point pertains to the reported occurrence of RSD following fractures of the extremities. The numbers ranged from as low as 0.01% in one series that included all limbs,[1] to as high as 35% in another series that was a prospective study of Colles' fracture.[2]

Clearly, reported incidence is determined by the inclusion criteria of the researcher. This remains an area of controversy because each author tended to adopt a different subgroup as the minimum requirement. Characteristic features most commonly included are severe pain, burning, swelling, vasospasm, temperature changes, loss of motor function, trophic changes of the skin and its appendages, and increased sweating. Typically, patients are included when any two or more of these features are found.

In a series of 829 patients presenting with symptoms that fulfilled a fairly rigid criteria for RSD, Veldman et al.[3] reported 41% lower-extremity involvement. No further differentiation was made to separate the foot from the knee. Wilder et al.[4] reviewed 70 children and adolescents with RSD, and reported a surprising 87% lower extremity involvement. Of these, the foot, the ankle, and the knee are affected in roughly equal numbers. Although most of Wilder's et al. cases resulted from injuries sustained during supervised sports activities, that is, under special circumstances, such data do refute the long-held impression that RSD of the lower extremities are much less common than in the upper limbs.

Within the setting of a sports medicine and knee injury practice, Tietjen[5] reported 14 patients who fit the criteria of RSD in a retrospective review of 67 patients with unexplained persistent knee pain. The RSD cases constituted 21% of this subset of patients who initially presented with symptoms that defied anatomic analyses and progressed to unsatisfactory outcomes. In turn, the subset came from a cohort of 3,000 knee conditions considered over the review period, thus yielding an overall RSD prevalence of 0.5%.

RSD in the knee has been most frequently associated with a history of direct or indirect trauma. Other etiologic factors mentioned include chondromalacia, infection, and total knee arthroplasty. It is notable that all authors agree there is a female preponderance in their RSD patient populations. However, no one has evaluated the significance of this fact.

Brief Historic Review

Mitchell et al. first described the syndrome of severe lancinating, burning pain in a limb showing varying degrees of dystrophy in victims of the American Civil War, who sustained bullet injuries to their peripheral nerves.[6] He also named the condition *causalgia.*

Since then, several similar conditions, not necessarily the result of penetrating injuries but sharing the common features of pain with dystrophy, have been recognized. In many of them, evidence of sympathetic hyperactivity such as vasospasm, hyperhidrosis, and decreased skin temperature are also present. These "causalgic" conditions were given different names, including Sudeck's atrophy, posttraumatic pain dysfunction syndrome, shoulder hand syndrome, minor causalgia, and algoneurodystrophy. These labels make long, interesting lists but they also reflect the disagreement regarding their underlying mechanisms.

Recently, in an effort to avoid semantics that emphasize differences and to turn towards a simplicity that highlights similarities that will promote focusing on the treatment of this family of conditions, clinicians in the field have generally adopted the term *sympathetically maintained pain* (SMP) as Roberts proposed.[7] RSD is now considered a member of SMP. The original term *causalgia,* which also comes under the SMP umbrella, is now applicable exclusively to cases in which major nerve injuries exist.

Pathophysiology

Where RSD and other SMP are concerned, this is a situation when more means less. As more knowledge is gained from clinical observations and experimental studies, there is less agreement in a single common pathophysiologic mechanism. Since the manifestations of the somatosensory and motor disorders coupled with autonomic dysfunctions and tissue structural changes are so variable, scientists are loathed to accept any one animal model or hypothesis that purports to explain them all.

Indeed, this state of affairs is reflected by a "Consensus statement on the Reflex Sympathetic Dystrophy syndrome" issued by the VIth World Congress on Pain,[8] which defined *RSD* as

> a descriptive term referring to a complex disorder or group of disorders that may develop as a consequence of trauma affecting the limbs, with or without obvious nerve lesion. RSD may also develop after visceral diseases and central nervous system lesions or, rarely, without an obvious antecedent event. It consists of pain and related sensory abnormalities, abnormal blood flow and sweating, abnormalities in the motor system, and changes in structure of both superficial and deep tissues (trophic changes).

It is not necessary that all components are present. It is agreed that the name "reflex sympathetic dystrophy" is used in a descriptive sense and does not imply specific underlying mechanisms.

When neuropathic pain symptoms such as constant burning pain and touch-evoked allodynia (which means pain sensation induced by stimuli not normally painful) are blocked by sympathetic nerve blocks, thus indicating that they are maintained by sympathetic activity, it does not follow that the other symptoms such as numbness, dysesthesia, and heat-evoked hypalgesia/hyperalgesia are also produced by the same neuropathic mechanism. Price et al. came to this conclusion after conducting psychophysical observations in patients with chronic SMP symptoms. They stated that it is possible that the sensory neuropathic symptoms may be produced by a different neuropathic mechanism, and that these separate mechanisms may coexist. Moreover, in different patients, the same symptoms may be produced by different mechanisms. Lastly, there is even the logical possibility that several different neuropathic mechanisms may simultaneously produce the same symptom in a single patient.[9] This possibility will certainly explain why sympathectomies often are followed by recurrence of the same symptoms.

Given the aforementioned caveat, there is now generally accepted experimental evidence which suggests that partial injury to a mixed peripheral nerve may be responsible for at least some of the features found in RSD. Under normal conditions, sympathetic nerve stimulation does not excite the nociceptors (pain receptors) at the endings of an uninjured nerve. Within days after partial nerve injury, changes occur that render the nociceptors excitable by sympathetic stimulation. They now also respond to intra-arterially injected norepinephrine. If the nociceptors were already sensitized by tissue injury and inflammation, their responses will be further augmented by sympathetic nerve activities.

At the spinal cord level, a class of dorsal horn neurons that are multireceptive, the wide-dynamic-range neurons (WDR) contribute to painful sensations. Chronic stimulation of the WDR by nociceptors causes hyperexcitability and plasticity of the WDR, resulting in expansion of their receptive fields.[10] This may explain why innocuous stimulations are now perceived as painful (hyperalgesia).

The question of a diasthesis or personality predisposition towards developing RSD has often been raised. The patient's exaggerated response to mild stimulation naturally led physicians to suspect psychologic disorders. There is literature on both adults and children that hypothesizes the presence of psychologic disorders, particularly anxiety and depression, which predisposes one to develop RSD. On the other hand, it is only obvious that chronic pain and suffering will produce a host of psychologic complications of their own. In a review, Bruehl and Carlson concluded that the question of a premorbid predisposing disorder cannot be answered from existing literature because of methodologic weakness.[11] They do stress the importance of psychologic factors in the progression and maintenance of the disease.

Diagnosis

Symptoms and Signs

The classical features of RSD are well known and tend to be reproduced in most texts. However, the familiar picture of a discolored, swollen, and distorted limb held in a protective cover rarely occurs in the knee except in the late chronic stages. The usual presentation is a patient who complains of excessive pain with walking and other weight-bearing activities. Often there is a history of seemingly minor trauma followed by disproportionate disabilities including startling loss of the range of motion. If there was a previous operation, it would be associated with a protracted recovery period during which the patient poorly tolerated all rehabilitative efforts. History such as this should raise a high index of suspicion and should prompt the search for more specific RSD features.

Burning and hypersensitivity to light clothing that causes an unpleasant feeling (dysesthesia) over the patella and often the lower thigh are frequently noticed. Heat intolerance, especially to sunburns, may be a prominent feature. The knee may be warmer or cooler than the opposite side in an unpredictable manner. By contrast, the feet are usually cold. It is almost pathognomonic when patients are seen in cold weather wearing long pants with "cut outs" over their knees or wearing shorts and thick socks on their feet.

Vasomotor instability may be present either as skin mottling or larger areas of erythema. Characteristically, color patterns change over several minutes when the skin is exposed to room temperature. It is more frequently observed in young females with fair skin and may appear anywhere from the feet to the thighs. In our experience, this physical sign is sometimes associated with features of Raynaud's phenomenon, although this impression has not been confirmed by any reported series.

Tissue edema without joint effusion and muscle atrophy without hyperhidrosis are consistent features in RSD of the knee; so is mechanical allodynia along the margins of the patella and along the tibial joint lines. Frequently, the symptoms extend beyond the confines of the knee joint but not in a clearly stocking/glove distribution. The anterior aspects of the limb are much more likely involved than the popliteal fossa.

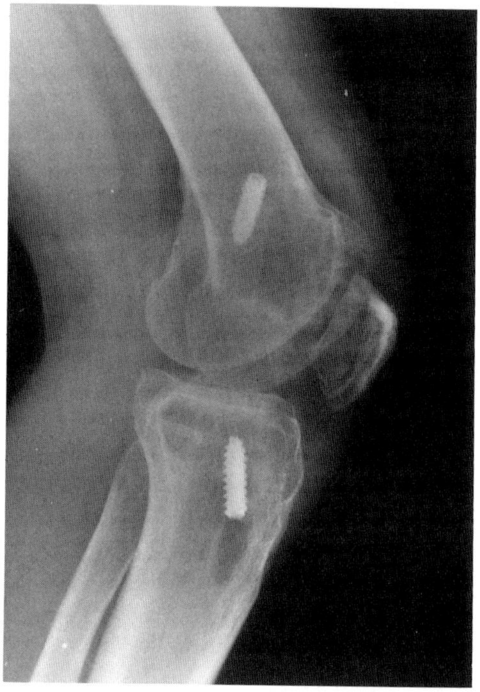

FIGURE 17.1 Localized osteoporosis in a post-anterior cruciate ligament reconstruction patient who developed RSD.

Diagnostic Aids

Thermography, x-rays, and bone scans may show temperature changes; localized or patchy osteoporosis (Figure 17.1); and a unilateral, diffusely increased (Figure 17.2) or decreased uptake, respectively. Each finding, when present in isolation, tends to be nonspecific and impossible to distinguish from other inflammatory conditions.

The "gold standard" has been symptomatic relief from a sympathetic nerve block. In fact, in many cases, the sympathetic nerve block is used as the diagnostic test. RSD is confirmed only after a positive response to a diagnostic sympathetic block is obtained. Care must be taken that somatic nerves are not anesthetized during the diagnostic sympathetic block, or the result cannot be interpreted. However, even a "pure" block can be confounded by placebo effects. To circumvent this, phentolamine, an alpha adrenergic receptor blocker has been used as a diagnostic agent. The patient's reaction to this drug infused intravenously can be observed in a blinded fashion.[12]

Treatment

Naturally, treatment must be targeted towards relief of suffering; preservation of function; and ultimately, a return of normal function. Suffering is not just limited to the pain sensation but also includes the fear of pain, which may be a potent force that prevents adequate rehabilitation.

To minimize fear of motion, patients should be given only active or actively assisted therapy within their limits of tolerance. "Aggressive" therapy usually leads to patient noncompliance and delayed progress. It is inappropriate, especially in the early stages of RSD. Instead, modalities that are tolerated and effective such as cryotherapy and transcutaneous electrical nerve stimulation (TENS) should be used liberally.

When analgesics are needed, a nonnarcotic agent should be the first choice. Ketorolac (Toradol), a nonsteroidal anti-inflammatory agent with analgesic properties, has gained popular-

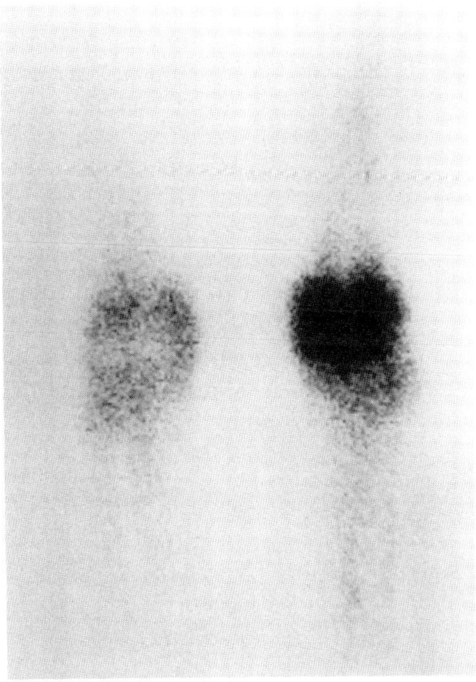

FIGURE 17.2 Typical bone scan in RSD showing diffuse increased uptake in affected knee.

ity recently. It is often given with a tricyclic antidepressant such as amitriptyline. This agent is used for its antiserotonin reuptake properties, which have shown effectiveness in reducing some of the neuropathic symptoms.

When narcotics have to be used, they should be given in adequate doses to enable patients to get over severe episodes, and then tapered. Transdermal fentanyl patches provide a more constant blood level. This is a welcomed feature by most patients. Be aware that even though the stigmata of "taking narcotics" is avoided this way, patients are still receiving a potent narcotic and tolerance will build up in time the same way as other more traditional drugs.

Intermittent sympathetic nerve blocks done in the early stages can be effective in achieving remission. Even in established cases, they are valuable as an option in offering periodic "breaks" to the patient. The procedure is not without risk and repeated blocks tend to lose efficacy. When judiciously done at the crest of periods of exacerbations, intermittent sympathetic nerve blocks can usually abort the need to resort to narcotics or an escalation in the narcotic dosage. Of course, this is applicable only to those who respond to sympathetic blockade. Nerve blocks can either be done at the lumbar sympathetic chain with local anesthetics, or regionally in the limb with intravenous infusion of an alpha adrenergic blocker such as guanethidine, reserpine, or bretylium. Currently, the intravenous forms of the first two agents are not available in the United States. There is controversy regarding exactly how often the blocks should be done. At our institution, in a series of 38 patients treated this way, 90% have achieved satisfactory control without the need of chronic narcotics over a followup period of six months to two years. The number of blocks received by this group ranged from three to 30. Typically, blocks were done closely, up to three times per week for two weeks in early cases, then tapered off to once or less weekly when symptoms subside or response becomes stabilized.[13] If anticipated favorable response is not obtained following initial "diagnostic" or "prognostic" blocks, other methods are used instead.

When there are coexisting correctable anatomic lesions, they will need to be dealt with. However, any surgical intervention will lead to acute and prolonged exacerbation of the preexisting symptoms. Therefore, operations should be done only when clearly indicated and with the greatest of precautions. To an RSD patient, there is no minor surgery. A "simple" arthroscopy can lead to loss of ground gained by months of hard work. Indeed, arthroscopy was the most common antecedent event in our patient series.

When manipulation or surgery must be done, patients are usually given a continuous epidural anesthetic and opiate infusion for several days in a manner similar to that described by Cooper et al.[14] This will create a pain-free window of time to regain or maintain range of motion. The same opportunity is also used for tapering the patient's narcotic requirements.

Surgical sympathectomy is usually not recommended, except when definitely indicated. The following case report illustrate the point.

A 25-year-old woman with established RSD of the right knee developed cellulitis of the same leg that required fasciotomy to relieve an anterior compartment syndrome. Postoperative wound healing was delayed secondary to a constant serosanguineous discharge. While undergoing lumbar sympathetic blockade as part of her ongoing RSD treatment, it was observed that with each nerve block, oozing from the wound would cease until the effect of the block had dissipated. When the patient's blood count dropped to the point that she required repeated transfusions, the decision was made to undergo surgical sympathectomy. Her leg wound healed within a week postsympathectomy. Four years later, she noted recurrence of mild RSD symptoms in the same leg.

Psychologic examination and ongoing counseling for the patients and their immediate family members must be an integral part of the treatment regimen. Chronicity invariably generates a sense of hopelessness in the patient and frustration both in the patient's family and the treating physician. Because formal psychiatric treatment is seldom needed at the initial examination phase and patient's reluctance to see a psychiatrist can be anticipated in most cases. This topic is usually brought up after rapport is established. Considerable anguish can be avoided if the therapist is introduced as a consultant who helps with developing individual and family coping skills. It is better yet if ancillary techniques such as biofeedback can be taught by the same professional.

For any patient, treatment should follow a preplanned algorithm to effect minimum time lost between each chosen method. Obviously, flexibility must be built into the steps, allowing for individual variations. The emphasis is oriented towards the multidisciplinary approach, which ensures that important aspects of the patient's care is not overlooked.

Conclusion

In the minds of many physicians, RSD continues to remain a diagnosis of exclusion, a label of failure reluctantly accepted when all else has failed. This unfortunate mind-set tends to perpetuate the clinical impression that no satisfactory outcome can be expected from such cases. While this is certainly true in some, there is still a majority that can maintain a reasonable quality of life. Early diagnosis and specific, goal-directed treatments buttressed by a supportive social milieu can succeed in keeping or even returning the patient to a meaningful existence. Clearly, this can only be achieved when health care providers remain vigilant by keeping the condition high on their differential diagnosis lists.

References

1. Smith D, Campbell S: Reflex sympathetic dystrophy syndrome. Diagnosis and management. *West J Med* 1987;147:342–345.
2. Atkins R, Duckworth T, Kanis J: Features of algodystrophy after Colles' fracture. *J Bone Joint Surg Br* 1990;72(1):105–110.
3. Veldman P, Reynen H, Arntz I, et al.: Signs and symptoms of reflex sympathetic dystrophy: Prospective study of 829 patients. *Lancet* 1993; 342:1012–1016.
4. Wilder R, Berde C, Wolohan M, et al.: Reflex sympathetic dystrophy in children. *J Bone Joint Surg Am* 1992;74A(6):910–919.
5. Tietjen R: Reflex sympathetic dystrophy of the knee. *Clin Orthop* 1986;209:234–243.
6. Mitchell W, Morehouse G, Keen W: *Gunshot Wounds and Other Injuries of Nerves.* Philadelphia, JB Lippincott, 1964.
7. Roberts W: A hypothesis on the physiological basis for causalgia and related pains. *Pain* 1986; 24:297–311.
8. Janig W, Blumberg H, Boas R, et al.: The reflex sympathetic dystrophy syndrome. Consensus statement and general recommendations for diagnosis and clinical research, in Bond M, Charlton J, Woolf C (eds.): *Pain Research and Clinical Management.* Proceedings VIth World Congress on Pain. Amsterdam, Elsevier, 1991, pp. 373–376.
9. Price D, Bennett G, Raffii A: Psychophysical observations on patients with neuropathic pain relieved by a sympathetic block. *Pain* 1989;36: 273–288.
10. Woolf C, King A: Dynamic alterations in the cutaneous mechanoreceptive fields of dorsal

horn neurons in the rat spinal cord. *J Neurosci* 1990;10:2717–2726.

11. Bruehl S, Carlson C: Predisposing psychological factors in the development of reflex sympathetic dystrophy. *Clin J Pain* 1992;8:287–299.
12. Arner S: Intravenous phentolamine test: Diagnostic and prognostic use in reflex sympathetic dystrophy. *Pain* 1991;46:17–22.
13. O'Brien S, Ngeow J, Gibney M, et al.: Reflex sympathetic dystrophy of the knee: Etiology, diagnosis and treatment, *Orthop Trans* 1991; 15:747 (Abstracts).
14. Cooper D, DeLee J, Ramamurthy S: Reflex sympathetic dystrophy of the knee: Treatment using continuous epidural anesthesia. *J Bone Joint Surg Am* 1989;71A(3):365–369.

Index

ISBN 0-387-94371-4

9 780387 943718